Medicinal Plants

Edited by Sanjeet Kumar

Published in London, United Kingdom

Medicinal Pl
http://dx.do
Edited by San

Contributors
Kaj Winther,
Fereche Itob
Bee, Mohamm
Islam, Lysia
Nnadozie, S
I.P. Tripat
Ganga Rao B
Afonne, Eme
Gangopadhya
Abiele Hilda
Sheridan, M
Pawirodihar
Zhao-Huang
Elnawasany

First pu
IntechO
registr

British
A catal

Additio

Medici
Edited
p. cm.
Print I
Onlin
eBook

For EU product safety concerns:
IN TECH d.o.o., Prolaz Marije Krucifikse Kozulić 3, 51000 Rijeka, Croatia,
info@intechopen.com or visit our website at intechopen.com.

Meet the editor

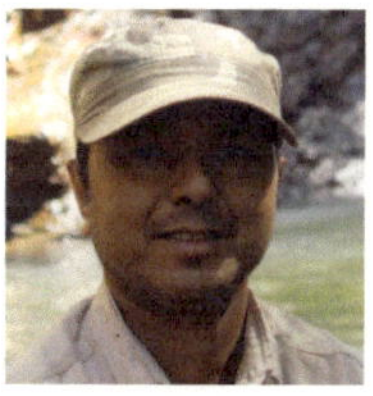

Sanjeet Kumar is the founder and CEO of Ambika Prasad Research Foundation (APRF) and the Institute of Biological Sciences (IBS), India. He has experience working with many Indian organizations and institutes, including the Regional Plant Resource Center (RPRC), Regional Institute of Education (RIE), Institute of Bioresources and Sustainable Development (IBSD), National Institute of Technology (NIT), and Forest and Environment Department, Odisha. His research interests are plant taxonomy, medicinal plants, biodiversity and conservation, restoration of floral wealth, phytochemistry, and microbiology. He has published about 120 research papers in national and international journals, 16 books, and several book chapters and scientific articles. He is currently supervising MSc and Ph.D. students.

Contents

Preface

Although we are currently in an advanced scientific era where we have sound technologies to solve healthcare problems, the world is still experiencing microbial infections, antimicrobial resistance, drug failures, disorders, and pandemics due to malpractices of drugs, natural mutation, and urban lifestyles. The major causes of therapeutic failure depend on a complex interplay of socio-cultural and clinico-medical factors, which can be observed at every step of the therapeutic chain. Even though vaccines are available to protect against polio, tetanus, flu, hepatitis B, hepatitis A, rubella, measles, rotavirus, chickenpox, and more, there is still a need for medicinal food and agents from nature. Medicinal plants are rich resources of ingredients that can be used in drug formulation, whether pharmaceutical, non-pharmaceutical or synthetic. They also play a critical role in the development of human cultures around the world.

The use of medicinal plants goes back to ancient times. Egyptian papyrus and Chinese manuscripts describe the uses of many local herbs. Evidence shows that Unani hakims (traditional medicine practitioners in South Asia), Indian traditional healers, and European and Mediterranean travelers were using plants as medicinal agents for more than 4000 years. Ancient cultures like the Indus Valley, Mesopotamian, Egyptian, and Huanghe civilizations used plants as medicines, as shown by archeological evidence. Among the ancient civilizations, India has been known to have a rich diversity of medicinal plants. Indigenous traditional knowledge (ITK) and the forest of India are full of therapeutic information and medicinal wealth, respectively, both of which provide raw materials for drug formulation. About 8,000 herbal remedies have been codified in Ayurveda, Yoga, Naturopathy, Unani, Siddha, and Homeopathy (AYUSH) systems. The World Health Organization (WHO) estimated that about 80% of people worldwide rely on local herbal medicines for their primary healthcare needs and identified 21,000 plant species as having medicinal value. After the COVID-19 pandemic, the world is going back to nature and readopting traditional practices, ITK, and old therapeutic systems. Readopting is difficult but not impossible. As such, this book provides a glimpse into plants and their traditional uses as well as their contemporary utilization for treating, managing, and even curing health problems. It is a useful resource for researchers, academicians, intellectuals, and interested readers.

Sanjeet Kumar
Biodiversity and Conservation Lab.,
Ambika Prasad Research Foundation,
Cuttack, India

Section 1

Medicinal Plants and Their Traditional Therapeutic Values

Chapter 1

The Use of Native Flora/Herbal Products in Human Papilloma Virus (HPV) Infection: A Global Perspective Study

Franca Nneka Alaribe Nnadozie, Sidonie Tankeu and Daisy Nwaozuzu

Abstract

Human papilloma virus (HPV) is associated with 99% cause of cervical cancer with 20.2 million women at risk of having it in South Africa. Vaccine is the major way to prevent HPV infection. However, the vaccination program is not within easy reach for all that need it. Plants are an important source of medicines for African people, some herbal medicines are widely used for many ailments such as malaria, respiratory problems, pains, infection, and inflammation. There is limited information regarding the efficacy of medicinal plant use as there lack human studies, and no proper dosing measures are available. This study evaluated the global perspective of people over using medicinal plant products/plant-derived bio-therapeutics in the management of HPV infection. A survey method (Survey Monkey) distributed through social media was used for 3 months. 117 people participated and data realized from the study indicated their approval and readiness to use medicinal plant products.

Keywords: human papillomavirus, infection, cervical cancer, medicinal plants, efficacy

1. Introduction

In South Africa and other Sub-Sahara countries, cervical cancer (CC) is the most prevalent type of cancer disease suffered by women, with 20.2 million women at risk and 12.983 cases diagnosed annually [1]. Management of CC requires access to health care systems. Due to the stage of progression, the affected persons by this disease would require surgery, radiotherapy, and chemotherapy in order to increase their chances of survival. However, if CC is left unmanaged death may result [2].

In Low Middle-Income Countries (LMICs), the unaffordability of therapeutic resources and negligence of palliative care are among the factors hampering the fight against CC. Most women often consult health care providers at an advanced stage of cervical cancer due to financial hardship. The partial resources available for treatment are not adequate to provide effective surgical, radiotherapy, and chemotherapeutic services [2].

Studies [3, 4] have shown that among HIV positive women, there is consistent higher incidence of human papilloma virus (HPV) infection (the major cause of CC), persistent HPV infection with high-risk types, multiple types of HPV, and cervical cancer precursors (CIN or SIL). An estimate as high as 20–40% has been made for the prevalence of CIN in HIV-positive women. Many studies have shown that HIV-positive women are more likely to have persistent HPV infections than HIV-negative women [3]. South Africa is among countries in the world with a very high HIV prevalence. Zhang et al. [3] in their study recorded nearly half (41/83, 43%) of HIV-infected women co-infected with carcinogenic HPV genotypes [3]. Similarly, Temmerman et al. [4] reported a five-fold increased risk of high-grade SIL among 513 HIV-positive women in a family planning clinic in Kenya. Other reports from the region show that women with HIV develop cervical cancer at an earlier age than women who are HIV-negative [4]. Statistically, cervical cancer in South Africa is at a prevalence of 22.8 and 27 per 100,000 women when compared with the global average of 15.8. A total of 5743 new cases are encountered annually with an approximately 3000 mortalities. About 99% of these mortalities are associated with HPV, HPV strains 16 and 18 being responsible for 70% of the cases [1, 5].

Currently, in most of these sub-Sahara African countries, a vaccination program is either ongoing [1] or not yet incorporated into the eradication/screening policy [6, 7]. In South Africa, there is a vaccination of Cervarix®, which is provided for protection against HPV-16 and HPV-18 strains [1]. However, this vaccination program is either expensive, not efficient, or not within easy reach for all that need it. Furthermore, not much effort has been observed in HPV eradication and cervical cancer status in spite of the vaccination efforts in all the locations where it is operating.

Traditional medicines or herbal medicines have always been recorded as an important component of the health care system of the African people [8]. Medicinal plants/extracts involved in this practice are becoming a worldwide topic, drawing an impact on world health. They are still being administered by traditional practitioners in some parts of the health care system, especially in the rural areas of developing countries [9, 10] for the treatment of various illnesses, including viral infection, cancer, osteoarthritis, asthma, heart disease, tuberculosis, swollen ankles, bone fracture, malaria, convulsion, piles, hypertension, typhoid fever, diabetes, and anemia [8, 11, 12]. Additionally, extracted compounds of medicinal plants are being employed as inputs in toxicology, phytochemicals, pharmaceuticals, and other chemical industries [8, 13]. Furthermore, [14] has shown that medicinal plants are a source of bioactive agents employed in the preparation of synthetic medicine, therefore, function in the discovery of drugs like antiviral, antidiabetic, anticancer, antifungal, antiasthma, antibacterial, anti-HIV, and antimalarial [14]. This study evaluates how people see the use of native floral-derived products and bio-therapeutics in the management of HPV infection.

2. Materials and methods

2.1 Study design

A mixed-method, including both qualitative and quantitative methods, was used by means of an electronic survey setup (Survey monkey) conducted between December 2020 and March 2021 to assess people's notions about the use of medicinal plant extract or bio-therapeutics in the treatment/management of HPV infection. A total of 117 participants took part in the online survey monkey questionnaire.

2.2 Data collection

Data collection was predominantly close-ended questions and a few open-ended questions were compiled in the form of an electronic survey/questionnaire on the Survey monkey Google platform. A link to the survey was disseminated via social media platforms along with an information leaflet. Participants accessed the survey and participated voluntarily and anonymously. Implied consent was assumed by the act of participating in the survey.

2.3 Data analysis

The quantitative data was subjected to data preparation for validation. Data was prepared and statistically analyzed using Excel for comprehensive data presentation. The significance level was established as $p < 0.05$.

3. Results

3.1 Demographical characteristics

Demographically, gender (**Figure 1a**), race (**Figure 1b**), age group (**Figure 1c**), and country of residence (**Figure 1d**) were the characteristics used. Under gender, 93 females and 21 males participated in the study questionnaire. 3 of the participants preferred not to say. The number of females that participated was statistically significant (P-Value = 0.001347 < 5%) compared to the number of males (**Figure 1a**). Data under race (**Figure 1b**) indicated participation of races from Black/African (96), White/Caucasian (6), Asian/Asian America (6), Hispanic/Latino (0), American India (0), Native Hawaiian, or other Pacific Islander (0). Other races not included in the list indicated a total score of 9.0. Black/African participants showed the highest score of 96, which is statistically significant compared to participants from other race groups. **Figure 1c** depicts the age group of participants, which ranged from 18 years to 65 and above. Participants from 18 to 24 were 3, 25–34 (6), 35–44 (18), 45–54 (72), 55–64 (15), and 65 and above were 3 participants. Age group 45–54 indicated the highest group of age that participated in the survey with 72 people that responded, followed by age group 35–44 with 18 respondents. In order to know people's notions using location on the use of plant extracts for the treatment of HPV, participants' countries of residence were requested in the survey. The number of participants residing in Nigeria was 51, in South Africa was 12, and those residing in other countries were 51 similar to those in Nigeria (**Figure 1d**).

3.2 Knowledge of HPV infection and the type of cancers it can cause

HPV infection is the most sexually transmitted infection (STI). There are over 100 types of HPV and more than 40 can infect humans [15]. HPV is known to be the cause of 70% of cervical cancer and other cancers such as vulva cancer, Papillomas/Carcinomas, vagina, penis, and oropharynx cancers. Additionally, 630,000 cases of HPV-related cancers are diagnosed each year [1, 16–18].

For the above reasons, it was necessary to ascertain the knowledge of participants about HPV infection and other cancers it can cause. Data realized from this survey question (**Figure 2**) indicates that 78 participants are aware of HPV infection and

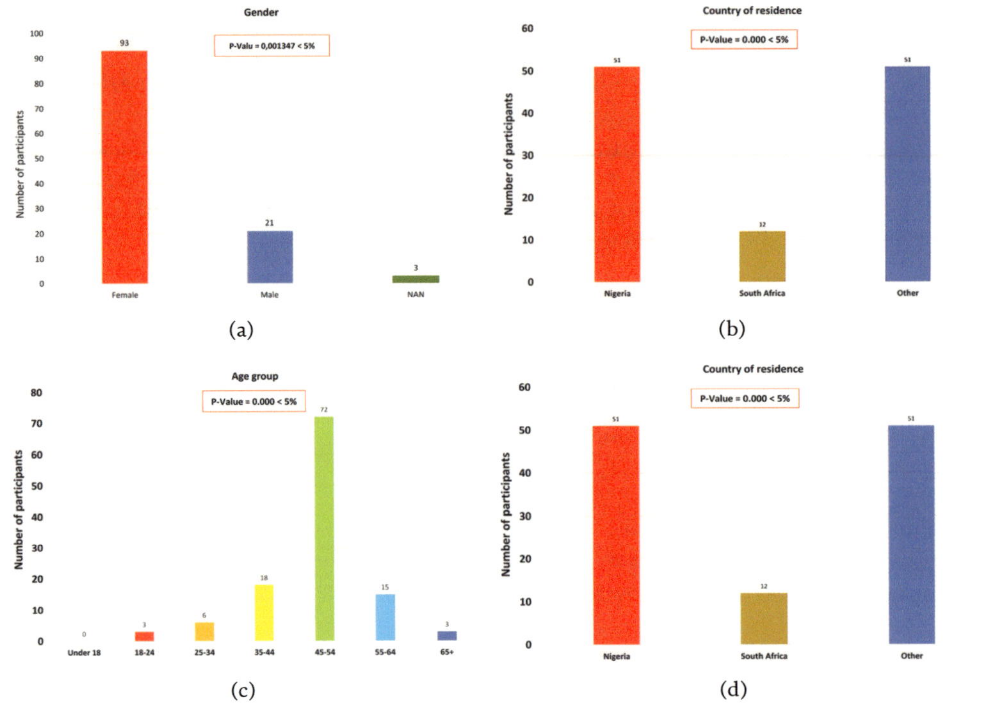

Figure 1.
Used demographic characteristics in the study. Gender (a), race (b), age group (c), and country of residence (d). Any parameter with the highest score in each group was statistically significant (P-value = <5%) compared to others.

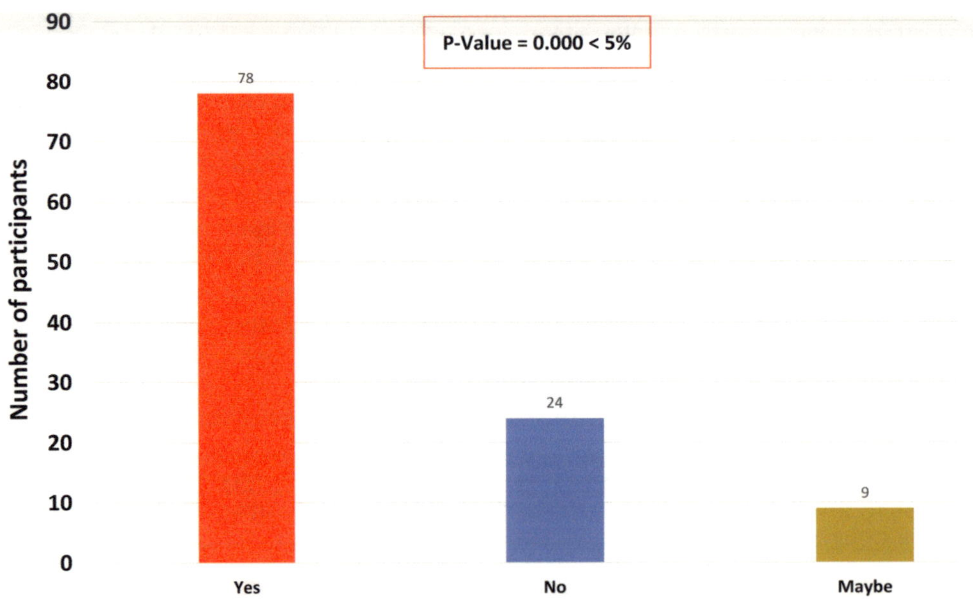

Figure 2.
Participants with knowledge of HPV infection and the types of cancers it can cause. The level of awareness was highly statistically significant at P-value = 0.000 < 5% for 78 participants. However, 24 participants declared their lack of awareness of HPV infection and the type of cancers it can cause.

other types of cancers it can cause while 24 participants are ignorant of this. 9 participants are not sure (maybe) of their level of awareness to this. This shows that most people are aware of HPV infection and other types of cancer.

3.3 Knowledge of relative suffering or have suffered from any HPV-related cancers

As cervical cancer had earlier been indicated as the second most prevalent type of cancer suffered by women in developing countries [19] and with the nature of HPV infection as indicated in [15], we tried to have the knowledge of participants with relatives suffering or have suffered HPV-related cancers. On the question, do you have a family member, friend, or relative suffering or has suffered from cancer that HPV is one of its causes? Data from this survey question indicated that only 15 people have either friends, relatives, or family members suffering or have suffered HPV-related cancer while 93 (P-Value = 0.000 < 5%) people have not had such experience and 3 were not sure (**Figure 3**). This figure shows that although most participants are aware of HPV infection as well as other types of cancer, they do not have many relatives affected by HPV-related cancer. Financial burden of these HPV cancers sickness was also included in the survey question. Results indicated that 15 participants showed bad financial effects/burdens on them due to these HPV cancers while 39 showed neutral burden over the HPV cancer sickness. No participant indicated the financial burden to have a good effect (figure not shown).

3.4 Use of herbal products for any purpose

Question to find out if participants have in any way used herbal or plant medicinal products for any purpose showed that 63 participants know and have used herbal products for one purpose or the other. A total of 43 participants indicated that they have never employed herbal products for any purpose while 6 participants were not sure if they have (**Figure 4**). The majority of participants demonstrated that they have already used herbal products for their health.

3.5 Awareness of some herbal products being used effectively either singly or in combination for the treatment of different ailments

Currently, many herbal products or medicinal plant extracts have been showcased for the treatments of different sicknesses [8, 10]. This study also evaluated the level of awareness of participants regarding the single-use or a combination of herbal products for the treatment of different diseases effectively. Data from participants' responses showed that 96 participants were aware of the effective use of herbal products for the treatment/management of different ailments. This value was highly significant (P-Value = 0.000 < 5%) compared to the number of participants (3) that declared ignorant of the use of herbal products. 12 participants responded maybe to this effect (**Figure 5**).

3.6 Future use of herbal products for HPV management/treatment

Readiness of the participants to patronize/support the use of any native flora/herbal discovered for the management/treatment of HPV infection was evaluated. Data from this showed that 93 participants indicated their interest in the

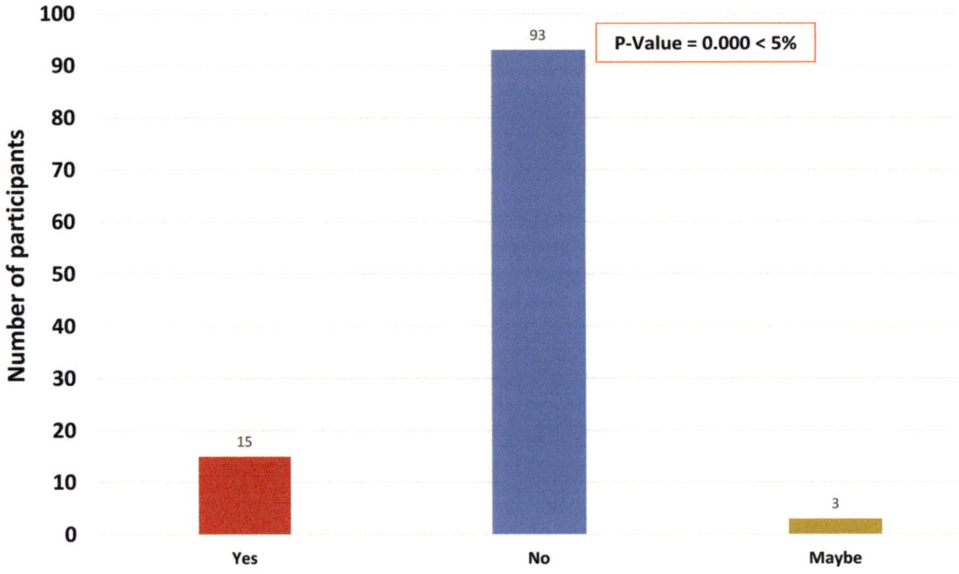

Figure 3.
Response to survey question indicating some participants with relatives and friends suffering from any HPV-related cancers.

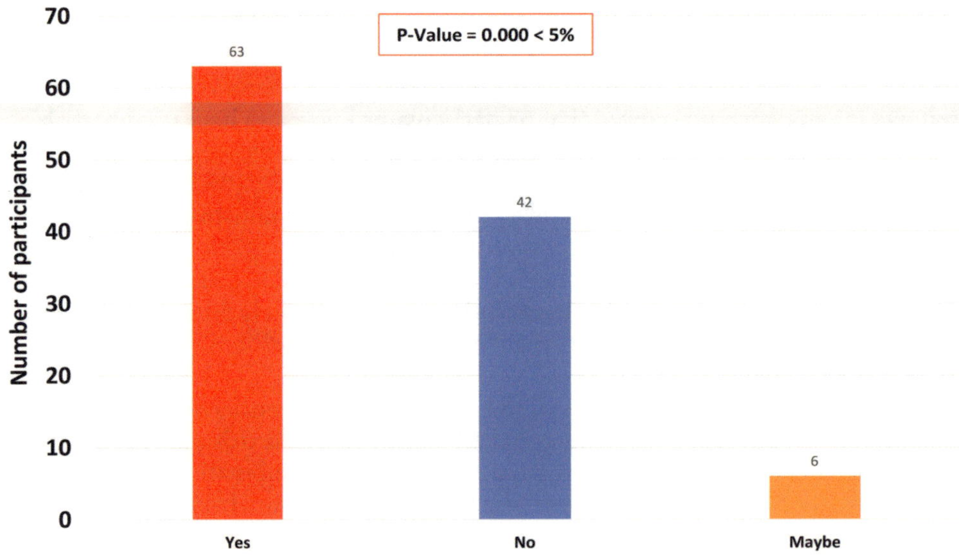

Figure 4.
Number of participants that have employed herbal products for any purpose.

future use of herbal products. 3 participants did not approve the future use of herbal products while 18 participants' opinions were uncertain (**Figure 6**). Most participants were willing to use any future herbal products that may be produced to manage HPV. This is in agreement with previous observation where most participants indicated that they have previously used herbal products to improve their health.

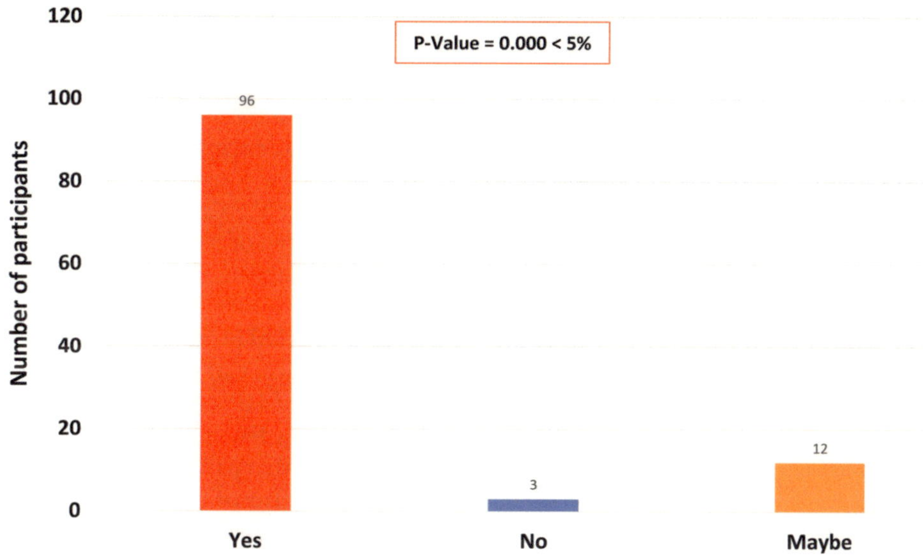

Figure 5.
Number of participants with knowledge of effective use of herbal products either singly or in combination for the treatment of different diseases.

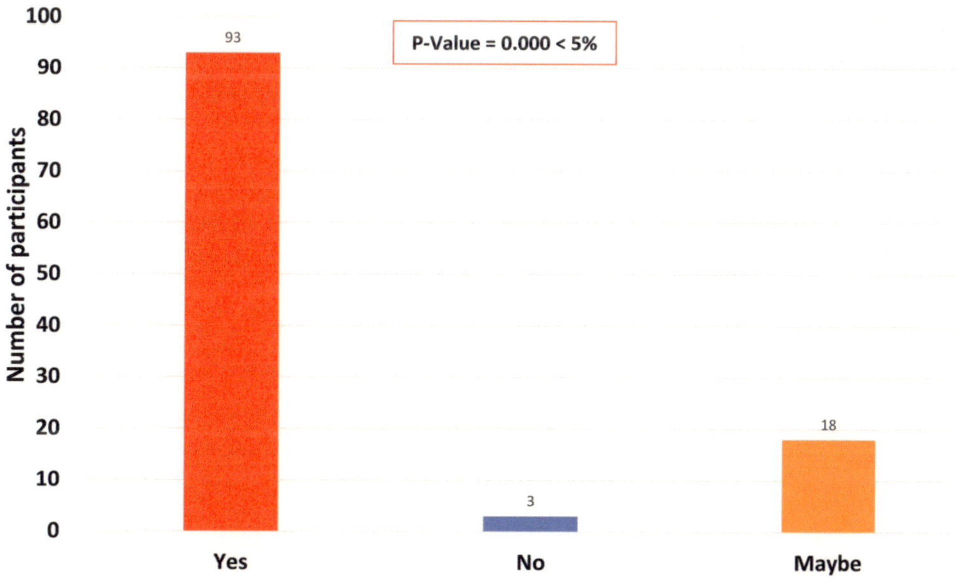

Figure 6.
Number of participants showing their readiness to support or buy any native flora/herbal product discovered for the treatment or management of HPV infection.

4. Discussion

The higher incidence of HPV infection, especially in HIV-positive women, and the higher prevalence of cervical cancer in LMICs call for urgent attention. Despite all the efforts of the government to ameliorate HPV infection through immunization and cervical cancer screening measures, yet not much has been achieved in HPV infection level and reduction in CC prevalence, especially in sub-Sahara Africa [1, 3, 6].

HPV is known to be the most sexually transmitted infection and 40 types of HPV can infect humans. HPV is also implicated in the proliferation of not only CC but other types of cancers [1, 16]. Therefore, eradication or ameliorating of HPV infection becomes imperative and necessary.

Currently, the importance of medicinal plant extracts has been showcased severally in the literature due to their involvement in the production of different drugs, herbal products, and bio-therapeutics for the treatment/management of different diseases.

This study evaluated people's notions of future use of herbal products for the treatment/management of HPV infection. **Table 1** exhibits some of the medicinal plants/active compounds evaluated for antiviral/inhibition of HPV by previous studies with **Figure 7** depicting photographs of some of the plants listed in **Table 1**.

In this study, demographically, the number of females (93) that participated was highly statistically significant (**Figure 1a**) compared to the number of males (21). The reason may be perhaps due to CC cancer being discussed here is one of the women gynecological cancers or questionnaire was more distributed among women online groups. However, HPV infection affects both females and males and can cause other cancers rather than CC. Similar incidence also occurred in the age group (**Figure 1c**) where ages from 35 to 44, 45–54, and 55–64 were the age group that participated. The score value from the age group 45–54 was very high and statically significant compared to other age groups. This is perhaps due to the screening stage of cervical cancer falling in these age groups. Again, the survey questionnaire was mostly distributed among women groups than men groups. For the race, Africans was the most participated (**Figure 1b**). This could be a result of influence due to location and execution of study questionnaire. However, studies have observed that traditional medicine/herbal products are being practiced and used mostly by poor African black communities for their wellbeing [11, 23].

It is quite interesting that a high number of participants (78) already have the knowledge of HPV infection and its impact on the associating types of cancer (**Figure 2**).

Medicinal Plants	Active compounds	References
Hedyotis diffusa	Rutin	Song et al., 2020 [20]
Rheum emodi	Croyophanol	Salaria et al., 2022 [21]
Thymus serpyllum	Apigenin	Salaria et al., 2022
Moringa oleifera	Glucomoringin	"
Brassica Oleracea	—	Yarnell Eric, 2015 [22]
Astragalus membranaceus	—	"
Platycodon grandiflorus	—	"
Wolfiporia cocos	—	"
Angelica sinensis	—	Yarnell Eric, 2015
Berberis aristata	Berbamine	Salaria et al., 2022
Zanthoxylum armatum	Armatamide	"
Oxalis corniculata	Isovitexin	Salaria et al., 2022

Table 1.
Some medicinal plants/phytoconstituents that have been evaluated for anti-carcinogenicity for HPV.

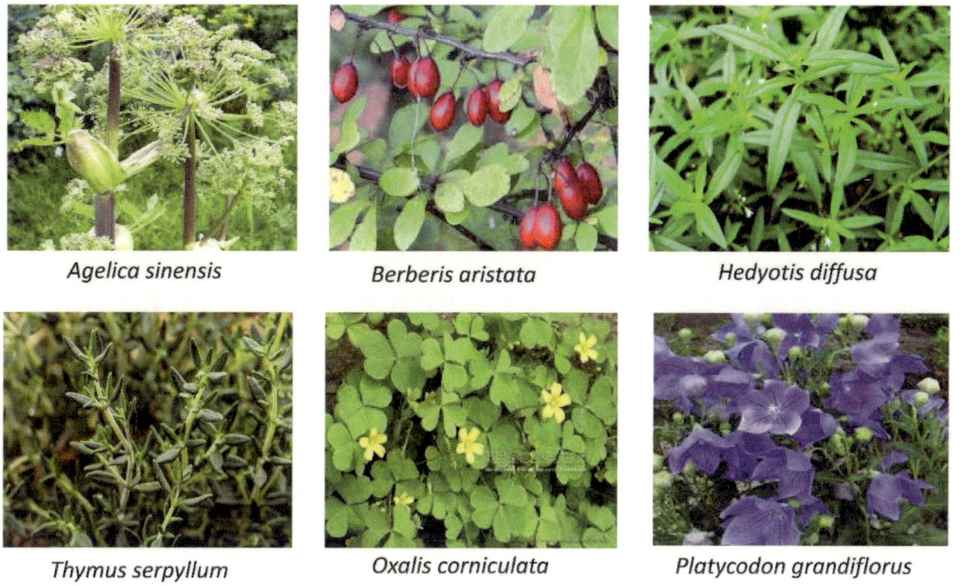

Figure 7.
Photographs of some of the plants listed in ***Table 1.***

Only few participants (15) revealed that their relatives had experienced a type of cancer disease due to HPV infection. Consequently, the number of participants recorded with financial burdens was small/few (**Figure 3**).

Additionally, many participants (63) indicated that they have used herbal products for different purposes. However, 43 participants showed that they have never used herbal products for any purpose. This study impressively indicated that almost all the participants (96) know that herbal products can be effectively used singly or in combination for the treatment of diseases (**Figure 5**). This number is highly statistically significant (P-Value = 0.000 < 5%) compared to those without awareness. Furthermore, **Figure 6** of this study indicated the willingness of the participants to support or patronize the use of any native flora/herbal product discovered for the management/treatment of HPV infection.

5. Conclusion

Knowing people's reaction over the therapeutic capacity of these herbal products will not only help in the production of herbal products for HPV infection and reduce the prevalence of cervical cancer/other HPV implicated cancers but it will be of economic importance to agriculture and health sector. It will also address the gap of unemployment and good propagation of medicinal plants species that are on the verge of being wiped off. The knowledge will also attract more research in the field of agriculture, biomedical sciences, pharmaceuticals, chemistry, biotechnology, etc. This study could perhaps serve as a common interaction between people's notions and the use of medicinal plant extracts and herbal products for the treatment of HPV infection and other related diseases.

For future work, we intend to work on already identified medicinal plants found to have antiviral effects with HPV up to the prototype stage and further.

Challenges encountered: Study should have the survey for a longer period of time so as to get more people involved and a more generalizable result. Our current study is for a short period of time and with a small population. Our survey was not widely distributed and the links sometimes were not easily accessed. Some of the survey questions were not completely answered so many questionnaires were eliminated.

Acknowledgements

The authors like to thank the Foundation for women's health promotion and welfare initiatives (FWHPWI) members for assisting in the filling and dissemination of the online survey questionnaire links to the public, and Prof David Katerere and group, Department of Pharmaceutical Sciences, Faculty of Science, Tshwane University of Technology for their encouragement.

Conflict of interest

No conflict of interest.

Author details

Franca Nneka Alaribe Nnadozie[1,2]*, Sidonie Tankeu[1,2] and Daisy Nwaozuzu[1,3]

1 Foundation for Women's Health Promotion and Welfare Initiatives, Pretoria, Gauteng, South Africa

2 Department of Pharmaceutical Sciences, Tshwane University of Technology, Faculty of science, Pretoria, Gauteng, South Africa

3 Coventry University, Coventry, United Kingdom

*Address all correspondence to: foundationforwomenshealth@gmail.com; chisara5@hotmail.com

References

[1] Bruni L, Albero G, Serrano B, Mena M, Gómez D, Muñoz J, et al. ICO/IARC Information Centre on HPV and Cancer (HPV Information Centre). Human Papillomavirus and Related Diseases in South Africa: In Cancer Association of South Africa (CANSA) Position Statements and Fact Sheet on Cervical Cancer 2020. 2019. https://cansa.org.za/ what-cansa-believes/

[2] Burt LM, McCormak M, Lecuru F, Kanyike DM, Bvochora-Nsingo M, Ndlovu N, et al. Cervix cancer in sub-Saharan Africa: An assessment of cervical cancer management. An American Society of Clinical Oncology Journal. 2021;**2**:173-182

[3] Zhang HY, Tigglaac SM, Sahascabuddhe W, Smith JS, Jiang CQ, Mei RB, et al. HPV prevalence and cervical intraepithelial neoplasia among HIV-infected women in Yunnan Province, China: A pilot study. Asian Pasific Journal of Cancer Prevention. 2012;**13**(1):91-96. DOI: 10.7314/APJCP.2012.13.1.091

[4] Temmerman M, Tyndall MW, Kidula N, Claeys P, Muchiri L, Quint W. Risk factors for human papillomavirus and cervical precancerous lesions, and the role of concurrent HIV-1 infection. International Journal of Gynecology & Obstetrics. 1999;**65**:171-181. DOI: 10.1016/S0020-7292(99)00043-0

[5] Human papilloma virus vaccine. Available from: https://www.westerncape.gov.za/general-publication/hpv-vaccinations [Accessed December 10, 2021]

[6] Braimoh O, Dim CC, Nwagha HU, Ezegwui U. The need to incorporate routine cervical cancer counselling and screening in the management of women at outpatient clinics in Nigeria. Annals of African Medicine. 2014;**11**(2):201

[7] Mensah KB, Mensah ABB. Cancer control in Ghana: A narrative review in global context. Cell Press. 2020;**6**(8):e04564. DOI: 10.1016/j.heliyon.2020

[8] Alaribe FN, Motaung KSCM. Medicinal plants in tissue engineering and regenerative medicine in the African continent. Tissue Engineering. Part A. 2019;**25**(11-12):827-829. DOI: 10.1089/ten.TEA.2019.0060 PMID: 30838937

[9] Sulaiman FA, Kazeem MO, Waheed AM, Temowo SO, Azeez IO, Zubair FI, et al. Antimicrobial and toxic potential of aqueous extracts of Allium sativum, Hibiscus sabdariffa and Zingiber officinale in Wistar rats. Journal of Taibah University for Science. 2014;**8**(4):315-322. DOI: 10.1016/j.jtusci.2014.05.004

[10] Ullah R, Alqahtani AS, Noman OMA, Alqahtani AM, Ibenmoussa S, Bourhia M. A review on ethno-medicinal plants used in traditional medicine in the Kingdom of Saudi Arabia. Saudi Journal of Biological Sciences. 2020;**27**(10):2706-2718. DOI: 10.1016/j.sjbs.2020.06.020

[11] Alaribe FN, Maepa MJ, Mkhumbeni N, Motaung SCKM. Possible roles of Eucomis autumnalis medicinal plant in bone and cartilage regeneration: A review. Tropical Journal of Pharmaceutical Research. 2018;**17**:741

[12] Bisi-Johnson MA, Obi CL, Hattori T, Oshima Y, Li S, Kambizi L, et al. Evaluation of the antibacterial and anticancer activities of some south African medicinal plants. BMC

Complementary and Alternative Medicine. 2011;**11**:14

[13] Hensel A, Kisseih E, Lechtenberg M, Petereit E, Agyare C, Asase A. In: Heinrich EM, Jager AK, editors. From Ethnopharmacological Field Study to Phytochemistry and Preclinical Research: The Example of Ghanaian Medicinal Plants for Improved Wound Healing. 1st ed. Chichester, UK: John Wiley & Sons, Ltd.; 2015. pp. 179-197

[14] Moshi MJ. Current and future prospects of integrating traditional and alternative medicine in the management of diseases in Tanzania. Tanzania Health Research Bulletin. 2005;7:159

[15] Healthline. Everything you need to know about human papillomavirus infection, 2017. Available from: https://www.healthline.com/health/hpv-in-the-mouth#prevention [Accessed July 15, 2021]

[16] Ayat P, Sharif S, Hewitt K, Grigorian A, Goldman SA, McFarlane IM. Vulvar squamous cell carcinoma in a patient with AIDS: A case study. American Journal of Medical Case Reports. 2020;**8**:522-527

[17] BMC. Mapping evidence on the distribution of human papillomavirus-related cancers in sub-Saharan Africa: scoping review protocol. Available from: https://systematicreviewsjournal.biomedcentral.com/articles/10.1186/s13643-017-0623-3

[18] American Association for Cancer Research (AACR). Lets End HPV Related Cancers. Available from: https://www.aacr.org/professionals/policy-and-advocacy/science-policy

[19] Nigeria: Human Papillomavirus and Related Cancers. Fact Sheet. 2021. https://hpvcentre.net/statistics/reports/NGA_FS.pdf

[20] Salaria D, Rolta R, Mehta J, Awofisayo O, Fadare OA, Kaur B, et al. Phytoconstituents of traditional Himalayan herbs as potential inhibitors of human papillomavirus (HPV-18) for cervical cancer treatment: An *In silico* approach. PLoS One. 2022;**17**(3):e0265420. DOI: 10.1371/journal.pone.0265420

[21] Song Y-C, Huang H-C, Chang CY-Y, Lee H-J, Liu C-T, Lo H-Y, et al. A potential herbal adjuvant combined with a peptide-based vaccine acts against HPV-related tumors through enhancing effector and memory T-cell immune responses. Frontiers in Immunology. 2020;**11**:62. DOI: 10.3389/fimmu.2020.00062

[22] Eric Y. Herbs against Human Papillomavirus. Alternative and Complementary Therapies. 2015;**21**:2. DOI: 10.1089/act.2015.21205

[23] Alaribe FN, Razwinani M, Makwese M, Motaung KSC. The potential effect of medicinal plants for cartilage regeneration. In: Nikolopoulos DD, Safos GK, Dimitrios K, editors. Cartilage Tissue Engineering and Regeneration Techniques. London, UK: IntechOpen; 2019. DOI: 10.5772/intechopen.84780

Chapter 2

Paris polyphylla: An Important Endangered Medicinal Plants of Himalayan Foothills

Arunkumar Phurailatpam and Anju Choudhury

Abstract

Paris polyphylla is an important threatened medicinal plants found mainly in the north eastern parts of India. These rhizomatic plants are in great demands and extracted injudiciously from the wild. The rhizome is the economic part which is used for its various medicinal properties. The present article gives an account of updated information on its phytochemical and pharmacological properties and its ethno medicinal uses on account of the tale from the local people and veds, literature and their conservation aspects in the region. The review reveals that wide numbers of phytochemical constituents have been isolated from these plants. The rhizomes of the several species of the genus *Paris* have been used as haemostatic and anti-inflammatory agent to treat traumatic injuries, snake bites, abscess, parotitis and mastitis. For the last few decades or so, extensive research work has been done to prove its biological activities and pharmacology of its extracts. Excessive injudicious collection and harvesting from the wild has pushed these species towards extinction. Domestication, cultivation and strict laws are the need of the hour to save these species from extinction.

Keywords: medicinal plants, *Paris polyphylla*, conservation, threatenened, North East India

1. Introduction

The knowledge of using of plants and herbs as medicines and for the treatment of many kinds of diseases and for healthy living is handed over from generation to generation in all the communities. Numerous traditional uses of plants and herbs for medicinal purposes have been documented and published time by time. Mankind has been continuously using the medicinal plants in several ways for treating of various ailments and for cosmetics purposes. In India, the sacred Vedas dating back between 3500 B.C and 800 B.C gave many references of medicinal plants. "Virikshayurveda is one of the oldest works in traditional herbal medicine in India, which is compiled even before the beginning of Christian era and it formed the basis of medicinal studies in ancient India. Knowledge of herbs has been handed down from generation to generation for thousands of years and herbal drugs constitute a major part in all traditional systems of medicines. Plants have been used for medicine from time immemorial because they are easily accessible and cheap and above all they were the only means for healthcare. Recently, there has been a tremendous increase in the use of herbal products in many countries, both developing and developed, which resulted in an exponential growth of herbal products globally. Herbal medicines have a strong traditional or conceptual base and the potential for them to be useful as drugs in terms of safety and effectiveness, leads for treating different diseases. Many of the population in the developing and underdeveloped countries still depend on herbal medicine where access to modern medicine is little [1]. Plants continue to serve as possible sources for developing new drugs from the chemicals derived from various parts of plants. In recent time there has been a marked shift towards herbal cures because of the adverse and noticeable side effects of modern drugs. However, due to increase in population, deforestation, roads and railways, urbanization and unsustainable harvesting and collection from the wild, many useful plant species along with their uses are disappearing every day. Unsustainable and injudicious extractions of these medicinal plants have pushed some of the important species towards extinction. An important anti cancerous plant, *Taxus wallichiana* Zuccarini was pushed towards endangerment due to injudicious harvesting and collection of Paclitaxel (Taxol), the most effective anti cancerous compound used for treating a variety of cancers [2, 3]. This species was extracted in large scale from the wild injudiciously for its anti-cancerous properties during 1980s which led endangered status at present [4]. It has become the most threatened species and has been categorized as endangered by the IUCN [5]. Today, history is again repeating for many other species, including *Paris polyphylla* Smith. In this context, I would like to bring forth an important threatened medicinal plant species (*Paris polyphylla*) found in North eastern part of India in the foothills of Himalayan which has been very less documented and evaluated but talking of its importance, it's a plant with varied medicinal uses and great demand in the market.

Paris polyphylla is a rhizomatous herbaceous species belonging to Melanthiaceae family. The genus comprises of 24 species, which are distributed in Bhutan, China, India, Japan, Korea, Laos, Mongolia, Myanmar, Nepal, Russia, Thailand, Vietnam and Europe [6]. China has the highest number of species (22 species) with 12 endemic species. In India the genus is represented by 2 species, *viz. P. polyphylla* and *P. thibetica* with about 6 intraspecific taxa (**Table 1**) [6].

As of May 2012 the World Checklist of Selected Plant Families (WCSP) recognizes several varieties [8, 9].

- *Paris polyphylla* var. *alba*
- *Paris polyphylla* var. *chinensis*
- *Paris polyphylla* var. *latifolia*
- *Paris polyphylla* var. *nana*
- *Paris polyphylla* var. *panxiensis*
- *Paris polyphylla* var. *polyphylla*
- *Paris polyphylla* var. *stenophyla*
- *Paris polyphylla* var. *yunnanensis*

State	District	Village/region	Local name
Arunachal Pradesh	Kameng, Subansiri, Kurung Kume, Siang, Lohit, Tirap and Changlang	—	Do-Tala
Manipur	Senapati	Hengbung, Maram, Purul and Ma-kui regions	Singpan
	Tamenglong	Puilong Village	
Uttarakhand	—	—	Satwa
Himachal Pradesh	—	—	—
Jammu & Kashmir	—	—	—
Mizoram	—	—	—
Sikkim	—	—	—
Nagaland	Tuensang	Pangsha village	—
	Phek	Chida region	
	Kohima	Arudara region	
	Mokokchung	Longkum village	
Meghalaya	West Khasi Hill	Nongstoin region	Sohbsein

Source: [7].

Table 1.
Geographical distribution and availability of P. polyphylla *in India.*

The Flora of China recognizes five additional varieties, three of which are placed in different species by the WCSP:

- *P. polyphylla* var. *appendiculata* = *P. thibetica*
- *P. polyphylla* var. *brachystemon* = *P. polyphylla* var. *stenophyla*
- *P. polyphylla* var. *kwantungensis* = *P. polyphylla* var. *polyphylla*
- *P. polyphylla* var. *minor* = *P. delavayi*
- *P. polyphylla* var. *pseudothibetica* = *P. delavayi*

2. Taxonomic classification

Common Name—PARIS
Botanical Name—*Paris polyphylla* Sm.
Family—Melanthiaceae
Part Used—Rhizome

P. polyphylla is a shade loving herbaceous, perennial plant usually found in temperate and subtropical regions. It grows well in shady moist forest thickets and bamboo forests with moist soil. It bears rhizomes which is the economical part and has medicinal properties. It has a single unbranched stem and 2–3 whorls of leaves are present on the nodes. It flowers during the month of April. It has odd flowers with long yellow radiating anthers [10]. The morphological characteristics of the herb are given below (**Figure 1**):

Habit: Aerial, erect plant, herb, rhizomatous,.

Stem: Unbranched, non woody, smooth, 50–100 cm tall, 1–2.5 cm thick.

Leaf: Simple type, arranged in whorls and petiolate; lanceolate, reticulate with three primary veins, smooth margin, spider-like flowers.

Inflorescence: At the initial growth stage It forms a closed whorl

Flower: blooms at terminal. Flowers are solitary, yellowish green; monoecious; sepaloid outer is larger and inner is smaller, tepal 3–5.

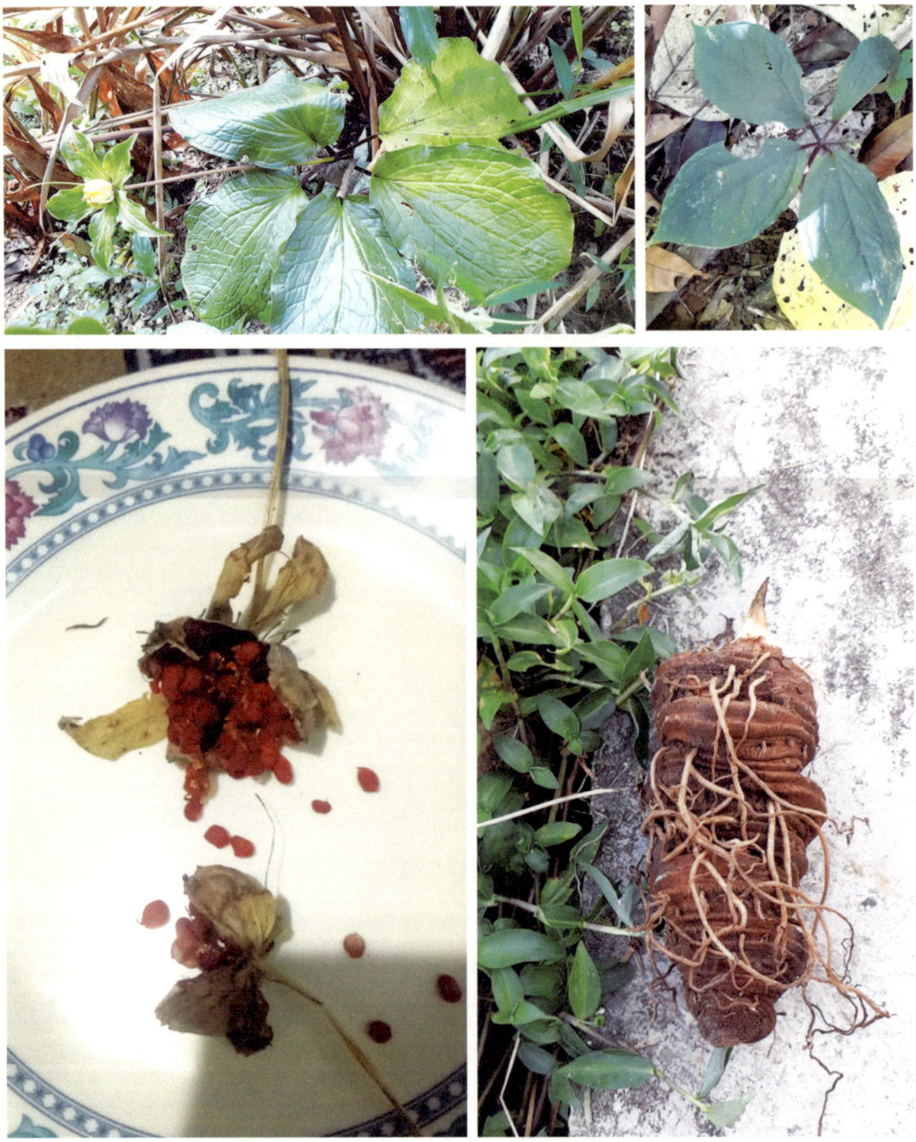

Figure 1.
Arunkumar Phurailatpam, College of Horticulture and Forestry, Central Agricultural University, Pasighat, Arunachal Pradesh, India.

Androecium: Stamens-free and 6–11 in numbers.
Gynoecium: 1 pistil, 3–5 carpels, syncarpous (carpels fused), ovary superior.
Seed: Reddish orange in colour; a mature fruit contains about 50–60 seeds.

3. Habitat

P. polyphylla grows luxuriantly under the shade with a good canopy closure at an altitude of 1300–2500 m above sea level as forest under storey. It grows mainly in a forest with bamboo groves, grassy or rocky slopes, stream-sides, mixed conifer forests and scrub thickets [6]. It is a slow germinating herb and takes about seven to eight months to sprout from the seed. It thrives well inside the deep forest cover in nature. It grows best in humus-rich and well-drained soil and waterlogging is found to be lethal for this herb. Plants that lack inflorescences are usually shorter in height. It has been reported that the plants when taken out of the natural habitat failed to either flower or set seed. This plant is a very slow growing herb and almost takes a year to increase it rhizome size from one node to another and this is one important reason for the fast disappearance of this species from the natural habitat. The rhizomes are the economic part of this plant and they are harvested from the wild injudiciously.

4. Morphology

P. polyphylla is a perennial, rhizomatous, herbaceous plant with green and unbranched aerial parts which grows upto 50–100 cm. It has a erect smooth stems with a rhizome. The leaves are arranged in whorl and usually 6–7 in numbers. The leaves has parallel reticulate venation and lanceolate in shape. The flowers are borne above the leaves whorl and are yellow green in colour. The Inflorescence is solitary. Flowers are bisexual and the perianth is of two series. The outer sepaloid is larger as compared to the inner one. The tepals may be 3, 4 or 5. It contains 6–11 Androceum and the stamens are free. It contains one gynoecium and a pistil with 3–5 carpels. The

Variety	Description
P. polyphylla var. *alba*	Style and apical part of ovary white
P. polyphylla var. *chinensis*	Anthers about twice as long as filaments
P. polyphylla var. *kwantungensis*	Filaments can grow to about 10 mm; stigma lobes
P. polyphylla var. *latifolia*	Ovary and capsule tuberculate Ovary and capsule smooth
P. polyphylla var. *minor*	Filaments 1–2 mm; anthers around 6 mm
P. polyphylla var. *nana*	Plants about 10 cm tall; free portion of anther connective inconspicuous
P. polyphylla var. *polyphylla*	Leaf blade oblong, elliptic, or obovate—lanceolate, 2.5–5.0 cm wide
P. polyphylla var. *stenophylla*	Leaf blade lanceolate to linear-lanceolate; 1.5–2.5 cm wide
P. polyphylla var. *yunnanensis*	Inner tepals are 3–5 mm wide; distally widened sometimes; narrowly spatulate

Source: Flora of China (online), eFloras.org, retrieved 11 February 2015.

Table 2.
Different varieties of P. polyphylla.

ovary is superior. It blooms in the month of April–June in the region and flowering may last up to 3–4 months. The capsules split when it got ripened in late summer. A mature fruit contains 50–60 red seeds.

Different varieties of *P. polyphylla* have been identified. Some of them are given below (**Table 2**).

5. Ethno medicinal uses

This plant has many uses in traditional health care in many countries especially in China and Nepal. Some of the uses are as/in analgesic, removes heat, antispasmodic, antitussive, depurative, snake bites, boils and ulcers, diphtheria and epidemic Japanese B encephalitis, stomach ache, appendicitis, tonsillitis, insect bites, boils. It also counteracts toxicity, causes the subsidence of swelling, alleviates pain and relieves convulsions, boils, carbuncles, sore throat, traumatic pain, convulsions. It also has anti-tumor action.

6. Pharmacology

6.1 Anti tumour activity

Lee et al. [11] of the Department of Biochemistry, the Chinese University of Hong Kong reported that the steroidal saponin of *Paris polyphylla,* polyphyllin D, could served as a candidate for breast cancer treatment. It was found that treatment of MCF-7 and MDA-MB-231 cells with polyphyllin D resulted in the inhibition of viability and induction of apoptosis in a dose dependent manner. Mechanistically, polyphyllin D dissipates the mitochondrial membrane potential, induces a down regulation of anti-apoptotic Bcl 2 expression and an up-regulation of pro-apoptotic Bax-expression and activate caspase 9.

Yan et al. [12] of Tianjin University, China has reported that (Diosgenin-3-α-L-arabinfuranosyl (1-4)-[α-L-rhamnopyanosyl (1-2)]-β-D-Glycopyranoside), the main steroidal saponin of *Paris polyphylla* showed remarkable cytotoxicity and caused typical apoptosis in a dose dependent manner. Rhizoma Paridis saponins showed anti-cancer activity against lung adenocarcinoma cell lines, both *in-vivo* and *in-vitro*.

While investigating the anti-cancer activity of 15 traditional Chinese medicines which are usually used for tumour patients in China, using MTT(methyl thiazolylt diphenyl-tetrazolium bromide) method on 6 human digestive tumour cell lines-human liver carcinoma cell lines ($HepG_2$) and SMMC-7721), human gastric cancer cell lines (BGC-823), human colon adenocarcinoma cell line (LoVo and W-116) and oesophagus adenocarcinoma cell line (CaEs-17), it was found t ha t *Paris polyphyll a* showed a predominant inhibitory effect on all the cell lines with IC50 values ranging from 10 μg/mL to 30 μg/mL. The finding suggested the potential of *Paris polyphylla* Smith against digestive cancer [13].

Anti tumour constituents from *Paris polyphylla* var. yunanensis isolated by column chromatography with silica gel and purified by Sephadex LH20 column chromatography and reverse phase preparative HPLC [14] are:

1. Diosgenin-3-O-α-L-arabinofuranosyl (1-4) β-D-glycopyranoside

2. Pennogenin-3-O-α-L-arabinofuranosyl (1-4) β-D-glycopyranoside

3. Isorhamn etin-3-O-β-D-glycopyranoside
4. Ethyl-α-D-fructofuranoside
5. Pennogenin-3-O-α-L-rhamnopyranosyl (1-4)[α-L-rhamnopyranosyl(1-2)] β-D-glycopyranoside, and
6. 6.Pennogenin-3-O-α-L-rhamnopyranosyl (1-4) [α-L-rhamnopyranosyl (1-4)] α-L-[α-L-rhamnopyranosyl(1-2)] β-D-glycopyranoside.

6.2 Immuno-stimulating properties

In the study of three diosgenyl saponin compounds is olated from *Paris polyphylla* i.e. **(1)** 3-O-α-1-rhamnopyranosyl (1-4)-α-1-rhamnopyranosyl (1-4)-[α-1-rhamnopyranosyl (1-2)-α-d-glucopyranoside, **(2)** Diosgenin-3-O-α-1-rhamnopyranosyl (1-2)-α-1-arabinofuranosyl-β-d-glucopyranoside and **(3)** Diosgenin on the immuno-modulatory activity about phagocytosis, respiratory burst and nitric oxide (NO) production, it was found that **(1)** and **(2)** exhibited significant enhancement of phagocytosis, respiratory burst and NO product ion in RAW 264.7 cells (mouse macrophage cells) but **(3)** only showed great augmentation of phagocytotic function. **(3)** Neither showed respiratory burst response nor increases the production of NO. It was concluded that the presence of glucoside moieties of diosgenyl saponins is essential for the activation of immunological reactions, especially during the period of oxygen consumption such as in the process including inflammation and microbial activity although diosgenin **(3)** could only stimulate the macrophages phagocytosis including elimination of foreign or denatured substance [15].

7. Anti-bacterial action

The roots have shown anti bacterial action against *Bacillus dysentery, B. typhi, B. paratyphi, E. coli, Staphylacoccus aureas, Haemolytic streptococci, Meningococci* etc. [16].

8. Spermicidal action

The plant extract showed effective spermicidal activity against rat and human sperms. The vaginal application of the plant's extract (100 mg/animal) prevented pregnancy up to 60% of the rabbits tested [17].

9. Anti fungal

Deng et al. in 2008 evaluated the anti-fungal activity of *Paris polyphylla* saponin against *Cladosporium cladosporioides* and *Candida species* and showed comparable activity to chemicals used in some commercial products.

10. Others

The rhizome of the plant contains sugars (7.9%) and two glycosides viz a-paridin (m.p. 244–46°) and a-paristypnin (m.p. 147–49°) which produces a tingling sensation on the tongue. α-Paristypnin has a depressant action on carotid pressure, myocardium and respiratory movements. It produces vasoconstriction in kidney, vasodilation in the spleen and limbs and stimulates the intestines [17].

11. Chemical composition

Devkota [17] isolated 6 (six) compounds from *Paris polyphylla* collected from Parbat district Nepal.

The compounds are

1. Przewalskinone B (1,5-Dihydroxy-7-methoxy-3-methylanthraquinone) which has a anthraquinone skeleton

2. Polyphyllin C (Diosgenin-3-O[α-Lrhamnopyanosyl(1-3)-β-D-glucopyranoside) which has a steroidal skeleton.

3. Polyphyllin D (Diosgenin-3-O[α-Lrhamnopyanosyl (1_{Rha}-2_{Glu})-α-Larabinofuranosyl (1_{Ara}-4_{Glu})]-β–D-Glucopyranoside) which has a steroidal skeleton

4. Saponin-1 (Diosgenin-3-O[α-L-rhamnopyanosyl (1_{Rha}-2_{Glu})-α-L-rhamnopyranosyl (1_{Ara}-4_{Glu})]-β-D-Glucopyranoside) which has a steroidal skeleton

5. Stigmasterol which is a steroid, and

6. Stigmasterol-3-O-β-D-glucoside.

A new saponin-polyphyllin A-H has been isolated from the rhizome of *Paris polyphylla* of which first six are spirostanol steroidal saponins and remaining two are furastanol steroidal saponins [18].

A novel steroidal saponin along with the 12 known compounds were separated from *Paris polyphylla* var. chinensis [19]. The novel compound was obtained as an amorphous solid and spectral data including two dimensional NMR showed the structure as 3b,21-dihydroxypregnane-5-en-20S-(22,16)-lactone-1-O-a-L-rhamnopyrnosyl(1®2)-[b-D-xylopyranosyl(1®3)]-b-D-glucopyranoside.The 12 known compounds are known steroids and their structures were identified by 13C NMR spectrum as

1. Diosgenin

2. Pennogenin

3. Diosgenin-3-*O*-a-L-rhamnopyranosyl(1→2)-b-D-glucopyranoside

4. Pennogenin-3-*O*-a-L-rhamnopyranosyl(1→2)-b-D-glucopyranoside

5. Diosgenin-3-*O*-a-L-rhamnopyranosyl (1→2)[a-Larabinofuranosyl(1→4)]-b-D-glucopyranoside

Plant species	Isolated compounds
P. polyphylla	Paris saponin I (diosgenin3-O-α-L-rha-(1→2)-[α-L-arab-(1→4)]-β-D-glu)
	Paris saponin I (diosgenin3-O-α-rha-(1→4)-α-L-rha-(1→4)-[α-L-rha-(1→2)]-β-D-glu)
	Paris saponin III (diosgenin 3-O-α-L-rhamnopyranosyl-(1→2)-[α-L-rhamnopyranosyl-(1→4)]-β-D-glucopyranoside)
	PolyphyllinVI (pennogenin-3-O-α-L-rhamnopyranosyl-(1→2)-β-D-glucopyranoside)
	Polyphyllin VII (pennogenin-3-O-α-L-rhamnopyranosyl-(1→4)-α-L-rhamnopyranosyl-(1→4)[O-β-D-glucopyranosyl-(1→2)]-β-D-glucopyranoside)
P. polyphylla	Saponin-1 (diosgenin-3-O[α-L-rhamnopyanosyl (1Rha-2Glu)-α-L-rhamnopyranosyl (1Ara-4Glu)]-β-glucopyranoside)
	Polyphyllin C (diosgenin-3-O[α-L-rhamnopyanosyl(1→3)-α-D-glucopyranoside)
	Polyphyllin D (diosgenin-3-O[α-L-rhamnopyanosyl (1Rha-2Glu)-α-L-arabinofuranosyl (1Ara-4Glu)]-β-D-glucopyranoside)
	Przewalskinone B (1,5-Dihydroxy-7-methoxy-3-methylanthraquinone)
	Stigmasterol
	Stigmasterol-3-O-β-D-glucoside
P. polyphylla var. chinensis	Diosgenin
	Pennogenin
	Diosgenin-3-O-α-L-rhamnopyranosyl (1→2)-β-D-glucopyranoside
	Pennogenin-3-O-α-L-rhamnopyranosyl(1→2)-β-D-glucopyranoside
	Diosgenin-3-O-α-L-rhamnopyranosyl(1→2) [-α-L-arabinofuranosyl(1→4)]-β-D-glucopyranoside
	Pennogenin-3-O-α-L-rhamnopyranosyl(1→2)[-α-L arabinofuranosyl (1→4)]-β-D-glucopyranoside
	Diosgenin-3-O-α-L-rhamnopyranosyl(1→2)-[β-D-glucopyranoside(1→3)]-β-D-glucopyranoside
	Diosgenin-3-O-α-L-rhamnopyranosyl (1→4)-α-L rhamnopyranosyl (1→4)[α-L-rhamnopyranosyl (1→2)]-β-D-glucopyranoside
	Pennogenin-3-O-α-L-rhamnopyranosyl(1→4)-α-L-rhamnopyranosyl (1→4)[α-L-rhamnopyranosyl (1→2)]-β-D-glucopyranoside
	3-O-α-L-arabinofuranosyl(1→4)[α-L-rhamnopyranosyl(1→2)]-β-D-glucopyranoside-β-D-chacotriosyl-26-O-β-D-glucopyranoside
	2β, 3β, 14α, 20β, 22α, 25β hexahydroxycholest-7-en-6-one
	2β,3β,14α, 20β,24β,25β hexahydroxycholest-7-en-6-one
P. polyphylla var. chinensis	3b, 21-dihydroxy pregnane-5-en-20S-(22,16)-lactone-1-O-α-L-rhamnopyranosyl (1→2)-[β-D-xylopyranosyl (1→3)]-β-D-glucopyranoside.
P. polyphylla Smith var. yunnanensis	(25R)-spirost-5-en-3b,7b-diol-3-O-α-L-arabinofuranosyl-(1→4)-[α-L-rhamnopyranosyl-(1→2)]-β-D-glucopyranoside
	(25R)-spirost-5-en-3b,7a-diol-3-O-α-L-arabinofuranosyl-(1→4)-[α-L-rhamnopyranosyl-(1→2)]-β-D-glucopyranoside
	26-O-β-D-glucopyranosyl-(25R)-$\Delta^{5(6)\ 17(20)}$-dien-16,22-dione-cholestan-3b,26-diol-3-O-α-L-arabinofuranosyl-(1→4)-[α-L-rhamnopyranosyl-(1→2)]-β-D-glucopyranoside

Plant species	Isolated compounds
P. polyphylla Smith var. yunnanensis	26-O-β-D-glucopyranosyl-(25R)-5-ene-furost-3β,17α, 22α, 26-tetrol-3-O-α-L-arabinofuranosyl-(1→4)-[α-L-rhamnopyranosyl-(1→2)]-β-D-glucopyranoside
	26-O-β-Dglucopyranosyl-(25R)-5, 20 (22)-diene-furost-3β, 26-diol-3-O-α-L-arabinofuranosyl-(1→4)-[α-L-rhamnopyranosyl-(1→2)]-β-D-glucopyranoside
	(25R)-spirost-5-ene-3β, 12α-diol-3-O-α-L-rhamnopyranosyl-(1→4)-α-L-rhamnopyranosyl-(1→4)-[α-L-rhamnopyranosyl-(1→2)]-β-D-glucopyranoside
P. polyphylla var. stenophylla	24-O-β-D-galactopyranosyl-(23S,24S,25S)-spirost-5-ene-1b,3b,21,23,24-pentol-1-O-α-L-rhamnopyranosyl-(1→ 2)-[β-D-xylopyranosyl-(1→3)]-β-D-glucopyranoside
	21-O-β-D-galactopyranosyl-24-O-β-D-galactopyranosyl-(23S,24S)-spirost-5,25(27)-diene-1b,3b,21,23,24-pentol-1-O-α-L-rhamnopyranosyl-(1→ 2)-[β-D-xylopyranosyl-(1→3)]-β-D-glucopyranoside

Source: [7].

Table 3.
Some chemical constituents isolated from the rhizomes of P. polyphylla.

6. Pennogenin-3-*O*-a-Lrhamnopyranosyl (1→2)-[a-Larabinofuranosyl(1→4)]-b-D-glucopyranoside
7. Diosgenin-3-*O*-a-L-rhamnopyranosyl (1→2) [b-Dglucopyranoside(1→3)]-b-D–glucopyranoside
8. *D*iosgenin-3-O-a-L-rhamnopyranosyl (1→4)-a-Lrhamnopyranosyl (1→4)[a-L-rhamnopyranosyl (1→2)]-b-D-glucopyranoside
9. Pennogenin-3-*O*-a-Lrhamnopyranosyl (1→4)-a-Lrhamnopyranosyl (1→4) [a-L–rhamnopyranosyl (1→2)]-b-D-glucopyranoside
10. 3-*O*-a-Larabinofuranosyl(1→4)[a-Lrhamnopyranosyl (1→2)]-b-D-glucopyranoside-b-D-chacotriosyl-26-*O*-b-D-glucopyranoside
11. 2b,3b,14a,20b,22a,25b hexahydroxycholest-7-en-6-one, and
12. 2b,3b,14a,20b,24b,25b hexahydroxycholest-7-en-6-one (**Table 3**).

12. Propagation

P. polyphylla grows well in humus-rich moist soil in full or partial shade. Prolonged seed dormancy and slow germination is the real challenge for regeneration through seed. It is mainly propagated by rhizomes though propagation by seed is also possible. Hence rhizomes from the wild are the only source for propagation as well as for medicinal purposes. Slow regeneration, long dormancy period, slow growth period along with over exploitation are the main reasons for decline in the population of *P. polyphylla* in the wild. It is on the verge of extinction due to its excessive illegal collection for many years [15]. Moreover, this perennial plant can only be harvested after growing for 5–7 years, which aggravates the shortage of its resource [20].

To preserve this natural resource and ensure a stable and renewable source of *P. polyphylla* for medicinal purposes, successful propagation is imperative [21].

This calls for an urgent need to discover alternate resources from which the continuous supply can be obtained. Domestication of this plant and cultivation in large scale in those areas similar to natural habitat is the only solution to save this plant from extinction. Propagation by tissue culture is another prospective for the propagation and conservation of this endangered plant species.

13. Conservation

Paris polyphylla Sm. (Satuwa) is one of the medicinal plants listed as vulnerable by the IUCN. Seed viability was found to be low and the seeds did not germinate in laboratory conditions even under different chemical treatments. The growth of the rhizome is very slow and takes almost a year to increase its node number. There seems to be a need for raising awareness amongst people living near the plant habitat on *Paris polyphylla* propagation. Scientists must make aware the sustainable use of the rhizome and its cultivation practice for the conservation of this plant. If some part of the rhizome containing the bud is left underground, the plant would become more sustainable and would help in conserving its population in the future. It was observed in a study done in Nepal, that overharvesting, unscientific collection of rhizomes, harvesting of plants before seed maturity, low viable seed production and long dormancy of seeds are some of the major threats to the plant's propagation. *Paris polyphylla* is considered to be a highly traded plant and have become less abundant in the past decade and this could be due to deforestation. It is found out that during the harvesting process, the whole plant is often uprooted to collect the rhizome, which leads to the destruction of the stock. During harvesting or collection from the wild the every plant is uprooted for its rhizomes irrespective of its maturity. This unsustainable harvesting practice, combined with illegal/cross-border trades of rhizome, and habitat destructions were common in their natural habitat. Old growth habitat decline and fragmentation were major threats to the population of *P. polyphylla*. Market driven collection resulted in rushed and premature collection and habitat degradation. Cultivation of the species coupled with *in-situ* conservation could be a solution to address the escalated herbal demand.

Local communities opined that the need of the risen market demand for its medicinal, biological and pharmaceutical purposes can be met once the *P. polyphylla* can be sustainably harvested and cultivated with the active involvement of local communities and application of sustainable harvesting guidelines. Works are progressed at College of Horticulture and Forestry, Central Agricultural University, Pasighat, Arunachal Pradesh, India for the conservation of this vulnerable species. Tissue cultured plants are produced in the laboratory from the rhizomes of *Paris polyphylla* collected from natural habitat. Then the tissue cultured plants are planted in the wild in their natural habitat or similar habitat so that it can grow and increases its population in nature without interference from human.

14. Conclusion

Paris polyphylla is an important medicinal plants found in the North Eastern part of India which are threatened by the over exploitation and lack in cultivation efforts. This species have many medicinal properties for the treatment of many ailments. Due to their less population and availability these plants fetch a very good price in the market. Most of these plants are sold in the black market and due to its great demand the plants are collected or harvested injudiciously from the wild which push them towards threaten stage. *P. polyphylla* usually grows in high altitude and temperate region as forest understory. In natural habitat the propagation of this species takes much long time which also makes difficulty in propagation and multiplication in nature. Due to its great demand in the world market the species is collected from the wild injudiciously and causes the decline in population. This species comes under threatened species under IUCN. There is also a great demand in the market for this plant and many of which is met from cultivation. It's the need of the hour for the policy makers and scientist to frame policies and research work for the conservation of these two species before it is too late.

Author details

Arunkumar Phurailatpam* and Anju Choudhury
College of Horticulture and Forestry, Central Agricultural University, Pasighat, Arunachal Pradesh, India

*Address all correspondence to: arunkumarph@gmail.com

References

[1] WHO. WHO Traditional Medicine Strategy 2002-2005. Switzerland: World Health Organization, Geneva; 2002. p. 61

[2] Cragg JG, Donald SG. Testing identifiability and specification in instrumental variable models. Econometric Theory. 1993;**9**(2):222-240

[3] Goldspiel BR. Clinical overview of the taxanes. Pharmacotherapy: The Journal of Human Pharmacology and Drug Therapy. 1997;**17**(5P2):110S-125S

[4] Paul A, Bharali S, Khan ML, Tripathi OP. Anthropogenic disturbances led to risk of extinction of *Taxus wallichiana* Zuccarini, an endangered medicinal tree in Arunachal Himalaya. Natural Areas Journal. 2013;**33**:447-454

[5] Thomas P, Farjon A. Taxus wallichiana. The IUCN Red List of Threatened Species 2011: e.T46171879A9730085. 2011. DOI: 10.2305/IUCN.UK.2011- 2.RLTS. T46171879A9730085. en

[6] Liang S, Soukup VG. *Paris Linnaeus*. In: Sing-chi C, Song-jun L, Jiemei X, Tamura MN, editors. Flora of China, Flagellariaceae through Marantaceae. Vol. 24. St. Louis, USA: Science Press, China and Missouri Botanic Garden Press; 2000. pp. 88-95

[7] Arcadius P, Shiny CT. An overview of *Paris polyphylla*, a highly vulnerable medicinal herb of Eastern Himalayan Region for sustainable exploitation. The Natural Products Journal. 2020;**10**(1):3-14

[8] Govaerts RHA. World checklist of selected plant families published update Facilitated by the Trustees of the Royal Botanic Gardens, Kew. Cited as *Paris polyphylla* var. polyphylla. 2011

[9] Liang S, Soukup VG. "Paris polyphylla", retrieved 2012-05-01. In: Wu Z, Raven PH, Hong D, editors. (1994 onwards), Flora of China (online). 2012. Available from: eFloras.org [Accessed: May 01, 2012]

[10] Shah AS, Mazumder PB, Choudhury MD. Medicinal properties of *Paris polyphylla* smith: A review. Journal of Herbal Medical Toxicology. 2012;**6**(1):27-33

[11] Lee MS, Yuet-Wa JC, Kong SK, Yu B, Eng Choon VO, Nai Ching HW, et al. Effects of polyphyllin D, a steroidal saponin in *Paris polyphylla*, in growth inhibition of human breast cancer cells and in xenograft. Cancer Biology & Therapy. 2005;**4**(11):1248-1254

[12] Yan LL, Zhang YJ, Gao WY, Man SL, Wang Y. *In vitro* and *in vivo* anticancer activity of steroid saponins of *Paris polyphylla* var. yunnanensis. Experimental Oncology. 2009; **31**:27-32

[13] Sun J, Liu BR, Hu WJ, Yu LX, Qian XP. In vitro anticancer activity of aqueous extracts and ethanol extracts of fifteen traditional Chinese medicines on human digestive tumor cell lines. Phytotherapy Research. 2007;**21**:1102-1104

[14] Wang Y, Zhang YJ, Gao WY, Yan LL. Anti-tumor constituents from *Paris polyphylla* var. yunnanensis. China Journal of Chinese Materia Médica. 2007;**32**(14):1425-1428

[15] Zhang M, Li YW, Li ZY, Huang XL, Zhu and Liu Q.S. Progress on studies of endangered ethno-medicine of Rhizoma Paris. Journal of Central University Natural (Nat Sci Ed). 2011;**20**:65-69

[16] Anonymous. Newsfinder. 2002. pp. 1-4

[17] Devkota KP. Bioprospecting studies on Sarcococca hookeriana Bail, Sonchus wightianus DC, Paris polyphylla Smith and related medicinal herbs of Nepal [PhD thesis]. Karachi-75270, Pakistan: HEJResearch Institute of Chemistry, International Centre for Chemical Science, University of Karachi; 2005

[18] Rastogi P, Mehrotra BN. Compedium of Indian Medicinal Plants: CDRI-Lucknow and National Institute of Science and Communication New Delhi. 1992. 1993;3:479-480

[19] Yun H, Lijian C, Wenhong Z, Yuhong D, Yongli W, Qiang W, et al. Chemistry of Natural Products. 2007;**43**(6):672-677

[20] Wen F, Yin H, Chen C, Liu X, Xue D, Chen T, et al. Chemical characteristics of saponins from *Paris fargesii* var. brevipetala and cytotoxic activity of its main ingredient, paris saponin H. Fitoterapia. 2012;**83**:627-635

[21] Jianjun Q, Zheng N, Zhang B, Sun P, Hu S, Xu W, et al. Mining genes involved in the stratification of *Paris polyphylla* seeds using high-throughput embryo transcriptome sequencing. BMC Genomics. 2013;**14**:358

Chapter 3

Ethnobotany

Jafer Siraj

Abstract

Ethnobotany is a life science which studies the interaction between human beings and flora in particular and broadly deals with the investigations, observations, and identifications of botanical diversity used for the prevention and treatment of human and livestock ailments. The current chapter reviews the history and development of ethnobotany and the involvement of this branch of science in the innovation and derivation of drug products which is originated from plants and claimed by the traditional healers and indigenous people used for the prevention and treatment of disease. This chapter also combines interdisciplinary and multidisciplinary methods that can lead to further productive, comprehensive, and systemic guesstimates in the investigation of the relationship between the plants and humans. Regardless of its various bottlenecks, ethnobotany becomes an attractive and hopeful area of research. It also covers ethnobotanical knowledge and modern science, ethnobotany research and their applications, plant conservation and sustainable management practices, taxonomy, and economic botany. The chapter also deals with the ways in which different societies and cultures have come to perceive, know, use, classify, and symbolically represent plants and animals.

Keywords: ethnobotany, ethnobiology, ethnoecology, ethnomedicine, herbal medicine, ethnopharmacology, natural products, medicinal plants

1. Introduction

1.1 Ethnobotanical terms and concepts

The word ethnobotany was first announced by American botanist John Harshberger in 1896 as "the study of interaction of human beings with flora." Ethnobotany is a life science which studies the interaction between human beings and flora in particular and broadly deals with the investigations, observations, and identifications of botanical diversity used for the prevention and treatment of human and livestock ailments [1]. It also studies about the indigenous people knowledge, beliefs, and practices (i.e. it may be cultural and religious practices) related with medicinal plants. Also it includes how human beings categorize, isolate, and associate with floras besides with joint relationships of floras and human beings. The ethnobotanists should have to discuss with native community to share their routine life and to respect their cultures in order to obtain valuable information about the plants used for the medicinal purpose. Ethnobotanists have an obligation both to the scientific civic and the native principles. The field of ethnobotany is a much comprehensive discipline which is concerned in all studies about the interaction between human and floras. In addition to medicinal plants, ethnobotany also give emphasis on other natural products including food, plants used in rituals, coloring agents, fiber plants, poisons, fertilizers, building materials for houses, household items, boat, etc. [2].

Botany is the science which deals with floras including physiology, morphology, genetics, ecology, distribution, taxonomy, and economic importance. Occasionally, fungi are included in botany [3]. **Ethnobiology** is a multidisciplinary ground that deals with the interaction of human with living things including plants and animals. Ethnobotany might be considered as a particular subdivision of ethnobiology. There is numerous specific division of ethnobotany that emphasizes one specific characteristic of the field [4]. **Ethnomedicine** focuses on complementary and alternative medicine including diagnostic and therapeutic along with herbal remedies. It is generally the comparison of the traditional medicines practiced by various ethnic groups, especially by indigenous people [5]. **Ethnopharmacology** is the study of the purposes, mechanism of action, efficacy, and safety of drugs which is herbal or plant origin, and it may include both stimulants and centrally active herbal remedies [6]. **Economic botany** emphasizes applied economic, agricultural, or marketable features of a plant that are used by people but does not intensely discover customary beliefs, the "ethno" side of ethnobotany. Economic botany deals with the aim of discovering novel products which are plant origin and which might be or might not be related with indigenous practices, while ethnobotany studies are documenting traditional use practices of plants by the indigenous people without considering the economic value of the plants. Ethnobotanists use different methods and materials for their ethnobotanical studies, including ancient writings, surveys, discussions with key informants, and field investigations of the relationship between the plants and human beings. They typically work together with native people or traditional healers who have knowledge about the plants to record the indigenous biodiversity including plants, and also for the identification of botanical diversity, parts used for the treatment of human and livestock diseases, and method of preparations and applications [7]. **Biocultural diversity** is the entire diversity demonstrated by the world's natural and cultural arrangements. It includes both the **biodiversity index** (the variety of florae, faunae, territories, and ecologies) and the **cultural diversity index** (variety of people customs and languages). Biodiversity is calculated by sharing the amount of diverse species in specific habitat by the entire digit of persons living in that specific habitat. Cultural diversity can be measured by dividing the quantity of diverse languages, religions, and tribal groups in specific habitat by the quantity of whole persons living in that specific habitat [8].

Ethnobotany covers various disciplines, including botany, biochemistry, pharmacognosy, toxicology, medicine, nutrition, agriculture, ecology, evolution, comparative religion, sociology, anthropology, linguistics, cognitive studies, history, and archeology, due to the fact that plants have significant purpose in day-to-day activity of human beings. The multidisciplinary habit of ethnobotany permits a widespread range of methods and uses and leads to the investigation of plants in various ways by the researchers [9]. But plants with medicinal importance are usually the focus area for the investigator under the field of ethnobotany, and the study of these medicinal plants has essential role for the development of ethnobotany field [2]. It is obvious that interdisciplinary and multidisciplinary methods can lead to further productive, comprehensive, and systemic guesstimates in the investigation of the relationship between the plants and humans. Regardless of its various bottlenecks, ethnobotany becomes an attractive and hopeful area of research [9].

1.2 Applied ethnobotany and ethnoecology

In addition to developing quantitative approach for the ethnobotanical assessment, ethnobotany has progressed along with broader method, including additional features of the natural environment. Ethnobotanists somewhat frequently categorize themselves more and more as ethnobiologists or ethnoecologists for the reason that these fields bargain more prospects to evaluate the relationship between the people and the whole surroundings in addition to the societies' interaction with the external environment including the effect of global trade on domestic economy and individual life. Since 1992, the interaction of human beings with plants has created a new term known as "applied ethnobotany" which in fact relates to studies and approaches which allow to work together with the indigenous people and traditional practitioners in an actual way, to investigate the knowledge of native people and develop a better management structures which shape specific use practices and social dynamics [10]. Applied ethnobotanies also made every effort to fill the gap between indigenous knowledge and modern practice and to recognize the association between indigenous practices and knowledge schemes and procedures, directions, and financial fashions at the nationwide and worldwide level [10]. In recent times, the term ethnoecology has been invented. Martine defines ethnoecology as a discipline which integrates many diverse academic fields. The term ethnoecology is used to incorporate all fields which designate the relationship between indigenous people and the ecosystem, including subdisciplines such as ethnobiology, ethnobotany, ethnoentomology, and ethnozoology [11]. In fact, ethnoecology is the discipline of how individuals comprehend the interaction between human beings and the living things, including animals, plants, and physical elements of a place [12].

2. Ethnobotany in history

Human being has been consuming floras meanwhile beforehand documented history. Our most primitive ancestors collected floras for foodstuff, medication, fibers, and construction supplies, momentary on their knowledge through oral customs. Farming, the exercise of generating yields and rising livestock, came about autonomously in diverse areas of the universe 10,000–15,000 years ago. Plant knowledge was an unlimited benefit in ancient societies, as it conversed a bigger opportunities of survival. Many ancient researchers took an extreme concern in botany, publishing herbals that enclosed plant information, and in addition also contained botanical importance. By using this baseline, an individual can identify and collect medicinal plants from the traditional healers own garden or from the forest and also can easily understand the method of preparations and applications. The term ethnobotany did not coin out as a discipline during the ancient civilization until earlier modern period. Despite the fact that individuals historically had a nearby relationship with the plants and various intellectuals investigated botany, rare scholars investigated the plant knowledge of an ethnic group till the twentieth century. The following are the rare leading ethnobotanical researchers and texts that aided disperse botanical knowledge all the way through the ages [8].

The ancient Egyptians (3000 B.C.) were specialists in using remedies for curative and preventive purposes. The curing of the sick was carried out by priest doctor and pharmacist "Son" who prescribed and prepared remedies. The crude drugs used for the plant derivation included Aloes, Gum, Myrrh, Poppy, Pomegranate,

Colocynth, Linseed, Squill, Coriander, Onion, Anise, Melon, Castor, etc. The *Ebers Papyrus* found in Egypt in the 1870s contains prescriptions written in hieroglyphics for over 700 preparations. This prescription for an asthma remedy is prepared by the combination of herbs heated on a brick so that the victim possibly will inhale their smokes. The **Babylonian medicine** was known as **Laws of Hamorabi** (772 B.C.). The medicines used were mostly of vegetable origin. The medications used include 250 constituents of plant and 180 constituents of animal origin. Several of these remedies were known to the ancient Egyptians. In the **Old Indian medicine,** the "Riveda" and Ayurveda (Acoko 2000 B.C.) contained the holy medicinal plants. The gathering of plant constituents was undertaken only by a guiltless, pure, and religious individual. The fresh plants were considered to be most effective. The most famous Indian remedies were sandalwood, clove, pepper, cardamom, caraway, ginger, benzoin, cannabis, castor oil, sesame oil, aloes, etc. Besides the well-known **acupuncture**, the Chinese medicine is very recognized for the herbal remedy. The **Pen Ts'ao Kang Moa** (1000 B.C.) contained an unbelievable amount of herbal medicines and preparations of animal source. Their book comprises many recipes for every ailment. Among the plants and minerals highly respected for its magic well-being power were ginseng, rhubarb, ephedra, star anise, pomegranate, and aconite. Opium is a very old Chinese drug for diarrhea and dysentery. **Pythagoras** (560 B.C.) used drugs such as mustard and squill. **Hippocrates** (466 B.C.) was familiar with abundant medicines and wrote "**Corpus Hipocraticum** 460 B.C." The Greek Empire was followed by that of the Romans **Dioscorides** who was a Greek by birth and was the first to define medicines, and his work "**Greek Herbal of Dioscorides**" included 5000 medicinal plants in addition to animal and mineral medicines. **Pliny,** who lived about the same time as **Dioscorides**, was also a renowned author of natural history. **Galen** (134–200 A.C.) was a physician and he is ascribed the use of "**Galenical preparations.**" Islamic literatures were found **the first beginnings of chemistry**, the name of which is derived from an Arabic word "Kemia," as were also such familiar words such as alcohol and alkali. The Arabs added several new plants and medicines to those previously recognized to the Greeks and Romans. In their days, pharmacy attained its maximum reputation and developed an independent branch of medicine. It is thought-provoking to note that the first dispensary was opened in Baghdad, the center of trade in those days. The dispensary was made of **sandalwood** and named **"Sandalia." Rhazey** (850–932 A.C.) who was born at Rai in Persia was the director of Baghdad hospital. He published a famous book **"Alhawi Kabeer"** [8].

3. Ethnobotanical knowledge and modern science

Out of the several plants biodiversity found on the earth surface, the plants which are used for the prevention and treatment of human and livestock disease are the significant ones due to the fact that those medicinal plants have secondary metabolites known as specialized metabolites [13]. Specialized metabolites with therapeutic possessions are dispersed throughout some plants genera, and these floras act as processing house for the natural products which are responsible for specialized metabolites [14]. The specialized metabolites have the potential biological activity that in turn used to protect the health and well-being of people and are the essential lead compounds for the modern medicines [15]. Study reported that medicinally important plants are the major source of treatment for up to 80% of the population until now, especially for underprivileged nations [16]. Also, the rest 20% of population living in higher-income countries still depends on complementary and alternative medicines which are especially plant origin and natural products [17]. Fascinatingly, out of the 25 dispensed drugs, about 12 of them are products which are plants origin [18, 19]. The role of ethnobotanists and researchers are incredible in the innovation of different present-day drugs, including artemisinin, aspirin, ephedrine, codeine and papaverine, colchicine, taxol, digoxin and digitoxin, capsaicin, tetrahydrocannabinol, and cannabidiol which are derived from Artemisia annua L., Filipendula ulmaria (L.) Maxim., Ephedra spp., Papaver somniferum L., Colchicum autumnale L., Taxus brevifolia Nutt., Digitalis purpurea L., Capsicum spp., and Cannabis sativa L., respectively [13, 20–22]. The uses of artemisinin in the modern medicine become acknowledged after a Chinese scientist (Tu Youyou) wins Nobel Prize in a year 2015 [23]. The results from the search of "medicinal plants" term on Google Scholar become more than 200,000 starting from the year 2000 until now.

Native people and ethnic groups use more than thousands of wild plants for the prevention and treatment of different human and livestock ailments, and even some of them are not identified and scientifically named still now, and hope several conventional medicines will be discovered from the plants and natural products in the future by the scientific community [24–26]. The well-known anthropologist David Maybury-Lewis had given emphasis to the role of indigenous people in supporting the invention of several plants which are medicinally important and used by this indigenous people for the treatment of different diseases [27]. Ethnobotanists can accelerate the proof of identity of plants which are medicinally important, and it is recommended that instead of conducting ethnobotanical assessment only, bioactive and lead compound can be extracted by mimicking the ethnobotanical information obtained from the indigenous people or traditional healers that can simplify the activity of bioprospecting of the plants [28]. Garnatje et al. [13, 29] advocated the term "ethnobotanical convergence" for the similar uses of plants included in the same node of a phylogeny. Although the term "ethnobotanical convergence" was condemned by Hawkins and Teixidor-Toneu [30], it is however assumed that connecting new technologies with the indigenous ethnobotanical information can accelerate the development of new modern drugs from the natural products and plants. Connecting ethnobotany with other fields such as phytochemistry, pharmacology, pharmacognosy, and molecular biology can support the botanical diversity identification and analysis of chemical constituents of medicinal plants which have the ability to prevent and treat human and livestock ailments [31]. Furthermore, approaches such as genomics and omics can also be employed to identify the genes underlying the (specialized) metabolites present in the plants characterized by high-throughput metabolomics approaches such as gas chromatography–mass spectrometry (GCMS), liquid chromatography-mass spectrometry (LCMS), and nuclear magnetic resonance (NMR) spectroscopy [32, 33]. The proper identification, utilization, and conservation of medicinal plants can assist in providing better alternative health care services in rural areas, especially in developing countries [34, 35]. Moreover, several medicinal plants collected from the traditional healers own garden or from the forest are majorly important, and high percent of individuals relay on these medicinal plants in order to get cure from their diseases [36]. The shortage of quality health care provisions that safeguard healthy lives and encourage safety of the individuals at all ages groups especially in the third-world nations of Asia and Africa strengthens the significance of medicinal plants used by the specific ethnic groups [34, 35]. In the past more than 10 years, the majority of population in the world depends on products derived from the plants which in turn shows the increasing demands of products derived from the natural resources, and it may lead to the over-increment of the need of medicinal plants. So, the scientific community and ethnobotanists should fasten the investigation related with the development of products from the plants by working together with the indigenous people and traditional healers who have the ability to collect those plants which are medicinally useful by considering the emerging number of both communicable and noncommunicable and population growth and global climate change.

4. Plant collection and identification

A **herbarium** is a process of collecting dried-out plant samples that used for study purposes. The key roles of a herbarium are to make available reference materials for botanical diversity identification of newly collected specimens, help as a supply for botanists and botany subjects, record the occurrence of a plant types in a specific area, decide taxonomy concerns, and store type and voucher samples. A **type specimen** is the exact specimen on which the name of a taxon is based. They are vastly valued and may be stored distinctly or attached onto different colored paper to escape loss or harm. A **voucher specimen** helps as the root for a scientific research. It is a consistent technique to authenticate the exact identity of the plant used for the research. Incase if questions are raised about the identity of the medicinal plants, the only way to answer this questions is by using the voucher numbers given for the specific plants. So, this shows whether the plants are correctly identified by the experts [37].

The person who collects the medicinal plant specimens are not allowed collecting endangered plant species or rare plants in a specific territory. And also, the individuals should respect the local regulations and need to obtain permission from the responsible bodies/officers. Incase if the medicinal plants were found only on individuals or traditional healers own gardens, verbal informed consent or permission should be obtained from the owner of plants to collect the specimens. After the plant specimens were collected from the traditional healers own garden or from the forest, the specimens should be put into the plastic bags, labeled, pressed, and transported to the national biodiversity centers. Then, the plant materials should be dried using the appropriate drying system and prepared for the botanical diversity identification using standard herbarium procedures. The identification mechanism is taken place by the botanists or taxonomists in the laboratory. But some botanical diversity identification processes can be taken place directly in the traditional healers own garden or in the forest if the owner or laws are not permitted to collect the plant specimens. The plant specimens should be deposited in the national herbarium or biodiversity laboratory by collecting them and immediately pressing between papers using a field press. Sticky specimens may be pressed between waxed paper. The pressing procedure in between newspaper should be carried out simultaneously by collecting the specimens due to the reason that once the specimens dried, they are difficult to press and arrange. The plant specimen should be arranged to show all the significant structures including lower and upper leaf, flower heads, and so on. Large specimens can be folded or cut into sections. Bulky fruit can be cut in half; large cones can be tagged to be stored in a box. Plant specimens should be dried as rapidly after it was collected and transported to the laboratory [38].

Sticks with good plants need to be gathered for the sample. The parts of the plants collected as sample should have to encompass pure phyllotaxy and the forking scheme. For small herb, collection of more specimens as could fix on the herbarium sheet is desirable. In common, cutters are used to cut the stems, whereas for a while tallness, pruner is used, and for spiny samples, such as *Berberis mucrifolia*, leather glove is mandatory. For leaves and aromatic plants, digger is useful to dig out underground part. Particular plants stems lie horizontally under the ground. In such cases, the underground part should be washed from the mud elements, etc. If it is stem, then samples have been placed in a branching manner. Marine floras are light or to some extent filamentous and are hard to be organized on the page. A sheet of mounting paper is located below the moving or submerged tiny floras, and then the paper is slowly raised till the sample lies on the paper and out of the water. Then paper is raised to create a slope prudently so that it enables water runoff. These floras need to be shaken well before placing them in flimsies. Certain floras can be placed in plastic bags. The flowers that straightforwardly damage or can be lost among higher flowers from the same gathering place can be positioned in small bags within the larger bag. Unhealthy flowers, depauperate samples, diseased branches, etc., should be escaped [39].

Details about the plant specimens geographic area with the help of Geographic Information Systems (GIS), specimen collection date, and collection number should be noted down at the period of the specimen collection in a field notebook or electronically. This information is necessary to arrange the label for the herbarium specimen sheet. The collection number should be written on the edge of the sheet of paper. After the exact botanical diversity of the specimen becomes identified, the scientific name of their plant can be written together with the collection number. Herbarium specimen labels are organized in several means, but they usually hold a heading with state or region, province or district, country, and name of institution related with the sample, followed by the scientific name (genus, species, and author), details about the area such as geographic types or distance from adjacent town or landmark, and locale specifics (soil, altitude, humidity, etc.), Collection date, name of the specimen collector, and collection number are also significant information. The label is located at the bottommost-right-hand corner of a herbarium mounting sheet and attached immediately. Glue is also applied to the back of the plant sample, and it is organized on the mounting sheet. Lesser weight may be located on the top of the specimen till the glue is dry. Fragments of plant material such as seeds or pollen can be located in a small folded pocket, which is also glued immediately to the sheet. Once dried, the herbarium stamps the sheet with its name and assigns it an accession number. It is then filed in the herbarium cabinets that are usually ordered alphabetically as per plant family, genus, and species. Some herbaria use numerical arrangement as per the Adolf Engler method of arrangement [37].

Knowledge of plant anatomy is essential for classifying plant species. Deprived of it, a plant may be not identified correctly, with possibly severe consequences. Botanical diversity identification keys are valuable tools if you have adequate information of plant anatomy to appropriately use them. A dichotomous key offers the user with two alternatives at each stage, while a polyclave key may offer quite a lot of choices at each stage. Electronic polyclaves usually let the user to effort some well-known features of the specimen, thus removing various species in the key. It may, moreover, offer the possibility or chance that the left behind species are the right choice and may quick the user to say other features to remove further species. There are little elementary rules to make a dichotomous key. The entries should initiate with a couplet that has same first words (e.g. Leaves opposite or Leaves alternate) but are opposing statements. A leaf cannot be both alternate and opposite so that the decision is perfect. To avoid misunderstanding, they should not have several entries in a row that start with the identical word and should not use overlying ranges of measurement. Negative statements (e.g. Leaves not opposite) should also be avoided. Couplets can be numbered, lettered, or a combination of both. Occasionally indented keys use no numbers or letters at all [38].

Even though this key is only a rare line, it comprises terms that need specialized knowledge of plant anatomy. If you do not know what "samaroid wings" or "perianth" are, the key is unusable. Field guides frequently enclose keys and illustrations to support the plant identification. They usually emphasize a restricted geographic area and compressed adequate to carry in the field. A field guide lets the user to compare the unidentified plant with identified plants that cultivate in the area. Even with a good field guide and key, it is often hard to identify a plant down to the species level, specifically if it is not flowering or fruiting. If possible, a botanist will gather a specimen to take back to the laboratory for an additional systematic investigation [40].

5. Ethnobotany research and their applications

Even though many new chemical constituents have been derived and identified from medicinal plants used by the multicultural ethnic group, there are no conventional drugs synthesized from these plants using ethnobotanical knowledge and regulated as pharmaceutical products in the United States in at least in the past 40 years [41]. This may look like astonishing, considering the amount of resources and materials invested during the investigation of ethnobotanical knowledge for the past 40 years. On the other hand, indigenous knowledge about the medicinal plant is still used by the scholars and researchers for the identification of new chemical constituents and structures [42] that can be used as the main points for the development of new chemicals that have biological activity. Nowadays, the jobs for scholars and researchers have become more difficult than the past. They did not focus on finding new cultures, rather they focused on previously invented more than 4000 cultures and knowledge. An essential problem challenged by researchers on medicinal plant is that the study on medicinal plant may not all the time result in perfect separation of mechanisms of action, rather they only show "in-vitro pharmacological activity" or "in-vivo pharmacological activity on different organ or "identification chemical constituents and suggesting that it may have such activity due to the presence of this functional groups," etc. A close relationship between ethnobotanists who conduct research for the assessment of medicinal plant use practices by the indigenous people and traditional healers and experimental pharmacologists who conduct study on the pharmacological activity of traditional medicinal plants claimed by the traditional healers is very important in order to add values on present health care system by discovering novel drugs from the natural products and plants [43].

Most of the scholars have related the current use of medicinal plants to their ancient civilization of ethnic groups by investigating the local names of the medicinal plants and uses in archival material and literature, but also more in recent times through past linguistic analysis of popular names [44, 45]. Investigation of the history of the use practices of *Rhododendron tomentosum* Harmaja in Norway by the indigenous people indicates continuity in vernacular names and the therapeutic indication of this medicinal plants from the first eighteenth to twentieth centuries, with only a loss in use as a salt substitute. The investigation of cognates to indigenous medicinal plant names offers us evidences to the past interaction between the medicinal plants and the native society, whereas the specific name of medicinal plants indicates some striking characteristics of the plant, color, their native uses, and views of the indigenous people [46]. Sabine Nebel's studied that the evaluation of names for edible greens among *Grecanico* speakers in Italy and Greek findings shows astonishing continuity of language and customs. For instance, *Portulaca oleracea* L. (purslane) is called *andracla* in Gallicianò and *andrakla* in Greece. The uses of several of these medicinal plants are the most persistent form of traditional healing practices in ancient Greek civilization [38]. Spanish ethnobotanists and researchers also try to relate historical-linguistic method to the Spanish use practices of medicinal plants called *manzanilla* (chamomile) in drinking teas since the ages of Moorish practices in the twelfth and thirteenth centuries, and even further back to Dioscorides in ancient Greece [46]. Also, other researchers present an infrequent sight into Lithuanian botanical diversity classification by tracing and certainly separating the roots of cognate native names for sycamore maple (*Acer pseudoplatanus* L.), plane tree (*Platanus* spp.), black poplar (*Populus nigra* L.), guelder rose (*Viburnum opulus* L.), and blessed wreaths prepared from collected rye. They show the importance and risks of using traditional texts and ethnographic data, such as melodies, mysteries, and children's verses, as botanical indication for rebuilding the etymology and figurative history of ethnobotanical naming [47].

Many scholars give emphasis on the present uses of higher plants collected from the forest or wild not only due to the continuous historical use practices by the indigenous people or recurrence in new markets but also due to the their significance nutritional values. Generally, wild plants are nutritive because of their high content of minerals and vitamins [48, 49]. Study show that the consumption of common golden thistle (*Scolymus hispanicus* L.) among poor farmers in Portugal has a long history, also stretching back to ancient Roman times, and has now become popular among tourists. Underlying the use of this particular thistle, though, is the fact that it manages to maintain its high nutritional value regardless of the quality of the soils in which it grows. Native agriculturalists have acknowledged this distinctiveness and thus ignore all other thistles that cultivate in the area [49]. Also, other characteristics like sex are also essential concern in the collection and preparation of wild plants for healing and foods in Europe. Even though the depth knowledge of collection and preparation of wild fruits and plants is considered as the characteristic of females in various countries [50], but thistles collection and preparation is the activity of males in Portugal [49]. Researchers identified and presented about females who become males in the Albanian Alps: in this ancient form of transgenderism, there is convergence of the ethnomedicinal knowledge of "typical" males, regarding food and plants used for the treatment livestock ailments (ethnoveterinary), wild greens, and the ethnomedicinal knowledge of females, regarding weedy food and medicinal plants [51].

Around 679 ethnobotanical surveys were accompanied in Latin America until 2012. Out of these surveys, 41% of ethnobotanical studies were carried out in Brazil, 22% of these studies were conducted in Mexico, 9% of these surveys were carried out in Peru, 8% were conducted in Argentina, 6% were conducted in Bolivia, and 14% of the studies were conducted in the rest of the countries of Latin American continent [52]. Apart from the infamous development of ethnobiology as a field in Latin America, the amount of ethnobotanical research conveyed for the scientific community look like to delay in various countries. From the results of research conducted on ethnobatanical information in Latin America especially in Brazil, Mexico, and Argentina, it is true that there is rapid increment of scientific studies on the ethnobotany fields in the continent. This condition could be improved by the integration of better funds for ethnobotanical studies by investing in human resources and economic capitals and through the formation of thematic areas and ethnobotanical cultures (as observed in Brazil and Mexico). The overall objective of these thematic areas are to promote and enlarge debates on the disciplines, build protocols, and create knowledge that may fulfill the existing gaps in various areas of ethnobotany. Ethnobotanical study may also be encouraged by an escalation in the number of scientific proceedings and journals to distribute the results obtained from the researches and by the design of undergraduate courses and master programs to teach scholars who will conduct quality researches on this field. These methods can fufill the existing gaps and intervals in ethnobotanical study and also lead to the alliance of ethnobotanical knowledge throughout the Latin America continent [52].

Ethnobotany seems to have appealed its correct place among the scientific field getting finance studies, but much task yet to be conducted. There is still a lot of ethnobotanical information yet to be recorded, especially in different parts of Africa like ethnobotanical knowledge of the Khoi, Ndebele, and Swazi, as well as the relationship of this ethnic group with traditional medicinal plants, wealth of unrecorded information, especially relating to the ethnobotany of the Khoi, Ndebele, and Swazi, as well as the interaction between plants and people, folk taxonomies, historical use practices of plants, uses of plants for the treatment of livestock ailments, and medicinal plant uses before the colonial period. In addition to these, medicinal plants used for the treatment of dental disease, plant parts used for the perfumes, cosmetics, insect repellents, colorant flowers, yeast plants, thatching plants, textile plants, musical instruments, as well as hunting, fishing, and other technologies. It is very important to isolate market-based research from indigenous knowledge-based research. Hence, market-based research may depend on the profit obtained from the study within reasonable time, but the former may be of more direct value in the short term, but indigenous knowledge-based research may be more urgent and important, as a consequence of their long period role on the way to a deeper identification of medicinal plants use practices by the traditional healers and native societies, especially in Africa. Study shows that urbanization and solid traditional effects from other parts of the globe are prominent to an extraordinary loss of indigenous knowledge in South Africa. Scholars and researchers should be stimulated to grasp the chances offered by ethnobotanical study and to document the aspects of their own historical-linguistic information and indigenous medicinal plant use practices by the different ethnic groups for the sake of future generations. It is obvious that once the traditional knowledge is documented well systematically, it is not adulterated for life time. It is truly accepted that each individuals and generations can understand and interpret indigenous knowledge in different angle. The sources of present-day technologies and discoveries by the scientists are the traditional and indigenous knowledge of our illiterate ancestors. However, the investigation of native knowledge concerning medicinal plants uses for the prevention and treatment of human and livestock diseases should be given emphasis especially in Africa. Hence, it is not feasible to give oral indigenous knowledge information for the scientific community without tangible and well-documented traditional knowledge about medicinal plants use practices in Africa [53].

Study conducted on ethnobotanical study in northern Angola showed that about 2390 medicinal plants were reported to be used by the traditional healers and community. Those medicinal plants were categorized under 358 species in 96 plant families, while just 3 out of 358 stated species are endemic to Angola and about one-fifth are neophytes. As the distance from where the medicinal plants collected increased, the number of use citations also higher. According to this study, large proportion of women (83%) was involved in the collection and preparation of medicinal plants from the forest and garden. The authors of this study discover new medicinal plants used for the treatment of different ailments by the indigenous people in the study, including Gardenia ternifolia which is claimed to have anti-measles, and ethnobotanical knowledge and the chemical constituents of Annona stenophylla subsp. cuneata medicinal plant have never been identified and documented elsewhere especially in the study area. Regardless of the long-term fighting in Angola, indigenous use practices of medicinal plants for the prevention and treatment of human and livestock disease remain a crucial part of traditional heritage. For that reason, plants are critical components in all parts of livelihood, particularly in the health care system. This condition is compounded by the still low-quality medical sectors in the Angola, particularly in countryside of the countries [54].

Another study conducted on hierarchies of knowledge; ethnobotanical knowledge, practices, and beliefs of the Vhavenda in South Africa for biodiversity conservation showed that 84 medicinal plant species were stated by the respondents which are categorized under 44 families. The majority of the stated medicinal plants were categorized under the fabaceae. The authors were identified 6 new species which are not reported before in Vhavenda ethnobotanical documents, also 68 medicinal plants claimed to have new indications and another 14 species have the similar uses with previously record. In this survey, high percent of plants reported were consumed as dietary supplements (36.0%) and used for the treatment of different human and livestock diseases (26.1%) and comprised mostly indigenous plants (73.8%) paralleled to nonnative plants (26.2%). The Vhavenda takes a variety of activities for the management of plant diversity that can be endorsed to taboos avoiding the usage of endangered and rare species, advertisement of sustainable collecting activities, and the proliferation of plant species for environmental refurbishment. Also, the authors reported about 48.4% of indigenous plant knowledge was transferred to generations through family/relatives, followed by studying about plants cultivation, collecting information by individual itself, through traineeships with traditional practitioners, and through learning in the schools and clan gatherings which constituted 16.1%, 9.7% 6.4%, and 19.4%, respectively. The reasons behind the difficulty in transferring knowledge about traditional plants use practices of Vhavenda are alterations in traditional knowledge platforms for information exchange, destruction of traditional organizations, and shifting value structures. The Vhavenda ethnic groups preserve a complex "knowledge-practice-belief" structure nearby for the use, control, and protection of plant biodiversity. The documentations of indication of new medicinal plants for the different purpose in this research and the expansion of the previously invented plants for the treatment of different human and livestock disease are valuable for providing an additional complete understanding into the indigenous plants use practices by this ethic groups in South Africa. The indigenous knowledge of medicinal plants use practices of this ethnic group is widespread comprising a variety of indigenous, exotic, wild, and cultivated plants. The indigenous people and traditional healers cultivate and gather a diversity of plants from the own garden, and from the wild and deciduous woodlands representing an all-embracing knowledge base conceivably imitating the sociocultural perspective of comparative separation and long-term settlement of the Vhavenda in the area. The domination of native plant diversity signified in ethnobotanical survey proposes that plant knowledge acclimatization may initiate with common and readily existing plants; conversely, the new popularity of nonnative plant diversity also reveals a form of adaptation to new acquired plant variety that has become integrated into the Vhavenda depository of valuable plant diversity. Native practices and organizations are also inserted in traditional settings and coded in cosmologies and belief systems that have safeguarded the sustainable utilization of plant biodiversity. Plant managing plans aim is to sustain consistent and continual supply of plant biodiversity for dietary purposes, medicinal use practices, and other uses through selective practices such as the prohibition of endangered and rare plants from use, the advertisement of sustainable collecting practices, and the proliferation of plant biodiversity [55].

A study review on medicinal plant use practices in Ethiopia showed that the country is rich in biodiversity and believed to have about 6000 higher plants diversity with about 10% of native higher plant species. This amount of biodiversity of plants species also includes most of the lower plant species. The genetic variety enclosed in the many biotic makeup is also great, consequently making the country a serious biodiversity homeland for plants. As one of the 12 Vavilovian midpoints of origin for home grown crops and their wild relatives, it is the country of various native crops and genetic stocks. Ethiopia is considered as the richest country in biodiversity since 5000 years ago when ancient Egyptians, Greeks, and Romans used it as a basis of exclusive merchandises like Frankincense, Myrrh, and other plant products, which are also used for the production of different drugs. Among the largest biodiversity of plant species found in Ethiopia, highest percent has medicinal purposes. With similar fashion with the rest of the world, most of the people of Ethiopia rely on medicinal plants for the treatment of human and livestock ailments. Accordingly, about 95% of traditional therapeutic synthesis are the products of plant source. It is not ambitious to say medicinal plants have been used as a basis for the traditional remedies in order to prevent and treat different human and livestock diseases in Ethiopia. Medicine preparation from the medicinal plants is an essential part of the tradition of Ethiopian people. Most Ethiopian indigenous healing knowledge is retained in stringent mystery; conversely, it is dynamic in that the traditional healers create every struggle to broaden their range by reciprocal transferring of traditional medicinal knowledge to each generations or by reading the traditional pharmacopeias. It is difficult to acquire indigenous healing information of the traditional practitioners for the reason that they claim that the knowledge is their own and only like to transfer their knowledge to their relatives, especially to the eldest son [56].

Traditional practitioners in Ethiopia use the medicinal plant existing in the biodiversity for the prevention and treatments of various human and livestock ailments. A study showed that around 800 plants diversity which is medicinally important in Ethiopia is used for treating around 300 diseases. As stated by several researchers, there are diverse kinds of plant diversity with their parts used for the treatment purposes, the place where they grow, and the type of conditions treated by using these medicinal plants. There are about 18 medicinal plant diversity with 63 genera, and they are used by the indigenous society for the prevention and treatment of different human diseases. According to the literature, the common medicinal plants used for the prevention and treatments of human conditions are *Aloe* species, *Eucalyptus globulus*, *Hagenia abyssinica*, *Cupressus macrocarpa*, *Buddleja polystachya*, *Acmella caulirhiza*, *Acacia* species, *Citrus* species, *Clematis* species, *Coffee Arabica*, *Croton macrostachyus*, *Euphorbia* species, *Ficus sycomorus*, and *Moringa stenopetala*. According to other reviews, all plant life forms were not in the same way used as therapies, for the reason that there is the dissimilarity in the distribution among the life forms. Therefore, the growth forms of medicinal plants were trees, shrubs, herbs, climbers, and others. The most predominant plant parts used for the prevention and treatments of different human and livestock ailments are herbs, followed by shrubs and trees [57].

A study conducted on ethnobotanical assessment and physicochemical properties of Commonly Used Medicinal Plants in Southwest Ethiopia showed that a total of 72 plants species were stated by the respondents for the treatment of different human and livestock ailments and classified under 61 genera and 39 families. Herbs constituted the predominant plant growth parts followed by shrubs, tree, and climbers. Leaves were the most frequently used medicinal plant parts by the traditional healers in the study followed by roots and seeds. Regarding the method of preparation of the medicinal plants, crushing, powdering, pounding, and pressing were used sequentially by the traditional healers [58].

6. Conservation of medicinal plants

Conservation of medicinal plants should have an objective of conserving biodiversity within specified place like by preparing botanical garden to confirm that all the plant species will be ready to use by the future generations [59]. Sustainable managing of indigenous medicinal plant diversity is very significant not only for the reason that their potential benefit as lead compound for new drug discoveries but also because of the large percent of people around the world still depends on traditional medicinal plants [60]. There is certain protection activities that have been carried out everywhere in the globe intended to keep endangered medicinal plants from additional harm [61]. This includes in situ and ex situ protection actions. Both in situ and ex situ protection efforts are applied to protect medicinal plant genetic biodiversity. In situ conservation is the protection of plant biodiversity in their natural territories. Certain indigenous medicinal plants have to be well kept in situ because of the difficulty for domestication and managing [62]. Medicinal plants can also be protected by confirming and inspiring their growth in different spaces, as they have been used traditionally [62]. This can be promising in the place of churches, mosques, graveyards, farm margin, river bank, and so on. An interpretation that has been made by the researcher showed that medicinal plant diversity grown around the religious sites is prohibited from collecting [60]. The second one is ex-situ conservations means conservation outside their natural habitats. This comprises gen bank, herbal gardens, and others. As it was stated, home gardens have an abundant influence for the protection of medicinal plant species in broad, and at the same time the biodiversity can also be well kept; thus, home gardens are strategic and best agricultural systems for the protection, production, and development of species that are medicinally important [62, 63]. Various efforts have been made to safeguard and encourage sustainable use of plants that are medicinally important in different country. In the field, biodiversity protection goes alongside with the protection of ethnobotanical and ethnopharmacological information. Ethnobotanical investigation can point out managing difficulties of biodiversity through interviews and market studies; moreover, it provides resolutions by encouraging indigenous knowledge and customs that had protection advantages [64, 65]. A study reported that the wise utilization of species that are medicinally useful wants the participation of diverse sectors and larger community support and for this, awareness formation is suggested [66].

7. Conclusion

Ethnobotany is a life science which studies the interaction between human beings and flora in particular and broadly deals with the investigations, observations, and identifications of botanical diversity used for the prevention and treatment of human and livestock ailments. It also studies about the indigenous people knowledge, beliefs, and practices (i.e. it may be cultural and religious practices) related with medicinal plants. Also, it includes how human beings categorize, isolate, and associate floras beside with joint relationships of floras and human beings. The ethnobotanists should have to discuss with native community to share their routine life and to respect their cultures in order to obtain valuable information about the plants used for the medicinal purpose. Ethnobotany might be considered as a particular subdivision of ethnobiology. Ethnobotanists use different methods and materials for their ethnobotanical studies including ancient writings, surveys, discussions with key informants, and field investigations of the relationship between the plants and human beings. They typically work together with native people or traditional healers who have knowledge about the plants to record the indigenous biodiversity including plants and also for the identification of botanical diversity, parts used for the treatment of human and livestock diseases, and method of preparations and applications.

Ethnobotanists somewhat frequently categorize themselves more and more as ethnobiologists or ethnoecologists for the reason that these fields bargain more prospects to evaluate the relationship between the people and the whole surroundings in addition to the societies' interaction with the external environment including the effect of global trade on domestic economy and individual life. Since 1992, the interaction of human beings with plants has created a new term known as "applied ethnobotany" which in fact relates to studies and approaches which allow to work together with the indigenous people and traditional practitioners in an actual way, to investigate the knowledge of native people and develop better management structures which shape specific use practices and social dynamics. Applied ethnobotanies also make every effort to fill the gap between indigenous knowledge and modern practice and to recognize the association between indigenous practices and knowledge schemes and procedures, and directions and financial fashions at the nationwide and worldwide level. In recent times, the term ethnoecology has been invented. Martine defines ethnoecology as a discipline which integrates many diverse academic fields. The term ethnoecology is used to incorporate all fields which designate the relationship between indigenous people and the ecosystem, including subdisciplines such as ethnobiology, ethnobotany, ethnoentomology, and ethnozoology. In fact, ethnoecology is the discipline of how individuals comprehend the interaction between human beings and the living things including animals, plants, and physical elements of a place.

Human being has been consuming floras meanwhile beforehand documented history. Our most primitive ancestors collected floras for foodstuff, medication, fibers, and construction supplies, momentary on their knowledge through oral customs.

DOI: http://dx.doi.org/10.5772/intechopen.104754

Farming, the exercise of generating yields and rising livestock, came about autonomously in diverse areas of the universe 10,000–15,000 years ago. Plant knowledge was an unlimited benefit in ancient societies, as it conversed a bigger opportunities of survival. Many ancient researchers took an extreme concern in botany, publishing herbals that enclosed plant information, and in addition also contained botanical importance. By using this baseline, an individual can identify and collect medicinal plants from the traditional healers own garden or from the forest and also can easily understand the method of preparations and applications. The term ethnobotany did not coin out as a discipline during the ancient civilization until earlier modern period. Despite the fact that individuals historically had a nearby relationship with the plants and various intellectuals investigated botany, rare scholars investigated the plant knowledge of an ethnic group till the twentieth century. The following are the rare leading ethnobotanical researchers and texts that aided disperse botanical knowledge all the way through the ages.

Even though many new chemical constituents have been derived and identified from medicinal plants used by the multicultural ethnic group, there are no conventional drugs synthesized from these plants using ethnobotanical knowledge and regulated as pharmaceutical products in the United States in at least in the past 40 years. This may look like astonishing, considering the amount of resources and materials invested during the investigation of ethnobotanical knowledge for the past 40 years. On the other hand, indigenous knowledge about the medicinal plant is still used by the scholars and researchers for the identification of new chemical constituents and structures that can be used as the main points for the development of new chemicals that have biological activity. Nowadays, the jobs for scholars and researchers have become more difficult than the past. They did not focus on finding new cultures, rather they focused on previously invented more than 4000 cultures and knowledge. An essential problem challenged by researchers on medicinal plant is that the study on medicinal plant may not all the time result in perfect separation of mechanisms of action, rather they only show “in-vitro pharmacological activity” or “in-vivo pharmacological activity on different organ” or “identification chemical constituents and suggesting that it may have such activity due to the presence of this functional groups,” etc. A close relationship between ethnobotanists who conduct research for the assessment of medicinal plant use practices by the indigenous people and traditional healers and experimental pharmacologists who conduct study on the pharmacological activity of traditional medicinal plants claimed by the traditional healers is very important in order to add values on present health care system by discovering novel drugs from the natural products and plants. On the assumption that there is a necessity for original, cautious, systematic, and cooperative records of the relationship of human beings with plant nature, for joining societal and environmental systems, for sustaining and improving biodiversity, and for recoupling health and well-being with traditional and ecological integrity, ethnobotany will be a discipline of significance and prominence in the globe.

Author details

Jafer Siraj
School of Pharmacy, College of Medicine and Health Sciences, Mizan-Tepi University, Mizan-Aman, Ethiopia

*Address all correspondence to: sirajjafer@gmail.com; jafersiraj@mtu.edu.et

References

[1] Balick MJ, Cox PA. People, Plants, and Culture: The Science of Ethnobotany. New York, NY, USA: Scientific American Library; 1996. p. 228

[2] Heinrich M, Barnes J, Gibbons S, Williamson EM. Fundamental Pharmacognosy Phytotherapy. London: Churchill Livingstone; 2004. pp. 24-25

[3] Fernald ML. Gray's manual of botany: A handbook of the flowering plants and ferns of the Central and Northeastern United States and Adjacent Canada. 8th ed. New York: American Book; 1950. p. 1632

[4] Alexiades MN, editor. Selected Guidelines for Ethnobotanical Research: A Field Manual. New York: The New York Botanical Garden; 1996. p. 306

[5] Collins M. Medieval Herbals: The Illustrative Traditions (British Library Studies in Medieval Culture). Scholarly Publishing Division, Toronto: University of Toronto Press; 2000

[6] Heinrich M, Edwards S, Moerman DE, Leonti M. Ethnopharmacological field studies: A critical assessment of their conceptual basis and methods. Journal of Ethnopharmacology. 2009;**124**:1-17

[7] Arber AR. Herbals: Their Origin and Evolution: A Chapter in the History of Botany. 3rd ed. Cambridge: Cambridge University Press; 1986

[8] Schmidt BM, Klaser Cheng DM. Ethnobotany: A Phytochemical Perspective. 1st ed. USA: John Wiley & Sons Ltd; 2017. pp. 3-4

[9] Ghorbani A, Naghibi F, Mosaddegh M. Ethnobotany, ethnopharmacology and drug discovery. Iranian Journal of Pharmaceutical Sciences. 2006;**2**(2):109-118

[10] Aumeeruddy-Thomas Y, Shengji P. Applied Ethnobotany: Casestudies from the Himalayan region. People and Plants Working Paper 12. Godalming, UK: WWF; 2003

[11] Martin GJ. Ethnobotany: A Methods Manual. London: Chapman & Hall; 1995

[12] Davidson-Hunt I. Ecological ethnobotany: Stumbling toward new practices and paradigms. MASA Journal Department of Anthropology. 2000;**16**:1-13

[13] Garnatje T, Peñuelas J, Vallès J. Ethnobotany, phylogeny, and 'omics' for human health and food security. Trends in Plant Science. 2017;**22**:187-191

[14] Zhu F, Qin C, Tao L, Liu X, Shi Z, Ma X, et al. Clustered patterns of species origins of nature-derived drugs and clues for future bioprospecting. Proceedings of the National Academy of Sciences of the United States of America. 2011;**108**:12943-12948

[15] Hussain MDS, Rahman MDA, Fareed S, Ansari S, Ahmad I, Mohd S. Current approaches toward production of secondary plant metabolites. Journal of Pharmacy and Bioallied Sciences. 2012;**4**:10

[16] Ekor M. The growing use of herbal medicines: Issues relating to adverse reactions and challenges in monitoring safety. Frontiers in Pharmacology. 2014;**4**:177

[17] Bussmann RW. Ethnobotany and biodiversity conservation. In: Ambasht NK, Ambasht RS, editors.

Modern Trends in Applied Terrestrial Ecology. Boston, MA, USA: Springer; 2002. pp. 343-360

[18] Baker JT, Borris RP, Carté B, Cordell GA, Soejarto DD, Cragg GM, et al. Natural product drug discovery and development: New perspectives on international collaboration. Journal of Natural Products. 1995;**58**:1325-1357

[19] Farnsworth NR, Akerele O, Bingel AS, Soejarto DD, Guo Z. Medicinal plants in therapy. Bulletin of the World Health Organization. 1985;**63**:965-981

[20] Rao KV. Taxol and related taxanes. I. Taxanes of Taxus brevifolia bark. Pharmaceutical Research. 1993;**10**:521-524

[21] Abourashed EA, El-Alfy AT, Khan IA, Walker L. Ephedra in perspective—A current review. Phytotherapy Research. 2003;**17**:703-712

[22] Sarpras M, Gaur R, Sharma V, Chhapekar SS, Das J, Kumar A, et al. Comparative analysis of fruit metabolites and pungency candidate genes expression between bhut jolokia and other capsicum species. PLoS One. 2016;**11**:e0167791

[23] Su XZ, Miller LH. The discovery of artemisinin and the Nobel prize in physiology or medicine. Science China. Life Sciences. 2015;**58**:1175-1179

[24] Alves RR, Rosa IM. Biodiversity, traditional medicine and public health: Where Do they meet? Journal of Ethnobiology and Ethnomedicine. 2007;**3**:14

[25] Uniyal SK, Singh K, Jamwal P, Lal B. Traditional use of medicinal plants among the tribal communities of Chhota Bhangal, Western Himalaya. Journal of Ethnobiology and Ethnomedicine. 2006;**2**:14

[26] Pan SY, Litscher G, Gao SH, Zhou SF, Yu Z-L, Chen HQ, et al. Historical perspective of traditional indigenous medical practices: The current renaissance and conservation of herbal resources. Evidence-Based Complementary and Alternative Medicine. 2014;**2014**:525340

[27] Wright RM, Kapfhammer W, Wiik FB. The clash of cosmographies: Indigenous societies and project collaboration—Three ethnographic cases (Kaingang, Sateré-Mawé, Baniwa). Vibrant Virtual Brazilian Anthropology. 2012;**9**:382-450

[28] Saslis-Lagoudakis CH, Savolainen V, Williamson EM, Forest F, Wagstaff SJ, Baral SR, et al. Phylogenies reveal predictive power of traditional medicine in bioprospecting. Proceedings of the National Academy of Sciences of the United States of America. 2012;**109**:15835-15840

[29] Garnatje T, Peñuelas J, Vallès J. Reaffirming 'ethnobotanical convergence'. Trends in Plant Science. 2017;**22**:640-641

[30] Hawkins JA, Teixidor-Toneu I. Defining Ethnobotanical Convergence, Trends in Plant Science. 2017;**22**:639-640

[31] Obakiro SB, Kiprop A, Kowino I, Kigondu E, Odero MP, Omara T, et al. Ethnobotany, ethnopharmacology, and phytochemistry of traditional medicinal plants used in the Management of Symptoms of tuberculosis in East Africa: A systematic review. Tropical Medicine and Health. 2020;**48**:68

[32] Schilmiller AL, Pichersky E, Last RL. Taming the hydra of specialized metabolism: How systems biology and comparative approaches are revolutionizing plant biochemistry. Current Opinion in Plant Biology. 2012;**15**:338-344

[33] Kumar A, Kumar S, Thomas TD, Ramchiary N, Swamy MK, Ahmad I. Linking omics approaches to medicinal plants and human health. in natural bio-active compounds. In: Akhtar MS, Swamy MK, editors. Biotechnology, Bioengineering, and Molecular Approaches. Vol. 3. Singapore: Springer; 2019. pp. 31-57 ISBN 9789811374388

[34] Sofowora A, Ogunbodede E, Onayade A. The role and place of medicinal plants in the strategies for disease prevention. African Journal of Traditional, Complementary and Alternative Medicines. 2013;**10**:210-229

[35] Karunamoorthi K, Jegajeevanram K, Vijayalakshmi J, Mengistie E. Traditional medicinal plants: A source of phytotherapeutic modality in resource-constrained health care settings. Evidence Based Complementary and Alternative Medicine. 2013;**18**:67-74

[36] Plotkin MJ. Tales of a Shaman's Apprentice: An Ethnobotanist Searches for New Medicines in the Amazon Rain Forest. New York, NY, USA: Viking Penguin; 1993. p. 318

[37] Jones SB, Luchsinger AE. Plant Systematics. 2nd ed. New York: McGraw-Hill Publishing Co.; 1986

[38] Judd WS, Campbell CS, Kellog EA, Stevens PF, Donoghue MJ. Plant Systematics: A Phylogenetic Approach. 4th ed. Sunderland: Sinauer Associates, Inc.; 2015

[39] Maden K. Plant collection and herbarium techniques. Our Nature. 2004;**2**:53-57

[40] Milliken W. Neotropical Juglandaceae. In: Milliken W, Klitgard B, Baracat A, editors. Neotropikey—Interactive Key and Information Resources for Flowering Plants of the Neotropics. Kew: Royal Botanic Gardens; 2009. Available from: http://www.kew.org/science/tropamerica/neotropikey/families/Juglandaceae.htm

[41] McClatchey W. Bioprospecting and ethnobotany research. Ethnobotany Research and Applications. 2005;**3**:189-190

[42] Do Q-T, Bernard P. Reverse pharmacognosy: A new concept for accelerating natural drug discovery. In: Khan MTH, Ather A, editors. Lead Molecules from Natural Products. Advances in Phytomedicine Series. Vol. 2. The Nederlands: Elsevier; 2006. pp. 1-19

[43] McClatcheya WC, Mahady GB, Bennett BC, Shiels L, Savo V. Ethnobotany as a pharmacological research tool and recent developments in CNS-active natural products from ethnobotanical sources. Pharmacology & Therapeutics. 2009;**123**(2):239-254. DOI: 10.1016/j.pharmthera.2009.04.002

[44] Blanco E, Morales R. Plants known as te in Spain: An Ethno-pharmaco-botanical review. Journal of Ethnopharmacology. 2005;**98**(1-2):1-19

[45] Nebel S, Pieroni A, Heinrich M. Ta chorta: Wild edible greens used in the Graecanic area in Calabria, southern Italy. Appetite. 2006;**47**(3):333-342

[46] Pardo-de-Santayana M. Estudios ethnobotanicos en Campoo (Cantabria). Madrid: Consejo Superior de Investigaciones Científi cas; 2008

[47] Šeškauskaitė D, Gliwa B. Some Lithuanian ethnobotanical taxa: A linguistic view on thorn apple and related plants. Journal of Ethnobiology and Ethnomedicine. 2006;**2**:13

[48] Ansari NM, Houlihan L, Hussain B, Pieroni A. Antioxidant activity of five

vegetables traditionally consumed by South-Asian migrants in Bradford, Yorkshire, UK. Phytotherapy Research. 2005;**19**:907-911

[49] Pardo-de-Santayana J, Tardío E, Blanco AM, Carvalho JJ, Lastra E, Miguel S, et al. Traditional knowledge of wild edible plants used in the northwest of the Iberian Peninsula (Spain and Portugal): A comparative study. Journal of Ethnobiology and Ethnomedicine. 2007;**3**:27

[50] Howard PL. Women and Plants: Case Studies on Gender Relations in Biodiversity Management and Conservation. London: Zed Press; 2003

[51] Kathe W, Honnef S, Heym A. Medicinal and aromatic plants in Albania, Bosnia-Herzegovina, Bulgaria, Croatia and Romania. In: Report by WWF Deutschland and TRAFFIC Europe-Germany. Bonn: German Federal Agency for Nature Conservation (BfN); 2003

[52] Albuquerque UP et al. The current status of ethnobiological research in Latin America: gaps and perspectives. Journal of Ethnobiology and Ethnomedicine. 2013;**9**(1):1-9. DOI: 10.1186/1746-4269-9-72

[53] Wyk V. A review of ethnobotanical research in southern Africa. South African Journal of Botany. 2002;**68**:1-13

[54] Lautenschläger T et al. First large-scale ethnobotanical survey in the province of Uíge, northern Angola. Journal of Ethnobiology and Ethnomedicine. 2018;**14**(1):1-73. DOI: 10.1186/s13002-018-0238-3

[55] Constant NL, Tshisikhawe MP. Hierarchies of knowledge: ethnobotanical knowledge, practices and beliefs of the Vhavenda in South Africa for biodiversity conservation. Journal of Ethnobiology and Ethnomedicine. 2018;**14**(1):1-28. DOI: 10.1186/s13002-018-0255-2

[56] Fenetahun Y, Eshetu G. A review on ethnobotanical studies of medicinal plants use by agro-pastoral communities in Ethiopia. Journal of Medicinal Plants Studies. 2017;**5**(1):33-44

[57] Moges A, Moges Y. Ethiopian Common Medicinal Plants: Their Parts and Uses in Traditional Medicine – Ecology. London: IntechOpen. DOI: 10.5772/intechopen.86202

[58] Siraj J, Belew S, Suleman S. Ethnobotanical assessment and physicochemical properties of commonly used medicinal plants in Jimma zone, Southwest Ethiopia. Journal of Experimental Pharmacology. 2020;**12**:605. DOI: 10.2147/JEP.S267903

[59] Demissie A. Biodiversity conservation of medicinal plants: and prospects. In: Zewdu M, Demissie A, editors. Conservation and Sustainable Use of Medicinal Plants in Ethiopia. 2001, 56-64. Preceding of the National Workshop on Biodiversity Conservation and Sustainable Use of Medicinal Plants in Ethiopia, 28 April- 01 May. Addis Ababa: IBCR; 1998

[60] Cunningham AB. African medicinal plants: Setting priorities at the interface healthcare between conservation and primary health care. In: Sample A, editor. People and Plants Working Paper. Paris: UNESCO; 1993. pp. 1-50

[61] Cunningham AB. People, Park and plants use recommendations for multiple use zones and development alternatives around Bwindi: Impenetrable National Park, Uganda. In: Sample A, editor. People and Plants, Working Paper. Vol. 4. Paris: UNESCO; 1996. pp. 18-25

[62] Asfaw Z. The role of homegarden in production and conservation of

medicinal plants. In: Conservation and Sustainable Use of Medicinal plants in Ethiopia. (Medhin Zewdu and Abebe Demissieeds.). Proceeding of the National Workshop on Biodiversity Conservation and Sustainable use of Medicinal Plants in Ethiopia. Vol. 2001. Addis Ababa: IBCR; 1998. pp. 76-91

[63] Asfaw Z, Nigatu A. Homegardens in Ethiopia: Characteristics and plant diversity. SINET: Ethiopian Journal of Science. 1995;**18**(2):235-266

[64] Gadgil M, Bekes F, Folke C. Indigenous knowledge for biodiversity conservation. Ambio. 1993;**22**:151-156

[65] Turner NJ. Ethnobotany: Future direction for the new millennium. Manitoba Anthropology Student's Journal. 2000;**16**:15-18

[66] Shanker D. Medicinal plants and biodiversities. Journal of Ethiopharmacology. 1993;**33**:100-119

Chapter 4

Traditional Medicinal Plants as the Potential Adjuvant, Prophylactic and Treatment Therapy for COVID-19 Disease: A Review

Moleboheng Emily Binyane
and Polo-Ma-Abiele Hildah Mfengwana

Abstract

Coronavirus disease 2019 (COVID-19) is a respiratory disease caused by a severe acute respiratory syndrome coronavirus-2 (SARS-CoV-2). In an effort to combat the pandemic caused by COVID-19 disease, researchers have identified several traditional medicinal plants (TMPs) as potential adjuvant, prophylactic, and treatment for COVID-19. TMPs reported in this paper were identified based on the findings of molecular docking research and the documented traditional use of these plants for COVID-19-related symptoms, such as fever, coughing, headaches, and tiredness. Secondary metabolites with antiviral, anti-inflammatory, and immunomodulatory activity against various SARS-CoV-2 proteases were also identified from the list of South African medicinal plants. This review discusses secondary metabolites of TMPs with pharmacological benefits, which contribute to the management of COVID-19, and these include *Acacia Senegal*, *Artemisia afra*, *Aspalathus linearis*, *Clerodendrum splendens*, *Dioscorea batatas* decne, *Echinacea purpurea*, *Hypoxis hemerocallidea*, *Xysmalobium undulatum*, *Tinospora crispa*, *Sutherladia frutescens*, and *Zingiber officinale*.

Keywords: traditional medicinal plants, COVID-19, adjuvant, antiviral, immunomodulatory

1. Introduction

Coronavirus disease 2019 (COVID-19) that caused pandemic started in December 2019 in Wuhan, China [1–3]. The novel coronavirus responsible for this respiratory disease was identified to be the member of the Coronaviridae family known to cause infections in humans called severe acute respiratory syndrome coronavirus-2 (SARS-CoV-2) [1]. SARS-CoV-2 is reported to be found in bats, and the infections occurred in humans because of the intermediate host, the pangolin [2]. SARS-CoV-2 is the third coronavirus reported to cause the respiratory disease pandemic after severe acute respiratory syndrome (SARS) and Middle East respiratory syndrome (MERS) [2]. COVID-19 disease spreads from human to human by respiratory droplets [4], and the symptoms include dry cough, fever, fatigue, body aches, dyspnea, chills and shivering, sputum production, diarrhea, nausea, nasal congestion, rhinorrhea, and loss of speech or movement [3, 5–7]. To date, COVID-19 is still the cause of morbidity and mortality worldwide, accounting to 409 confirmed positive cases and 5.8 million deaths between 7 and 13 February 2022 [8]. Among the African countries, South Africa (SA) reported the highest numbers of new mortality between 7 and 13 February 2022 [8].

Vaccines were quickly developed for the prevention of COVID-19 pandemic [9], but there is no specific treatment available [4] as vaccinated individuals can still contact and transmit the COVID-19 virus. COVID-19 symptom management is mainly supported with oxygen therapy, steroids, antivirals, antibiotics, and anti-inflammatory agents, including chloroquine and hydroxychloroquine [5, 6]. However, antibiotics, antiviral, and anti-inflammatory drugs are reported to be the cause of health problems due to their toxicities [6]. Africa has a long historic record on the use of traditional medicinal plants (TMPs), and phytomedicine is preferred as 80–90% of rural population rely on medicinal plants for primary healthcare [10]. Fortunately, the World Health Organization (WHO) promotes the use of traditional, complementary, and alternative medicine on condition that their efficacy, safety, and quality are scientifically reported [1, 11]. Therefore, considering the potential of TMPs as alternative and complementary conventional drugs for COVID-19 management is an important research topic during the current situation of COVID-19 pandemic [12]. Several studies were conducted on TMPs and their pharmacological activities against COVID-19 [10, 13–15], and this review is, therefore, aimed at the documentation of TMPs that can be used in adjuvant, prophylactic, and management therapy of COVID-19.

2. Potential use of TMPs in adjuvant, prophylactic, and management therapy for COVID-19 disease

TMPs have become the subject of interest in the era of COVID-19 pandemic, and various researchers have conducted studies based on selecting TMPs commonly used traditionally to treat fever, cold, and flu symptoms [13, 14]. *Echinacea purpurea* and *Zingiber officinale* were identified among TMPs with promising adjuvant symptomatic therapy [14]. A number of secondary metabolites isolated from TMPs were identified to have immunomodulatory, antiviral, and anti-inflammatory activities against SARS-CoV-2 [15]. TMPs with immunomodulatory effect could be used in COVID-19 patients as a prophylactic and treatment therapy [16]. Immunomodulation agents identified as potential therapy against infectious diseases, including COVID-19, are, among others, *Dioscorea batatas* decne, *Clerodendrum splendens,* and *Tinospora crispa* [17].

Active secondary metabolites of these TMPs have immunomodulatory effect and can reduce cytokine production against viral infections [6]. TMPs with potential antiviral activity against SARS-CoV-2 were identified as *Artemisia afra*, *Acacia Senegal*, *Aspolathus linerias*, *Hypoxis hemerocallidea, Sutherladia frutescens*, and *Xysmalobium undulatum* [15, 18, 19]. Madagascar's *Artemisia afra* was found to have inhibitory effect against SARS-CoV-2 [18]. Although the safety and dosage of this medicinal plant was determined *in vitro*, clinical studies must still be conducted to evaluate the use of this medicinal plant for COVID-19 prevention and treatment in COVID-19 patients [18]. Molecular docking research using the list of South African TMPs identified plants with antiviral activity against SARS-CoV-2 included *Acacia Senegal*, *Aspolathus linerias*, *Hypoxis hemerocallidea*, *Sutherladia frutescens*, *and Xysmalobium undulatum* [19].

TMPs reported in this review article target various stages in viral life cycle starting from the prevention of viral entry to the E6 cells, halting the fusion of the S protein, the inhibition of SARS-CoV-2 receptor-binding domain, the prevention of viral replication, and the transcription by targeting SARS-CoV-2 RNA-dependent RNA polymerase and major proteases [6, 15, 17, 19–25]. The diagrams in **Figure 1** show strategies for the prevention and management of COVID-19 using TMPs.

2.1 *Acacia senegal*

A. senegal (**Figure 2**), also known as white gum tree, belongs to the *Mimosoideae* family of plants and is widely distributed in Senegal, Cameroon, and Sudan [26–28]. Exotic *A. Senegal* is found in South Africa and is called siKhambophane and umKhala in isiZulu [29]. *A. senegal* is traditionally used to treat respiratory symptoms and infections, such as flu and sore throat (**Table 1**), and other conditions including, sinusitis, toothaches, stomach ulcer, colic, diarrhea, and dysentery [19, 26]. This medicinal plant has pharmacological activities, which include anti-inflammatory, antibacterial, antifungal, and antioxidant [26]. Secondary metabolites identified from *A. senegal's*

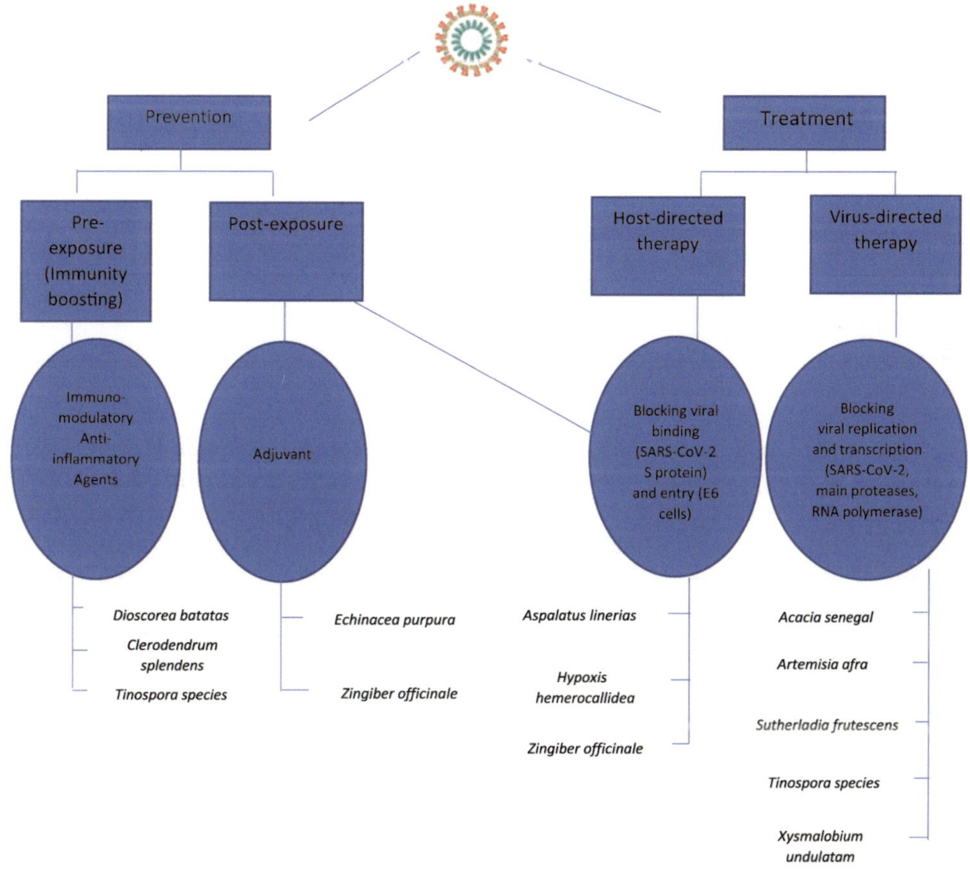

Figure 1.
Identified strategies for prevention and treatment of COVID-19 using TMPs.

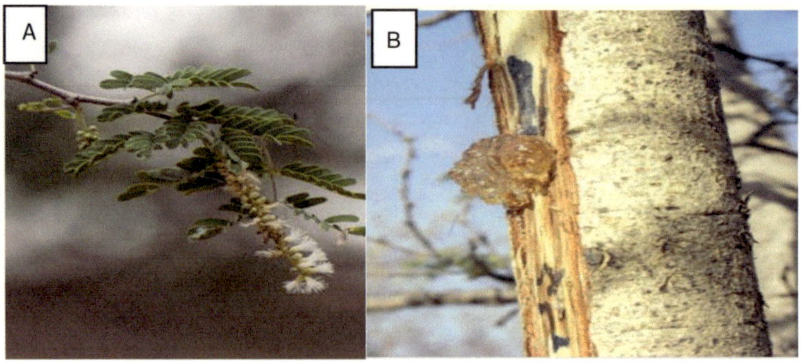

Figure 2.
Acacia Senegal *leaves in picture A and bark in picture B.*

TMPs	Traditional uses in respiratory symptoms and diseases
Acacia senegal	Flu, sore throat [19]
Artemisia afra	Cold, cough, headache, influenza, sore throat, asthma, pneumonia [30, 31]
Aspalathus linearis	Asthma [32]
Clerodendrum splendens	Asthma, cough, [20, 33]
Dioscorea batatas decne	Asthma [21]
Echinacea purpurea	Common cold [34]
Hypoxis hemerocallidea	Tuberculosis [35, 36]
Sutherladia frutescens	Influenza, fever [37]
Tinospora species	Fever [23]
Xysmalobium undulatum	Headache [19]
Zingiber officinale	Cold, cough, asthma, influenza, headache, fever, sore throat [14, 38–40]

Table 1.
Traditional uses of TMPs in respiratory symptoms and diseases.

plants extracts include glycosides, alkaloids, flavonoids, and arabic acid [15, 19, 26]. Arabic acid was determined to have a higher docking score (−5.2 kcal/mol) against 3CLpro, suggesting that *A. senegal* is a medicinal plant with antiviral activity against SARS-CoV-2 3C-like major protease (**Table 2**) [15, 19]. Thus, testing *A. senegal in vitro* might help to characterize new treatment and/or prophylactic strategies against SARS-CoV-2.

2.2 *Artemisia afra*

Artemisia afra (**Figure 3**), also known as African wormwood, belongs to the *Asteraceae* family [44, 45]. It is indigenous to Africa and is widely distributed in South Africa, Namibia, Zimbabwe, Kenya, Tanzania, Uganda, and Ethiopia [30, 44]. *Artemisia afra* is called Umhlonyane in Xhosa and Lengana in Sesotho [44]. It is used traditionally for the treatment of respiratory symptoms and diseases including cold, cough, headache, influenza, sore throat, asthma, and pneumonia (**Table 1**), and other disease conditions such as diabetes, colic, dyspepsia, bladder and kidney disorders,

TMPs	Secondary metabolites with a Adjuvant, prophylactic, and anti-COVID-19 activity
Acacia senegal	Arabic acid, Anti-SARS-CoV-2 3C-like major protease activity [15, 19]
Artemisia afra	Flavonoids, Anti-SARS-CoV-2 activity [15]
Aspalathus linearis	Flavonoids, quercetin, luteolin, Anti-SARS-CoV activity [41]
Clerodendrum splendens	Type II arabinogalactam, immuno modulatory activity [17, 20]
Dioscorea batatas decne	Allantoin, batatas, choline, dioscorin, diosgenin, gracillin, glycoproteins, L-arginine, mucopolysaccharides, prosapogenin, protein, polysaccharide, saponins, Immunomodulatory activity [17, 21, 22]
Echinacea purpurea	Chicoric acid, polysaccharide, alkamides, immunomodulatory activity [14] and Extracts, Anti-coronavirus activity [42]
Hypoxis hemerocallidea	Hypoxide, Anti-SARS-CoV-2 receptor binding domain activity [19]
Sutherladia frutescens	L-canavanine, Anti-SARS-CoV-2 3C-like main protease activity [19]
Tinospora crispa	hydroxy-5-cholen-24-oic acid, androstan-17-one, 3-ethyl-3-hydroxy-(5.alpha), camphenol, (−)-globulol, yangambin, nordazem, TMS derivative, benzene ethanamide, Anti-SARS-CoV-2 main protease activity [25]
Tinospora cordifolia	Amritoside, apigen-6-C-glucosyl7-O-glu-coside, 20a hydroxy ecdysone, tinosporine B, epicatechin, Anti-SARS CoV-2 main protease activity [6]
Xysmalobium undulatum	Uzarin, Anti-SARS-CoV-2 RNA dependent RNA polymerase activity [19]
Zingiber officinale	10-paradol, 8-paradol, scopoletin, 10-shogaol, 8-gingerol, 10-gingerol, Anti-SARS-CoV-2 activity [43]

Table 2.
Secondary metabolites of TMPs with adjuvant, prophylactic, and anti-COVID-19 activity.

constipation, malaria, and rheumatism [30, 31]. *Artemisia afra* contains secondary metabolites including tannins, alkaloids, terpenoids, cardiac glycosides, and saponins [30]. Pharmacological activities of *Artemisia afra* include antioxidant, antiviral, antiplamodial, antifungal, and antibacterial [30, 31, 44]. *Artemisia afra* aqueous and ethanolic extracts, as well as teas, were shown to inhibit SARS-CoV-2 plaque formation *in vitro* [15]. The antiviral activity of this medicinal plant is reported to have been as a result of flavonoids present in *Artemisia* species (**Table 2**) [15]. The extracts showed some toxicity at higher concentrations with the selectivity index of 10, which opened a therapeutic window that is required to be further investigated in clinical trial [15]. There is still a need to prove whether *Artemisia afra* extracts can reach the serum levels required to completely inhibit the virus in COVID-19 patients.

2.3 *Aspalathus linearis*

A. linearis (**Figure 4**), also known as Rooibos in Afrikaans, belongs to the *Fabaceae* family and is an endemic South African species cultivated to produce a tea [46–48]. It is used commonly for the treatment of respiratory disease such as asthma (**Table 1**) and other diseases including cardiac arrhythmias, colic, diarrhea, and hypertension [32]. Rooibos contains flavonoids including aspalathin, isoorientin,

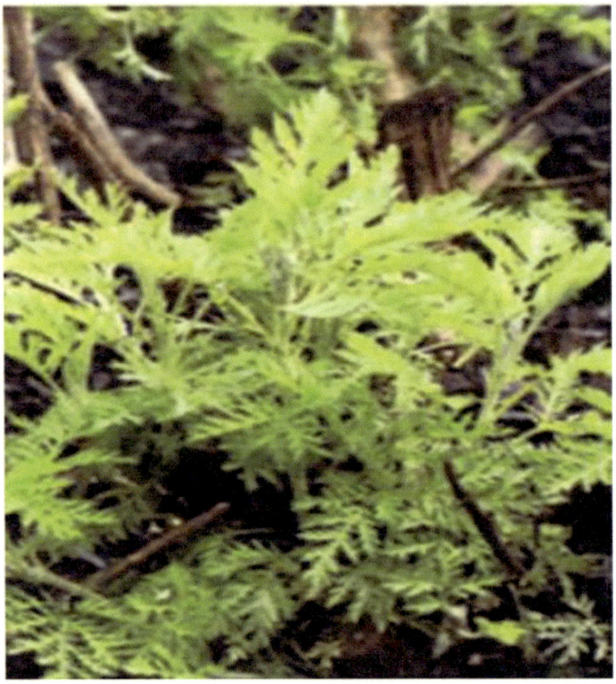

Figure 3.
Artemisia afra *leaves.*

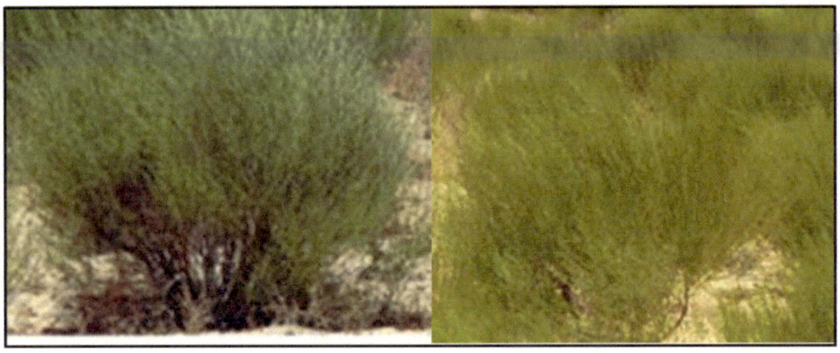

Figure 4.
Aspalathus linearis.

isovitexin, nothofagin, orientin, quercetin, rutin, and vitexin [41]. Other present secondary metabolites include polyphenols and phenolic compounds such as dihydro-chalcones, flavonols, flavonones, and proanthocyanadins [41, 46, 47]. Rooibos has pharmacological activities including antioxidant, antiviral, immunomodulatory, anti-inflammatory, cardioprotective, and nephroprotective effects [41]. Flavonoids, quercetin, and luteolin (**Table 2**) present in Rooibos were found to inhibit SARS-CoV infection by preventing entry of virus into E6 cells, and luteolin acts by binding to SARS-CoV S proteins, thereby interfering with the S protein function [41]. However, more experiments must be conducted to validate the clinical relevance of Rooibos in treating COVID-19 and other respiratory diseases [41]. Although other studies have highlighted the drug interactions associated with the

Rooibos derived phytochemicals [42], more research is required in determining the safety of Rooibos in patients.

2.4 *Clerodendrum splendens*

Clerodendrum splendens (**Figure 5**), also known as bag flower, bleeding-heart, and glory bower in English [33, 49], belongs to the *Lamiaceae* family of plants [20]. It is distributed in tropical Africa, Southern Asia, America, and Northern Australasia [33]. *Clerodendrum splendens* is used traditionally to treat respiratory diseases such as asthma and coughs (**Table 1**) and other diseases including anorexia, leucoderma, leprosy, malaria, skin diseases, ulcers, uterine fibroids, wounds, burns, and sexually transmitted diseases such as syphilis and gonorrhea [20, 33]. Phytochemical constituents present in *Clerodendrum splendens* include alkaloids, cyanogenic glycosides, diterpenes, flavonoids, phenolic compounds, saponins, steroids, tannins, terpenoids, and volatile compounds [17, 20]. It has pharmacological activities including antibacterial, antifungal, anti-inflammatory, antiproliferative, antioxidant, and hepatoprotective [17, 20, 33]. *Clerodendrum splendens* contains a polysaccharide, type II arabinogalactam (**Table 2**), that has been shown to have immunomodulatory activity both *in vitro and in vivo* [17, 20]. Its antiproliferative activity is reported to be as a result of clerodane diterpenes and phenyl propanoids found in aerial parts this plant [17]. The methanol extract of *Clerodendrum splendens* was reported to have *in vitro* anti-inflammatory activity (**Table 2**) [24]. The findings reported on *Clerodendrum splendens* form the basis for further research into the efficacy and safety of this plant as potential COVID-19 treatment and anti-inflammatory agents [17, 24].

2.5 *Dioscorea batatas* decne

D. batatas decne (**Figure 6**), commonly called Chinese yam [50, 51], belongs to the *Dioscoreaceae* family of plants [21, 52]. *Dioscoreaceae* plant species are widely distributed in West Africa, Southeast Asia, and Tropical America [52]. *D. batatas* decne is used traditionally for the treatment of respiratory disease such as

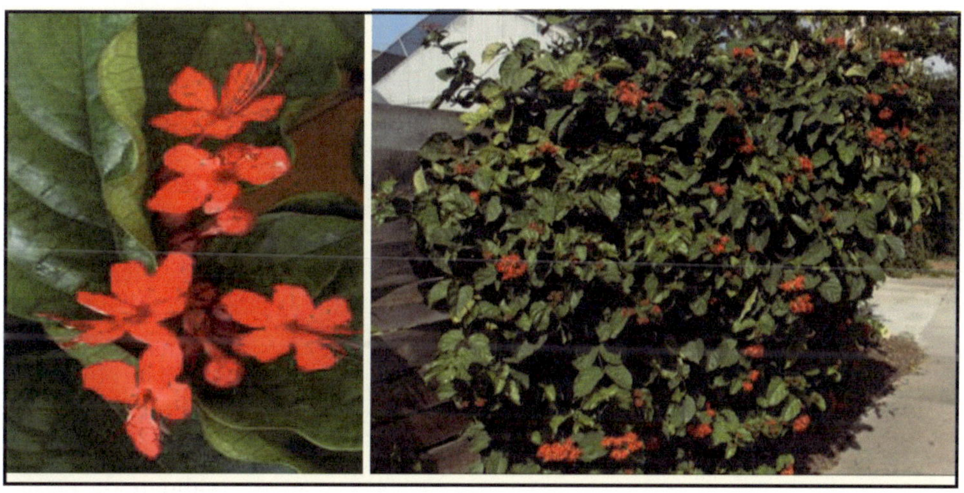

Figure 5.
Clerodendrum splendens *leaves and flowers.*

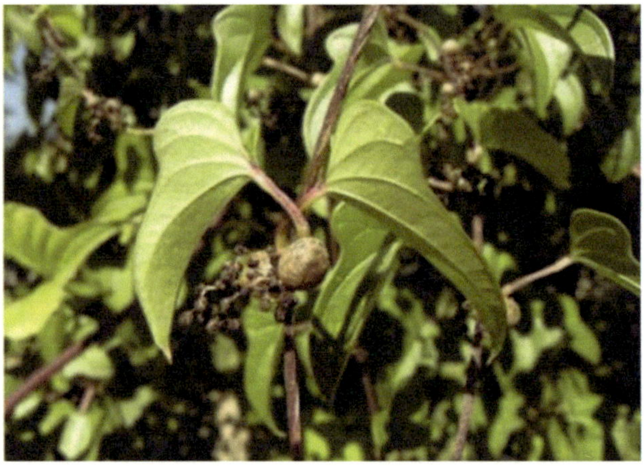

Figure 6.
Dioscorea batatas *decne leaves and fruits.*

asthma (**Table 1**) and other conditions including, abscesses, cancer, inflammation, hypertension, ulcer, chronic diarrhea, and diabetes [21]. It has antioxidant and anti-inflammatory activities [22, 50]. *D. batatas* decne contains various active components, such as allantoin, batatasins, choline, dioscorin, diosgenin, gracillin, glycoproteins, L-arginine, mucopolysaccharides, prosapogenin, protein, polysaccharides, and sapogenins (**Table 2**) with immunomodulation effects when orally administered [17, 21, 22]. The immunomodulatory activity of tuber protein and dioscorin occurs through the activation of TLR4-induced macrophage due to the stimulation of signaling molecules such as NF-kB, JNK, p38, and ERK, and by TNF-a and IL-6 cytokines expression [17, 21, 22]. The immunomodulation effect of tuber extract on inflamed and normal skin was reported to be due to the enhancement of granulocyte-macrophage colony-stimulating factor promoter [17]. The tuber extract of *D. batatas* was found to be the potent inhibitor of SARS-CoV (**Table 2**) at concentrations between 25 and 200 μg/mL [53].

2.6 *Echinacea purpurea*

E. purpurea (**Figure 7**), also known as Eastern Purple Coneflower, belongs to the *Asteraceae* family [54–56]. It is native to eastern North America [55]. *E. purpurea* is used for the treatment of respiratory conditions such as common cold (**Table 1**) and other conditions including pain, cancer, toothache, seizures, arthritis, and skin disorders [14, 34, 54]. *E. purpurea* has been approved by the European Medicine Agency Herbal Medicinal Product Committee to be used as prophylactic therapy for the maximum of 10 days for immunostimulation and to prevent cold and other respiratory infections [14]. Pharmacological activities of *E. purpurea* include antiviral, antioxidant, antibacterial, immunomodulatory, antitumor, and anti-inflammatory [54, 55]. *E. purpurea* contains phytochemicals such as alkamides, betaine, phenolic compounds, polysaccharides, lipoproteins, saponins, sesquiterpenes, and polyacetylene [55]. *Echinacea* species exerts a soothing effect and could be useful in the relief of respiratory symptoms and common cold [14]. The immunomodulatory activity of *E. purpurea* was reported to be as a result of chicoric acid, polysaccharide, and alkamides (**Table 2**) in a rat study [14]. The use of *Echinacea*

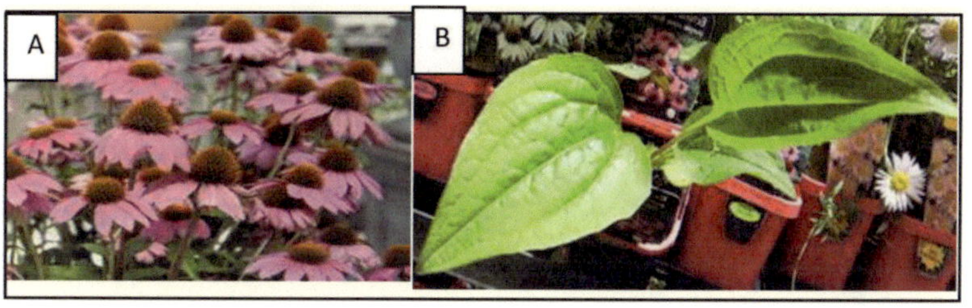

Figure 7.
Echinacea purpurea. *(A) Flowers and (B) leaves.*

for supplementation is reported to decrease the duration of acute respiratory tract infections and the severity of the disease [57]. The extract of *E. purpurea* (L.) Moench has shown direct antiviral activity against coronaviruses, and the preliminary published findings on human clinical trials covering antiviral activity of *Echinacea* against SARS-CoV-2 further support the use of this plant species against this particular coronavirus [58].

2.7 *Hypoxis hemerocallidea*

Hypoxis hemerocallidea (**Figure 8**), also known as African Potato, belongs to the *Hypoxidaceae* family [35, 36, 59]. It is called inkomfe in Zulu and Lotsane in Tswana [60]. *Hypoxis hemerocallidea* is widely distributed in Southern Africa including, South Africa, Lesotho, Mozambique, and Zimbabwe and is also found in East Africa [36]. It is used traditionally to treat HIV/acquired immunodeficiency syndrome, arthritis, diabetes mellitus, testicular tumors, cancers, infertility, urinary infection, cardiovascular diseases, and respiratory disease such as tuberculosis (**Table 1**) [35, 36]. *Hypoxis hemerocallidea* contain phytochemicals, such as sterols, sterolins, norlignan, daucosterol, and rooperol, responsible for its therapeutic benefits [35]. Hypoxide is the main glycoside isolated from *Hypoxis* species [36]. Molecular docking analysis identified hypoxide (**Table 2**) as a potent inhibitor of SARS-CoV-2 receptor-binding domain with the docking score of −6.9 kcal/mol [19]. The study conducted on rats has demonstrated that *Hypoxis hemerocallidea* has the ability to impair kidney function. There is a need for more *in vitro* and *in vivo* research on the toxicity, safety, and efficacy of *Hypoxis hemerocallidea* [61].

2.8 *Sutherladia frutescens*

Sutherlandia frutescens (**Figure 9**), also known as cancer bush, belongs to *Fabaceae* family of plants [6, 62]. It is an indigenous medicinal plant commonly used in South Africa to treat respiratory symptoms and disease such as fever and influenza (**Table 1**) and other diseases including cancers, diabetes, kidney and liver problems, rheumatism, depression, wounds, hemorrhoids, gonorrhea, urinary tract infections, and back pain [37]. Various *Sutherlandia* formulations are available in pharmacies and herbal shops and include capsules and tablets, gels, creams, liquid extracts, and ointments [37]. *S. frutescens* has been scientifically reported to have anticancer, antidiabetic, and anti-HIV properties [37, 62]. It has phytochemical constituents including sutherlandioside A, B, C and D, D-pinitol, gamma (γ) aminobutyric acid, and L-canavanine responsible for its biological

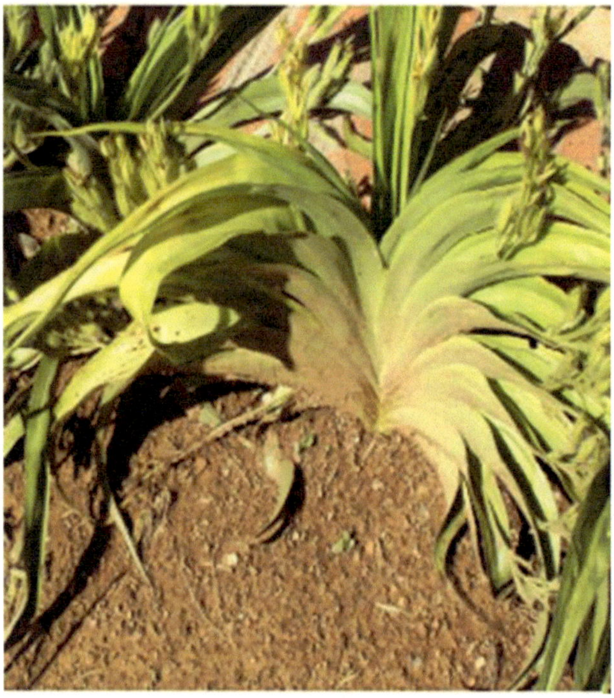

Figure 8.
Hypoxis hemerocallidea *leaves.*

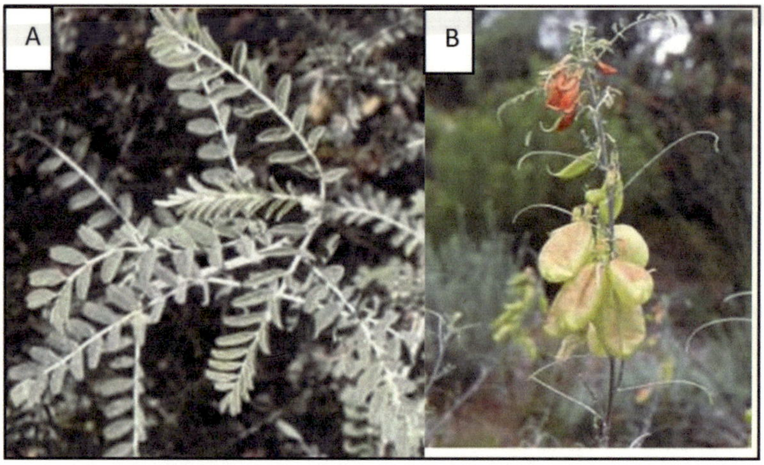

Figure 9.
Sutherlandia frutescens. *(A) Leaves and (B) flowers.*

activities [37]. The results of molecular docking analysis identified L-canavanine (**Table 2**) present in *S. frutescens* as a potential inhibitor of SARS-CoV-2 3C-like main protease [19]. The results of a randomized, double-blind, placebo-controlled trial of *Sutherlandia* leaf powder in healthy adults revealed that 800 mg/day of *Sutherlandia* leaf powder capsules were safe for consumption twice per day for three months in healthy adults [63].

2.9 *Tinospora species*

Tinospora crispa (**Figure 10A**) is also known as Seruntum in Malaysia, Brotawali in Indonesia, Makabuhay in Philippines, Boraphet in Thailand, Da ye ruanjinteng in China, Banndol Pech in Cambodia, Golonchi in Bangladesh, and Lyann span Zeb kayenn in Martinique island [23, 64]. *Tinospora cordifolia* (**Figure 10B** and **C**), also known as heart leaved Moonseed plant in English, Giloy in Hindi, and Guduchi in Sanskrit [65]. *Tinospora* species belongs to the family *Menispermaceae* [23, 65, 66]. *Tinospora crispa* is found in South East Asia and the Pacific [23, 66], and *Tinospora cordifolia* is found throughout India and certain parts in China [65]. Traditionally, *Tinospora* species are used to treat respiratory diseases and symptoms such as fever (**Table 1**) and other conditions including muscle pain, immune system associated inflammatory disorders, rheumatism, muscle pain, diabetes, and abdominal pain, septicemia, scabies, and ulcer-related disorders, hypertension, jaundice, paralysis, skin disease, leprosy, flatulence, dyspepsia, and diarrhea [6, 23, 66]. Phytochemical constituents of *Tinospora crispa* include alkaloids, flavonoids, furanoditerpenes, lignans, lactones, and steroids [66]. *Tinospora crispa* has pharmacological activity including antioxidant [23]. Active constituents such as boldine, cardioside, eicosenoic acid, quercetin, magnoflorin, and syringin are reported to have the antioxidant potential higher than that of ascorbic acid [23]. The same constituents are also reported to have the ability to increase the expression of IL-6, IL-8, and INF-g, thereby activating the immune system [17]. *Tinospora cordifolia* contains secondary metabolites including folioside A, tinocordiside, magnoflorine, and syringin with immunomodulatory activity [6]. The results of the molecular docking study on *Tinospora crispa* have revealed nine potential anti-SARS-CoV-2 lead molecules, namely, imidazolid-4-ne, 2-imino-1-(4-methoxy-6-dimethylamino-1,3,5-triazin-2-yl), spiro [4, 8] dec-6-en-1-ol, 2,6,10,10-tetramethyl, 3.beta-hydroxy-5-cholen-24-oic acid, androstan-17-one, 3-ethyl-3-hydroxy-(5.alpha), camphenol, (−)-Globulol, yangambin, nordazem, TMS derivative, and benzeneethanamide (**Table 2**). Three of these molecules have demonstrated some biological activity, which led to further optimization and drug development research for COVID-19 disease [25]. Molecular docking analysis also revealed that *Tinospora cordifolia* contains bioactive compounds, including amritoside, 20a hydroxy ecdysone, apigen-6-C-glucosyl7-O-glucoside, tinosporine B, and epicatechin (**Table 2**), with promising anti-SARS CoV-2 main protease activity [6]. The acute toxicity study conducted on rats has revealed that the ethanol extract of *Tinospora crispa* stem is not toxic and did not cause animal

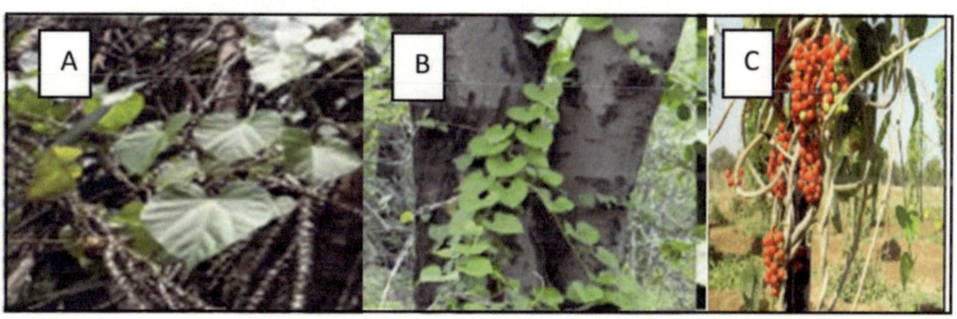

Figure 10.
(A) Tinospora crispa. (B) and (C) Tinospora cordifolia.

death at a dose of 4.0 g/kg of body weight (g/kg BW). However, six-month chronic toxicity study has reported hepatic and renal toxicities of the ethanol extract at a dose of 9.26 g/kg BW/day [64].

2.10 *Xysmalobium undulatum*

Xysmalobium undulatum (**Figure 11**) also known as Uzara wild cotton and milk bush, belongs to the family *Apocynaceae* [67–70]. Genus *Xysmalobium* is endemic to Africa and there are about 18 plant species occurring in SA [67]. Uzara is used traditionally to treat respiratory symptoms such as headaches (**Table 1**) and other disease conditions including, diarrhea, stomach cramps, afterbirth cramps, dysmenorrhea, wounds, sores, abscesses, and hysteria and has a diuretic effect [68]. Uzarin and its isomers allouzarin, xysmalorin, and alloxysmalorin are the main compounds isolated from Uzara [67]. Pharmacological activities of Uzara include antidiarrheal and antidepressant [68]. Uzarin (**Table 2**) was identified as the potential inhibitor of SARS-CoV-2 RNA-dependent RNA polymerase, and it showed favorable docking score of −3.5 kcal/mol in a molecular docking study conducted from the list of South African TMPs [19].

2.11 *Zingiber officinale*

Z. officinale (**Figure 12**), also known as Ginger, belongs to the *Zingiberaceae* family which comprises of close to two hundred species [38, 71]. *Z. officinale* is used for the treatment of respiratory symptoms and diseases including common cold, cough,

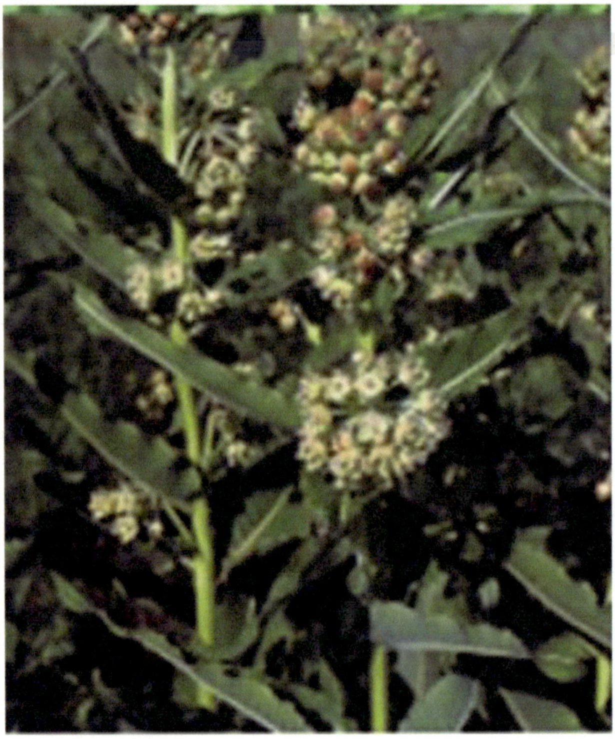

Figure 11.
Xysmalobium undulatum leaves and flowers.

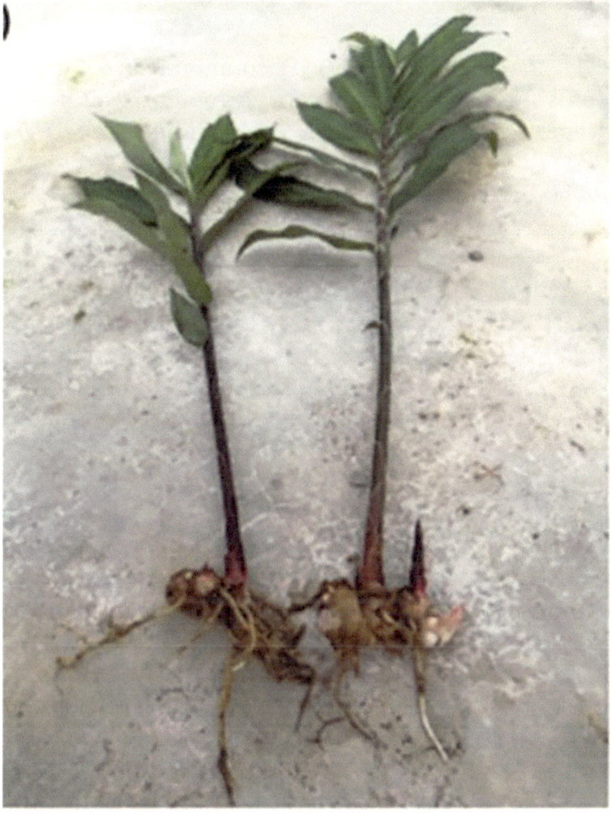

Figure 12.
Zingiber officinale *whole plant showing roots, stem, and leaves.*

asthma, influenza, headaches, sore throats, and fever (**Table 1**) and other diseases such as arthritis, rheumatism, nausea, flatulence, muscular aches, pains, cramps, constipation, hypertension, dementia, infectious diseases, helminthiasis, colic, and diarrhea [14, 38–40]. It has pharmacological activities including immunomodulatory, antitumorigenic, anti-inflammatory, antiapoptotic, antihyperglycemic, antilipidemic, antiemetic, antipyretic, antioxidant, antibacterial, and analgesic [38–40]. Active compounds in ginger include phenolic and terpene compounds, and phenolic compounds in ginger include gingerols, paradols and shogaols, and paradols [39]. The profile and chemistry of *Z. officinale* makes it a perfect anti-inflammatory therapy in the context of upper respiratory affections [39]. Molecular docking *in silico* studies suggested that phytochemical compounds, such as 10-Paradol, 8-Paradol, Scopoletin, 10-Shogaol, 8-Gingerol, and 10-Gingerol, in *Z. officinale* (**Table 2**) have potential in reducing viral load and detaching of SARS-CoV-2 in the nasal passages [43].

Future aspects include the extraction of the medicinal plants listed in **Table 1**, the isolation of pure compounds as well as their fingerprinting and identification, and the confirmation of their mechanisms of action [72]. Further testing of extracts in animal models and investigations of effective and safe dosages, route administration, drug administration intervals, pharmacokinetics, and mechanisms of action are required before the use of medicinal plants discussed in this review can be advocated to be used for COVID-19 patients [7].

3. Conclusions

The current review has summarized TMPs commonly used in the treatment of respiratory symptoms and diseases, which possess potential adjuvant, prophylactic, and therapeutic properties against SARS-CoV-2 including *Acacia Senegal*, *Artemisia afra*, *Aspalathus linearis*, *Clerodendrum splendens*, *D. batatas* decne, *E. purpurea*, *Hypoxis hemerocallidea*, *Xysmalobium undulatum*, *Tinospora crispa*, *Sutherladia frutescens,* and *Z. officinale*. Secondary metabolites present in selected TMPs are responsible for the pharmacological activities of these medicinal plants. TMPs identified by molecular docking analysis should be investigated experimentally as potential SARS-CoV-2 treatment. Further studies are warranted to isolate and test secondary metabolites with inhibitory properties against SARS-CoV-2. Safety and efficacy profiles of these TMPs must be explored *in vitro* and *in vivo*. Animal studies and human clinical trials are required for further testing of these TMPs before recommendations to use in COVID-19 patients.

Acknowledgements

We acknowledge the Central University of Technology, Department of Health Sciences and Walter Sisulu University, Department of Internal Medicine and Pharmacology.

Conflict of interest

The authors declare no conflict of interest.

Author details

Moleboheng Emily Binyane[1] and Polo-Ma-Abiele Hildah Mfengwana[2*]

1 Walter Sisulu University, Mthatha, South Africa

2 Central University of Technology, Bloemfontein, South Africa

*Address all correspondence to: pntsoeli@cut.ac.za

References

[1] Chali BU, Melaku T, Berhanu N, Mengistu B, Milkessa G, Mamo G, et al. Traditional medicine practice in the context of COVID-19 pandemic: Community claim in Jimma zone, Oromia, Ethiopia. Infection and Drug Resistance. 2021;**14**:3773-3783. DOI: 10.2147/IDR.S331434

[2] Wiersinga WJ, Rhodes A, Cheng AC, Peacock SJ, Prescott HC. Pathophysiology, transmission, diagnosis, and treatment of coronavirus disease 2019 (COVID-19): A review. Journal of the American Medical Association. 2020;**324**(8):782-793. DOI: 10.10 01/jama.2020.12839

[3] Seth S, Batra J, Srinivasan S. COVID-19: Targeting proteases in viral invasion and host immune response. Frontiers in Molecular Biosciences. 2020;**7**(215):1-9. DOI: 10. 3389/fm olb.2020.00215

[4] Keni R, Alexander A, Nayak P.G, Mudgal J, Nandakumar K. COVID-19: Emergence, spread, possible treatments, and global burden. Frontiers in Public Health. 2020;**8**(216):1-13. DOI:10.3389/fpubh.2020.00216

[5] Parasher A. COVID-19: Current understanding of its pathophysiology, clinical presentation and treatment. Postgraduate Medical Journal. 2021;**97**: 312-320. DOI: 10.1136/postgradmedj-2020-138577

[6] Murugesan SK, Kottekad S, Crasta I, Sreevathsan S, Usharani D, Perumal MK, et al. Targeting COVID-19 (SARS-CoV-2) main protease through active phytocompounds of ayurvedic medicinal plants - *Emblica officinalis* (amla), *Phyllanthus niruri* Linn. (Bhumi amla) and *Tinospora cordifolia* (Giloy) - a molecular docking and simulation study. Computers in Biology Medicine. 2021;**136**(104683):1-13. DOI: 10.1016/j.compbio med. 2021.104683

[7] Peter AE, Sandeep BV, Rao BG, Kalpana VL. Calming the storm: Natural immunosuppressants as adjuvants to target the cytokine storm in COVID-19. Frontiers in Pharmacology. 2021; **11**(583777):1-22. DOI: 10.3389/fphar. 2020.583777

[8] World Health Organization. COVID-19 Weekly Epidemiological Update. WHO Geneva, Switzerland. Available from: https://apps.who.int/iris/bitstream/handle/10665/345454/CoV-weekly-sitrep7Sep21-eng.pdf?sequence=2 [Accessed: February 23, 2022]

[9] Bruxvoort KJ, Sy LS, Qian L, Ackerson BK, Luo Y, Lee GS, et al. Effectiveness of mRNA-1273 against delta, mu, and other emerging variants of SARS-CoV-2: Test negative case-control study. British Medical Journal. 2021;**375**(e068848):1-15. DOI: 10.1136/bmj-2021-068848

[10] Attah AF, Fagbemi AA, Olubiyi O, Dada-Adegbola H, Oluwadotun A, Elujoba A, et al. Therapeutic potentials of antiviral plants used in traditional African medicine With COVID-19 in focus: A Nigerian perspective. Frontiers in Pharmacology. 2021;**12**(596855):1-15. DOI: 10.3389/fphar.2021.596855

[11] Mothibe ME, Sibanda M. African Traditional Medicine: South African Perspective. London: IntechOpen; 2019. pp. 1-27. DOI: 10.5772/intechopen.83790

[12] Turkson BK, Agyemang AO, Baidoo MF, Bayor MT. COVID- 19: The role of medicinal plants and research

institutions. International Journal of Pharmacognosy and Clinical Research. 2021;**3**(1):05-11

[13] Yimer G, Ekuadzi E, Fasinu P, Cristina de Melo A, Pillai GC. Traditional medicines for COVID-19: Perspectives from clinical pharmacologists. British Journal of Clinical Pharmacology. 2021;**87**:3455-3458. DOI: 10.1111/bcp.14981

[14] Silveira D, Prieto-Garcia JM, Boylan F, Estrada O, Fonseca-Bazzo YM, Jama CM, et al. COVID-19: Is there evidence for the use of herbal medicines as adjuvant symptomatic therapy? Frontiers in Pharmacology. 2020;**11**(581840):1-15. DOI: 10.3389/fphar.2020.581840

[15] Lall N. The potential of South African medicinal plants for the treatment of COVID-19. Annals of Phytomedicine. 2021;**10**(1):S1-S3. DOI: 10.21276/ap.covid19.2021.10.1.1

[16] Mphekgwana PM, Makgahlela M, Mothiba TM. Use of traditional medicines to fight COVID-19 during the South African nationwide lockdown: A prevalence study among university students and academic staff. The Open Public Health Journal. 2021;**14**:441-445. DOI: 10.2174/1874944502114010441

[17] Alhazmi HA, Najmi A, Javed SA, Sultana S, Bratty MA, Makeen HA, et al. Medicinal plants and isolated molecules demonstrating immunomodulation activity as potential alternative therapies for viral diseases including COVID-19. Frontiers in Immunology. 2021;**12**:1-24. DOI: 10.3389/fimmu.2021.637553

[18] Nie C, Trimpert J, Moon S, Haag R, Gilmore K, Kaufer BB, et al. *In vitro* efficacy of *Artemisia extracts* against SARS-CoV-2. Virology Journal. 2021;**18**:182-188. DOI: 10.1186/s12985-021-01651-8

[19] Dwarka D, Agoni C, Mellen JJ, Soliman ME, Baijnath H. Identification of potential SARS-CoV-2 inhibitors from South African medicinal plant extracts using molecular modelling approaches. South African Journal of Botany. 2020;**133**:273-284. DOI: 10.1016/j.sajb.2020.07.035

[20] Koffi Kouakou K, Schepetkin IA, Jun S, Kirpotina LN, Yapi A, Khramova DS, et al. Immunomodulatory activity of polysaccharides isolated from *Clerodendrum splendens*: Beneficial effects in experimental autoimmune encephalomyelitis. BioMedicine Central Complementary and Alternative Medicine. 2013;**13**(149):1-19. DOI: 10.1186/1472-6882-13-149

[21] Go H, Rahman MM, Kim G, Na C, Song C, Kim J, et al. Antidiabetic effects of yam (*Dioscorea batatas*) and its active constituent, allantoin, in a rat model of streptozotocin-induced diabetes. Nutrients. 2015;**7**:8532-8544. DOI: 10.3390/nu7105411

[22] Lim JS, Hahn D, Gu MJ, Oh J, Lee J, Kim J. Anti-infammatory and antioxidant effects of 2,7-dihydroxy-4, 6-dimethoxy phenanthrene isolated from *Dioscorea batatas* Decne. Applied Biological Chemistry. 2019;**62**(29):1-9. DOI: 10.1186/s13765-019-0436-2

[23] Ahmad W, Jantan I, Bukhari SNA. *Tinospora crispa* (L.) Hook. f. and Thomson: A review of its ethnobotanical, phytochemical, and pharmacological aspects. Frontiers in Pharmacology. 2016;**7**(59):1-19. DOI: 10.3389/fphar.2016.00059

[24] Okugbo OES, Oikeh OT, Oriakhi EI, Olubodun K, Omoigui S, Osarenren OP.

Phytochemical screening and *in vitro* anti-inflammatory activity of methanol extract of *Clerodendrum splendens* leaf. Nigerian Society for Experimental Biology. 2014;**14**(3):160-167

[25] Rakib A, Paul A, Chy NU, Sami SA, Baral SK, Majumder M, et al. Biochemical and computational approach of selected phytocompounds from *Tinospora crispa* in the management of COVID-19. Molecules. 2020;**28**(25):3917-3936. DOI: 10.3390/molecules25173936.9

[26] Magnini RD, Hilou A, Compaore S, Pagès J. A review on ethnobotanical uses, biological activities and phytochemical aspects of *Acacia senegal* (L.) Willd. and *Acacia seyal* Delile. (Fabaceae). International Journal of Plant Science and Horticulture. 2020;**15**:32-55. DOI: 10.36 811/ijpsh.2020.110023

[27] Heuzé V, Thiollet H, Tran G, Hassoun P, Bastianelli D, Lebas F. Gum arabic tree (*Acacia senegal*). Feedipedia, a programme by INRA, CIRAD, AFZ and FAO. Available from: http://www.feedipedia.org/node/342[Accessed: March 09, 2022]

[28] Harmand J, Ntoupka M, Mathieu B, Njiti CF, Tapsou J, Bois J, et al. Gum Arabic production in *Acacia senegal* plantations in the Sudanian zone of Cameroon: Effects of climate, soil, tapping date and tree provenance. Bois et Forêts des Tropiques. 2015;**311**:21-30. Available from: file:///C:/Users/Staff/Downloads/2012BFTHarmandetalgumarabic%20(1).pdf [Accessed: March 09, 2022]

[29] Orwa C, Mutua A, Kindt R, Jamnadass R, Anthony S. Agroforestree Database: A Tree Reference and Selection Guide Version 4.0. 2009. Available from: http://apps.world agro forestry.org/treedb/AFTPDFS/Acacia_senegal.PDF [Accessed: February 02, 2022]

[30] Kane NF, Kyama MC, Nganga JK, Hassanali A, Diallo M, Kimani FT. Comparison of phytochemical profiles and antimalarial activities of *Artemisia afra* plant collected from five countries in Africa. South African Journal of Botany. 2019;**125**:126-133

[31] Falowo AB, Mukumbo FE, Muchenje V. Phytochemical constituents and antioxidant activity of *Artemisia Afra* and *Bidens Pilosa* essential oil in ground pork. Journal of Essential Oil Bearing Plants 2019;**22**(1):176-186. DOI:10.1080/0972060X .2019.15 74 212.

[32] Khan A, Gilani AH. Selective bronchodilatory effect of rooibos tea (*Aspalathus linearis*) and its flavomoid, chysoeriol. European Journal of Nutrition. 2006;**45**:463-469. DOI: 10.1007/s00394-006-0620-0

[33] Wang J, Luan F, He X, Wang Y, Li M. Traditional uses and pharmacological properties of *Clerodendrum* phytochemicals. Journal of Traditional and Complementary Medicine. 2018;**8**:24-38. DOI: 10.1016/j.jtcme.2017.04.001

[34] Weber W, Taylor J, Van Der Stoep A, Weiss NS, Standish LJ, Calabrese C. Echinacea *purpurea* for prevention of upper respiratory tract infections in children. The Journal of Alternative and Complementary Medicine. 2005;**11**(6):1021-1026. DOI: 10.1089/acm.2005.11.2021

[35] Oguntibeju OO, Meyer S, Aboua YP, Goboza M. *Hypoxis hemerocallidea* significantly reduced hyperglycaemia and hyperglycaemic-induced oxidative stress in the liver and kidney tissues of streptozotocin-induced diabetic male wistar rats. Evidence-Based Complementary and Alternative Medicine. 2016;**1**:1-10. DOI: 10.1155/2016/8934362

[36] Matyanga CMJ, Morse GD, Gundidza M, Nhachi CFB. African potato (*Hypoxis hemerocallidea*): A systematic review of its chemistry, pharmacology and ethno medicinal Properties. BioMedicine Central Complementary Medicine and Therapies. 2020;**20**(182):1-12. DOI: 10.1186/s12906-020-02956-x

[37] Aboyade OM, Styger G, Gibson D, Hughes G. *Sutherlandia frutescens*: The meeting of science and traditional knowledge. The Journal of Alternative and Complementary Medicine. 2014;**20**(2):71-76. DOI: 10.1089/acm.2012.0343

[38] Rehman R, Akram M, Akhtar N, Jabeen Q, Saeed T, SMA S, et al. *Zingiber officinale* roscoe (pharmacological activity). Journal of Medicinal Plants Research. 2011;**5**(3):344-348

[39] Mao Q, Xu X, Cao S, Gan R, Corke H, Beta T, et al. Bioactive compounds and bioactivities of ginger (*Zingiber officinale* Roscoe). Foods. 2019;**8**(185):1-15. DOI: 10.3390/foods8060185

[40] Zhang S, Kou X, Zhao H, Mak K. Balijepalli M.K, Pichika M.R. *Zingiber officinale* var. *rubrum*: Red ginger's medicinal uses. Molecules. 2022;**27**(775):1-31. DOI: 10.3390/molecules27030775

[41] Abdul NS, Marnewick JL. Rooibos, a supportive role to play during the COVID-19 pandemic? Journal of Functional Foods. 2021;**86**(104684):1-15. DOI: 10.1016/ jjff.2021.104684

[42] Fantoukh OI, Dale OR, Parveen A, Hawwal MF, Ali Z, Manda VK, et al. Safety assessment of phytochemicals derived from the globalized south African rooibos tea (*Aspalathus linearis*) through interaction with CYP, PXR, and P-*gp*. Journal of Agricultural and Food Chemistry. 2019;**67**(17):4967-4975. DOI: 10.1021/acs.jafc.9b00846

[43] Haridas M, Sasidhar V, Nath P, Abhithaj J. Sabu1 A, Rammanohar P. Compounds of Citrus medica and *Zingiber officinale* for COVID-19 inhibition: In silico evidence for cues from Ayurveda. Future Journal of Pharmaceutical Sciences. 2021;**7**(13):1-9. DOI: 10.1186/s43094-020-00171-6

[44] Liu NQ, Van der Kooy F, Verpoorte R. Review *Artemisia afra* : A potential flagship for African medicinal plants? South African Journal of Botany. 2009;**75**:185-195. DOI: 10.1016/j.sajb.2008.11.001

[45] Cowan D, Pramlall S, Labuschagne K, Bruton M, Joubert A. Traditional medicine for COVID-19. Academy of Science of South Africa (ASSAf) Publications. Guest. 2020;**16**(3):26. DOI: 20.500.11911/154

[46] DL MK, Blumberg JB. A review of the bioactivity of South African herbal teas: Rooibos (*Aspalathus linearis*) and honeybush (*cyclopia intermedia*). Phytotherapy Research. 2007;**21**:1-16. DOI: 10.1002/ptr.1992

[47] Joubert E, de Beer D. Rooibos (*Aspalathus linerias*) beyond the farm gate: From herbal tea to potential phytopharmaceutical. South African Journal of Botany. 2011;**77**:869-886. DOI: 10.1016/j.sajb.2011.07.004

[48] Johnson R, de Beer D, Dludla PV, Ferreira D, Muller CJF, Joubert E. Aspalathin from Rooibos (*Aspalathus linearis*): A bioactive C-glucosyl dihydrochalcone with potential to target the metabolic syndrome. Planta Medica. 2018;**84**:568-583. DOI: 10.10 55/s-0.044-100622

[49] Top Tropicals. *Clerodendrum Splendens*. Fort Myers, Florida. Available

from: https://toptropicals .com/ catalog/ uid/clerodendrum_splendens.htm: Top Tropicals; 2021 [Accessed: March 10, 2022]

[50] Byeon S, Oh J, Lim JS, Lee JS, Kim J. Protective effects of *Dioscorea batatas* flesh and peel extracts against ethanol-induced gastric ulcer in mice. Nutrients. 2018;**10**(1680):1-14. DOI: 10.3390/ nu10111680

[51] Moro A. *Dioscorea batatas* decne. Trieste, Italy Available from: http://luirig. altervista.org/schedenam/fnam.php? tax on=27823: Department of Life Sciences, University of Trieste - Dryades Project; [Accessed: March 10, 2022]

[52] Kumar S, Das G, Shin H, Patra JK. *Dioscorea* spp. (a wild edible tuber): A study on its ethnopharmacological potential and traditional use by the local people of Similipal biosphere reserve, India. Frontiers in Pharmacology. 2017;**8**(5):1-17. DOI: 10.3389/ fph ar.2017.00052

[53] Wen C, Shyur L, Jan J, Liang P, Kuo C, Arulselvan P, et al. Traditional Chinese medicine herbal extracts of *Cibotium barometz*, *Gentiana scabra*, *Dioscorea batatas*, *Cassia tora*, and *Taxillus chinensis* inhibit SARS-CoV replication. Journal of Traditional and Complementary Medicine. 2011;**1**:41-50. DOI: 10.1016/s2225-4110(16)30055-4

[54] Manayi A, Vazirian M, Saeidnia S. *Echinacea purpurea*: Pharmacology, phytochemistry and analysis methods. Pharmacognosy Reviews. 2015;**9**(17):63-72. DOI: 10.4103/0973-7847.156353

[55] Coelho J, Barros L, Dias MI, Finimundy TC, Amaral JS, Alves MJ, et al. *Echinacea purpurea* (L.) Moench: Chemical characterization and bioactivity of its extracts and fractions. Pharmaceuticals. 2020;**13**(125):1-16. DOI: 10.3390/ph13060125

[56] Lim TK. Edible medicinal and non-medicinal plants: *Echinacea purpurea*. Economic Botany & Ethnobotany. 2013;7:340-371. DOI: 10.1007/ 978-94-007-7395-0_23

[57] Aucoina M, Cooleya K, Saundersa PR, Carèb J, Anheyerd D, Medinab DN, et al. The effect of *Echinacea* spp. on the prevention or treatment of COVID-19 and other respiratory tract infections in humans: A rapid review. Advances in Integrative Medicine. 2020;7:203-217. DOI: 10.1016 /j.aimed. 2020.07.004

[58] Nicolussi S, Ardjomand-Woelkart K, Stange R, Gancitano G, Klein P, Ogal M. *Echinacea* as a potential force against coronavirus infections? A mini-review of randomized controlled trials in adults and children. Microorganisms. 2022;**10**(211):1-11. DOI: 10.3390/microorganisms10 020211

[59] Zimudzi C. African potato (*Hypoxis* Spp): Diversity and comparison of the phytochemical profiles and cytotoxicity evaluation of four Zimbabwean species. Journal of Applied Pharmaceutical Science. 2014;**4**(4):79-83. DOI: 10.7324/ JAPS.2014.40414

[60] Random Harvest, *Hypoxis hemerocallidea*. Available from: https://www .random harvest.co.za/ South-African-Indigenous-Plants/ Show-Plant/Plant Id/355/Plant/Hypoxis-hemerocallidea [Accessed: January 03, 2022]

[61] Musabayane CT, Xozwa K, Ojewole JAO. Effects of *Hypoxis hemerocallidea* (Fisch. And C.a. Mey.) [*Hypoxidaceae*] corm (African potato) aqueous extract on renal electrolyte and

fluid handling in the rat. Renal Failure. 2005;**27**(6):763-770. DOI: 10.1080/0886 0220500244807

[62] Ntuli SBN, Gelderblom WCA, Katerere DR. The mutagenic and antimutagenic activity of *Sutherlandia frutescens* extracts and marker compounds. BioMedicine Central Complementary and Alternative Medicine. 2018;**18**(93):1-10. DOI: 10.1186/s12906-018-2159-z

[63] Johnson Q, Syce J, Nell H, Rudeen K, Folk WR. A randomized, double-blind, placebo-controlled trial of *Lessertia frutescens* in healthy adults. PLoS Clinical Trials. 2007;**2**(4):e16:0.001-e16:0.007. DOI: 10.1371/journal.pctr.0020016

[64] Ahmad W, Jantan I, SNA B. *Tinospora crispa* (L.) Hook F. and Thomson: A review of its ethnobotanical, phytochemical, and pharmacological aspects. Frontiers in Pharmacology. 2016;7(59):59. DOI: 3389/fphar.2016.00059

[65] Mittal J, Sharma MM, Batra A. *Tinospora cordifolia*: a multipurpose medicinal plant- A review. Journal of Medicinal Plants Studies. 2014;**2**(2):32-47

[66] Haque A, Jantan I, Harikrishnan H, Ahmad W. Standardized ethanol extract of *Tinospora crispa* upregulates pro-inflammatory mediators release in LPS-primed U937 human macrophages through stimulation of MAPK, NF-κB and PI3K-Akt signaling networks. BioMedicine Central Complementary Medicine and Therapies. 2020;**20**(245):1-13. DOI: 10.1186/s12906-020-03039-7

[67] Vermaak I, Enslin GM, Idowu TO, Viljoen AM. *Xysmalobium undulatum* (uzara) – Review of an antidiarrhoeal traditional medicine. Journal of Ethnopharmacology. 2014;**156**:135-146. DOI: 10.1016/j.jep.2014.08.016

[68] Kanama S, Viljoen A, Enslin G, Kamatou G. ChenW, Sandasi M, Idowu T. Uzara – A quality control perspective of *Xysmalobium undulatum*. Pharmaceutical Biology. 2016;**54**(7):1272-1279. DOI: 10.3109/13880209.2015.1073335

[69] Gouws C, Smit T, Willers C, Svitina H, Calitz C, Wrzesinski K. Anticancer potential of *Sutherlandia frutescens* and *Xysmalobium undulatum* in LS180 colorectal cancer mini-tumors. Molecules. 2021;**26**:6051-6069. DOI: 10.3390/molecules26030605

[70] van Wyk BE. A broad review of commercially important Southern African medicinal plants. Journal of Ethnopharmacology. 2008;**119**:342-355. DOI: 10.1016/j.jep.2008.05.02 95

[71] Zhang S, Kou X, Zhao H, Mak K, Balijepalli MK, Pichika MR. *Zingiber officinale* var. *rubrum*: Red Ginger's Medicinal Uses. Molecules. 2022;**27**(775):1-31. DOI: 10.3390/molecules27030775

[72] Soleymani S, Pharm D, Naghizadeh A, Karimi M, Zarei A, Mardi R, et al. COVID-19: General strategies for herbal therapies. Journal of Evidence-Based Integrative Medicine. 2022;**27**:1-18. DOI: 10.1177/2515690X2

Chapter 5

Diseases of Medicinal Plants Cultivated in Karnataka and Their Management

P. Swetha and R. Sundararaj

Abstract

A broad spectrum of fungal diseases infecting selected 10 medicinal plants surveyed in Karnataka, India, was studied in the present research. We present a detailed review on previously reported as well as our present investigation's details of fungal diseases, etiology, symptoms, and its management. Some of the commonly observed diseases are Anthracnose disease, Blight disease, Leaf spot, Root rot, Powdery mildew, Downy mildew, and Wilt disease. The detailed analysis of medicinal plants revealed that the medicinal plants are susceptible to diverse fungal phytopathogens. Therefore, sustainable management of the diseases is necessary for the successful cultivation of disease-free medicinal plants.

Keywords: diseases, medicinal plants, Karnataka

1. Introduction

India is a cradle for diverse medicinal plants and has an immense repository of traditional medicinal knowledge. There are valuable resources that aid in treating various illnesses. About 90% of the medicinal herbs in India are accessible only from the forest, and hence, there is an imminent need for the commercial cultivation of medicinal plants. Karnataka one of the Indian states is known for the major biodiversity hotspots of India, *viz.*, the Western Ghats, which boasts a huge diversity of medicinal plants in the country. Plant diseases create challenging problems in commercial plantations and pose economical threats. Medicinal plants are not an exception and are vulnerable to the attack and invasion of several pathogens resulting in huge crop loss as well as degradation of their medicinal properties. Toxins produced by these pathogens are also of a great concern in case of medicinal plants. Therefore, the prevention of the diseases of medicinal plants should be the utmost priority. In this context, diseases of the 10 important medicinal plants cultivated in Karnataka *viz.*, Sweet flag (*Acorus calamus* L.), Adosa (*Adhatoda vasica* (L.) Nees), Safed musli (*Chlorophytum borivilianum* Sant. & Fern.), Gurmar (*Gymnema sylvestre* (Retz.) Schult.), Hibiscus (*Hibiscus rosa-sinensis* L.), Noni (*Morinda citrifolia* L.), Velvet bean

(*Mucuna pruriens* (L.) DC.), Tulsi (*Ocimum sanctum* Linn.), Long pepper (*Piper longum* Linn.), and Crepe jasmine (*Tabernaemontana divaricata* & *Tabernaemontana coronaria* (L.) R. Br. ex Roem. & Schult.), and their management measures are reviewed and presented.

1.1 Sweet flag (*A. calamus* L.)

Rust caused by *Uromyces acori* [1]; leaf spot disease by unidentified pathogen [2] and bacterial leaf blight caused by *Xanthomonas campestris* P.V.O. *Oryzae* [3] have been reported on *A. calamus*. In this plant, rust disease caused by *U. acori* was prevalent in Tumkur district during the winter months, with the highest disease index of 69.4% in December, and the extent of infection ranged from 3 to 4% (**Figure 1**).

1.2 Adosa (*A. vasica* (L.) Nees)

There are relatively few reports of disease on *A. vasica;* these include leaf spot caused by *Rhizoctonia solani* [4, 5]; Alternaria blight [6] and rust by *Puccinia thwaitesii* [7]; leaf spot by *Alternaria alternata*, anthracnose disease by *Colletotrichum capsici,* leaf rust by *Aecidium adhatodae* [8]; leaf necrotic spots by *Colletotrichum gloeosporioides* [4, 9]; and wilt by *Fusarium oxysporum* Schlect [10]. Wilt disease by *F. oxysporum* occurs during high humidity conditions and the highest disease index and death of 7% of the plants were observed during the month of September and the extent of infection ranged from 3 to 7% in Bangalore (**Figure 2**).

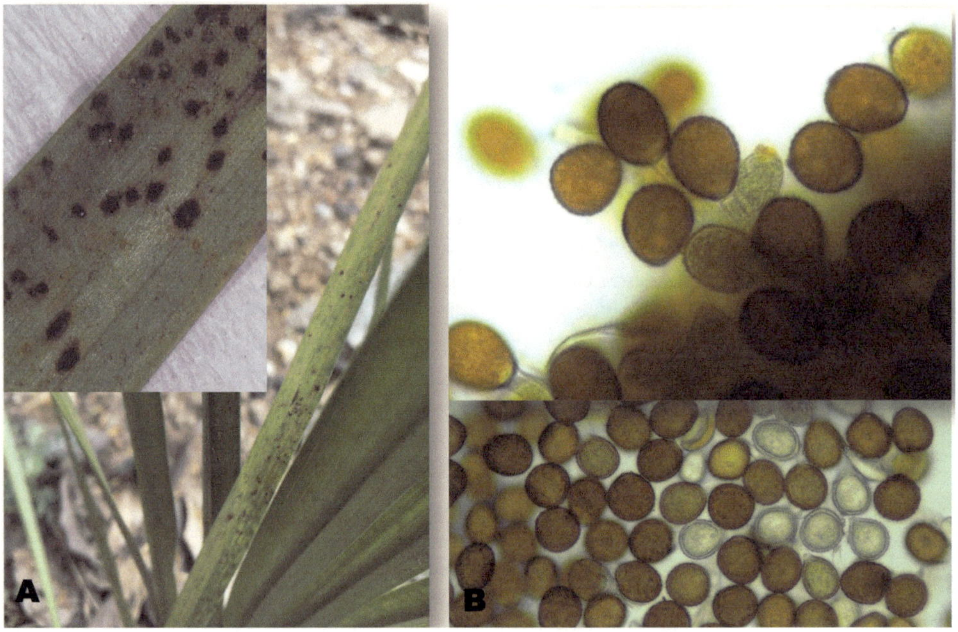

Figure 1.
Rust symptoms in Acorus calamus *(A) caused by* Uromyces acori *(B).*

DOI: http://dx.doi.org/10.5772/intechopen.104632

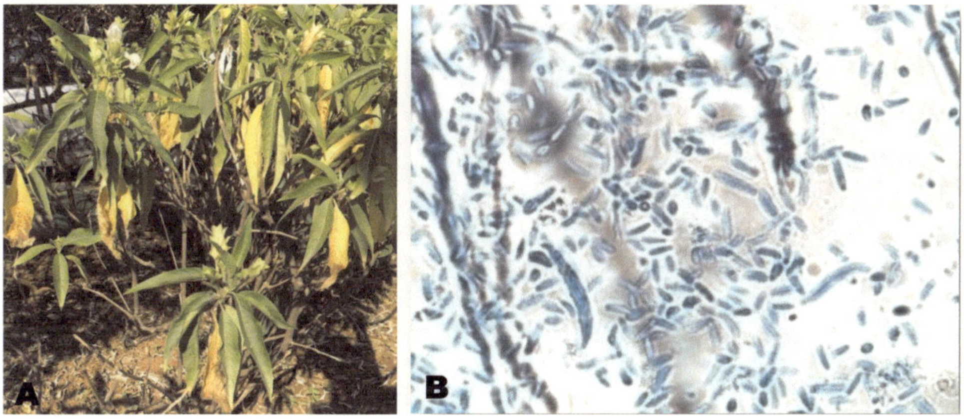

Figure 2.
Wilt symptoms in Adhatoda vasica *(A) caused by* Fusarium oxysporum *(B).*

1.3 Safed musli (*Chlorophytum borivilianum*)

Leaf blight disease caused by *A. alternata* [11] and *Colletotrichum chlorophytumi* [12]; red spot disease by unidentified pathogen [11]; root rot disease by a *Rhizoctonia solani*, *Aspergillus flavus*, *Fusarium oxysporum* complex [13] and *Haemofonectira haematococca* [14]; and anthracnose disease by *Colletotrichum chlorophyti* [15] are the major diseases reported so far in *C. borivilianum*. Leaf spot disease in this plant by the pathogen *A. alternata* was observed in Bangalore during March (**Figure 3**).

1.4 Gurmar (*G. sylvestre* (Retz.) Schult.)

Powdery mildew and leaf spot caused by *Colletotrichum* sp. [16] and *Pseudomonas syringae* [17] are the major diseases so far reported in *G. sylvestre*. Leaf

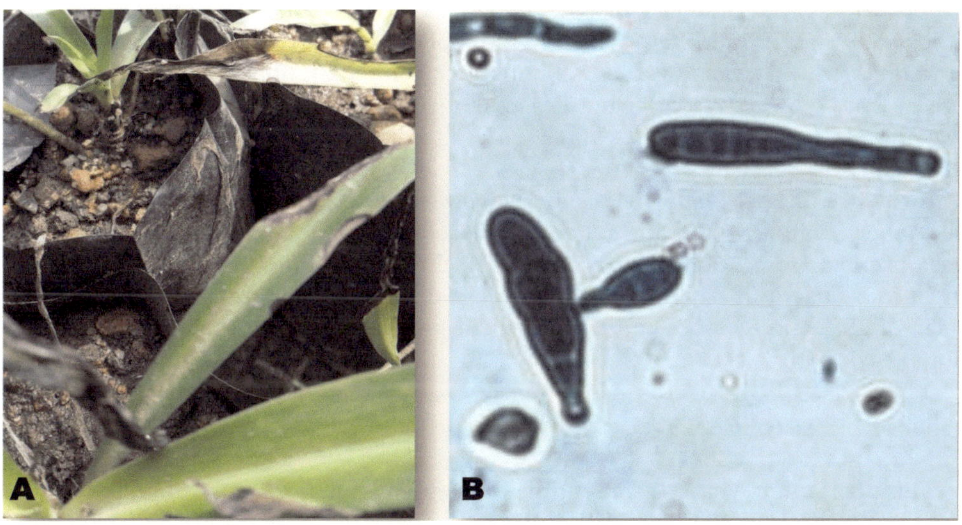

Figure 3.
Leaf blight symptoms in Chlorophytum borivilianum *(A) caused by* Alternaria alternata *(B).*

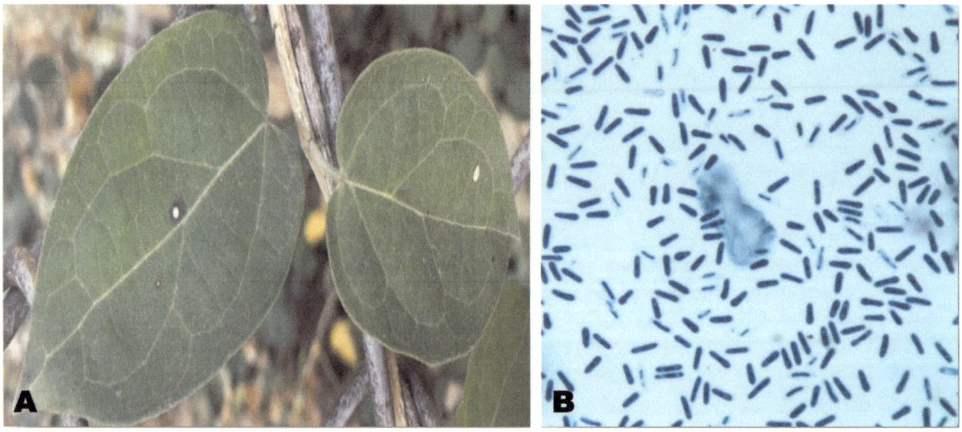

Figure 4.
Leaf spot symptoms in Gymnema sylvestre *(A) caused by* Colletotrichum gleosporoides *(B).*

spot symptoms due to the pathogen *C. gloeosporioides* occur during January in Bangalore (**Figure 4**).

1.5 *Hibiscus* (*H. rosa-sinensis* L.)

A number of fungal diseases commonly infect hibiscus plants; in addition, physiological disorders also occur [18]. Leaf spots caused by several species of fungi cause brown or black circular or irregular shaped spots on the leaves [18]. Sooty mold is a black fungus on the upper surfaces of leaves, growing in the secretion of aphids, mealybugs, many scales, and immature whiteflies. The mold spoils the appearance of foliage but is not particularly injurious to the plant [18]. Root rots and collar rots, one of several species of fungi causing soft rotting of roots and sometimes also stems. Infected plants often wilt as though they are short of water [18]. Anthracnose by *Colletotrichum gloeosporioides* (*Glomerella cingulata*) [19]; powdery mildew by *Podosphaera* sp. [20]; dieback disease by *Botrytis* sp. and *Erwinia* sp.; wilt disease by *Fusarium oxysporum* and *Verticillium*; Choanephora blight caused by *Choanephora infundibulifera* [21]; botrytis blight by *Botrytis cinerea* [22]; hibiscus witches broom disease caused by *Candidatus* Phytoplasma brasiliense [23]; Phytophthora disease by *Plagithmysus nicotianae* var. *nicotianae* [24] and rust by *Kuehneola malvicola* were also reported [25].

Incidence of Leaf blight disease by *Nigrospora sphaerica* was observed in December (**Figure 5**) and anthracnose disease by the pathogen *C. gloeosporioides* was observed from August that gradually declined in the month of December on *H. rosa-sinensis* in Bangalore. Anthracnose disease exhibited the highest disease index of 29.4% in October and the extent of infection ranged from 2 to 4% (**Figure 6**).

1.6 Noni (*M. citrifolia* L.)

This plant is known to be susceptible for some fungal diseases. Anthracnose caused by *C. gloeosporioides*, by which small brown-shaped spots of varying size (0.5–2.5 cm) appear on the leaves that gradually enlarge and coalesce. The center of the coalesced lesion turns grayish white leaving a shot hole symptom. Under humid conditions,

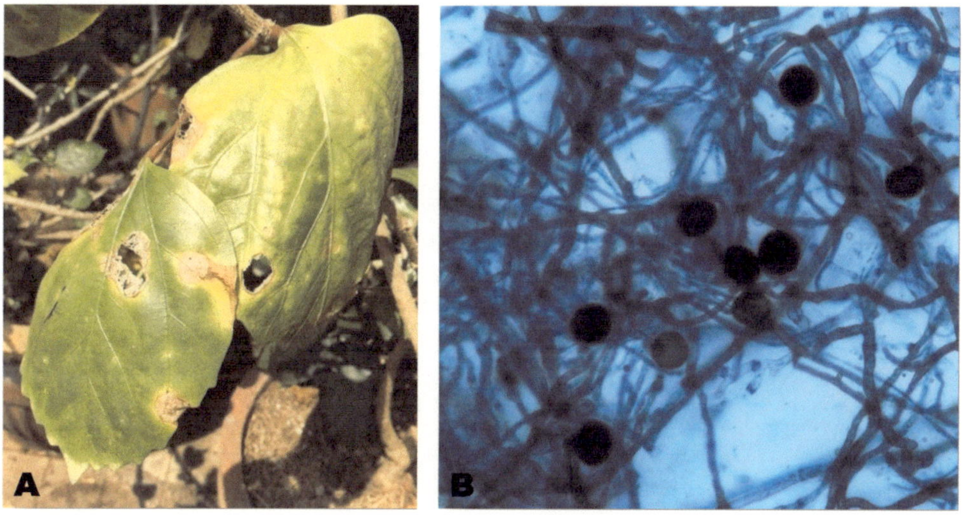

Figure 5.
Leaf blight symptoms in Hibiscus rosa-sinensis *(A) caused by* Nigrospora sphaerica *(B).*

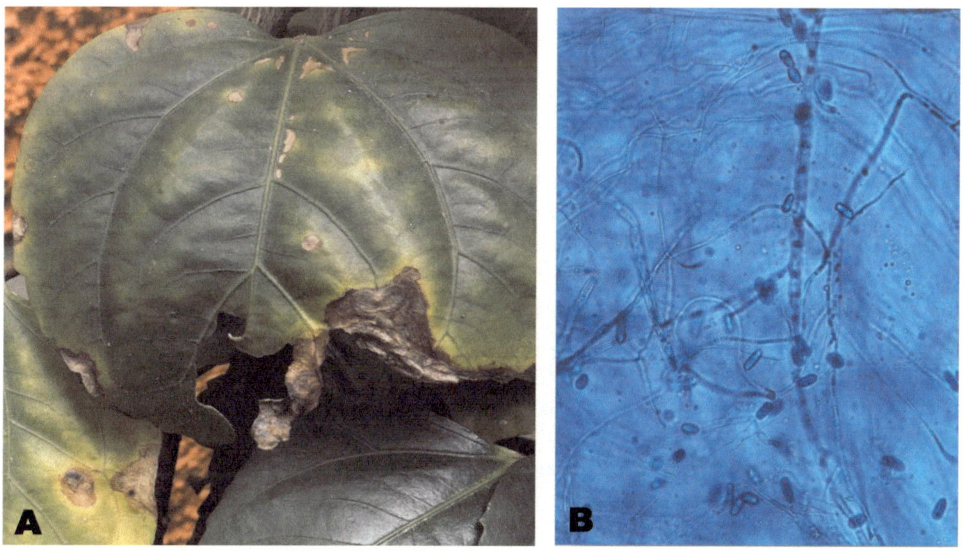

Figure 6.
Anthracnose symptoms in Hibiscus rosa-sinensis (A) caused by Colletotrichum gleosporoides (B).

acervuli with pink masses of spores emerged on the lesions [26, 27]. *C. gloeosporioides* infect all parts of the plant like twigs, flowers, and fruits irrespective of stages of the crop growth. Symptoms of the infection on the flowers appear as dull brown lesions, and the infected flowers dry off within 48 h after infection. The twigs infected by *C. gloeosporioides* are characterized by the presence of necrotic brown lesions with yellow halo. The necrotic lesions spread gradually toward fruits through peduncle that leads to the development of infection on flowers and fruits. Later, the infected fruits shrink, dry off, and get mummified. After mummification, the infected fruits are

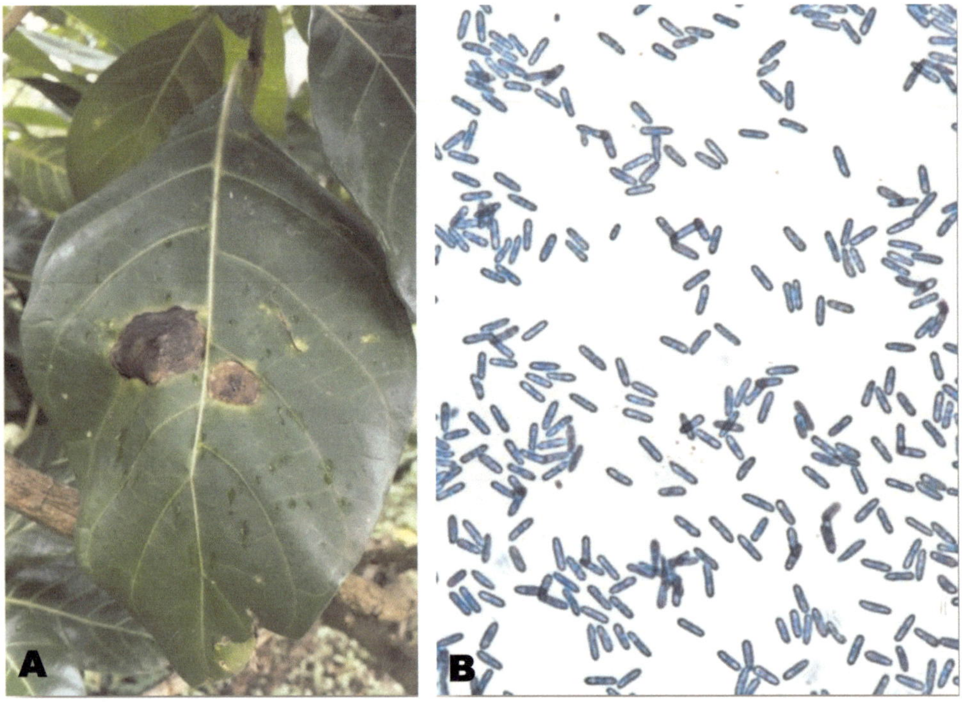

Figure 7.
Anthracnose symptoms in Morinda citrifolia *(A) caused by* Colletotrichum gleosporoides *(B).*

colonized by saprophytic molds like *Aspergillus* and *Penicillium* [26]. Tamil Nadu and Karnataka states in southern India witnessed a severe outbreak of leaf blight, during 2008–2009 by the infection of *A. alternata* [27]. The same pathogen was reported to cause dry fruit rot, which is characterized by the presence of black necrotic sunken spot of 2 to 3 mm diameter on the green unripe fruits [28]. *Pantoea agglomerans* causes soft rot of fruits with the typical symptoms of soft rot of fruits with brown water-soaked lesions on the surface of matured but unripe fruits. The lesion spread quickly within one or two days to the entire fruit, and the infected fruits emit a bad odor. The affected tissue becomes softened and rots subsequently [26]. It is also infected by a wide range of other fungal pathogens such as *Phytopthora* sp. and *Sclerotium rolfisii* (black flag and stem, leaf and fruit blights), *Guignardia morindae* (leaf spot), *Phellinus noxius* (brown root rot), *A. alternata* (dry fruit rot) and *Phytophthora morindae* [29]; *P. agglomerans* (wet fruit rot); and *Collectrotrichum* sp. (anthraconose) [28]. The pathogenic alga, *Cephaleuros minimus* has been reported to cause leaf spot and occurrence of mold infection by *Rhizopus* sp. in the post-harvested fruits [28]. Fusarium wilt disease by *Fusarium oxysporum* [30] and phytoplasma disease caused by phytoplasmas (mycoplasma like organisms or MLOs) [31] were also reported. Among these diseases, anthracnose disease by *C. gloeosporioides* was observed in *M. citrifolia* at Bangalore throughout the year with the highest disease index of 13.79% in December and the extent of infection ranged from 10 to 15% (**Figure 7**). Wilt disease on *M. citrifolia* by *F. oxysporum* is prevalent in Bangalore during high humidity conditions and the highest disease index and death of 10% of the plants during September and the extent of infection ranged from 8 to 10% (**Figure 8**).

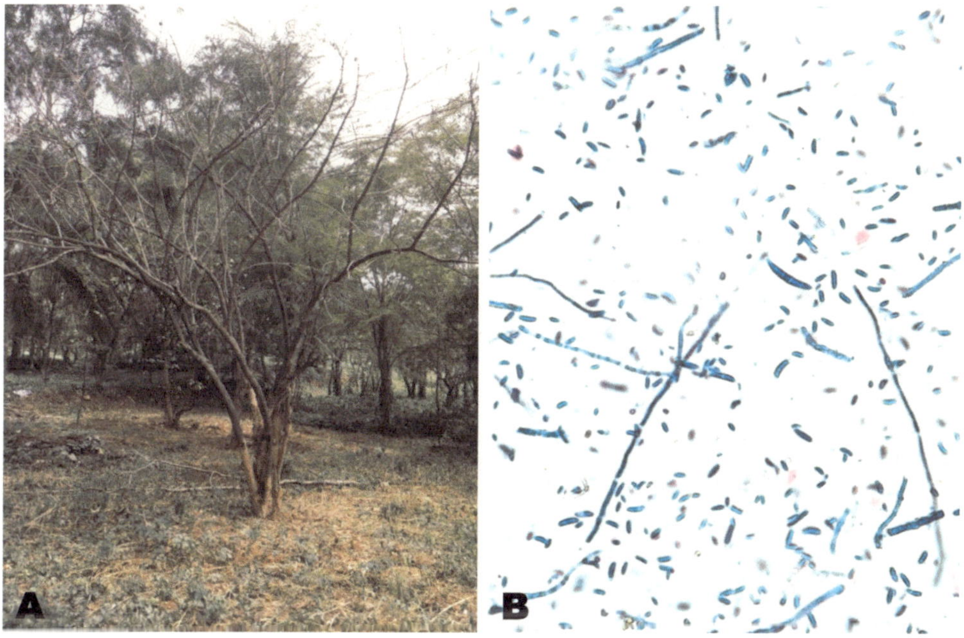

Figure 8.
Wilt symptoms in Morinda citrifolia *(A) caused by* Fusarium oxysporum *(B).*

1.7 Velvet bean (*M. pruriens* (L.) DC.)

Necrotic crowns and numerous necrotic lesions along the roots and runners of *M. pruriens* caused by *Macrophomina phaseolina* are considered as a serious threat in Nigeria [32]. Foliar fungal diseases (*Cercospora* leaf spot and angular leaf spot, *Phaeoisariopsis griseola*) were also reported in the USA as substantially reducing the biomass of *Mucuna* [33]. Charcoal rot caused by *Modiolula phaseolina* was reported by [34]. Incidence of Leaf blight disease caused by *C. gloeosporioides* occurs in Bangalore in September while in December in Gadag (**Figure 9**). Also, incidence of Rust disease caused by *Uromyces mucunae* was observed in the month of January in Gadag district (**Figure 10**).

1.8 Tulsi (*O. sanctum* L.)

There are several diseases that could cause leaf damage leading to yield loss, such as Fusarium wilt (*Fusarium oxysporum f.* sp. *basilicum*) [35]. Other destructive diseases include bacterial leaf spot (*Pseudomonas cichorii*), gray mold (*Botrytis cinerea*), fungal leaf spot by *Alternaria* sp., *Cercospora ocimicola* and *C. gloeosporioides* and damping off or root rot (*Rhizoctonia solani; Pythium* sp.), root rot by *Rhizoctonia solani* and *Pythium* sp. [36]; leaf blight by a species of *Alternaria* [37]; *Gray mold caused* by *Botrytis cinerea* [38]; and powdery mildew caused by *Erysiphe biocellata* [39]. Downy mildew (*Peronospora belbahrii*) is also very destructive and widespread disease in this plant [35].

Wilt disease of Tulsi by *F. oxysporum* is severe during December causing complete mortality in January in Bangalore, and the extent of infection of this disease ranged

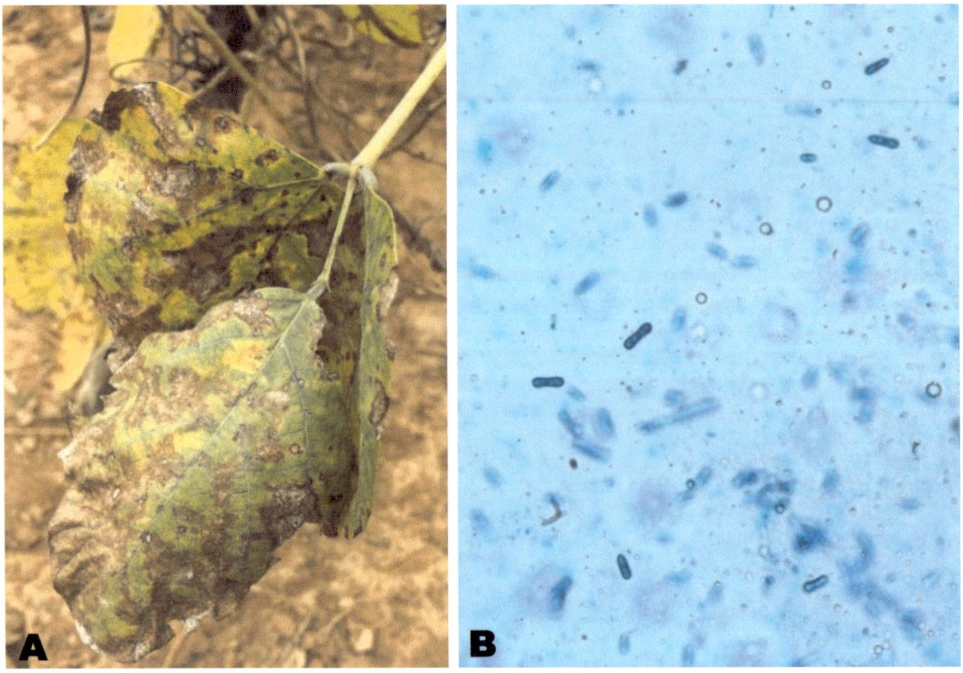

Figure 9.
Leaf blight symptoms in Mucuna pruriens *(A) caused by* Colletotrichum gleosporoides *(B).*

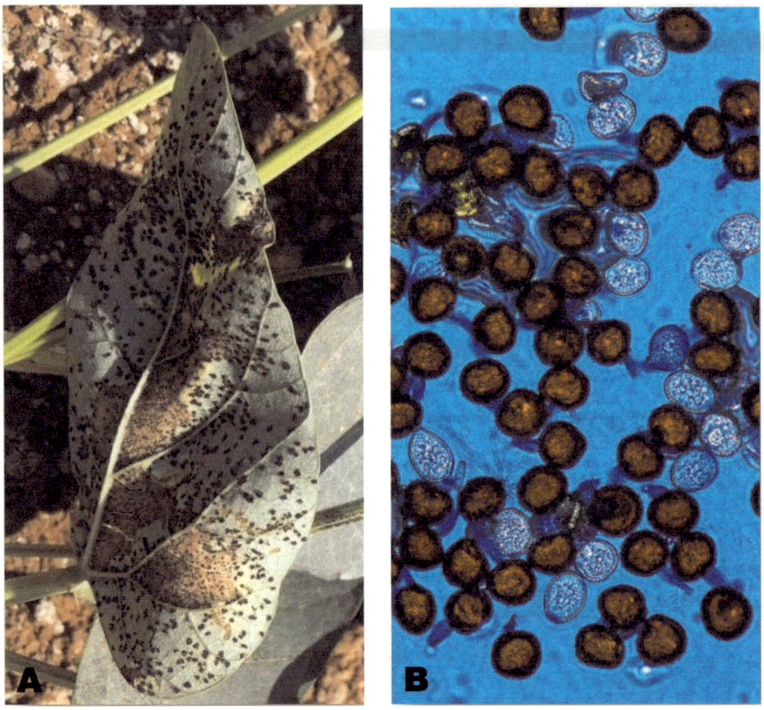

Figure 10.
Rust symptoms in Mucuna pruriens *(A) caused by* Uromyces mucunae *(B).*

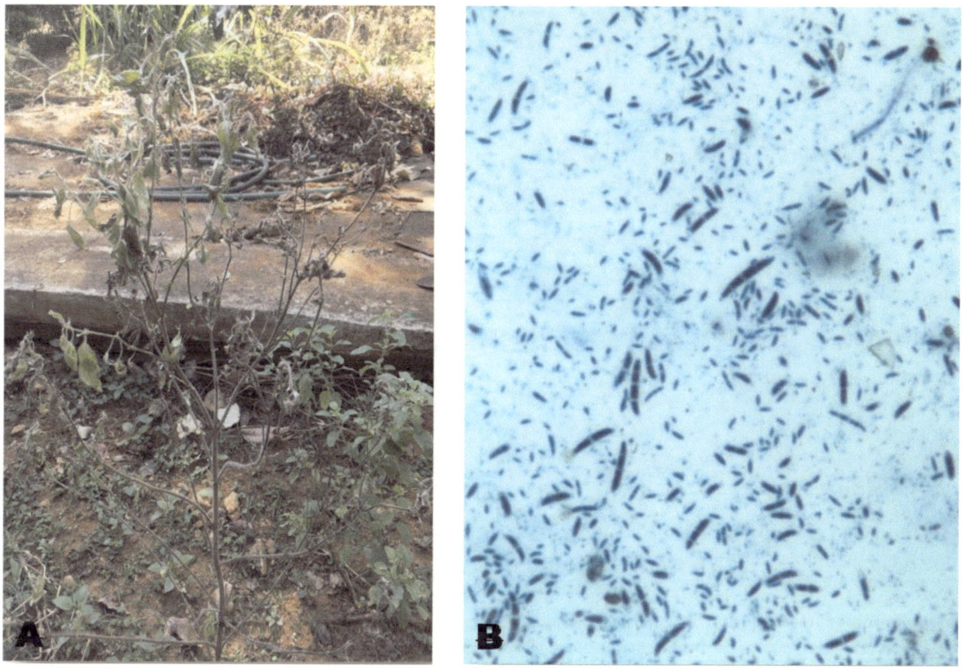

Figure 11.
Wilt symptoms in Ocimum sanctum *(A) caused by* Fusarium oxysporum *(B).*

from 80 to 100% with the death of most of the plants (**Figure 11**). Incidence of powdery mildew by *Erysiphe biocellata* occurs in January causing complete mortality in March, and the extent of infection of this disease ranged from 70 to 100% with the death of 100% of the plants (**Figure 12**). Fungal leaf spot disease by *C. gloeosporioides* is noticed in August (**Figure 13**).

1.9 Long pepper (*P. longum* L.)

Known to be affected by the number of fungal diseases like showing symptoms of rotting of leaves and vines and by *C. gloeosporioides* [40], necrotic spots and blights on leaves by *Collectotrichum* sp. and *Cercospora* sp. [41]; leaf spot by *Botryodiplodia theobromae*, leaf rot by *Fusarium pallidoroseum* [42] and *Rhizocotonia solani* [40]; Cercospora leaf spot by *C. piperata* [43, 44] and Phytophthora rot by *Phytophthora capsici,* basal wilt by *Sclerotium rolfisii*, Phytophthora Foot rot by *Phytophthora capsici*, and phyllody disease by phytoplasma [40]. In Bangalore, the onset of the anthracnose disease caused by *Colletotrichum boninense* was observed in June with the highest disease index of about 17.5% in September. It gradually decreased during the subsequent months and was found vanish during April and May and the extent of infection of this disease ranged from 29 to 35% (**Figure 14**).

1.10 Crepe jasmine (*T. divaricata/coronaria* (L.)

Leaf brown or black spots caused by *Phytophthora citrophthora* in which brown or black spots and patches may be either ragged or circular, with a water-soaked or

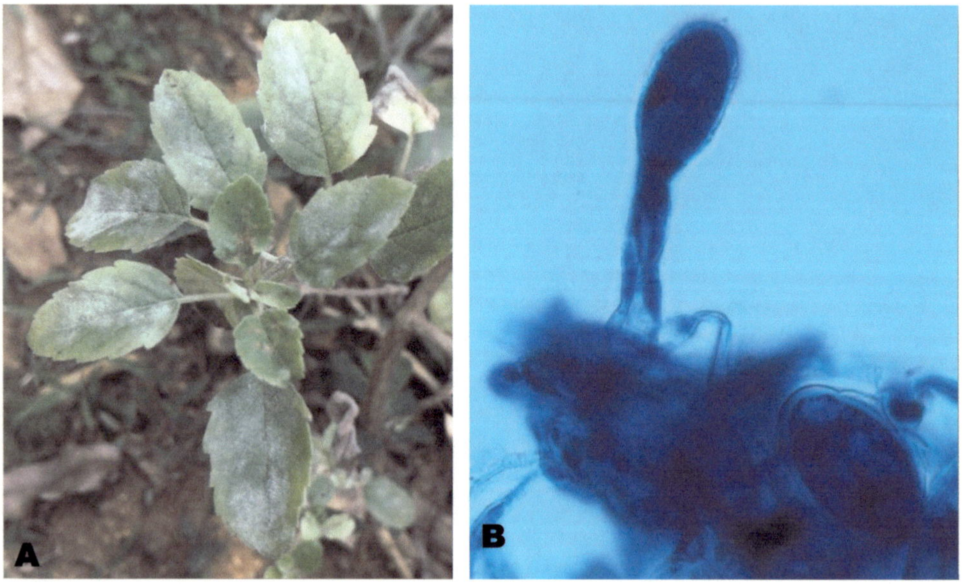

Figure 12.
Powdery mildew symptoms in Ocimum sanctum *(A) caused by* Erysiphe biocellata *(B).*

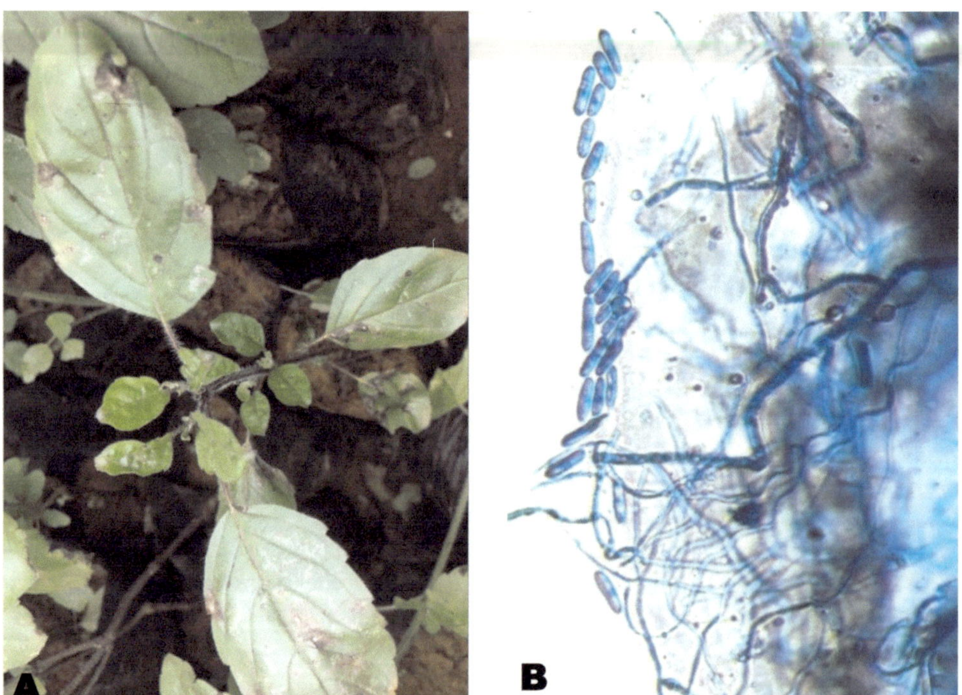

Figure 13.
Leaf spot symptoms in Ocimum sanctum *(A) caused by* Colletotrichum gleosporoides *(B).*

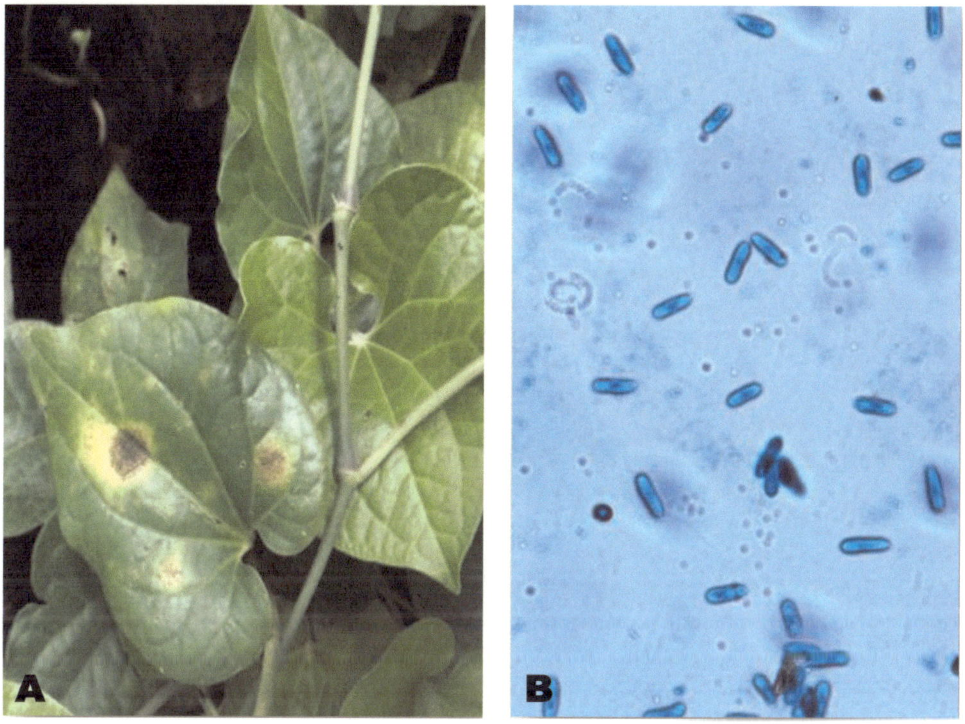

Figure 14.
Leaf spot symptoms in Piper longum *(A) caused by* Colletotrichum boninense *(B).*

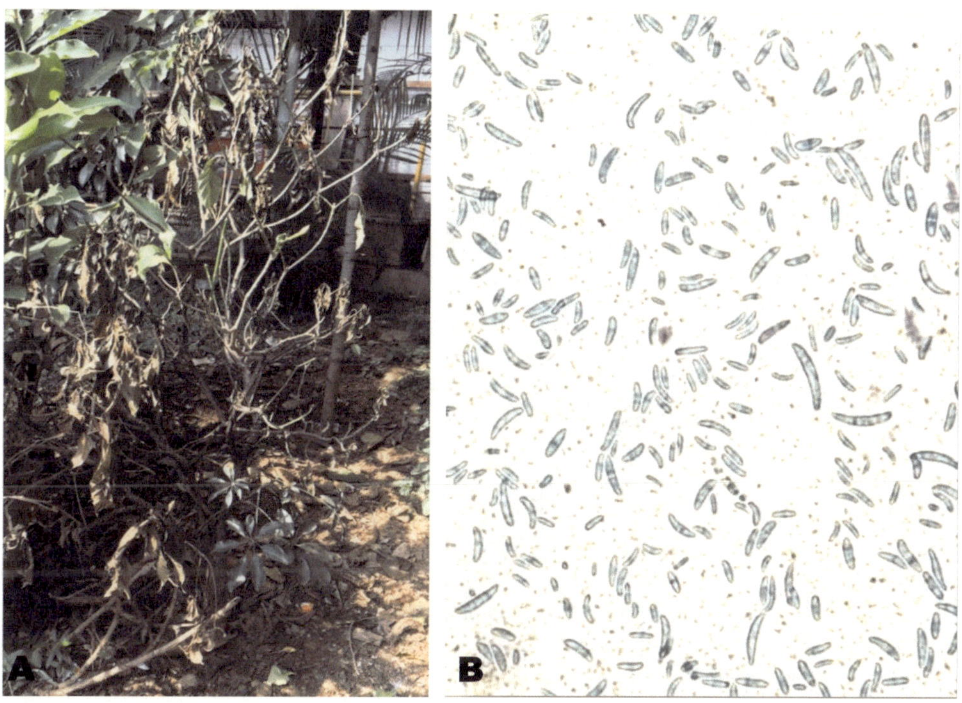

Figure 15.
Wilt symptoms in Tabernaemontana divaricata (A) caused by Fusarium oxysporum (B).

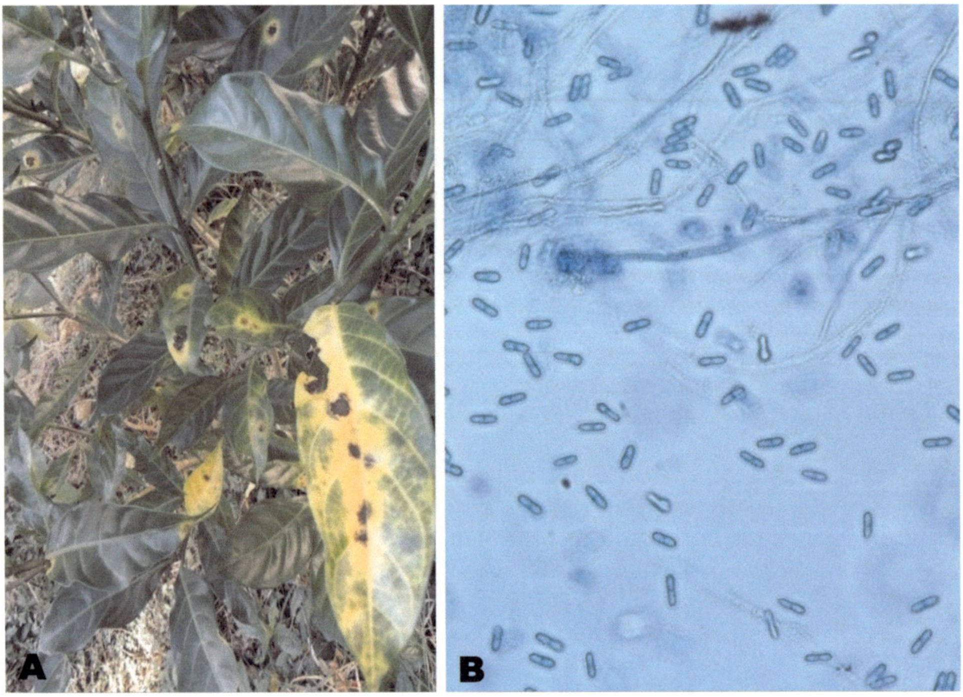

Figure 16.
Leaf spot symptoms in Tabernaemontana coronaria (A) caused by Colletotrichum boninense (B).

yellow-edged appearance. Insects, rain, dirty garden tools, or even people can help its spread of this disease [44]. *T. divaricata* is also affected by wilt disease by *Fusarium oxysporum* [45] and rust disease by *Uredo manilensis* [46]. It was found to be affected by *Fusarium oxysporum* with wilting symptoms from September to November, causing death of plants in November and the extent of infection of this disease ranged from 10 to 20% (**Figure 15**). *T. coronaria* with leaf spot disease caused by *Colletotrichum gloeosporioides* was observed from November to January with the highest disease index of 9.7% in the month of January and the extent of infection of this disease ranged from 40 to 50% (**Figure 16**).

2. Management of diseases

On the basis of the experiments conducted and the results obtained in our studies and the reports of earlier researchers the following management measures are recommended for the economically important diseases of medicinal plants in Karnataka.

#Disease recorded in Karnataka for the first time.

*Disease recorded for the first time on the host plant.

Diseases of *A. calamus*.

Disease and its pathogen	Symptoms	Management practices
Rust disease [1] *Uromyces acori*	• Infected leaves shows reddish brown pustules on both surface of leaves with ruptured epidermis. • Severe infection consisting of yellow brown-coalesced pustules at the center, circular rings of brown pustules at the periphery and brown to black-coalesced raised spots at the center was observed. • Formation of yellow and brown pustules in a scattered pattern in advanced stages. • On stems, affected tissues showed necrosis and death of plants [1].	**Cultural method** [46] • Removal of weeds from bunds and channels. • Avoid application of excess nitrogen. • Apply N in three doses (50% during basal, 25% during the tillering phase and 25% N in panicle initiation stage). **Chemical Method** [46] • Application of Carbendazim 50WP @ 500 g/ha (or) Tricyclozole 75 WP @ 500 g/ha (or) Metominostrobin 20 SC @ 500 ml/ha (or) Azoxystrobin 25 SC @ 500 ml/ha. **Biological control** [46] • Dipping seedling root, soil application, and foliar spray with with TNAU Pf 1liquid formulation (500 ml for one-hectare seedlings) are recommended [47, 48].
Leaf spot disease [2] Unidentified	• Occurrence of discolored spots on the leaves of the plant [2].	• Application of Captan @10 g and Chlorpyrifos @20 ml/10 L will help in the mitigation of the disease [2].
Bacterial leaf blight disease [3] *Xanthomonas campestris* P.V. O. *Oryzae*	• Bacterial leaf blight produces tannish-gray to white lesions along the veins and characteristic symptoms of yellow lesions with wavy margins on leaf blades that may extend to the sheath. • Symptoms are observed at the tillering stage, disease incidence increases with plant growth, peaking at the flowering stage. • Leaves of the entire plant turn pale yellow and wilt during resulting in a partial or total crop failure. • Occurrence of bacterial ooze from infected leaves has been observed in warm and humid climates, which contributes to the spread of this disease [3].	• Application of Bordeaux mixture with or without sugar, copper-soap mixture, copper-mercury fungicides, copper oxychloride and streptomycin solution. Spraying synthetic organic bactericides such as nickel dimethyl dithiocarbamate, dithianone, phenazine and N oxide techlofthalam [3]. • Chlorinating irrigation water with stable bleaching powder.

Diseases of *A. vasica.*

Disease and its pathogen	Symptoms	Management practices
Wilt Disease#* *Fusarium oxysporum* Schlect. emend. [10]	• The leaves slowly wilt and die; they usually do not turn yellow, the leaves tend to stay green they begin to darken and turn brown, or blackish color and chlorosis occur and the plant dies [10].	• Use Safer Yard & Garden Insect Killer to control many garden insects. • Avoid application of excess nitrogen fertilizers that may increase susceptibility to the disease. • Deweeding using a weed flamer or natural herbicide.

Disease and its pathogen	Symptoms	Management practices
		• Application of Mycostop (1–2 g/ 100 sq. ft.), biological fungicide that with sufficient watering protect crops against wilt caused by *Fusarium*. • If the disease persists, removal of the entire plant and solarization of the soil before planting again is essential [49].
Leaf spot disease [4, 5] *Rhizoctonia solani* & *Colletotrichum gloeosporioides*	• Initially, symptoms appear as minute, round, light brown spots but later the spots grow and acquire a round to irregular shape with coalescence of some spots. • Fully developed spots are water-soaked dark brown to blackish, scattered all over the leaf lamina with margins of the spots diffusing and at the center. • Severe infection resulted in defoliation [5]. • Concentric grey-brown spots appear on the leaves and join together to create large necrosed patch. Fruiting fungal bodies are observed in the middle of the spots [50].	• Spraying with Benomyl 0.1% (or) Mancozeb 0.2% (or) Carbendazim 0.1% is recommended [51].
Leaf spot disease [8] *Alternaria alternata*	• Initially, symptoms appear as minute, round, light brown spots but later the spots grow and acquire a round to irregular shape with coalescence of some spots. • Fully developed spots are water-soaked dark brown to blackish, scattered all over the leaf lamina with margins of the spots diffusing and at the center. • Severe infection resulted in defoliation [5]. • Concentric grey-brown spots appear on the leaves and join together to create large necrosed patch. Fruiting fungal bodies are observed in the middle of the spots [50].	• Spraying with Benomyl 0.1% (or) Mancozeb 0.2% (or) Carbendazim 0.1% is recommended [52].
Anthracnose disease [8] *Colletotrichum capsici*	• Large expanding leaf spots with dark to tan centers and diffuse, irregular margins. • Expansion of individual lesions results in their "target spot" appearance; that is, concentric rings become visible in the lesions as the lesions grow each day. • Lesions may coalesce to form large, blighted areas on leaves, often at	• Sanitation by removal of severely diseased leaves of the plant and destruction of fallen infected leaves is recommended. • Management of moisture and humidity by ensuring good drainage, deweeding, adequate plant spacing, pruning, minimize leaf wetness, and overhead irrigation.

Disease and its pathogen	Symptoms	Management practices
	leaf margins. Infected leaves may abscise (drop) prematurely. • Symptoms are often most severe within dense noni canopies and/or on the lower leaves. • Fruits and stems are not susceptible to infection [53].	• Avoid mechanical spread of the pathogen on hands and tools during harvesting operations [53]. • Spraying of *P. fluorescens, Bacillus subtilis* were found to be effective [54]. • Most studies have evaluated the leaf extracts of various plants to control *C. capsici*. Leaf extracts of neem, Datura, *Ocimum*, Polyalthia, *Vinca rosea* were found fungitoxic against *C. capsici* [55]. • Yeasts strains isolated from rhizosphere were found to be antagonistic to *C. capsici* by inhibiting the mycelia growth of *C. capsici* to the extent of 40.6 to 43.1%, which intern found to control the anthracnose to the tune of 60% [56]. • There are several species of *Trichoderma*, of which the major ones are *Trichoderma asperellum*, *T. viridae*, *T. harzianum*, and *T. longibrachiatum*. Isolates of T. longibrachiatum found to inhibit the mycelia growth of Colletotrichum capsici up to 66% due to the volatile compounds released by *Trichoderma* [57]. • Use disease-free seeds. • Seed treatment with thiram 2 kg/ha or zineb 2.5 kg/ha. • Spraying of captan 0.2% with sufficient interval. • Essential oil of *Nigella sativa* is shown to have antimicrobial activity [51].
***Alternaria* blight** [6] *A. alternata*	• The *Alternaria* leaf blight infects all aerial parts of plant. • Initially, the disease appears in the form of small, scattered brown spots on the leaf lamina, which later increases in size and coalesces covering the entire area with dark brown margin and yellow halo. • Linear necrotic lesions appear on stem, petioles, and sepals. In severe cases, the head and seeds also get infected [58].	• The fungicide Indofil M-45, Ridomil at 0.5% and bio agents like *Trichoderma harzianum, T. viride, T. pseudokoningii, T. koningii, Aspergillus niger*, and *A. flavus* reduced the growth of *A. alternata* [59].
Leaf rust [7] *Puccinia thwaitesii*	• The disease starts as circular brown or reddish brown, granular. • Sori or a group of sori were observed in chlorotic areas, which soon die.	• *Trichoderma harzianum* was found to be effective against rust pathogen *Puccinia thwaitesii* [60].

Disease and its pathogen	Symptoms	Management practices
	• As the disease advances, the red pustules become black spots circular and small and later coalesce to form large patches [7].	
Leaf rust [8] *Aecidium adhatodae*	• The postules are circular or elliptical, smaller than those of stem rust, and they do not coalesce and contain masses of orange-brown Urediospores. • Infection sites primarily are found on the upper surfaces of leaves and leaf sheaths and occasionally on the neck. • They survive on stubbles and volunteer crops [61].	• Mixed cropping with suitable crops is recommended. • Avoid application of excess dose of nitrogenous fertilizers. • Spraying of Zineb at 2.5 kg/ha or Propioconazole @ 0.1% is recommended [61].

Diseases of *Chlorophytum borivilianum.*

Disease and its pathogen	Symptoms	Management practices
Leaf blight [11] *Alternaria alternata*	• Initially, reddish-brown lesions on the leaves, forming longitudinal streaks along the midrib, veins and margin of the infected leaves. Finally, rotting and death of leaves is observed [11].	• Spraying biocontrol agents like *Trichoderma* sp. • Spraying with Benomyl 0.1% (or) Mancozeb 0.2% (or) Carbendazim 0.1% IS recommended [52].
Colletotrichum chlorophytumi [12]	• Yellowing of leaves leading to withering and ultimately death of the whole leaf [12].	• Application of Bavistin solution @1 g in 1 liter of water at the interval of 25 days twice [12].
Red spot [11] Unidentified	• Occurrence of red, orange, and yellow leaf spots on plants [11].	• Application of Bavistin solution @1 g in 1 liter of water at the interval of 25 days twice [11].
Root rot disease [13] *Rhizoctonia solani, Aspergillus flavus,Fusarium oxysporum* [13]	• Initially gradual drying of leaves of affected plants. • The basal portion of the root appears watery and soft and root system is very much reduced and its tissues are also affected. In advanced stages, the infection spreads to roots, and the roots decompose and turn into a decaying mass of tissues resulting in poor and stunted development of roots [62].	• Fungicides, neem-based formulations, organic cakes and a biocontrol agent *Trichoderma viride.* • Application of mancozeb 63% + carbendazim 12% (SAAF-75WP), carbendazim 50WP, propiconazole 25EC, 0.1% tebuconazol (250EC), and hexaconazole 5EC are highly effective. • Root dipping for 15 min. in a mixture of 0.3% thiram (80WP) + 0.15% carbendazim (50 WP). • Application of *Trichoderma viride* at 5 g kg^{-1} soil before planting. • Field application of a mixture of NC + mustard cake (1:1) before planting at the rate of 4 q h^{-1}.

Disease and its pathogen	Symptoms	Management practices
		• Soil drenching 45 days after sowing (DAS), with a mixture of 0.3% thiram +0.15% carbendazim +0.5% *T. viride* + 0.4% NC + 0.4% mustard cake. • Spraying of 0.2% carbendazim (50WP). • Neem-based formulations and six oil cakes extracts, neem oil, neem formulation no 2 at 3% and neem, jatropha cakes extract at 40% were highly inhibitory to *Rhophitulus solani* [13].
Haemofonectira haematococca sp. nov. [14]	• Initially gradual drying of leaves of affected plants. • The basal portion of the root appears watery and soft and root system is very much reduced and its tissues are also affected. In advanced stages, the infection spreads to roots, and the roots decompose and turn into a decaying mass of tissues resulting in poor and stunted development of roots [62].	• Root dipping for 15 min. in a mixture of 0.3% thiram (80WP) + 0.15% carbendazim (50 WP). • Application of *Trichoderma viride* at 5 g kg^{-1} soil before planting and field application of a mixture of NC + mustard cake (1:1) before planting at the rate of 4 q h^{-1}. • Soil drenching 45 days after sowing (DAS), with a mixture of 0.3% thiram +0.15% carbendazim +0.5% *T. viride* + 0.4% NC + 0.4% mustard cake. • Spraying of 0.2% carbendazim (50WP) [14].
Anthracnose [15] *Colletotrichum chlorophyti*	• Initially, small brownish spots on lamina, more prominent on margin or tip, are observed. • Typical symptoms of Anthracnose like sunken lesion that range from dark red to tan black [15].	• Spraying Bordeaux mixture 1% or carbendazim + mancozeb 0.1% is recommended. • Shade regulation and adopting integrated nutrition management practices in the plantation are essential. • Spraying *P. fluorescens* (FP 7) at 3 weeks interval [63].

Diseases of *G. sylvestre*.

Disease and its pathogen	Symptoms	Management measures
Leaf spot # [16] *Colletotrichum gloeosporioides*	• Appearance of minute black or brown points surrounded by a pale green ring visible on both the surfaces of the leaf. • As the spots enlarge, the center turns pale brown and then greyish-white surrounded by a deep brown band. • The fructifications of the fungus appear as tiny black dots in the white center. • The diseased spots are scattered over the leaf and are roundish when young but may become irregular when mature.	• Spraying 3 g of water soluble sulfur in one liter of water at an interval of 10–15 days [16].

Disease and its pathogen	Symptoms	Management measures
	• Leaf tissue withers and large brown patches of dried leaf may result [16].	
Leaf spot [17] *Pseudomonas syringae*	• Initial symptoms were small, angular, water-soaked lesions observable on both adaxial and abaxial surfaces. • Lesions enlarged, became tan to light brown, and were often surrounded by chlorotic haloes [64].	• Extracts of seaweeds (*Sargassum wightii, Turbinaria conoides, Ulva lactuca*) possess an antimicrobial activity against the pathogen [17].
Powdery mildew [16] *Unknown*	• Typical mildew growth is generally confined to the under-surface of the leaf. • Severe infection leads to infection on the upper-surface [16].	• Spraying 3 g of water soluble sulfur in one liter of water at an interval of 10–15 days [65].

Diseases of *H. rosa-sinensis.*

Disease and its pathogen	Symptoms	Management practices
Blight*# *Nigrospora sphaerica*	• Initial symptoms were yellow-to-brown, irregular-shaped lesions on the leaf margin, or tip later lesions expanded along the mid-vein until the entire leaf was destroyed. • Blighted leaves turn grayish to dark brown and wither, and ultimately affected plants died.	• In areas where the disease may cause yield loss, applying captan, captafol, fentin hydroxide, and mancozeb can inhibit conidial germination and carbendazim fungicide and copper base fungicide can effectively control the disease. • Spraying with Mancozeb 1 kg or Iprobenphos 500 ml or Carbendazim 250 g/ha is recommended [66].
Anthracnose # *Colletotrichum gloeosporioides* [*Glomerella cingulata*] [19]	• Appearance of yellowish brown to dark brown irregular spots present with a chlorotic yellow halo on leaves. • Progression of the disease leads the spots to coalesce and the leaves dry up. • The center of the lesions was covered by black acervuli [19].	• Spray Bordeaux mixture 1%, such that the spray solution reaches the lower surface of the leaves. • Spray Bordeaux mixture 1% or carbendazim + mancozeb 0.1% with the onset of pre-monsoon showers on the new foliage and spikes. • Regulate shade in the plantation with the onset of pre-monsoon showers. • Adopt integrated nutrition management practices in the plantation. • Spray *P. fluorescens* (FP 7) at 3-week interval. • Before storage, treat with hot water, (50–55°C) for 15 minutes or dip in Benomyl solution (500 ppm) or Thiobendazole (1000 ppm) for 5 minutes [63].
Bacterial Leaf Spot *Pseudomonas cichorii* [67]	• Lesions range from 2 to 10 mm in diameter and are usually surrounded by a two-color border with necrotic lesion center surrounded by yellowish halo.	• Starting new plants using pathogen-free cuttings and • Application of fertilizer affect severity of many bacterial diseases of ornamental plants.

Disease and its pathogen	Symptoms	Management practices
	• The central necrotic portions of the lesions are tan to whitish and sometimes fall out, creating a "shot-hole" appearance. • Severe spotting may cause premature defoliation. • Other parts of the hibiscus plant (e.g., flowers, petioles, stems) are not susceptible to the disease [67].	• Sanitation and removal of diseased plant organs such as leaves from the vicinity of healthy leaves is recommended. • Routine pruning and destroying branches with heavily diseased leaves. • Minimizing leaf wetness and relative humidity in the plant canopy can manage the disease effectively. • Ensure that soil is completely aerated. • Trim weeds around hibiscus plants to reduce relative humidity ensure plant spacing, intercropping, non-host plants between hibiscus plants to block the spread of bacteria between plants [67].
Powdery Mildew [20] *Podosphaera* sp. [20]	• Initially begins as white spots that turn gray or tan as the fungus grows and covers more of the foliage. • The fungus causes stunted growth and in severe cases, the leaves may wither and fall off the plant [68].	• Watering hibiscus at the base of the plants and not directly on the leaves is recommended. • Avoid high-nitrogen fertilizers and ensure proper spacing. • Trim affected growth immediately and dispose of diseased plant material carefully. • A mixture of neem oil and water is a safe, at a rate of 2 tablespoons neem oil to 1 gallon of water has shown to effectively manage the disease [68].
Dieback Disease *Botrytis* sp., *Erwinia* sp. [69]	• The rot will cause a change of color on the stem and sometimes it appears as a light brown dry rot. • The leaves begin to wilt as water does not progress in rotted stem [69].	• Removal of infected part of the stem from the plant and early spotting of the disease will help in mitigating the disease. • Application of diluted Phyton (Copper biocide) on the wound is recommended [69].
Wilt Disease *Fusarium oxysporum* and *Verticillium* [69]	• Characteristic symptoms of leaves slowly wilting and death of the entire plant are observed. • Initially, leaves will tend to stay the green and later may slowly darken as they wilt to a dark green, brown, or blackish color. • Wilt disease affects the entire plant, not just one tip or branch [69].	• Application of 1 pint of household bleach with 2 quarts of warm water is recommended. • Sanitation and removal of the wilted plant will ensure the prevention of the spread [69].
***Choanephora* Blight** *Choanephora infundibulifera* [21]	• Initial symptoms began as reddish purple spots at the tip of flowers and expanded to encompass entire flowers. • Infected lesions appeared water-soaked, reddish brown, and were followed by rapid rotting of infected tissues [21].	• Good sanitation practices including grooming the plants and removing spent or senescing flowers can minimize the potential for infection. • It is also important to avoid wetting the flowers when watering and crowding plants.

Disease and its pathogen	Symptoms	Management practices
		• Adequate spacing between the plants can promote good air circulation. • Use of potassium bicarbonate, mancozeb, copper hydroxide, and thiophanate-methyl is recommended [70].
***Botrytis* blight** *Botrytis cinerea* [22]	• Lesions initially occur on the tips of stems and rapidly moved downward when environmental conditions are cool and humid. • No lesions are observed on leaves; however, flowers became blighted, turn brown, and abscise prematurely. • Diseased stems occasionally are colonized by *C. gloeosporioides* is reported [22].	• Sanitation and aeration reduce humidity levels around plants and appropriate fungicide applications are recommended for disease control. • Fallen leaves and petals should be carefully removed from production areas. • Regular fungicide applications will reduce losses on especially susceptible hosts grown in humid environments [71].
***Hibiscus* witches' broom disease** *Candidatus Phytoplasma brasiliense* [23]	• Witches' brooms disease affected leaves and shoots display distorted, dwarfed, and discolored symptoms. • This disease results from a multitude of diseases such as powdery mildew or rusts, mistletoe, or from insect and mite feeding [72].	• Providing plants with proper cultural control and pruning will manage the disease [72].
Viral disease Rhabdovirus-like particles and hibiscus ring spot virus [73]	• Chlorosis along with vein yellowing mottling, vein banding and clearing vein enation, rosetting, leaf distortion, flower abortion, distortion, and stunting are the characteristic symptoms [73].	• The best way is the prevention of the disease. • Selection of virus free seed should be done from credible sources. This includes Cuttings, bulls, rhizomes, tubers, and seeds. • Eradication of the diseased plant will eliminate the inoculum from the field. • Insect vectors must be efficiently managed though eradication of weeds that harbor them and *via* sowing of trap crops. • Similarly, soil fumigation and nematicides can be applied against nematode-transmitted viruses to control nematodes [74].
***Phytophthora* disease** *Plagithmysus nicotianae* var. *nicotianae* [24]	• Production of brownish to black lesions [24].	• Chemical control includes the use of metalaxyl or its near-identical twin mefenoxam used in single or multiple applications. • The use of soil fumigants such as chloropicrin may reduce pathogen populations, and fumigant nematicides such as 1,3-dichloropropene reduce nematode populations that enhance black shank incidence and severity [75].

Disease and its pathogen	Symptoms	Management practices
Rust *Kuehneola malvicola* [25]	• Initially, minute orange-brown pustules typical of most rusts develop on the underside of leaves. • Upper leaf surface appear slightly larger yellow-orange spots and do not develop pustules. Premature defoliation may occur [25].	• Appropriate chemicals may be tried on prized plant specimens [76]. • Sanitation measures, including removal of dead fallen foliage and pruning infected flowering branches following bloom, should provide adequate control in many cases [25].

Diseases of *M. citrifolia.*

Disease and its pathogen	Symptoms	Management measures
Noni anthracnose *Colletotrichum gleosporoides* [27]	• Large expanding and diffusing leaf spots with dark to tan centers with irregular margins are observed. • Expansion of individual concentric lesion rings results in the "target spot" appearance. • Lesions coalesce to form large, blighted areas on leaves and leaf margins. Infected leaves may abscise prematurely. • Symptoms are severe within dense noni canopies and/or on the lower leaves; however, fruits and stems are not susceptible to infection [53].	• Sanitation by removal of severely diseased leaves of the plant and destruction of fallen infected leaves is recommended. • Management of moisture and humidity by ensuring good drainage, deweeding, adequate plant spacing, pruning, minimize leaf wetness, and overhead irrigation. • Avoid mechanical spread of the pathogen on hands and tools during harvesting operations [53]. • Spraying of *P. fluorescens, Bacillus subtilis* was found to be effective [54]. • Most studies have evaluated the leaf extracts of various plants to control *C. capsici*. Leaf extracts of neem, Datura, *Ocimum*, Polyalthia, *Vinca rosea* were found fungitoxic against *C. capsici* [55]. • Yeast strains isolated from rhizosphere were found to be antagonistic to *C. capsici* by inhibiting the mycelia growth of *C. capsici* to the extent of 40.6 to 43.1% which interns found to control the anthracnose to the tune of 60% [56]. • There are several species of *Trichoderma*, of which the major ones are *Trichoderma asperellum*, *T. viridae*, *T. harzianum*, and *T. longibrachiatum*. Isolates of T. longibrachiatum found to inhibit the mycelia growth of Colletotrichum capsici up to 66% due to volatile compounds released by *Trichoderma* [57]. • Use disease-free seeds.

Disease and its pathogen	Symptoms	Management measures
		• Seed treatment with thiram 2 kg/ha or zineb 2.5 kg/ha. • Spraying of captan 0.2% with sufficient interval. • Essential oil of *Nigella sativa* is shown to have antimicrobial activity [51].
Wilt disease# *Fusarium oxysporum* Schl.f.sp.*morindae* [30]	• The leaves slowly wilt and die; they usually do not turn yellow, the leaves tend to stay green they begin to darken and turn brown, or blackish color and chlorosis occurs, and the plant dies [10].The fungal disease develops during hot weather and is most destructive when soil temperatures approach 80°F. • Dry weather and low soil moisture encourage this plant disease [77].	• Use Safer Yard & Garden Insect Killer to control many garden insects. • Avoid application of excess nitrogen fertilizers that may increase susceptibility to the disease. • Deweeding using a weed flamer or natural herbicide. • Application of Mycostop (1–2 g/ 100 sq. ft.), biological fungicide that with sufficient watering protect crops against wilt caused by *Fusarium*. • If the disease persists, removal of the entire plant and solarization of the soil before planting again is essential [49, 77].
Black Flag disease [78] (Presently recorded) *Phytophthora* species, *Phytophthora morindae* [29]	• Severely diseased plants have characteristic "black flags," which describes the blackened, wilted, withered, or completely necrotic leaves hanging from blackened petioles and stems. • Initially, infection of the leaves, petioles, and stems may have blackened streaks or stripes along the veins. • Later, entire stems and petioles may collapse after being girdled by black lesions. • Fruit symptoms, common at the stem end, consist of a progressive soft rot with a water-soaked appearance and chocolate-brown or dark brown to black color. • Advanced stages of fruit infections result in dry, shriveled fruit "mummies" that may have a fuzzy or silvery surface [29].	• Disease can be controlled by following integrated cultural and preventive methods such as pruning, sanitation, avoidance, and an appropriate cropping system. • Regular monitoring for black flag disease must be carried out during periods of extended rain. • Pruning, removal, and destroying symptomatic foliage and fruits will reduce the pathogen inoculum levels and disease incidence. • Promoting good air circulation within the noni plant canopy will ensure rapid drying of leaves and fruits. • Reduction of relative humidity within the noni canop, ensuring adequate soil drainage and controlling weeds around the noni plants are recommended. • Maintain good plant nutrition with foliar sprays of fertilizers derived from phosphorus acid, such as Phosgard® [29].
Algal leaf spot [53] *Cephaleuros minimus*	• Initial leaf spots are characterized by a light brown color and surrounded by a conspicuous, diffuse, yellow halos.	• Sanitation and removal of severely diseased leaves from the plant and destruction of fallen-infected leaves.

Disease and its pathogen	Symptoms	Management measures
	• The effect of these symptoms may be minor; the disease is not fatal but some premature defoliation may occur [53].	• Moisture and humidity management ensuring good drainage, controlling weeds, adequate plant spacing, pruning, minimizing leaf wetness, and overhead irrigation. • Growing noni in full sun is recommended [53].
Noni shot hole [53] Unidentified	• Initial spots are tiny, maroon-colored specks on leaves and bracts that develop into lesions (2–10 mm diameter) with bleached or tan centers and maroon margins, often surrounded by or accompanied by yellowing of leaf tissue around lesions. • As the lesions mature the centers drop out, leaving the typical "shot hole" appearance. Infected leaves may abscise prematurely. However, stems and fruits display no symptoms [53].	• Sanitation and removal of severely diseased leaves from the plant and destruction of fallen infected leaves. • Moisture and humidity management ensuring good drainage, controlling weeds, adequate plant spacing, pruning, minimizing leaf wetness and overhead irrigation. • Protective spray applications of approved fungicides and avoiding spreading of the pathogen on hands and tools during harvesting operations are recommended [53].
Noni stem canker Unidentified [53]	• Initial characteristic symptom observed is rot of stem at the interface between woody and green stem tissues. • Stem may be girdled and collapsed, leading to plant death. • Stem lesions are irregular in shape with roughened, dark borders and an overall corky appearance [53].	• Pruning the diseased stem at least 1 inch below the stem canker is recommended. • For humidity management through plant spacing and pruning, weed control, good drainage is recommended. • Applications of protective or therapeutic fungicides will help mitigating the disease [53].
Noni stem blight *Sclerotium rolfsii*, and root-knot nematodes [53]	• Foliar chlorosis, wilting, stem girdling at or near soil line; internal stem necrosis, stem rot, defoliation leading to plant death [53].	• Avoid planting in low-lying areas with poor drainage, undue plant stresses. • Avoid plant-parasitic nematodes, injuring stems with weed-whackers. • Do not pile rocks around the base of noni plants, as they may injure the stem [53].
Sooty mold Sooty mold is caused by a ubiquitous, airborne fungus [53].	• Sooty mold consists of a black, powdery growth, usually on the upper surface of noni leaves. • The black growth is not pathogenic and exists as a thin layer [53].	• To control sooty mold, one must control the sap-feeding insects (scales, aphids) which infest the noni plant. • Sooty mold may in some cases be washed off noni leaves with a strong spray of soapy water [53].
Phytoplasma disease Phytoplasmas (mycoplasma-like organisms or MLOs) [31]	• Diseased plants usually express various growth and flowering abnormalities, together with chlorosis, stunting, and sometimes dieback symptoms [31].	• Controlling phytoplasma diseases usually begins with controlling insect vectors that starts with good weed removal practices and clearing brush that can host insect vectors.

Disease and its pathogen	Symptoms	Management measures
		• Removal of an infected plant is necessary to contain the pathogen. • Dry weather seems to increase leafhopper activity, so it is important to keep the plant watered. • Good cultural care and practices will increase plant resistance and spread of the disease [79].
Root rot disease [80] *Fusarium proliferatum*	• Initially, typical yellowing and root rot symptoms are observed. • Dark brown to black, discolored, decaying or completely rotted roots is observed [80].	**Chemical/Biological Control** • Seed is treated with fungicide may protect seedlings from root rot for a short time. **Cultural Practices** • Rotating crops may help reduce the severity of Fusarium root rot. • Herbicide injury, foliar diseases, hail damage, or drought may make it more susceptible to root rot [81].

Diseases of *M. pruriens.*

Disease and its pathogen	Symptoms	Management measures
Leaf blight*# *Colletotrichum gleosporioides*	• The symptoms on leaves began as dark brown lesions surrounded by chlorotic halos, and later became larger, round or irregular spots with gray to off-white centers surrounded by dark brown margins.	• Destroy all affected branches and spray the plants with 0.5% Bordeaux mixture or Mancozeb 0.25%.
Rust disease # *Uromyces mucunae* [47, 48]	• Small, irregular black spots occur on mature leaves covering the lower surface. • Yellow brown-coalesced pustules at the center, severe infection consisting of circular rings of brown pustules at the periphery and brown to black-coalesced raised spots at the center. • On stems, affected tissues showed softening, necrosis, and death of plants [47, 48].	**Cultural method** [46] • Removal of weeds from bunds and channels. • Avoid application of excess nitrogen. • Apply N in three doses (50% during basal, 25% during tillering phase and 25% N in panicle initiation stage). **Chemical Method** [46] • Application of Carbendazim 50WP @ 500 g/ha (or) Tricyclozole 75 WP @ 500 g/ha (or) Metominostrobin 20 SC @ 500 ml/ha (or) Azoxystrobin 25 SC @ 500 ml/ha. **Biological control** [46] • Dipping seedling root, soil application, and foliar spray with with TNAU Pf 1liquid formulation (500 ml for one hectare seedlings) are recommended [47, 48].

Disease and its pathogen	Symptoms	Management measures
Collar rot of seedling Unidentified [82]	• Localized lesion at or about the collet between the stem and the root is observed. • The lesions develop around the stem eventually forming a "collar" [82].	• Applications of 2 kg Trichorich (a formulation of *Trichoderma* in neem cake) and 2 kg *Pseudomonas fluorescens* mixed with 500 kg FYM to the root region is recommended [82].
Velvet bean severe mosaic virus disease. Velvet bean severe mosaic virus (VbSMV) [83]	• Naturally infected velvet bean plants shows diffused yellow spots on the young leaves, which turn into severe mosaic and yellowing symptoms in the older leaves. • Seeds from diseased plants showed poor germination. • The symptoms succession included chlorosis of the primary veins on the abaxial leaf surface, extending gradually to the secondary and tertiary veins to form a network of dark green veins [83].	• The use of insecticides for vector control and resistant cultivars is recommended [83].
Charcoal rot *Macrophomina phaseolina* [34, 84]	• Diseased plants are wilted and dead pre-maturely with patches similar to those of sudden death syndrome (SDS). • Discoloration in cortex tissues of taproot and lower stems is typical and when stems are split, piths of diseased plants have brown stem rot like browning in the lower part of the stem. • In some plants, however, no pith browning can be found [34, 84].	• Crop rotation with small grain, such as wheat or barley, helps to reduce population levels of the fungus. • Excessive seeding rates should be avoided so that plants do not compete for moisture, which increases disease risk during a dry season [34, 84].

Diseases of *O. sanctum*.

Disease and its pathogen	**Symptom**	**Management measures**
Wilt disease # *Fusarium oxysporum* [35]	• The affected plants had stunted growth with wilting symptoms. • Chlorosis of leaves with brown spots and streaks on the stem, vascular discoloration of roots, severely twisted stems, and leaf drop was observed [35].	• There is no remedy for *Fusarium* wilt of basil. Destroy infected plants and do not plant basil or other mint plants in that area for two to three years [35].
Powdery mildew disease # *Erysiphe biocellata* [39]	• The white mycelia covered leaves and stems are observed on the upper surface of lower leaves. • These white patches soon joined together to form larger white greyish powdery coating discernible on the severely affected leaves.	• Spraying NSKE 5% or neem oil 3% twice at 10-day interval from initial disease appearance, eucalyptus leaf extract 10% at initiation of the disease, and 10 days later and Carbendazim 500 g or wettable sulfur 1500 g/ha is recommended [85].

Disease and its pathogen	Symptom	Management measures
	• Leaves finally show necrosis resulting in withering, drying, and defoliation [39].	
Fungal Leaf Spots # *Colletotrichum gloeosporioides* and a complex of three fungal pathogens: *Alternaria* spp., *Cercospora* spp., and *Colletotrichum* spp. [86]	• These leaf spots show brown to black in color, with yellow halo around it. • The spots are irregular in shape and as the disease progressed, the spots coalesced and the entire leaves turned necrotic. • They occur when the leaves stay wet or damp for an extended period [86].	• Removing all diseased foliage, avoiding overhead watering, treating the holy basil plant weekly with a potassium bicarbonate fungicide will help prevent the fungal pathogen from spreading. • Some brands of potassium bicarbonate fungicide recommend mixing 2 teaspoons of the product with 1 gallon of water and applying the solution thoroughly to the foliage with a pump sprayer [86].
Bacterial Leaf Spot or Basil Shoot Blight *Pseudomonas cichorii* [87]	• Black or brown spots that appear on the leaves and streaking on the stems of the plant [87].	• While there is no fix for bacterial leaf spot, you can minimize the damage by making sure that your basil plants have plenty of air circulation and avoiding overhead watering is recommended [87].
Downy Mildew [87] *Peronospora belbaharii*	• Symptoms include yellow leaves that have fuzzy, grey growth on the undersides of the leaves [87].	• In the United States, mono- and dipotassium salts of phosphorous acid provided the best control, whereas moderate disease suppression was provided by mandipropamid, cyazofamid, and fiuopicolide [88]. • One of the most effective measures for disease control is *via* genetic manipulation of the host, namely introgression of resistant genes. The objectives of this study were to expand on what others have reported on potential sources of resistance to BDM in some species of *Ocimum* [89, 90]. • Downy mildew is aggravated by overly wet conditions, so ensuring avoiding overhead watering and ensuring the basil plants have good drainage and good air circulation is recommended. • Spraying with 0.3% wettable sulfur is recommended [87].
***Cercospora* leaf spot** *Cercospora ocimicola* [36]	• Circular to irregular dark spots on leaves with light centers is observed [36].	• Avoid overhead irrigation and splashing plants with water, instead water plants from the base and apply a layer of mulch

Disease and its pathogen	Symptom	Management measures
		around the plants to reduce water splash, removal and destroying any symptomatic leaves; minor infections can be controlled by spraying weekly with a fungicide containing potassium bicarbonate [36].
Root rot *Rhizoctonia solani*, *Pythium* spp. [36]	• Failure of seeds to germinate, germinated seedlings collapses brown, shriveled area at base of stem, roots brown, and water-soaked. • Disease promoted by high humidity and poor air circulation [36].	• Complete control of root rot caused by infection of *Rhophitulus solani* in *Ocimum* sp. was achieved with seed treatment of tolclofos-methyl (50SC) at 3 g kg^{-1}. Soil solarization and drenching of dazomet (98G) at 40 g active ingredient per m^2 around plants reduced incidence of root rot from 70.6% to 4.1% [91]. • Root rot can be controlled by drenching the nursery beds with a 0.1 per cent solution of mercurial fungicide and adopting phytosanitory measures [36].
Viral disease Yellow mosaic virus [92]	• Symptoms included leaf mosaic or mottling, yellowing, ring spots, stunting, and distortion of leaves, flowers, and fruits are observed [92].	• Seeds are to be treated with insecticides like carbosulfon at 30gm or monocrotophos at 5 ml per one kg seed before sowing. • Follow crop rotation and maintain soil health management. Grow suitable region wise resistant varieties. Use seeds collected from disease-free plants. • Infected plants should be removed and destroyed. • Control of white fly by spraying insecticides *viz.*, dimethoate 0.03 per cent or monocrotophos 1.6 per cent or metasystox (0.1 per cent) or triazophos 1.25 ml/l at the initial stage of disease proves effective. • Foliar sprays of methyl demeton 2 ml/l also control the vector spread [93].
Leaf blight *Alternaria* sp. [37]	• Early blight is first observed on the plants as small, black lesions mostly on the older foliage. • Spots enlarge, and by the time they are one-fourth inch in diameter or larger, concentric rings in a bull's eye pattern can be seen in the center of the diseased area.	• *L. lactis* subsp. *lactis* LABW4 can be used as a prospective agent to control leaf blight disease of *Ocimum* plant and to increase its medicinal properties [37].

Disease and its pathogen	Symptom	Management measures
	• Tissue surrounding the spots may turn yellow. • The fungus also infects the fruit, generally through the calyx or stem attachment. • Lesions attain considerable size, usually involving nearly the entire fruit; concentric rings are also present on the fruit [37].	
Gray mold *Botrytis cinerea* [38]	• Infected organs produce profuse off-white to gray mycelia covered with dark conidia disseminated in wind currents or by rain splashing from plant to plant. • The disease then progresses, killing all leaves and secondary buds leading to the death of the entire plant. • *B. cinerea* may also develop on the packed bunches during shipment to market, resulting in rot of the entire package [38].	• Cultural methods, particularly reduction of relative humidity and leaf wetness, and reduce black spot and gray mold incidence. • Thiram reduces gray mold incidence, which also controls black spot. • A formulation based on *Trichoderma harzianum*, which is active against gray mold, soon will be registered, possibly for basil [38].

Diseases of *P. longum.*

Disease and its pathogen	Symptoms	Management measures
Anthracnose # *Colletotrichum boninense*	• Initially, the lush green color of healthy leaves gradually changed to pale yellow. • These symptomatic leaves primarily showed brown concentric ring shaped spots, which later developed yellow halo around it. • Subsequently in the later stages, the leaves wilt and abscise.	• Spraying Bordeaux mixture 1% or carbendazim + mancozeb 0.1% is recommended. • Regulation of shade and adoption of integrated nutrition management practices in the plantation is recommended. • Spraying *P. fluorescens* (FP 7) at 3-week interval [63].
Leaf spot *Botryodiplodia theobromae [Lasiodiplodia theobromae]* [42]	• Oval, round to irregular or angular, necrotic, surrounded with the concentric rings. • Later, these spots increase in size and coalesce covering larger leaf area with dark brown margin and yellow halo [42].	• Collection and removal of fallen leaves. • Spraying with Carbendazim 0.1% and Mancozeb 0.25% [42].
Rot *Fusarium pallidoroseum* [42]	• Occur in patches • on the Leaves—turn yellow and then dry up slowly • Entire plant shows complete drying of the foliage • Whitish mold growth is observed [42].	• Field sanitation by destruction of infected plant debris. • Soil drenching—COC—0.25% and Pre planting treatment of bulbs with benomyl 15% + mancozeb 60% is recommended. • Local Bellary, Poona Red Globe, Patna Red, White Large—resistant varieties are recommended [42].

Disease and its pathogen	Symptoms	Management measures
***Cercospora* leaf spot** *Cercospora piperata* [43, 94]	• Round or irregular greyish spots • Dark brown or blackish borders appear on older leaves [43, 94].	• Remove and destroy the infected plant residues. • Spray Mancozeb or Copper oxychloride at 2 kg/ha at the intimation of the disease. • Two to three sprays may be given at 15-day interval [43, 94].

Diseases of *Tabernaemonta divaricata*.

Disease and its pathogen	Symptoms	Management measures
Anthracnose Leaf blight disease*# *Colletotrichum gloeosporioides*	• Primarily, blight start as minute, round, light brown spots, and the spots grow and acquire a round to irregular shape and some spots coalesce. • Fully developed spots were water soaked, dark brown to blackish, scattered all over the leaf lamina. • The spots were equally visible on lower and upper leaf surfaces. • Grey-brown spots made up of concentric markings appear on the leaves and can join together to create large dead patches.	• Spraying biocontrol agents like *Trichoderma virens* chemical fungicides like Benomyl 0.1% (or) Mancozeb 0.2% (or) Carbendazim 0.1% is recommended [52].
Wilt disease*# *Fusarium oxysporum*	• *Fusarium* sp. clogs the vascular tissues in roots and stem restricting water flow causing the foliage to wilt and turn yellow. • Chlorosis often appear later in the growing season and are first noticed on the lower (older) leaves. • As the disease progresses, the younger leaves will also be affected and the plant eventually dies.	• Use Safer Yard & Garden Insect Killer to control many garden insects. • Avoid application of excess nitrogen fertilizers that may increase susceptibility to the disease. • Deweeding using a weed flamer or natural herbicide. • Application of Mycostop (1–2 g/ 100 sq. ft.), biological fungicide that with sufficient watering protect crops against wilt caused by *Fusarium*. • If the disease persists, removal of the entire plant and solarization of the soil before planting again is essential [49].
Leaf blight disease *Phytophthora citrophthora* [44]	• Brown or black spots and patches may be either ragged or circular, with a water soaked or yellow-edged appearance [95].	• Use disease-free planting material. • Removal of infected leaves when the plant is dry. • Leaves that collect around the base of the plant should be raked up and disposed. • Overhead irrigation must be avoided. • Treatment of the seed with benomyl + thiram 1 g each per kg of seed is recommended [95].

Disease and its pathogen	Symptoms	Management measures
Wilt disease *Fusarium oxysporum* f. sp. *tabernaemontanae* [45]	• *Fusarium* sp. clogs the vascular tissues in roots and stem restricting water flow causing the foliage to wilt and turn yellow. • Chlorosis often appears later in the growing season and is first noticed on the lower (older) leaves. • As the disease progresses, the younger leaves will also be affected and the plant eventually dies.	• Use Safer Yard & Garden Insect Killer to control many garden insects. • Avoid application of excess nitrogen fertilizers that may increase susceptibility to the disease. • Deweeding using a weed flamer or natural herbicide. • Application of Mycostop (1–2 g/ 100 sq. ft.), biological fungicide that with sufficient watering protect crops against wilt caused by *Fusarium*. • If the disease persists, removal of the entire plant and solarization of the soil before planting again is essential [49].
Viral infection Plant Virus [96]	• Disrupts the cell's functionality, outward signs of a viral infection result in a plant disease with symptoms such as abnormal or stunted growth, damaged fruit, discolorations, or spots [96].	• Keep vectors such as aphids, leafhoppers, and thrips under control. • Viruses can also be introduced by infected pollen or through plant openings (as when pruning). • New plants should be checked, as well as tools and existing plants. • Use of certified seed that is deemed disease-free is recommended [96].
Viral disease Tobacco mild green mosaic virus [97]	• Symptoms on naturally infected *T. divaricata* are highly varied and include chlorotic ringspots, chlorotic banding, vein clearing, oak-leaf patterns, and mosaic on the younger leaves. • During the late winter, after the cold season, the yellow spots usually become necrotic and, as the surrounding tissue expands, the leaves become buckled and distorted. • The necrotic zones, in severely affected fully expanded leaves, disintegrate, leaving "shot holes" from which small or large areas of necrotic tissue have fallen out • Severely affected leaves wither, leaving the plant naked [97].	• Keep vectors such as aphids, leafhoppers, and thrips under control. • Viruses can also be introduced by infected pollen or through plant openings (as when pruning). • New plants should be checked, as well as tools and existing plants. • Use of certified seed that is deemed disease-free is recommended [96, 97].
Rust disease *Uredo manilensis* [98]	• Leaf lesions began as chlorotic flecks that expanded into necrotic spots with orange-to-reddish brown, sub epidermal uredinia. • Brown telia developed on the abaxial side of leaves [45].	• Select rust-resistant plant varieties when available. • Removal and destruction of infected leaves and fallen debris are recommended. • Drip irrigation and soaker hoses can be used to help keep leaves dry. • Use a slow-release, organic fertilizer on crops and avoid excess nitrogen.

Disease and its pathogen	Symptoms	Management measures
		• Apply copper sprays or sulfur powders to prevent infection of susceptible plants. For best results, apply early or at first sign of disease. • Effectively treat fungal diseases with SERENADE Garden®. • Containing sulfur and pyrethrins. • Removal of weeds to improve air circulation is recommended. • Use a thick layer of mulch or organic compost to cover the soil after you have raked and cleaned it well. • Burn or bag-infected plants after the growing season and do not compost [99].

3. Conclusion

The review and our study on the diseases of medicinal plants cultivated in Karnataka endorsed the fact that the medicinal plants are not free from diseases. Among the medicinal plants cultivated in Karnataka maximum of 12 diseases are reported in *H. rosa-sinensis* followed by 10 diseases each in *M. citrifolia* and *O. sanctum*, 7 diseases each in *A. vasica* and *T. divaricate/T. coronaria*, 5 diseases each in *C. borivilianum* and *M. pruriens*, 4 diseases in *P. longum*, and 3 diseases each in *A. calamus* and *G. sylvestre*. It includes 12 diseases that were recorded for the first time in Karnataka and 5 diseases recorded for the first time on the respective host plant. Since medicinal plants are for human consumption and animal welfare the usage of chemical pesticides for the management of diseases should be strictly avoided. The option of the extraction and purification of the secondary metabolites produced by the fungal antagonists for their biocontrol activities against fungal diseases to be explored. The genes conferring to antagonistic effect toward the pathogen could be genetically engineered into medicinal plants thereby producing resistant varieties or transgenic plants that are resistant to diseases. The biocontrol agent *T. virens* can be scaled-up for talc-based formulations and mass production of fungal bio pesticides for controlling fungal diseases of medicinal plants. All such efforts will pave way to produce medicinal plants in a more sustainable eco-friendly way and will prove to be beneficial not only to the producers but also to the consumers.

Author details

P. Swetha* and R. Sundararaj
Forest Protection Division, Institute of Wood Science and Technology, Bangalore, Karnataka, India

*Address all correspondence to: swetha.purushotham@gmail.com

References

[1] Rangaswami G. *Uromyces acori* Ramakrishnan and Rangaswami sp. nov. on *Acoras calamus* L. Ramakrishnan, T. S. Current Science. 1948;**17**(8):240-241

[2] ApniKheti. Sweet Flag [Internet]. Available from: https://www.apnikheti.com/en/pn/agriculture/horticulture/medicinal-plants/sweet-flag [Accessed: February 22, 2022]

[3] Vanitha S, Kandaswami M. Occurrence of bacterial leaf blight in vasambu (*Acorus calamus* Linn) caused by *Xanthomonas campestris* P.V.O. *Oxyzae* - A new report. South-Indian-Horticulture. 1998;**46**(3/6):366-367

[4] Gautam A, Avasthi S. *Colletotrichum gloeosporioides* on *Adhatoda vasica* in India. Journal of Agricultural Technology. 2013;**9**:581-587

[5] Verma OP, Singh N, Sharma P. First report of *Rhizoctonia solani* causing leaf spot of *Adhatoda vasica*. India Plant Pathology. 2007;**56**:726

[6] Singh N, Verma OP. Epidemiology of *Alternaria blight* of *Adhatoda vasica* caused by *Alternaria alternata*. Indian Journal of Agricultural Science. 2009;**79**:945-948

[7] Yadav VK, Sharma ND. Rust of *Justicia gendarussa*: A new record from Central, India. Journal of Mycology and Plant Pathology. 2006;**36**:40-41

[8] Manisha S, Kareppa BM. Studies on fungal diseases of *Adathoda zeylanica* Medic. International Journal of Plant Protection. 2010;**3**(1):132-134

[9] Ajay G, Shubhi A. *Colletotrichum gloeosporioides* on *Adhatoda vasica* in India. Journal of Agricultural Technology. 2013;**9**:581-587

[10] Snyder WC, Hansen HW. The species concept in *Fusarium*. American Journal of Botany. 1940;**27**:64-67

[11] ApniKheti. Safed Musli [Internet]. Available from: https://www.apnikheti.com/en/pn/agriculture/horticulture/medicinal-plants/safed-musli [Accessed: February 22, 2022]

[12] Chandra S, Tandon RN. Two new leaf spot fungi. Current Science. 1965;**34**: 565-566

[13] Pokhar R, Pinki S, Dodiya NS, Arunabh J. Evaluation of fungicides, neem bio-formulations and biocontrol agent for the management of root rot of safed musli caused by *Rhizoctonia solani*. Journal of Mycology and Plant Pathology. 2013;**43**(3):297-305

[14] Sharma JR, Singh P, Saini SS, Gill BS. Root rot of safed musli (*Chlorophytum borovillianum*) and its management. PAU Agricultural Research Journal. 2010;**47**(1–2):20-21

[15] Tetarwal JP, Rawal P, Singh V, Kantwa SL. Distribution and Severity of Anthracnose in Safed Musli (*Chlorophytum borivilianum* Santapau & Fernandez) In Southern Rajasthan. International Journal of Agriculture Sciences. 2017;**9**(8):3880–3885

[16] Krishnamurthi KK. Organic Agriculture for Sustainability. Chennai, India: Notion Press; 2016. p. 384

[17] Chinnadurai SK, Dronamraju VLS, Ramasamy R. Seaweed extracts control the leaf spot disease of the medicinal plant *Gymnema sylvestre*. Indian Journal of Science and Technology. 2008;**1**(3):1-5

[18] Hibiscus world. Pests and Diseases of Hibiscus by F.D. Hockings [Internet].

Available from: http://www.hibiscusworld.com/BeersBook/5-Pests.htm [Accessed: February 22, 2022]

[19] Rivera MC, Wright ER, Carballo S. First report of *Colletotrichum gloeosporioides* on Chinese Rose in Argentina. The American Phytopathological Society. 2000;**84**(12):1,345.2-1,345.2

[20] Pankaj BAC, Satish CA, Rajesh K, Ngachan ASV, Munda GC. First report of powdery mildew caused by *Podosphaera* sp. on *Hibiscus sabdariffa* in India. Australasian Plant Disease Notes. 2010;**5**:123-125

[21] Park JH, Cho SE. First report of Choanephora Blight caused by *Choanephora infundibulifera* on *Hibiscus rosa-sinensis* in Korea. Plant Disease. 2014;**98**(9):1275

[22] Rivera MC, Wright ER. First report of Blight caused by *Botrytis cinerea* on China Rose in Argentina. Plant. Health Progress. 2002;**3**(1):22

[23] Montano HG, Davis RE, Dally EL, Hogenhout SA, Pimentel JP, Brioso PS. *Candidatus* Phytoplasma brasiliense', a new phytoplasma taxon associated with hibiscus witches' broom disease. International journal of systematic and evolutionary microbiology. 2001;**51**(3): 1109-1118

[24] Thankamma L. *Phytophthora* species on eight indigenous host species in south India and their pathogenicity on rubber. Indian Phytopathology. 1983;**36**(1):17-23

[25] McRitchie JJ. Hibiscus Rust, *Kuehneola malvicola*. Florida: Florida Department of Agriculture & Consumer Services. Plant Pathology Circular No. 378; 1996

[26] Nakkeeran S, Marimuthu T, Raguchander T. Exploring DAPG and phenazine producing PGPR strains and fungal antagonists for the management of diseases of Noni (*Morinda citrifolia* L.). WNRF Technical Bulletin-11. World Noni Research Foundation. 2013;**329**:289-312

[27] Manjunath H, Nakkeeran S, Raguchander T. First report of anthracnose on noni caused by *Colletotrichum gloeosporioides* in India. Archives Of Phytopathology And Plant Protection. 2012;**45**:276-279

[28] Kavitha PG, Umadevi M. Medicinal properties and pests and diseases of Noni. Research Journal of Pharmacognosy and Phytochemistry. 2016;**8**(1):41-48

[29] Scot CN, Zoila A. *Phytophthora morindae*, a new species causing black flag disease on noni (*Morinda citrifolia* L) in Hawaii. Mycologia. 2010;**102**:122-134

[30] Luo SB, Chen ZX. Studies on the *Fusarium* wilt disease of medicinal Indian mulberry. II. A study on the comparison of physiological characteristics isolated from Fujian, Guangdong and Guangxi provinces. Wuyi-Science-Journal. 1987;**7**:243-251

[31] Davis RI, Jones P, Holman TJ, Halsey K, Amice R, Tupouniua SK, et al. *Phytoplasma* disease surveys in Tonga, New Caledonia and Vanuatu. Australasian Plant Pathology. 2006; **35**(3):335-340

[32] Berner DK, Killani E, Aigbokhan E, Couper DC. *Macrophomina phaseolina* on the tropical crop *Mucuna pruriens* var. utilis. Plant Disease. 1992;**76**:1283

[33] Keinath AP, Harrison HF, Niarino PC, Jackson DM, Pullaro TC. Increase in populations of *Rhioctonia solani* and wirestem of collard with velvet bean cover crop mulch. Plant Disease. 2003;**87**:719-725

[34] Abhinav A, Dinesh KM, Shrivardhan D, Mohit A, Ramesh CD, Vivek KB. Plant growth promotion and suppression of charcoal-rot fungus (*Macrophomina phaseolina*) in velvet bean (*Mucuna pruriens* L.) by root nodule bacteria. Journal of Phytopathology. 2017;**165**(7–8):463-478

[35] Gardening Know How. Treating Root Rot-Gardening Tips For Houseplants [Internet]. Available from: https://www.gardeningknowhow.com/plant-problems/disease/treating-root-rot-gardening-tips-for-housplants.htm [Accessed: February 22, 2022]

[36] Plant village. Basil [Internet]. Available from: https://plantvillage.psu.edu/topics/basil/infos [Accessed: February 22, 2022]

[37] Soma B, Ranjan G, Debalika D, Narayan CM. Suppression of leaf blight of *Ocimum sanctum* L. using lactic acid bacteria as novel bio-control agent. Proceedings of the National Academy of Sciences, India Section B: Biological Sciences. 2017;**88**(4):1389-1397

[38] Sharabani G, Shtienberg D, Elad Y, Dinoor A. Epidemiology of *Botrytis cinerea* in sweet basil and implications for disease management. The American Phytopathological Society: Plant Disease. 1996;**83**:554-560

[39] Sharma YR, Chaudhary KCB. Powdery mildew of *Ocimum sanctum* - A new record. Indian Phytopathology. 1980;**33**(4):627-629.2

[40] Suseela BR. Pest and diseases of pepper and their control. In: Annual Report: Indian Institute of Spices Research, Calicut, Annual Report 2008–09. Coimbatore, India: Natural Resources Management And Organic Farming Of Pepper; 2008. p. 90

[41] Kurian A, Shankar MA. Medicinal plants. Horticulture Science Series-2. Delhi: Jai Bharat Printing Press; 2007

[42] Anupam K, Jha PK. Piper longum—a new host of two fungal pathogens. Journal of Mycology and Plant Pathology. 2014;**44**(2):212-213

[43] Asthana RP, Mahmud KA. Cercospora leaf-spot on Piper longum Linn. Magazine of the Agricultural College of Nagpur. 1947;**21**(3–4):58-59

[44] Sushma N, Sharma ND. A new leaf blight disease of *Tabernaemontana coronaria*. Journal of Mycopathological Research. 1999;**37**(1):45-46,2

[45] Alaka P, Rao VG. Wilt disease of *Tabernaemontana coronaria* Willd. Biovigyanam. 1990;**16**(1):58-61,7

[46] TNAU Agritech Portal. Diseases of Paddy [Internet]. Available from: http://agritech.tnau.ac.in/crop_protection/crop_prot_crop%20diseases_cereals_paddy.html [Accessed: February 22, 2022]

[47] Chavan PB, Patil SK. Studies on rust fungi from Maharastra, India. Sydowia. 1972;**26**:277-281

[48] Pande A, Rao VG. A Compendium of Fungi on Legumes from India. Jodhpur: Scientific Publishers; 1998

[49] Planet Natural Research Center. Fusarium Wilt [Internet]. Available from: https://www.planetnatural.com/pest-problem-solver/plant-disease/fusarium-wilt/ [Accessed: February 22, 2022]

[50] Crocus. Fungal Leaf spot [Internet]. Available from: https://www.crocus.co.uk/pestsanddiseases/_/top12/Fungal%20leaf%20spot/ArticleID.1170 [Accessed: February 22, 2022]

[51] TNAU Agritech Portal. Crop Protection [Internet]. Available from: http://agritech.tnau.ac.in/crop_protection/chilli_phdiseases_2.html [Accessed: February 22, 2022]

[52] TNAU Agritech Portal. Crop Protection [Internet]. Available from: http://www.agritech.tnau.ac.in/crop_protection/crop_prot_crop%20diseases_flowers_crossandra.html [Accessed: February 22, 2022]

[53] The Noni Website. College of Tropical Agriculture and Human Resources, University Of Hawaii at Manoa [Internet]. Available from: https://www.ctahr.hawaii.edu/noni/algal.asp [Accessed: February 22, 2022]

[54] Rajavel R. Seed Borne *Colletotrichum capsici* (Syd). Butter and Bisby and its Management [Thesis]. Coimbatore: Tamil Nadu Agricultural University; 2000

[55] Shivapuri A, Sharma OP, Jhamaria SL. Fungi-toxic properties of plant extracts against pathogenic fungi. Journal of Mycology and Plant Pathology. 1997;**27**:29-31

[56] Chaisemsaeng P, Mongkolthanaruk W, Bunyatratchata W. Screening and potential for biological control of anthracnose disease (*Colletotrichum capsici*) on chilli fruits by yeast isolates. Journal of Life Sciences and Technologies. 2013;**1**(4):201-204

[57] Mishra A, Trivedi VS, Dabbs MR, Dixit S, Srivastava Y. Identification and evaluation of potential Trichoderma strains against *Colletotrichum capsici* and *Fusarium oxysporum* f. sp. *capsici* causing anthracnose and wilt disease in chilli. International Journal of Current Microbiology and Applied Sciences. 2017;**6**(9):1159-1166

[58] Tubaki K, Nishihara N. *Alternaria helianthi* (Hansf.) Comb Nov. Transactions of British Mycological Society. 1969;**53**:147-149

[59] Zarger SA, Rizvi G, Parashar R. Studies on leaf spot disease of mango and its management. International Journal of Pharma and Bio Sciences. 2015;**6**(1):769-776

[60] Ragi PR, Sivan VV, Joseph J, Sujana KA, Anil KN. Management of leaf rust disease of medicinal plant *Justicia gendarussa* Burm. F. with antagonistic fungi (*Trichoderma harzianum*). Journal of Horticultural Science & Ornamental Plants. 2013;**50**(2):68-70

[61] TNAU Agritech Portal. Crop Protection [Internet]. Available from: http://agritech.tnau.ac.in/crop_protection/wheat/crop_prot_crop%20diseases_cereals_wheat_1.html [Accessed: February 22, 2022]

[62] Shodhganga. [Internet]. Available from: http://shodhganga.inflibnet.ac.in/bitstream/10603/80251/12/12_chapter-3.pdf [Accessed: February 22, 2022]

[63] TNAU Agritech Portal. Crop Protection [Internet]. Available from: http://agritech.tnau.ac.in/crop_protection/mango_1.html [Accessed: February 22, 2022]

[64] Koike ST, Alger EI, Sepulveda LR, Bull CT. First report of bacterial leaf spot Caused by *Pseudomonas* syringae pv. tomato on Kale in California. Plant Disease. 2017;**101**(3):504,3

[65] TNAU Agritech Portal. Crop Protection [Internet]. Available from: http://agritech.tnau.ac.in/horticulture/horti_medicinal%20crops_gymnema.html [Accessed: February 22, 2022]

[66] TNAU Agritech Portal. Crop Protection. [Internet]. Available from:

http://agritech.tnau.ac.in/expert_system/paddy/cpdisgraindis.html [Accessed: February 22, 2022]

[67] Scot CN. Bacterial leaf spot of hibiscus in Hawai'i. Plant Disease. 2011;**72**

[68] Gardening Know How. Hibiscus Has White Fungus – How To Get Rid Of Powdery Mildew On Hibiscus Plants [Internet]. Available from: https://www.gardeningknowhow.com/ornamental/flowers/hibiscus/hibiscus-has-white-fungus.htm

[69] Hidden Valley Hibiscus. Dieback [Internet]. Available from: http://www.hiddenvalleyhibiscus.com/care/dieback.htm [Accessed: February 22, 2022]

[70] The Connecticut Agricultural Experiment Station. Plant Pest Handbook-A Guide [Internet]. Available from: http://www.ct.gov/caes/cwp/view.asp?a=2823&q=377734 [Accessed: February 22, 2022]

[71] Michigan State University. Botrytis blight [Internet]. Available from: https://www.canr.msu.edu/resources/botrytis_blight [Accessed: February 22, 2022]

[72] University of California Agriculture & Natural Resources. Garden plants diseases [Internet]. Available from: http://ipm.ucanr.edu/PMG/GARDEN/PLANTS/DISEASES/witch.html [Accessed: February 22, 2022]

[73] Plavšic B, Milicic D, Eric Z. Rhabdovirus-like particles In *Hibiscus rosa - sinensis* L. Acta Horticulture. 1985; **164**:41-44

[74] Waqar I. Management of plant virus diseases; farmer's knowledge and our suggestions. Hosts and Viruses. 2017; **4**(2):28-33

[75] Gallup CA, Sullivan MJ, Shew HD. Black Shank of Tobacco. The Plant Health Instructor. Saint Paul, Minnesota, United States: APS; 2006

[76] Pirone PP. Diseases and Pests of Ornamental Plants. New York, Chichester, United States: John Wiley & Sons Inc.; 1978. p. 566

[77] Planet Natural. Fusarium wilt [Internet]. Available from: https://www.planetnatural.com/pest-problem-solver/plant-disease/fusarium-wilt/ [Accessed: February 22, 2022]

[78] Scot CN. Black flag of Noni (*Morinda citrifolia*) caused by a *Phytophthora* species. Published by the College of Tropical Agriculture and Human Resources (CTAHR) and issued in furtherance of Cooperative Extension work. Plant Disease. 2004;**19**:1-4

[79] Gardening Know How. Phytoplasma disease [Internet]. Available from: https://www.gardeningknowhow.com/plant-problems/disease/phytoplasma-disease-plants.htm [Accessed: February 22, 2022]

[80] Thi ND, Chi HN, Thi BTH, Hoat T. First report of molecular characterisation of Fusarium proliferatum associated with root rot disease of Indian mulberry (Morinda officinalis How.) in Viet Nam. Archives of Phytopathology and Plant Protection. 2019;**52**:1-18

[81] Crop Watch. Fusarium Root Rot [Internet]. Available from: https://cropwatch.unl.edu/plantdisease/corn/fusarium-root-rot [Accessed: February 22, 2022]

[82] Vikaspedia. *Mucuna pruriens* [Internet]. Available from: http://vikaspedia.in/agriculture/crop-production/package-of-practices/medicinal-and-aromatic-plants/mucuna-pruriens-2

[83] Zaim M, Kumar Y, Hallan V, Zaidi AA. Velvet bean severe mosaic

virus: A distinct begomovirus species causing severe mosaic in *Mucuna pruriens* (L.) DC. Virus. Gene. 2011;**43**: 138-146

[84] Iowa State University. Charcoal Rot Is A Hidden Threat to Soybean Yield [Internet]. Available from: https://crops.extension.iastate.edu/charcoal-rot [Accessed: February 22, 2022]

[85] TNAU Agritech Portal. Crop Protection [Internet]. Available from: http://agritech.tnau.ac.in/crop_protection/greengram_disease/greengram_d7.html [Accessed: February 22, 2022]

[86] Home Guides. Basil [Internet]. Available from: http://homeguides.sfgate.com/brownish-yellow-spots-holy-basil-plant-71343.html [Accessed: February 22, 2022]

[87] Gardening Know How. Basil [Internet]. Available from: https://www.gardeningknowhow.com/edible/herbs/basil/basil-diseases.htm [Accessed: February 22, 2022]

[88] Homa K, Barney WP, Ward DL, Wyenandt CA, Simon JE. Evaluation of fungicides for the control of *Peronospora belbahrii* on sweet basil in New Jersey. Plant Disease. 2014;**98**:1561-1566

[89] Farahani-Kofoet RD, Römer P, Grosch R. Selecting basil genotypes with resistance against downy mildew. Scientific Horticulture. 2014;**179**:248-255

[90] Wyenandt CA, Simon JE, McGrath MT, Ward DL. Susceptibility of basil cultivars and breeding lines to downy mildew (*Peronospora belbahrii*). Horticulture Science. 2010;**45**: 1416-1419

[91] Varghese S, Manivel P. Cultivation of Ocimum. Ext. Bull. Boriavi, Anand, Gujarat, India. Gujarat, India: Directorate of Medicinal and Aromatic Plants Research; 2014

[92] Deshattiwar A. Studies On Yellow Mosaic Virus Disease On Leguminous Plants [Thesis]. Jabalpur: Jawaharlal Nehru Krishi Vishwa Vidyalaya; 2013

[93] The Hindu. Management of yellow mosaic virus in greengram [Internet]. Available from: https://www.thehindu.com/sci-tech/agriculture/management-of-yellow-mosaic-virus-in-greengram/article6335350.ece [Accessed: February 22, 2022]

[94] Rao PN. Fungi from Hyderabad. Indian Phytopathology. 1962;**15**(2): 112-122

[95] Rana MK. Vegetable Crop Science. Boca Raton: CRC Press; 2017. p. 472

[96] Backyard Gardner. *Tabernaemontana divaricate* [Internet]. Available from: https://www.backyardgardener.com/plantname/tabernaemontana-divaricata-flore-pleno-tabernaemontana/ [Accessed: February 22, 2022]

[97] Cohen J, Rosner A, Kagan S, Lampel M, Maslenin L, Zeidan M, et al. A new disease in *Tabernaemontana* associated with Tobacco mild green mosaic virus. Annals of Applied Biology. 2001;**138**:153-159

[98] Martínez-de la Parte E, Cantillo-Pérez T, García D, Guerrero-Barriel D. Crepe jasmine rust caused by *Uredo manilensis* newly reported in Cuba. New Disease Reports. 2011;**23**:32

[99] Planet Natural. Common rust [Internet]. Available from: https://www.planetnatural.com/pest-problem-solver/plant-disease/common-rust/ [Accessed: February 22, 2022]

Chapter 6

Complementary and Alternative Medicine in COVID-19 Infection, an Old Weapon against a New Enemy

Sally Elnawasany

Abstract

COVID-19 is a running story with an unexpected end. Despite the large effort to provide effective treatment and prophylaxis, many people are still getting infected. This may be explained by the continuous virus mutations, and hence, the attenuation of the vaccine's efficacy. Therefore, long-life boosting of the body's immunity is a hopeful way against SARS-CoV-2 infection. Medicinal plants and other complementary and alternative remedies were used effectively in treating numerous mankind's health problems. Recently, a lot of studies have confirmed the effect of natural products, cupping therapy, and acupuncture against SARS-CoV-2. The aim of this chapter is to remind ourselves of the natural pharmacy that God gave us, by shedding the light on the importance of some herbs and traditional remedies in the management of SARS-CoV-2 infection.

Keywords: SARS-CoV-2, medicinal plants, cupping therapy, acupuncture, complementary and alternative medicine

1. Introduction

Coronavirus disease 2019 (COVID-19) was reported by the World Health Organization (WHO) as a pandemic in 2020 [1]. The spread of the infection is still ongoing in spite of the hard trials to provide potent drugs and vaccines [2]. There is a growing concern about the importance of complementary and alternative medicine (CAM) in treating many infectious diseases [3, 4]. The effect of CAM on the improvement of the symptoms and outcome of SARS-CoV-2 infection was highlighted in multiple reviews [5–8].

2. Severe acute respiratory syndrome coronavirus 2 (SARS-CoV-2)

Severe acute respiratory syndrome coronavirus 2 (SARS-CoV-2) has aroused the attention of the world since 2019 [9]. It is the third severe epidemic of

 IntechOpen

beta-coronavirus (β-CoV) after the severe acute respiratory syndrome (SARS) and the middle east respiratory syndrome (MERS) [10]. SARS-CoV-2 is an enveloped, positive single-stranded RNA virus [11]. Its genome consists mainly of open reading frames (ORF). ORF1ab represents 67% of the viral genome which encodes the synthesis of polyproteins (nonstructural proteins) in the infected cell (1a, 1ab). The viral structural proteins are synthesized from the last 33% ORFs [12–14]. SARS-CoV-2 has four structure proteins: spike (S) glycoprotein, envelope glycoprotein (E), membrane glycoprotein (M), and nucleocapsid protein (N) [15–17]. The pathogenesis of SARS-CoV-2 starts by binding the spike protein (S) with angiotensin-converting enzyme 2, (ACE2). Then synthesis of different viral structural, nonstructural, and extra proteins take place in the infected cells. This is associated with inhibition of the host innate immunity at the early phase of the infection. Then the virus acts against adaptive immunity and spreads in the whole body with subsequent acute and chronic complications. Autoinflammation, immunosuppression, and hyperimmune response may occur [18]. The virulence of SARS-CoV-2 is mediated by the downregulation of pattern recognition receptors (PRRs), which triggers the anti-viral innate immunity mainly interferons (IFNs) release [18, 19]. In addition, the virus stimulates polyclonal activation and apoptosis of lymphocytes leading to pathological activation of macrophages, and immunosuppression [20]. The rapid replication rate of the RNA genome increases the incidence of mutations due to replication errors mediated by RNA polymerase or reverse transcriptase [21, 22]. Mutations in S-protein significantly alter viral pathogenesis [23]. This may impair the immune response to vaccines [24]. Treatment of SARS-CoV-2 has two pathways: the first is to overcome the viral infection either by blocking cell binding, replication, or direct viral effect on tissues. The second pathway is to counteract the overwhelming viral-induced immune response [25]. For blocking viral entry, many agents coexist, such as umifenovir [26, 27], soluble recombinant hACE2, and specific monoclonal antibodies [28, 29]. Several drugs were tried to inhibit viral replication, such as remdesivir [30] favipiravir [31], ribavirin, lopinavir, and ritonavir [32]. For immune modulation, a lot of drugs were introduced, such as dexamethasone [33], tocilizumab, interleukin-6 (IL-6) receptor-specific antibody [34, 35], Eculizumab, a complement 5 inhibitor [36], INF [37, 38], baricitinib, protein kinases inhibitors [39], and imatinib the Abl tyrosine kinase inhibitor (ATKI) [40]. Multiple COVID-19 vaccines have been developed and others are undergoing clinical validation. Despite improving disease morbidity, the vaccines failed to prevent SARS-CoV-2 infection [41, 42]. The drop in anti-SARS-CoV-2 neutralizing antibodies level explains the postvaccination reinfection [43]. Currently, there is no curative anti-SARS-CoV-2 treatment.

3. Complementary and alternative medicine in COVID-19 infection

3.1 Medicinal plants

3.1.1 Boswellia serrata (B. serrata)

B. serrata is an ancient traditional plant that was used in the treatment of cough, asthma, and other inflammatory lung conditions. *B. serrata* and its abundant active ingredients downregulate pro-inflammatory cytokines, 5-lipoxygenase, and leukotriene [44, 45]. Boswellic acids and *B. serrata* extract inhibited human leukocyte elastase (HLE), the claimed agent of the pathogenesis of cystic fibrosis, chronic bronchitis, and emphysema [46–49]. Moreover, alpha-keto-beta-boswellic acids (AKBA) stimulated the production of anti-inflammatory LOX-isoform-selective modulators and inhibited 5-lipoxygenase [50]. *B. serrata* can help in pulmonary fibrosis, which is a common complication of SARS-CoV-2 infection [51]. It antagonized the effect of bleomycin-induced injury by reducing collagen accumulation and airway dysfunction in rats [52]. The anti-asthmatic potential of *B. serrata* was investigated in many studies [53–55]. Furthermore, boswellic acid and AKBA induced anti-platelet aggregation effect, anti-profibrotic mechanisms, and hastened vascular remodeling by the TGFβ1/Smad3 pathway [56, 57]. Immune modulation is a promising property of boswellic acids [58], which is an important element in SARS-CoV-2 treatment. In small doses, boswellic acids enhanced lymphocyte proliferation, while higher doses had a blocking action. Similarly, at the level of the humoral response, primary antibody titers were decreased at big doses of boswellic acids, but lower doses elevated secondary antibody titers. Boswellic acids stimulate the phagocytosis of macrophages, as well [47, 59–61]. The anti-viral property of *B. serrata* was strongly emphasized against many viruses. It inhibited wild-type and a clinical isolate of HSV-1 via downregulation of nuclear factor-κB (NF-κB) [62]. In another study, the total Boswellia extract exerted a more potent anti-herpes activity than other compounds [63]. HIV, HCV, and influenza [64]. In a computational study on *B. serrata* bioactive ligands (compounds) against SARS-CoV-2 Mpro protein. Among the examined compounds, euphane, ursane, α-amyrin, phytosterols, and 2,3-dihydroxyurs-12-en-28-oic acid were found to have the ability of Mpro inhibition [65]. A clinical trial investigated the effect of combined glycyrrhizin (GR) capsule (60 mg) and boswellic acids (BA) (200 mg) versus placebo twice daily for 14 days in 50 patients with moderate SARS-CoV-2 or COVID-19 variants hospitalized. The group of GR + BA showed a significant shorter cure time, amelioration of clinical condition, and decrease in CRB compared to the placebo group [66].

3.1.2 Pomegranate *(Punica granatum* L.*)*

It is an old fruit that is cultivated in many parts of the world. Its pharmacological activities are mediated mainly by phenolic compounds [67]. Anti-viral action is demonstrated against many viruses [25, 68, 69]. The immune modulation activity of pomegranate was illustrated in several studies. It inhibited phorbol-12-myristate 13-acetate plus calcium ionophore A23187 (PMACI) induced inflammatory gene expression and the release of interleukin (IL)-6 and IL-8 in the myeloid precursor cell line KU812 cells [70]. Pomegranate extract attenuated the activation of NF-κB/p65 in human chondrocyte by counteracting the IL-1β-mediated phosphorylation of IKKβ, expression of IKKβ mRNA, and degradation of IκBα [71]. In another *in vitro* study, pomegranate flower (PFE) ethanol extracts reduced IL-6, IL-1β, and TNF-α production in lipo-poly saccharides (LPS)-induced RAW264.7 macrophages [72]. Baricitinib is a janus kinase (JAK) inhibitor and is a numb-associated kinase (NAK) inhibitor that inhibits AP2-associated protein kinase-1 (AAK1), this protein enhances endocytosis of the virus [73, 74]. Pomegranate possessed a janus kinase inhibitory action. These findings encourage the use of pomegranate in SARS-CoV-2 treatment [75, 76]. The anti-SARS-CoV-2 activity of pomegranate was demonstrated by a computational study where ellagic acid, gallic acid and mainly punicalagin, punicalin interacted with SARS-CoV-2 spike glycoprotein, angiotensin-converting enzyme 2, furin and transmembrane serine protease2 [77]. Pomegranate peel extract interfered with the binding between SARS-CoV-2 spike glycoprotein and ACE2 receptor and showed a possible anti-replication action by inhibition of the virus 3-chymotrypsin-like cysteine protease

($3CL^{Pro}$) [78]. Moreover, anti-replication potential was demonstrated in tannins, which are pomegranate compounds via binding ($3CL^{Pro}$) catalytic site in a virtual study [79]. Triterpenoids, other pomegranate compounds blocked the spike protein binding site of SARS-CoV-2 [80]. Pomegranate was investigated with other herbs in 184 patients with SARS-CoV-2 infection plus standard care for 7 days. There was a significant reduction in hospital duration and improvement of clinical symptoms in comparison to 174 patients in the standard-care group [81].

3.1.3 Curcumin (*Curcuma longa*)

C. longa is known as turmeric, which is a common spice that was traditionally used to treat many health disorders. Curcumin, a secondary metabolite has a potent antioxidative, anti-inflammatory [82], and anti-viral activities [83, 84]. Which is mediated by its effect on multiple molecular targets and signaling pathways of apoptosis and inflammation. It inhibits viral replication by interfering with NF-κB, PI3K/Akt signaling, post-transcriptional, and post-translational modifications. Moreover, it blocks viral attachment [85–88]. In silico docking study, curcumin interacted with SARS-CoV-2 protease, spike glycoprotein-RBD, and PD-ACE2, receptors that are vital in virus infection [89]. Curcumin also showed attenuation ability to SARS-CoV-2 protease (Mpro) in another study [90]. Stimulation of innate immunity, and hence, IFN production at the early stage of SARS-CoV-2 infection was investigated to reduce the fatality rate of the diseases [91, 92]. Immune modulation activity of curcumin was demonstrated in PEDV model of coronavirus where viral reproduction was hindered after treatment with cationic carbon dots based on curcumin. This effect was mediated by the activation of the innate immunity with subsequent production of interferon-stimulating genes (ISGs) and cytokines (IL-8 and IL-6) [93]. In addition to the anti-viral action of curcumin, its anti-inflammatory and anti-fibrotic potentials provide some help in pulmonary damage. It reduced the expression of IFN-γ, MCP-1, IL-6, and IL-2, which are involved in lung inflammation and fibrosis [94]. Curcumin decreased collagen in experimental models of pulmonary fibrosis, as well [95]. Furthermore, curcumin reduced pulmonary edema in hypoxic rats via attenuation of NF-κB activity and stabilizing hypoxia-inducible factor 1-alpha (HIF1-α) [96]. Many clinical trials have investigated the possible efficacy of curcumin on SARS-CoV-2 patients. Two studies used nanocurcumin 40 mg in a dose of 2 soft gels twice daily for 2 weeks in mild to moderate patients compared with the placebo group. Curcumin improved the clinical symptoms with a significant lowering of CRP level, elevation of lymphocyte count [97], and shortened the hospital duration [98]. In addition, nanocurcumin significantly reduced IL-6, IL-1β gene expression when it was given to 20 patients with SARS-CoV-2 in comparison to 20 patients in the placebo group [99]. Nanocurcumin 80 mg in a dose of 2 soft gels twice daily was introduced to 40 patients with mild and severe SARS-CoV-2 for 21 days versus placebo. Curcumin decreased the count of Th17 cells and the level of IL-17, IL-21, IL-23, and GM-CSF [100]. In another study, there was an increase in Treg cells count, expression levels of FoxP3, IL-10, IL-35, TGF-β, and cytokines serum level in the Nanocurcumin-treated group compared to the placebo [101]. Treg cells maintain the balance between inflammatory and regulatory responses. Dysfunction of Treg cells and related cytokines leads to hyperinflammation in SARS-CoV-2 patients [102, 103]. A combination of piperine (2.5 mg) and curcumin (252 mg) was introduced to 70 mild to severe SARS-CoV-2 patients twice daily in comparison with probiotics given group for two weeks. Rapid cure, less deaths, and short hospital stays were achieved by curcumin therapy [104].

3.1.4 Glycyrrhizin (*Glycyrrhiza glabra*)

Glycyrrhizin is an active constituent isolated from *G. glabra L. (Fabaceae), (licorice)* root, a common medicinal plant that grows in Mediterranean areas [105]. It has abundant phytochemicals, flavonoids, and triterpenoids [106]. The anti-viral action of licorice is mediated mostly by two triterpenoids, glycyrrhizin, and 18β-glycyrrhetinic acid [105, 107]. Glycyrrhizin exhibited an anti-viral effect against RNA and DNA viruses by acting on casein kinase II, protein kinase II and transcription factors [108–110]. Interestingly, glycyrrhizin and licorice extract have the ability to block SARS-CoV-2 and cell entry [111, 112]. Moreover, it has the ability to decrease the expression of type 2 transmembrane serine proteases (TMPRSS2), and hence, interfere with the virus entry and stimulate mineralocorticoid receptor (MR), by decreasing ACE2 expression [113]. In addition, glycyrrhizin interferes with receptor-binding domain (RBD) of SARS-COV2 and ACE2 [114]. Glycyrrhizic acid (GA) nanoparticles inhibited murine coronavirus MHV-A59 replication and attenuated pro-inflammatory cytokine release caused by MHV-A59 or the N protein of SARS-CoV-2 [115]. Regarding immunomodulation activity, glycyrrhizin upregulated lymphocytic proliferation in viral infection [116] which may help to manage SARS-CoV-2 associated lymphopenia. Licorice extract in a dose-dependent manner, induced an immune modulation of cell-mediated and humeral responses [117]. The antioxidative and anti-inflammatory potentials of licorice can protect against acute lung injury by inhibition of NF-κB and can increase the expression of peroxisome proliferator-activated receptor gamma (PPAR-γ), which decreases the inflammatory response [118]. Glycyrrhetinic acid derivative, diammonium glycyrrhizinate combined with vitamin C improved the clinical symptoms in severe suspected COVID-19 patients [119]. A clinical trial recorded amelioration of clinical state in SARS-CoV-2 patients who received glycyrrhizin and boswellic acids combined therapy [66].

3.1.5 Nigella sativa (N. sativa)

N. sativa is known as black cumin seed, black seed, Habbatul Barakah [120]. Since ancient times, It was widely used in traditional medicine for the treatment of asthma, common cold, headache, nasal congestion, and rheumatic diseases [121]. The Holy Bible mentioned it as "Curative black seed." Prophet Muhammad (PBUH) said that "In the black cumin, there is a cure for every disease except death." [122–124]. Among several pharmacological effects, antioxidant, anti-inflammatory, anti-viral, anticoagulant, and immunomodulatory properties make *N. sativa* an appropriate therapeutic agent in SARS-CoV-2 management [123, 125, 126]. *In vitro* and molecular docking studies reported the anti-SARS-CoV-2 potential of many *N. sativa* compounds; thymohydroquinone and dithymoquinone [127, 128], nigellidine α-hederin [129] thymol and thymoquinone [130]. The immunomodulatory importance of *N. sativa* to overcome cytokine storm was highlighted in a docking study where nigellidine showed affinity to TNFR1, IL1R, and TNFR2 [131]. In a multicenter, placebo-controlled, randomized clinical trial honey (1 gm/Kg/day), and *N. sativa* seeds (80 mg/Kg/day) were administrated to moderate or severe SARS-CoV-2 patients versus placebo group for 13 days along with standard care. *N. sativa* and honey-treated patients showed significant symptoms alleviation, rapid viral clearance and a decrease in mortality compared to placebo [132]. In another clinical trial, *N. sativa* oil was administered in a dose of 500 mg twice daily for 10 days to 86 patients compared to 87 patients as a control. A significant higher percentage of recovered patients and shorter recovery time were observed in *N. sativa* treated group [133].

3.1.6 Thyme *(Thymus Vulgaris)*

Thymus vulgaris was commonly used for its flavoring and medicinal advantages for centuries [134]. Thyme contains variable flavonoids and phenolic antioxidants, such as zeaxanthin, lutein, pigenin, naringenin, luteolin, and thymonin. The anti-oxidant property of thyme is mainly attributed to thymol, a phenolic component [135]. Through its anti-viral potential, thyme attenuated the cytopathic effect of the influenza virus in a dose-dependent manner [136]. Thymol showed the ability of viral spike protein inhibition in a computational study [137]. Moreover, carvacrol, a monoterpenoid phenol of thyme oil blocked the attachment of SARS-CoV-2 spike (S) glycoprotein to the cell and inhibited the viral protease [138]. Furthermore, the essential oil of thyme improved the clinical symptoms and caused a significant rise in lymphocyte count and calcium level along with a lowering of neutrophil count and blood urea nitrogen (BUN) in SARS-COV-2 patients [139].

3.1.7 Ginger *(the rhizome of Zingiber officinale)*

Ginger has been widely used for thousand years due to its numerous benefits. It was recorded in Chinese, Roman and Arabic medical literature [140]. It is mentioned in Holy Quran as one of Heaven's drinks [141]. Ginger contains many active ingredients, terpene and phenolic are mainly responsible for its pharmacological activities [142, 143]. Ginger has anti-inflammatory, antioxidative, immunomodulatory, antimicrobial, anti-fungal, anticancer, hepatoprotective, antidiabetic, cardiovascular protective, respiratory protective, anti-obesity, anti-nausea, and anti-emetic activities [144]. Ginger also exhibits a direct anti-viral potential [145–147]. A molecular docking study defined the inhibitory effect of 8-gingerol, 10-gingerol, 6-gingerol, and another class of the ginger's ingredients on SARS-CoV-2-related papain-like protease (PLpro) such protease is vital for viral survival and replication [148–150]. In addition, 6-gingerol showed interaction with some SARS-CoV-2 proteins which are crucial for replication, such as protease, SARS-CoV3C-like molecule, and cathepsin K [151] 6-gingerol binds with S protein as well [152]. Another docking study reported the affinity of gingerol, geraniol, shogaol, zingiberene, zingiberenol, and zingerone to the SARS-CoV-2 MPro [153]. A clinical study demonstrated that consumption of Echinacea tablet with *Zingiber officinalis* improved the clinical symptoms in COVID-19 outpatients. There was an alleviation of cough, dyspnea, and muscle pain without recorded side effects [154]. Consumption of ginger with other herbs improved the disease outcomes in COVID-19 patients [155–157].

3.1.8 Saussurea costus (S. costus)

S. costus, is a perennial, aromatic plant that is native to the Himalayan region [158]. For centuries, S. *costus* was applied in folk medicine to treat numerous health disorders, mainly lung problems [159]. It is mentioned in Islamic literature. Prophet Muhammad (PBUH) said that "Treat with the Indian incense, for it has healing for seven diseases; it is to be sniffed by one having throat trouble and to be put into one side of the mouth of one suffering from pleurisy." [124] *S. costus* has a lot of ingredients the most effective are terpenes, anthraquinones, alkaloids, flavonoids, costunolide, and dehydrocostus lactone [160]. These compounds have a variety of pharmacological effects: antifungal activity anthelmintic, antidiabetic, antitumor, antimicrobial, immunostimulant, antiulcer, anti-inflammatory, and antihepatotoxic [161–167]. Moreover, the anti-viral activity recommended the use of *S. costus* to treat many viruses [160]. Silico with a molecular docking study reported that dehidrocostus lactone showed better binding potential with SARS-CoV-2 S protein than other compounds of *S.costus* [168]. An animal experiment showed that *S. costus* with *N. sativa* and honey induced a significant elevation of Th2, Th17 along with a rise in humoral immunity markers (TGF-β, sIgA,, IL-4, B-def, and IgG) in rat treated group versus placebo [169].

3.2 Cupping therapy

Cupping therapy (Al-Hijamah) is an ancient part of CAM that was widely practiced in the world and mentioned in every culture [170, 171]. It is mentioned in the book of medicine of Sahih Al-Bukhari where Prophet Muhammad (PBUH) stated that "If there is any healing in your medicines, then it is in cupping, a gulp of honey or branding with fire (cauterization), (one of three) according to that suits the ailment, but I do not like to be (cauterized) branded with fire." [124] Cupping therapy is a procedure where cups are placed on the skin and induce suction, hence, a negative pressure is created. This allows toxic substances to get out of the body [172]. There are a lot of types of cupping therapy, dry and wet cupping are the two main types [173]. Dry cupping is done without skin laceration, however, in wet cupping, the skin is scarified, so that blood is drawn into the cup [174]. Cupping therapy acts via many mechanisms, it elevates the level of endogenous opioids in the brain, hence, improves pain control with subsequent comfort and relaxation [175]. Other mechanism is to improve blood circulation and clear the blood from toxins substances [176]. This mechanism is mediated by the enhancement of microcirculation, angiogenesis, and capillary endothelial cell repair [172, 177]. Muscle relaxation and parasympathetic activity due to blood loss and vasodilation is other mechanisms [178]. A lot of studies reported the possible preventive and therapeutic advantages of cupping therapy in variable diseases, such as lung disorders, type 2 diabetes mellitus, autoimmune diseases, cardiac diseases, and chronic fatigue syndrome [179–183]. Cupping therapy is highly recommended in patients with COVID-19 infection for health improvement and to boost the sensation of well-being [184]. The Immunomodulation effect was recorded in 30 patients with rheumatoid arthritis when cupping therapy was combined with conventional therapy versus 20 patients who received conventional treatment only. NK-cell was significantly increased while soluble interleukin-2 receptor (SIL-2R) insignificantly lowered after combined treatment [181]. In a randomized controlled trial, cupping therapy increased the arterial O_2 saturation when applied to smokers and enhanced breathing after 12 hours of application [185]. Cupping therapy and acupuncture helped in ameliorating the clinical severity in a case of COVID pneumonia and relieved the complications of respiratory disorders [186]. In a clinical study, warm cupping of the posterior thorax was applied with conventional treatments for 7 days in 8 patients who suffered from COVID-19 with acute respiratory destress syndrome (ARDS). Improvement of the symptoms severity scores was reported in all patients who were discharged without the need for mechanical ventilation [187].

3.3 Acupuncture

Acupuncture is a type of traditional Chinese medicine. It is commonly used in the treatment of respiratory diseases [188, 189]. Acupuncture is supposed to be an effective agent in treating the breathlessness of chronic obstructive pulmonary diseases (COPD) [190]. This encourages its utility to improve dyspnea and enhance the quality of life in COVID-19 patients [191]. Headache is a common symptom of COVID-19 infection. Acupuncture is widely used in pain and headache treatment [192, 193]. In China, it was added to COVID-19 patients' routine regimens [194]. Acupuncture-induced analgesia through opioid peptides and dopamine receptors. Where acupuncture activates dopamine and β-endorphin, which in turn downregulates cytokine production via type 1 dopamine receptors, so inhibit systemic inflammation [195–198]. This effect may help in the cytokine storm of COVID-19 infection. Despite having good potential for COVID-19 treatment, there is not enough high-quality evidence to support acupuncture [199].

4. Conclusion

Based on the previous studies, complementary and alternative remedies are needed to potentiate the effect of standard therapy and prophylaxis in COVID-19 patients. This will alleviate the symptoms, boost immunity and induce the sensation of well-being, especially in patients who are not eligible for the vaccines.

Acknowledgements

Gratitude and praise to God who sprouted man and plants from the earth to benefit each other.

Author details

Sally Elnawasany[1,2]

1 Tanta University, Egypt

2 AL-Rayan Collages, KSA

*Address all correspondence to: elnawasany_s@hotmail.com

References

[1] WHO CO. World health organization. Responding to community spread of COVID-19. Interim Guidance 7 March. Mar 2020:1-6

[2] Lam CS, Koon HK, Chung VC-H, Cheung YT. A public survey of traditional, complementary and integrative medicine use during the COVID-19 outbreak in Hong Kong. PLoS One. 2021;**16**(7):e0253890

[3] Liu X, Zhang M, He L, Li Y. Chinese herbs combined with Western medicine for severe acute respiratory syndrome (SARS). Cochrane Database Syst Rev. 17 Oct 2012;**10**(10):CD004882 (pp. 1-49). DOI: 10.1002/14651858.CD004882.pub3. PMID: 23076910; PMCID: PMC6993561

[4] Arora R, Chawla R, Marwah R, Arora P, Sharma R, Kaushik V, et al. Potential of complementary and alternative medicine in preventive management of novel H1N1 flu (swine flu) pandemic: Thwarting potential disasters in the bud. Evidence- Based Complementary and Alternative Medicine. ID 586506, pp. 16. DOI: 10.1155/2011/586506

[5] Fan AY, Gu S, Alemi SF. Chinese herbal medicine for COVID-19: Current evidence with systematic review and meta-analysis. Journal of Integrative Medicine. 2020;**18**(5):385-394

[6] Liu M, Gao Y, Yuan Y, Yang K, Shi S, Zhang J, et al. Efficacy and safety of integrated traditional Chinese and western medicine for corona virus disease 2019 (COVID-19): A systematic review and meta-analysis. Pharmacological Research. 2020;**158**:104896

[7] Xiong X, Wang P, Su K, Cho WC, Xing Y. Chinese herbal medicine for coronavirus disease 2019: A systematic review and meta-analysis. Pharmacological Research. 2020;**160**:105056

[8] Ng JY. Global research trends at the intersection of coronavirus disease 2019 (COVID-19) and traditional, integrative, and complementary and alternative medicine: A bibliometric analysis. BMC Complementary Medicine and Therapies. 2020;**20**(1):1-9

[9] Malik YS, Sircar S, Bhat S, Sharun K, Dhama K, Dadar M, et al. Emerging novel coronavirus (2019-nCoV)—Current scenario, evolutionary perspective based on genome analysis and recent developments. Veterinary Quarterly. 2020;**40**(1):68-76

[10] Dhama K, Khan S, Tiwari R, Sircar S, Bhat S, Malik YS, et al. Coronavirus disease 2019–COVID-19. Clinical Microbiology Reviews. 2020;**33**(4): e00028-e00020

[11] Hu B, Guo H, Zhou P, Shi Z-L. Characteristics of SARS-CoV-2 and COVID-19. Nature Reviews Microbiology. 2021;**19**(3):141-154

[12] Chilamakuri R, Agarwal S. COVID-19: characteristics and therapeutics. Cells. Jan 21, 2021;**10**(2):206

[13] Peng Q, Peng R, Yuan B, Zhao J, Wang M, Wang X, et al. Structural and biochemical characterization of the nsp12-nsp7-nsp8 core polymerase complex from SARS-CoV-2. Cell Reports. 2020;**31**(11):107774

[14] Kumar R, Verma H, Singhvi N, Sood U, Gupta V, Singh M, et al. Comparative genomic analysis of rapidly evolving SARS-CoV-2 reveals mosaic pattern of phylogeographical

distribution. mSystems. 2020;**5**:e00505-e00520

[15] Gorkhali R, Koirala P, Rijal S, Mainali A, Baral A, Bhattarai HK. Structure and function of major SARS-CoV-2 and SARS-CoV proteins. Bioinformatics and Biology Insights. 2021;**15**:11779322211025876

[16] Cui J, Li F, Shi Z-L. Origin and evolution of pathogenic coronaviruses. Nature Reviews Microbiology. 2019;**17**(3):181-192

[17] Aldaais EA, Yegnaswamy S, Albahrani F, Alsowaiket F, Alramadan S. Sequence and structural analysis of COVID-19 E and M proteins with MERS virus E and M proteins—A comparative study. Biochemistry and Biophysics Reports. 2021;**26**:101023

[18] Gusev E, Sarapultsev A, Solomatina L, Chereshnev V. SARS-CoV-2-specific immune response and the pathogenesis of COVID-19. International Journal of Molecular Sciences. 2022;**23**(3):1716

[19] Okamoto M, Tsukamoto H, Kouwaki T, Seya T, Oshiumi H. Recognition of viral RNA by pattern recognition receptors in the induction of innate immunity and excessive inflammation during respiratory viral infections. Viral Immunology. 2017;**30**(6):408-420

[20] Renner K, Schwittay T, Chaabane S, Gottschling J, Müller C, Tiefenböck C, et al. Severe T cell hyporeactivity in ventilated COVID-19 patients correlates with prolonged virus persistence and poor outcomes. Nature Communications. 2021;**12**(1):1-11

[21] Huang S-W, Wang S-F. SARS-CoV-2 entry related viral and host genetic variations: Implications on COVID-19 severity, immune escape, and infectivity. International Journal of Molecular Sciences. 2021;**22**(6):3060

[22] Santacroce L, Charitos IA, Carretta DM, De Nitto E, Lovero R. The human coronaviruses (HCoVs) and the molecular mechanisms of SARS-CoV-2 infection. Journal of Molecular Medicine. 2021;**99**(1):93-106

[23] Jiang C, Li X, Ge C, Ding Y, Zhang T, Cao S, et al. Molecular detection of SARS-CoV-2 being challenged by virus variation and asymptomatic infection. Journal of Pharmaceutical Analysis. 2021;**11**(3):257-264

[24] Harvey WT, Carabelli AM, Jackson B, Gupta RK, Thomson EC, Harrison EM, et al. SARS-CoV-2 variants, spike mutations and immune escape. Nature Reviews Microbiology. 2021;**19**(7):409-424

[25] Elnawasany S. Could Pomegranate Fight against SARS-CoV-2? Pomegranate. London, UK: IntechOpen; 2021

[26] Wang X, Cao R, Zhang H, Liu J, Xu M, Hu H, et al. The anti-influenza virus drug, arbidol is an efficient inhibitor of SARS-CoV-2 in vitro. Cell Discovery. 2020;**6**(1):1-5

[27] Zhu Z, Lu Z, Xu T, Chen C, Yang G, Zha T, et al. Arbidol monotherapy is superior to lopinavir/ritonavir in treating COVID-19. Journal of Infection. 2020;**81**(1):e21-ee3

[28] Monteil V, Kwon H, Prado P, Hagelkrüys A, Wimmer RA, Stahl M, et al. Inhibition of SARS-CoV-2 infections in engineered human tissues using clinical-grade soluble human ACE2. Cell. 2020;**181**(4):905-13.e7

[29] Tian X, Li C, Huang A, Xia S, Lu S, Shi Z, et al. Potent binding of 2019 novel coronavirus spike protein by a SARS

coronavirus-specific human monoclonal antibody. Emerging Microbes & Infections. 2020;**9**(1):382-385

[30] Wang M, Cao R, Zhang L, Yang X, Liu J, Xu M, et al. Remdesivir and chloroquine effectively inhibit the recently emerged novel coronavirus (2019-nCoV) in vitro. Cell Research. 2020;**30**(3):269-271

[31] Agrawal U, Raju R, Udwadia ZF. Favipiravir: A new and emerging antiviral option in COVID-19. Medical Journal Armed Forces India. 2020;**76**(4):370-376

[32] Chen Y-K, Huang Y-Q, Tang S-Q, Xu X-L, Zeng Y-M, He X-Q, et al. Comparative effectiveness and safety of ribavirin plus interferon-alpha, lopinavir/ritonavir plus interferon-alpha and ribavirin plus lopinavir/ritonavir plus interferon-alpha in patients with mild to moderate novel coronavirus pneumonia: Results of a randomized, open-labeled prospective study. 2020. Available at SSRN: https://ssrn.com/abstract=3576905 or http://dx.doi.org/10.2139/ssrn.3576905

[33] Ahmed MH, Hassan A. Dexamethasone for the treatment of coronavirus disease (COVID-19): A review. SN Comprehensive Clinical Medicine. 2020;**2**(12):2637-2646

[34] Xu X, Han M, Li T, Sun W, Wang D, Fu B, et al. Effective treatment of severe COVID-19 patients with tocilizumab. Proceedings of the National Academy of Sciences. 2020;**117**(20):10970-10975

[35] Alzghari SK, Acuña VS. Supportive treatment with tocilizumab for COVID-19: A systematic review. Journal of Clinical Virology. 2020;**127**:104380

[36] Diurno F, Numis F, Porta G, Cirillo F, Maddaluno S, Ragozzino A, et al. Eculizumab treatment in patients with COVID-19: Preliminary results from real life ASL Napoli 2 Nord experience. European Review for Medical and Pharmacological Sciences. 2020;**24**(7):4040-4047

[37] Stockman LJ, Bellamy R, Garner P. SARS: Systematic review of treatment effects. PLoS Medicine. 2006;**3**(9):e343

[38] Mantlo E, Bukreyeva N, Maruyama J, Paessler S, Huang C. Antiviral activities of type I interferons to SARS-CoV-2 infection. Antiviral Research. 2020;**179**:104811

[39] Jorgensen SC, Tse CL, Burry L, Dresser LD. Baricitinib: A review of pharmacology, safety, and emerging clinical experience in COVID-19. Pharmacotherapy: The Journal of Human Pharmacology and Drug Therapy. 2020;**40**(8):843-856

[40] Mulgaonkar N, Wang H, Mallawarachchi S, Ruzek D, Martina B, Fernando S. Bcr-Abl tyrosine kinase inhibitor imatinib as a potential drug for COVID-19. BioRxiv. 2020. DOI: 10.1101/2020.06.18.158196

[41] Cohn BA, Cirillo PM, Murphy CC, Krigbaum NY, Wallace AW. SARS-CoV-2 vaccine protection and deaths among US veterans during 2021. Science. 2022;**375**(6578):331-336

[42] Salvagno GL, Henry BM, Pighi L, De Nitto S, Gianfilippi G, Lippi G. The pronounced decline of anti-SARS-CoV-2 spike trimeric IgG and RBD IgG in baseline seronegative individuals six months after BNT162b2 vaccination is consistent with the need for vaccine boosters. Clinical Chemistry and Laboratory Medicine (CCLM). 2022;**60**(2):e29-e31

[43] Klompas M. Understanding breakthrough infections following mRNA SARS-CoV-2 vaccination. Journal

of the American Medical Association. 2021;**326**(20):2018-2020

[44] Ammon H, Mack T, Singh G, Safayhi H. Inhibition of leukotriene B4 formation in rat peritoneal neutrophils by an ethanolic extract of the gum resin exudate of Boswellia serrata. Planta medica. 1991;**57**(03):203-207

[45] Rashan L, Hakkim FL, Idrees M, Essa M, Velusamy T, Al-Baloshi M, et al. Boswellia gum resin and essential oils: Potential health benefits– an evidence based review. International Journal of Nutrition, Pharmacology, Neurological Diseases. 2019;**9**(2):53-71

[46] Safayhi H, Rall B, Sailer E-R, Ammon HPT. Inhibition by boswellic acids of human leukocyte elastase. Journal of Pharmacology and Experimental Therapeutics. 1997;**281**(1):460-463

[47] Siddiqui M. Boswellia serrata, a potential antiinflammatory agent: An overview. Indian Journal of Pharmaceutical Sciences. 2011;**73**(3):255

[48] Zhang Y, Yu Y-l, Tian H, Bai R-y, Bi Y-N, Yuan X-M, et al. Evaluation of anti-inflammatory activities of a triterpene β-elemonic acid in frankincense in vivo and in vitro. Molecules. 2019;**24**(6):1187

[49] Roy NK, Parama D, Banik K, Bordoloi D, Devi AK, Thakur KK, et al. An update on pharmacological potential of boswellic acids against chronic diseases. International Journal of Molecular Sciences. 2019;**20**(17):4101

[50] Gilbert NC, Gerstmeier J, Schexnaydre EE, Börner F, Garscha U, Neau DB, et al. Structural and mechanistic insights into 5-lipoxygenase inhibition by natural products. Nature Chemical Biology. 2020;**16**(7):783-790

[51] Rodriguez-Morales AJ, Cardona-Ospina JA, Gutiérrez-Ocampo E, Villamizar-Peña R, Holguin-Rivera Y, Escalera-Antezana JP, et al. Clinical, laboratory and imaging features of COVID-19: A systematic review and meta-analysis. Travel Medicine and Infectious Disease. 2020;**34**:101623

[52] Ali EN, Mansour SZ. Boswellic acids extract attenuates pulmonary fibrosis induced by bleomycin and oxidative stress from gamma irradiation in rats. Chinese Medicine. 2011;**6**(1):1-14

[53] Gupta I, Gupta V, Parihar A, Gupta S, Lüdtke R, Safayhi H, et al. Effects of Boswellia serrata gum resin in patients with bronchial asthma: Results of a double-blind, placebo-controlled, 6-week clinical study. European Journal of Medical Research. 1998;**3**(11):511-514

[54] Houssen ME, Ragab A, Mesbah A, El-Samanoudy AZ, Othman G, Moustafa AF, et al. Natural anti-inflammatory products and leukotriene inhibitors as complementary therapy for bronchial asthma. Clinical Biochemistry. 2010;**43**(10-11):887-890

[55] Al-Jawad FH, Al-Razzuqi RA, Hashim HM, Al-Bayati NJ. Glycyrrhiza glabra versus Boswellia carterii in chronic bronchial asthma: A comparative study of efficacy. Indian Journal of Allergy, Asthma and Immunology. 2012;**26**(1):6

[56] Tawfik MK. Anti-aggregatory effect of boswellic acid in high-fat fed rats: Involvement of redox and inflammatory cascades. Archives of Medical Science. 2016;**12**(6):1354-1361

[57] Shang P, Liu W, Liu T, Zhang Y, Mu F, Zhu Z, et al. Acetyl-11-keto-β-boswellic acid attenuates prooxidant and profibrotic mechanisms involving transforming growth factor-β1, and improves vascular remodeling in

spontaneously hypertensive rats. Scientific Reports. 2016;**6**(1):1-12

[58] Badria FA, Mikhaeil BR, Maatooq GT, Amer MM. Immunomodulatory triterpenoids from the oleogum resin of Boswellia carterii Birdwood. Zeitschrift für Naturforschung C. 2003;**58**(7-8):505-516

[59] Mikhaeil BR, Maatooq GT, Badria FA, Amer MM. Chemistry and immunomodulatory activity of frankincense oil. Zeitschrift für Naturforschung C. 2003;**58**(3-4):230-238

[60] Pungle P, Banavalikar M, Suthar A, Biyani M, Mengi S. Immunomodulatory activity of boswellic acids of Boswellia serrata Roxb. Indian Journal of Experimental Biology. Dec 2003;**41**(12):1460-1462. PMID: 15320503

[61] Ammon H. Modulation of the immune system by Boswellia serrata extracts and boswellic acids. Phytomedicine. 2010;**17**(11):862-867

[62] Goswami D, Mahapatra AD, Banerjee S, Kar A, Ojha D, Mukherjee PK, et al. Boswellia serrata oleo-gum-resin and β-boswellic acid inhibits HSV-1 infection in vitro through modulation of NF-κB and p38 MAP kinase signaling. Phytomedicine. 2018;**51**:94-103

[63] Badria FA, Abu-Karam M, Mikhaeil BR, Maatooq GT, Amer M. Anti-herpes activity of isolated compounds from frankincense. Biosciences Biotechnology Research Asia. 2016;**1**(1):1-10

[64] Xiao S, Tian Z, Wang Y, Si L, Zhang L, Zhou D. Recent progress in the antiviral activity and mechanism study of pentacyclic triterpenoids and their derivatives. Medicinal Research Reviews. 2018;**38**(3):951-976

[65] Roy A, Menon T. Evaluation of bioactive compounds from Boswellia serrata against SARS-CoV-2. Vegetos. 2022;**35**(2):404-414

[66] Gomaa AA, Mohamed HS, Abd-Ellatief RB, Gomaa MA, Hammam DS. Advancing combination treatment with glycyrrhizin and boswellic acids for hospitalized patients with moderate COVID-19 infection: A randomized clinical trial. Inflammopharmacology. 2022;**30**(2):477-486

[67] Ismail T, Akhtar S, Riaz M. Pomegranate peel and fruit extracts: A novel approach to avert degenerative disorders–pomegranate and degenerative diseases. In: Shekhar US, Howlader ZH, Kabir Y (Ed.). Exploring the Nutrition and Health Benefits of Functional Foods. Hershey, PA: IGI Global; 2017. pp. 165-184

[68] Howell AB, D'Souza DH. The pomegranate: effects on bacteria and viruses that influence human health. Evidence-Based Complementary and Alternative Medicine. Oct 2013. pp. 11, Article ID 606212. DOI: 10.1155/2013/606212

[69] Elnawasany S. Clinical Applications of Pomegranate. Breeding and Health Benefits of Fruit and Nut Crops. Nov 5, 2018. pp. 127-148

[70] Rasheed Z, Akhtar N, Anbazhagan AN, Ramamurthy S, Shukla M, Haqqi TM. Polyphenol-rich pomegranate fruit extract (POMx) suppresses PMACI-induced expression of pro-inflammatory cytokines by inhibiting the activation of MAP kinases and NF-κB in human KU812 cells. Journal of Inflammation. 2009;**6**(1):1-12

[71] Haseeb A, Khan NM, Ashruf OS, Haqqi TM. A polyphenol-rich pomegranate fruit extract suppresses NF-κB and IL-6 expression by blocking the activation of IKKβ

and NIK in primary human chondrocytes. Phytotherapy Research. 2017;**31**(5):778-782

[72] Xu J, Zhao Y, Aisa HA. Anti-inflammatory effect of pomegranate flower in lipopolysaccharide (LPS)-stimulated RAW264. 7 macrophages. Pharmaceutical Biology. 2017;**55**(1):2095-2101

[73] Stebbing J, Phelan A, Griffin I, Tucker C, Oechsle O, Smith D, et al. COVID-19: Combining antiviral and anti-inflammatory treatments. The Lancet Infectious Diseases. 2020;**20**(4):400-402

[74] Richardson P, Griffin I, Tucker C, Smith D, Oechsle O, Phelan A, et al. Baricitinib as potential treatment for 2019-nCoV acute respiratory disease. Lancet (London, England). 2020;**395**(10223):e30

[75] Sarithamol S, Pushpa V, Manoj K. Comparative study on Janus kinase enzyme activity of pomegranate leaf extract and its active component Ellagic acid for asthma. Oriental Journal of Chemistry. 2018;**34**(2):1041

[76] Martin H, Burgess EJ, Smith WA, McGhie TK, Cooney JM, Lunken RC, et al. JAK2 and AMP-kinase inhibition in vitro by food extracts, fractions and purified phytochemicals. Food & Function. 2015;**6**(1):304-311

[77] Frank B, Conzelmann C, Weil T, Groß R, Jungke P, Eggers M, et al. Antiviral activity of plant juices and green tea against SARS-CoV-2 and influenza virus *in vitro. bioRxiv [Preprint]*. 2020. DOI: 10.1101/2020.10.30.360545

[78] Tito A, Colantuono A, Pirone L, Pedone E, Intartaglia D, Giamundo G, et al. Pomegranate peel extract as an inhibitor of SARS-CoV-2 spike binding to human ACE2 receptor (in vitro): A promising source of novel antiviral drugs. Frontiers in Chemistry. 2021;**9**:638187

[79] Khalifa I, Zhu W, Mohammed HHH, Dutta K, Li C. Tannins inhibit SARS-CoV-2 through binding with catalytic dyad residues of 3CLpro: An in silico approach with 19 structural different hydrolysable tannins. Journal of Food Biochemistry. 2020;**44**(10):e13432

[80] Gowtham HG, Monu DO, Ajay Y, Gourav C, Vasantharaja R, Bhani K, et al. Exploring structurally diverse plant secondary metabolites as a potential source of drug targeting different molecular mechanisms of Severe Acute Respiratory Syndrome Coronavirus-2 (SARS-CoV-2) pathogenesis: An in silico approach. Scientific Reports 2020;**2**:1-38. DOI: 10.21203/rs.3.rs-27313/v1

[81] Karimi M, Zarei A, Soleymani S, Jamalimoghadamsiahkali S, Asadi A, Shati M, et al. Efficacy of Persian medicine herbal formulations (capsules and decoction) compared to standard care in patients with COVID-19, a multicenter open-labeled, randomized, controlled clinical trial. Phytotherapy Research. 2021;**35**(11):6295-6309

[82] Padmanaban G, Nagaraj VA. Curcumin from turmeric as an adjunct drug? Studies in Natural Products Chemistry. 2018;**57**:179-202

[83] Yang M, Lee G, Si J, Lee S-J, You HJ, Ko G. Curcumin shows antiviral properties against norovirus. Molecules. 2016;**21**(10):1401

[84] Hesari A, Ghasemi F, Salarinia R, Biglari H, Tabar Molla Hassan A, Abdoli V, et al. Effects of curcumin on NF-κB, AP-1, and Wnt/β-catenin signaling pathway in hepatitis B virus infection. Journal of Cellular Biochemistry. 2018;**119**(10):7898-7904

[85] Vajragupta O, Boonchoong P, Morris GM, Olson AJ. Active site binding modes of curcumin in HIV-1 protease and integrase. Bioorganic & medicinal chemistry letters. Jul 15, 2005;**15**(14):3364-3368

[86] Mathew D, Hsu W-L. Antiviral potential of curcumin. Journal of Functional Foods. 2018;**40**:692-699

[87] Praditya D, Kirchhoff L, Brüning J, Rachmawati H, Steinmann J, Steinmann E. Anti-infective properties of the golden spice curcumin. Frontiers in Microbiology. 2019;**10**:912

[88] Colpitts CC, Schang LM, Rachmawati H, Frentzen A, Pfaender S, Behrendt P, et al. Turmeric curcumin inhibits entry of all hepatitis C virus genotypes into human liver cells. Gut. 1 Jul 2014;**63**(7):1137-1149

[89] Utomo RY, Ikawati M, Meiyanto E. Revealing the Potency of Citrus and Galangal Constituents to Halt SARS-CoV-2 Infection. Preprints. Org. 2020;**2**:1-8

[90] Khaerunnisa S, Kurniawan H, Awaluddin R, Suhartati S, Soetjipto S. Potential inhibitor of COVID-19 main protease (Mpro) from several medicinal plant compounds by molecular docking study. Preprint. 2020;**2020**:2020030226

[91] Kumaki Y, Salazar AM, Wandersee MK, Barnard DL. Prophylactic and therapeutic intranasal administration with an immunomodulator, Hiltonol (poly IC: LC), in a lethal SARS-CoV-infected BALB/c mouse model. Antiviral Research. 2017;**139**:1-12

[92] Zhao J, Wohlford-Lenane C, Zhao J, Fleming E, Lane TE, McCray PB Jr, et al. Intranasal treatment with poly (I· C) protects aged mice from lethal respiratory virus infections. Journal of Virology. 2012;**86**(21):11416-11424

[93] Ting D, Dong N, Fang L, Lu J, Bi J, Xiao S, et al. Multisite inhibitors for enteric coronavirus: Antiviral cationic carbon dots based on curcumin. ACS Applied Nano Materials. 2018;**1**(10):5451-5459

[94] Avasarala S, Zhang F, Liu G, Wang R, London SD, London L. Curcumin modulates the inflammatory response and inhibits subsequent fibrosis in a mouse model of viral-induced acute respiratory distress syndrome. PLoS One. 2013;**8**(2):e57285

[95] Chen B, Zhang D-P, Gao W. Effect of curcumin on the expression of collagen type I protein and transforming growth factor-beta1 mRNA in pulmonary fibrosis rats. Zhonghua lao dong wei sheng zhi ye bing za zhi= Zhonghua laodong weisheng zhiyebing zazhi= Chinese Journal of Industrial Hygiene and Occupational Diseases. 2008;**26**(5):257-261

[96] Sagi S, Mathew T, Patir H. Prophylactic administration of curcumin abates the incidence of hypobaric hypoxia induced pulmonary edema in rats: a molecular approach. Journal of Pulmonary and Respiratory Medicine. 2014;**4**(1): pp.1000164, 12 pages

[97] Ahmadi R, Salari S, Sharifi MD, Reihani H, Rostamiani MB, Behmadi M, et al. Oral nano-curcumin formulation efficacy in the management of mild to moderate outpatient COVID-19: A randomized triple-blind placebo-controlled clinical trial. Food Science & Nutrition. 2021;**9**(8):4068-4075

[98] Saber-Moghaddam N, Salari S, Hejazi S, Amini M, Taherzadeh Z, Eslami S, et al. Oral nano-curcumin formulation efficacy in management of mild to moderate hospitalized coronavirus disease-19 patients: An open label nonrandomized clinical trial. Phytotherapy Research. 2021;**35**(5):2616-2623

[99] Valizadeh H, Abdolmohammadi-Vahid S, Danshina S, Gencer MZ, Ammari A, Sadeghi A, et al. Nano-curcumin therapy, a promising method in modulating inflammatory cytokines in COVID-19 patients. International Immunopharmacology. 2020;**89**:107088

[100] Tahmasebi S, El-Esawi MA, Mahmoud ZH, Timoshin A, Valizadeh H, Roshangar L, et al. Immunomodulatory effects of Nanocurcumin on Th17 cell responses in mild and severe COVID-19 patients. Journal of Cellular Physiology. 2021;**236**(7):5325-5338

[101] Tahmasebi S, Saeed BQ, Temirgalieva E, Yumashev AV, El-Esawi MA, Navashenaq JG, et al. Nanocurcumin improves Treg cell responses in patients with mild and severe SARS-CoV2. Life Sciences. 2021;**276**:119437

[102] Chen G, Wu D, Guo W, Cao Y, Huang D, Wang H, et al. Clinical and immunological features of severe and moderate coronavirus disease 2019. The Journal of Clinical Investigation. 2020;**130**(5):2620-2629

[103] Qin C, Zhou L, Hu Z, Zhang S, Yang S, Tao Y, et al. Dysregulation of immune response in patients with coronavirus 2019 (COVID-19) in Wuhan, China. Clinical Infectious Diseases. 2020;**71**(15):762-768

[104] Pawar KS, Mastud RN, Pawar SK, Pawar SS, Bhoite RR, Bhoite RR, et al. Oral curcumin with piperine as adjuvant therapy for the treatment of COVID-19: a randomized clinical trial. Frontiers in pharmacology. 2021:1056-1063

[105] Pastorino G, Cornara L, Soares S, Rodrigues F, Oliveira MBP. Liquorice (Glycyrrhiza glabra): A phytochemical and pharmacological review. Phytotherapy Research. 2018;**32**(12):2323-2339

[106] Li W, Asada Y, Yoshikawa T. Flavonoid constituents from Glycyrrhiza glabra hairy root cultures. Phytochemistry. 2000;**55**(5):447-456

[107] Wang H-L, Li Y-X, Niu Y-T, Zheng J, Wu J, Shi G-J, et al. Observing anti-inflammatory and anti-nociceptive activities of glycyrrhizin through regulating COX-2 and pro-inflammatory cytokines expressions in mice. Inflammation. 2015;**38**(6):2269-2278

[108] Fiore C, Eisenhut M, Krausse R, Ragazzi E, Pellati D, Armanini D, et al. Antiviral effects of Glycyrrhiza species. Phytotherapy Research: An International Journal Devoted to Pharmacological and Toxicological Evaluation of Natural Product Derivatives. 2008;**22**(2):141-148

[109] Batiha GE-S, Beshbishy AM, El-Mleeh A, Abdel-Daim MM, Devkota HP. Traditional uses, bioactive chemical constituents, and pharmacological and toxicological activities of Glycyrrhiza glabra L. (Fabaceae). Biomolecules. 2020;**10**(3):352-471

[110] Baltina L, Kondratenko R, Plyasunova O, Pokrovskii A, Tolstikov G. Prospects for the creation of new antiviral drugs based on glycyrrhizic acid and its derivatives (a review). Pharmaceutical Chemistry Journal. 2009;**43**(10):539-548

[111] Zhang L, Liu Y. Potential interventions for novel coronavirus in China: A systematic review. Journal of Medical Virology. 2020;**92**(5):479-490

[112] Luo P, Liu D, Li J. Pharmacological perspective: Glycyrrhizin may be an efficacious therapeutic agent for COVID-19. International Journal of Antimicrobial Agents. 2020;**55**(6):105995

[113] Murck H. Symptomatic protective action of glycyrrhizin (licorice) in COVID-19 infection? Frontiers in Immunology. 2020;**11**:1239

[114] Yu S, Zhu Y, Xu J, Yao G, Zhang P, Wang M, et al. Glycyrrhizic acid exerts inhibitory activity against the spike protein of SARS-CoV-2. Phytomedicine. 2021;**85**:153364

[115] Zhao Z, Xiao Y, Xu L, Liu Y, Jiang G, Wang W, et al. Glycyrrhizic acid nanoparticles as antiviral and anti-inflammatory agents for COVID-19 treatment. ACS Applied Materials & Interfaces. 2021;**13**(18):20995-21006

[116] Soufy H, Yassein S, Ahmed AR, Khodier MH, Kutkat MA, Nasr SM, et al. Antiviral and immune stimulant activities of glycyrrhizin against duck hepatitis virus. African Journal of Traditional, Complementary and Alternative Medicines. 2012;**9**(3):389-395

[117] Hussain K, Iqbal Z, Zahid Abbas R, Kasib Khan M, Kashif SM. Immunomodulatory activity of Glycyrrhiza glabra extract against mixed Eimeria infection in chickens. International Journal of Agriculture and Biology. 2017;**19**(4):928-932

[118] Zhang W, Wang G, Zhou S. Protective effects of isoliquiritigenin on LPS-induced acute lung injury by activating PPAR-γ. Inflammation. 2018;**41**(4):1290-1296

[119] Ding H, Deng W, Ding L, Ye X, Yin S, Huang W. Glycyrrhetinic acid and its derivatives as potential alternative medicine to relieve symptoms in nonhospitalized COVID-19 patients. Journal of Medical Virology. 2020;**92**(10):2200-2204

[120] AlAttas SA, Fat'heya MZ, Turkistany SA. Nigella sativa and its active constituent thymoquinone in oral health. Saudi Medical Journal. 2016;**37**(3):235

[121] Mollazadeh H, Afshari AR, Hosseinzadeh H. Review on the potential therapeutic roles of nigella sativa in the treatment of patients with cancer: Involvement of apoptosis:- black cumin and cancer. Journal of Pharmacopuncture. 2017;**20**(3):158

[122] Khan MA. Thymoquinone, a constituent of prophetic medicine-black seed, is a miracle therapeutic molecule against multiple diseases. International Journal of Health Sciences. 2019;**13**(1):1

[123] Maideen NMP. Prophetic medicine-nigella Sativa (black cumin seeds)–potential herb for COVID-19? Journal of Pharmacopuncture. 2020;**23**(2):62

[124] Khan MM. The Translation of the Meanings of Sahih Al-Bukhari (Arabic---English). Vol. 7. Kingdom of Saudi Arabia: Darussalam Publishers and Distributors: Riyadh; 1997

[125] Gholamnezhad Z, Havakhah S, Boskabady MH. Preclinical and clinical effects of Nigella sativa and its constituent, thymoquinone: A review. Journal of Ethnopharmacology. 2016;**190**:372-386

[126] Haq A, Lobo PI, Al-Tufail M, Rama NR, Al-Sedairy ST. Immunomodulatory effect of Nigella sativa proteins fractionated by ion exchange chromatography. International journal of immunopharmacology. Apr 1, 1999;**21**(4):283-295

[127] Esharkawy ER, Almalki F, Hadda TB. In vitro potential antiviral SARS-CoV-19-activity of natural product thymohydroquinone and dithymoquinone from Nigella sativa. Bioorganic Chemistry. 2022;**120**:105587

[128] Ahmad S, Abbasi HW, Shahid S, Gul S, Abbasi SW. Molecular docking, simulation and MM-PBSA studies of nigella sativa compounds: A computational quest to identify potential natural antiviral for COVID-19 treatment. Journal of Biomolecular Structure and Dynamics. 2021;**39**(12):4225-4233

[129] Bouchentouf S, Missoum N. Identification of Compounds from Nigella Sativa as New Potential Inhibitors of 2019 Novel Coronasvirus (Covid-19): Molecular Docking Study. 2020. DOI: 10.20944/preprints202004.0079.v1

[130] Shaikh YI, Shaikh VS, Ahmed K, Nazeruddin GM, Pathan HM. The revelation of various compounds found in Nigella sativa L.(black cumin) and their possibility to inhibit COVID-19 infection based on the molecular docking and physical properties. Engineered Science. 2020;**11**(2):31-35

[131] Maiti S, Banerjee A, Nazmeen A, Kanwar M, Das S. Active-site Molecular docking of Nigellidine to nucleocapsid/ Nsp2/Nsp3/M Pro of COVID-19 and to human IL1R and TNFR1/2 may stop viral-growth/cytokine-flood, and the drug source *Nigella sativa* (black cumin) seeds show potent antioxidant role. Research Square. DOI: 10.21203/rs.3.rs-26464/v1

[132] Ashraf S, Ashraf S, Ashraf M, Imran MA, Kalsoom L, Siddiqui UN, et al. Honey and Nigella Sativa against COVID-19 in Pakistan (HNS-COVID-PK): A Multi-center Placebo-Controlled Randomized Clinical Trial. medRxiv. 2020. DOI: 10.1101/2020.10.30.20217364

[133] Koshak AE, Koshak EA, Mobeireek AF, Badawi MA, Wali SO, Malibary HM, et al. Nigella sativa for the treatment of COVID-19: An open-label randomized controlled clinical trial. Complementary Therapies in Medicine. 2021;**61**:102769

[134] Stahl-Biskup E and Venskutonis RP. 27-Thyme. In: Peter KV, (ed.). Handbook of Herbs and Spices (Second Edition). Woodhead Publishing. 2012. p. 499-525

[135] Dauqan EM, Abdullah A. Medicinal and functional values of thyme (Thymus vulgaris L.) herb. Journal of Applied Biology and Biotechnology. 2017;**5**(2):17-22

[136] Walther C, Döring K, Schmidtke M. Comparative in vitro analysis of inhibition of rhinovirus and influenza virus replication by mucoactive secretolytic agents and plant extracts. BMC Complementary Medicine and Therapies. 2020;**20**(1):1-12

[137] Kulkarni SA, Nagarajan SK, Ramesh V, Palaniyandi V, Selvam SP, Madhavan T. Computational evaluation of major components from plant essential oils as potent inhibitors of SARS-CoV-2 spike protein. Journal of Molecular Structure. 2020;**1221**:128823

[138] Javed H, Meeran MFN, Jha NK, Ojha S. Carvacrol, A plant metabolite targeting viral protease (Mpro) and ACE2 in host cells can be a possible candidate for COVID-19. Frontiers in Plant Science. 2021:2237-2246

[139] Sardari S, Mobaiend A, Ghassemifard L, Kamali K, Khavasi N. Therapeutic effect of thyme (Thymus vulgaris) essential oil on patients with covid19: A randomized clinical trial. Journal of Advances in Medical and Biomedical Research. 2021;**29**(133):83-91

[140] Marwat SK, Shoaib M, Khan E, Rehman F, Ullah H. Phytochemistry and bioactivities of Quranic plant, zanjabil-ginger (Zingiber officinale roscoe): A review. American-Eurasian Journal of Agricultural & Environmental Sciences. 2015;**15**(5):707-713

[141] Al-Hilali M, Khan MM. The Noble Ouran: English Translation of the Meaning and Commentary. Madinah, KSA: King Fahd Complex for the printing of Holy Ouran; 1985. p. 817

[142] Kiyama R. Nutritional implications of ginger: Chemistry, biological activities and signaling pathways. The Journal of Nutritional Biochemistry. 2020;**86**:108486

[143] Mao Q-Q, Xu X-Y, Cao S-Y, Gan R-Y, Corke H, Beta T, et al. Bioactive compounds and bioactivities of ginger (Zingiber officinale roscoe). Food. 2019;**8**(6):185

[144] Jafarzadeh A, Nemati M. Therapeutic potentials of ginger for treatment of multiple sclerosis: A review with emphasis on its immunomodulatory, anti-inflammatory and anti-oxidative properties. Journal of Neuroimmunology. 2018;**324**:54-75

[145] Denyer CV, Jackson P, Loakes DM, Ellis MR, Young DA. Isolation of antirhinoviral sesquiterpenes from ginger (Zingiber officinale). Journal of Natural Products. 1994;**57**(5):658-662

[146] Ahmed I, Aslam A, Mustafa G, Masood S, Ali MA, Nawaz M. Anti-avian influenza virus H9N2 activity of aqueous extracts of Zingiber officinalis (ginger) and Allium sativum (garlic) in chick embryos. Pakistan Journal of Pharmaceutical Sciences. 2017;**30**(4):1341-1344

[147] Klaywong K, Khutrakul G, Choowongkomon K, Lekcharoensuk C, Petcharat N, Leckcharoensuk P, et al. Screening for lead compounds and herbal extracts with potential anti-influenza viral activity. Southeast Asian Journal of Tropical Medicine and Public Health. 2014;**45**(1):62

[148] Shin D, Mukherjee R, Grewe D, Bojkova D, Baek K, Bhattacharya A, et al. Papain-like protease regulates SARS-CoV-2 viral spread and innate immunity. Nature. 2020;**587**(7835):657-662

[149] AlAjmi MF, Azhar A, Owais M, Rashid S, Hasan S, Hussain A, et al. Antiviral potential of some novel structural analogs of standard drugs repurposed for the treatment of COVID-19. Journal of Biomolecular Structure and Dynamics. 2021;**39**(17):6676-6688

[150] Goswami D, Kumar M, Ghosh SK, Das A. Natural Product Compounds in Alpinia Officinarum and Ginger Are Potent SARS-CoV-2 Papain-like Protease Inhibitors. 2020. DOI: 10.26434/chemrxiv.12071997

[151] Oso BJ, Adeoye AO, Olaoye IF. Pharmacoinformatics and hypothetical studies on allicin, curcumin, and gingerol as potential candidates against COVID-19-associated proteases. Journal of Biomolecular Structure and Dynamics. 2022;**40**(1):389-400

[152] Rathinavel T, Palanisamy M, Palanisamy S, Subramanian A, Thangaswamy S. Phytochemical 6-Gingerol–a promising drug of choice for COVID-19. International Journal on Advanced Science, Engineering. 2020;**6**(4):1482-1489

[153] Ahkam AH, Hermanto FE, Alamsyah A, Aliyyah IH, Fatchiyah F. Virtual prediction of antiviral potential of ginger (Zingiber officinale) bioactive compounds against spike and MPro of SARS-CoV2 protein. Berkala Penelitian Hayati Journal of Biological Researches. 2020;**25**(2):52-57

[154] Mesri M, Saber SSE, Godazi M, Shirdel AR, Montazer R, Koohestani HR, et al. The effects of combination of Zingiber officinale and Echinacea on

alleviation of clinical symptoms and hospitalization rate of suspected COVID-19 outpatients: A randomized controlled trial. Journal of Complementary and Integrative Medicine. 2021;**18**(4):775-781

[155] Aldwihi LA, Khan SI, Alamri FF, AlRuthia Y, Alqahtani F, Fantoukh OI, et al. Patients' behavior regarding dietary or herbal supplements before and during COVID-19 in Saudi Arabia. International Journal of Environmental Research and Public Health. 2021;**18**(10):5086

[156] Azam MNK, Al Mahamud R, Hasan A, Jahan R, Rahmatullah M. Some home remedies used for treatment of COVID-19 in Bangladesh. Journal of Medicinal Plants Studies. 2020;**8**(4):27-32

[157] Wannes WA, Tounsi MS. Can medicinal plants contribute to the cure of Tunisian COVID-19 patients. Journal of Medicinal Plants Studies. 2020;**8**(5):218-226

[158] Pandey MM, Rastogi S, Rawat AKS. Saussurea costus: Botanical, chemical and pharmacological review of an ayurvedic medicinal plant. Journal of Ethnopharmacology. 2007;**110**(3):379-390

[159] Hassan R, Masoodi MH. Saussurea lappa: A comprehensive review on its pharmacological activity and phytochemistry. Current Traditional Medicine. 2020;**6**(1):13-23

[160] Zahara K, Tabassum S, Sabir S, Arshad M, Qureshi R, Amjad MS, et al. A review of therapeutic potential of Saussurea lappa-an endangered plant from Himalaya. Asian Pacific Journal of Tropical Medicine. 2014;7:S60-SS9

[161] Barrero AF, Oltra JE, Mr Á, Raslan DS, Saúde DA, Akssira M. New sources and antifungal activity of sesquiterpene lactones. Fitoterapia. 2000;**71**(1):60-64

[162] Ko SG, Kim H-P, Jin D-H, Bae H-S, Kim SH, Park C-H, et al. Saussurea lappa induces G2-growth arrest and apoptosis in AGS gastric cancer cells. Cancer Letters. 2005;**220**(1):11-19

[163] Khalid A, U R, Sethi A, Khilji S, Fatima U, Khan MI, et al. Antimicrobial activity analysis of extracts of Acacia modesta, Artimisia absinthium, Nigella sativa and Saussurea lappa against gram positive and gram negative microorganisms. African Journal of Biotechnology. 2011;**10**(22):4574-4580

[164] Kulkarni S. Immunostimulant activity of inulin isolated from Saussurea lappa roots. Indian Journal of Pharmaceutical Sciences. 2001;**63**(4):292

[165] Sutar N, Garai R, Sharma US, Singh N, Roy SD. Antiulcerogenic activity of Saussurea lappa root. International Journal of Pharmacy and Life Sciences. 2011;**2**(1):516-520

[166] Sunkara Y, Robinson A, Babu K, Naidu V, Vishnuvardhan M, Ramakrishna S, et al. Anti-inflammatory and cytotoxic activity of chloroform extract of roots of Saussurea lappa Clarke. Journal of Pharmacy Research. 2010;**3**(8):1775-1778

[167] Yaeesh S, Jamal Q, Shah AJ, Gilani AH. Antihepatotoxic activity of Saussurea lappa extract on D-galactosamine and lipopolysaccharide-induced hepatitis in mice. Phytotherapy Research. 2010;**24**(S2):S229-SS32

[168] Agung MK. Potensi senyawa seskuiterpenoid Saussurea costus (Falc.) Lipsch dalam menghambat reseptor spike protein sebagai antivirus SARS-COV-2 secara In silico. UIN Sunan Gunung Djati

Bandung. 2021. Available online: http://digilib.uinsgd.ac.id/id/eprint/47154

[169] Prawiro SR, Anam K, Prabowo B, Fitrianingsih AA, Hidayati DYN, Imawati S, et al. Generating the responses immune with honey, Saussurea costus, and nigella Sativa in cellular and humoral may resolve COVID-19? Systematic Reviews in Pharmacy. 2021;**12**(5):1501-1506

[170] Aboushanab TS, AlSanad S. Cupping therapy: An overview from a modern medicine perspective. Journal of Acupuncture and Meridian Studies. 2018;**11**(3):83-87

[171] Mehta P, Dhapte V. Cupping therapy: A prudent remedy for a plethora of medical ailments. Journal of Traditional and Complementary Medicine. 2015;**5**(3):127-134

[172] Cui S, Cui J. Progress of researches on the mechanism of cupping therapy. Zhen ci yan jiu=. Acupuncture Research. 2012;**37**(6):506-510

[173] Al-Bedah AM, Aboushanab TS, Alqaed MS, Qureshi NA, Suhaibani I, Ibrahim G, et al. Classification of cupping therapy: A tool for modernization and standardization. Journal of Complementary and Alternative Medical Research. 2016;**1**(1):1-10

[174] Kim J-I, Lee MS, Lee D-H, Boddy K and, Ernst E. Cupping for Treating Pain: A Systematic Review. Evidence-Based Complementary and Alternative Medicine. 2011;**467014**,7

[175] Subadi I, Nugraha B, Laswati H, Josomuljono H. Pain relief with wet cupping therapy in rats is mediated by heat shock protein 70 and ss-endorphin. Iranian Journal of Medical Sciences. Jul 2017;**42**(4):384

[176] Yoo SS, Tausk F. Cupping: East meets west. International Journal of Dermatology. 2004;**43**(9):664-665

[177] Lauche R, Materdey S, Cramer H, Haller H, Stange R, Dobos G, et al. Effectiveness of home-based cupping massage compared to progressive muscle relaxation in patients with chronic neck pain—A randomized controlled trial. PLoS One. 2013;**8**(6):e65378

[178] Vaskilampi T, Hänninen O. Cupping as an indigenous treatment of pain syndromes in the Finnish cultural and social context. Social Science & Medicine. 1982;**16**(21):1893-1901

[179] Yingdong L. Cupping therapy for 103 cases of high fever due to infection of the upper respiratory tract. The Journal of Chinese Medicine. 2002;**70**:38-40

[180] Baghdadi H, Abdel-Aziz N, Ahmed NS, Mahmoud HS, Barghash A, Nasrat A, et al. Ameliorating role exerted by Al-Hijamah in autoimmune diseases: Effect on serum autoantibodies and inflammatory mediators. International Journal of Health Sciences. 2015;**9**(2):207

[181] Ahmed SM, Madbouly NH, Maklad SS, Abu-Shady EA. Immunomodulatory effects of blood letting cupping therapy in patients with rheumatoid arthritis. The Egyptian Journal of Immunology. 2005;**12**(2):39-51

[182] Arslan M, Yeşilçam N, Aydin D, Yüksel R, Dane Ş. Wet cupping therapy restores sympathovagal imbalances in cardiac rhythm. The Journal of Alternative and Complementary Medicine. 2014;**20**(4):318-321

[183] Guo H-r, Q-y Z, Li X, Chen Y, Li M-Y, Zhuo X-M, et al. The effectiveness of cupping therapy on chronic fatigue syndrome: A single-blind randomized controlled trial. Complementary

Therapies in Clinical Practice. 2020;**40**:101210

[184] Rosyanti L, Hadi I. The Effectiveness of Complementary "Cupping Therapy" On The Community's Routine Blood Hematology Status During The COVID-19 Pandemic. International Conference on Health Practice and Research. Jun 30, 2022;**1**(1):1-11

[185] Hekmatpou D, Moeini L, Haji-Nadali S. The effectiveness of wet cupping vs. venesection on arterial O2 saturation level of cigarette smokers: A randomized controlled clinical trial. Pakistan Journal of Medical Sciences. 2013;**29**(6):1349

[186] Cheng SI. Medical acupuncture as a treatment for novel COVID-19-related respiratory distress: Personal experience from a frontline Anesthesiologist. Medical Acupuncture. 2021;**33**(1):83-85

[187] Karimi M, Kazemi AH, Asadi A, Zarei A, Zargaran A, SAA-h M, et al. Warm cupping of the posterior thorax in combination with standard conventional therapy for ARDS in COVID-19 patients in ICU: A case series. Journal of Acupuncture and Meridian Studies. 2022;**15**(3):194-200

[188] von Trott P, Oei SL, Ramsenthaler C. Acupuncture for breathlessness in advanced diseases: A systematic review and meta-analysis. Journal of Pain and Symptom Management. 2020;**59**(2):327-38.e3

[189] Zhang K, Li Y, Tang Q. Acupuncture for breathlessness in advanced diseases: Methodological issues. Journal of Pain and Symptom Management. 2020;**59**(3):e3-e4

[190] Huang ET-Y, Di PhD YM. Acupuncture therapies for chronic obstructive pulmonary disease: A systematic review of randomized, controlled trials. Alternative Therapies in Health and Medicine. 2014;**20**(6):10

[191] Zhang B, Zhang K, Tang Q, Sun K, Han Z. Acupuncture for breathlessness in COVID-19: A protocol for systematic review and meta-analysis. Medicine (Baltimore). Jul 2, 2020;**99**(27):e20701. DOI: 10.1097/MD.0000000000020701. PMID: 32629642; PMCID: PMC7337514

[192] Zhang R, Lao L, Ren K, Berman BM. Mechanisms of acupuncture–electroacupuncture on persistent pain. Anesthesiology. 2014;**120**(2):482-503

[193] Millstine D, Chen CY, Bauer B. Complementary and integrative medicine in the management of headache. BMJ. May 16, 2017;**357**:j1805. PMID: 28512119

[194] Badakhsh M, Dastras M, Sarchahi Z, Doostkami M, Mir A, Bouya S. Complementary and alternative medicine therapies and COVID-19: A systematic review. Reviews on Environmental Health. Apr 12, 2021;**36**(3):443-450. DOI: 10.1515/reveh-2021-0012. PMID: 33838089

[195] Han Z, Zhang Y, Wang P, Tang Q, Zhang K. Is acupuncture effective in the treatment of COVID-19 related symptoms? Based on bioinformatics/network topology strategy. Briefings in Bioinformatics. 2021;**22**(5):bbab110

[196] Torres-Rosas R, Yehia G, Peña G, Mishra P, del Rocio T-BM, Moreno-Eutimio MA, et al. Dopamine mediates vagal modulation of the immune system by electroacupuncture. Nature Medicine. 2014;**20**(3):291-295

[197] Chang S, Kim DH, Jang EY, Yoon SS, Gwak YS, Yi YJ, et al. Acupuncture attenuates alcohol dependence through

activation of endorphinergic input to the nucleus accumbens from the arcuate nucleus. Science Advances. 2019;**5**(9):eaax1342

[198] Zhao Z-Q. Neural mechanism underlying acupuncture analgesia. Progress in Neurobiology. 2008;**85**(4):355-375

[199] Chen C, Zhan J, Wen H, Wei X, Ding L, Tao C, et al. Current state of research about acupuncture for the treatment of COVID-19: A scoping review. Integrative Medicine Research. 2021;**10**:100801

Chapter 7

Annona muricata (Graviola): Nutraceutical in COVID-19

Lysiane Marèse Atcham Amougou

Abstract

Plants that possess therapeutic characteristics have been used in medicine from the beginning of time. Indigenous medicine has been practiced as a preventative approach in tropical areas to combat general infections, including viral infections. The family of Annonaceae species of plants, broadly distributed in these areas, is dedicated to one such plant-based medication. *Annona muricata* realistically is among the most well-known of these. A novel coronavirus (2019-nCoV) was typically identified as the reliable source of a viral pneumonia outbreak in January 2020 in Wuhan, China. Traditional medicine is reasonably believed to represent a possible opportunity in the successful fight against COVID-19. The Cameroonian response strategy has been properly implemented in outstanding community services without much practical efficiency on transmission rates. The reason for this is that people did not follow the government's prescriptions. As a direct result, local people would knowingly employ self-prescribed herbal medications to aggressively combat the COVID-19 spread. Local health officials should take action and recognize the value of species diversity mostly in the fight against the COVID 19 pandemic, making it available to the concerned public with the support of scientific and ethno pharmacological local institutions. The potential therapeutic usage of *Annona muricata* as an antiviral agent to powerfully aid in the possible fight against COVID 19 has been carefully investigated in this paper.

Keywords: *Annona muricata*, soursop fruit, health benefits, traditional uses, COVID 19

1. Introduction

The products of African traditional medicine have been used as the main sources of healthcare for the majority of the population despite the integration of conventional medicine in our healthcare system according to the West Africa Health Organization.

Traditional medicine is crucial for primary health care and in this chapter, we will focus on a particular plant specimen which has a therapeutic potential in the fight against the COVID 19 pandemic due to its phytochemicals constituents.

One such plant with an extensive use in herbal medicine is *Annona muricata*.

Annona muricata is a tropical medicinal plant which is recognized for its utility in many diseases such as malaria and cancer. These plants are natural sources of anti-inflammatory, and anti-cancer agents.

It belongs to the annonaceae family and also known as guanabana, soursop and graviola.

The management of various health conditions in west Africa such as food borne disease, malaria worm infections, bacterial infections, has been supported by herbal medicine for ages since people have limited access to modern medicine in developing countries. These plants are widely distributed worldwide especially in west Africa and have helped people into the preservation of health for decades.

In Cameroon, central African region, there is a rich biodiversity with almost 9000 plant species, some of which are commonly used to treat microbial infections and some other diseases as malaria, diabetes, and parasitic infections.

Annona plant species are widely studied for their biological activities including anti-tumor, anti-parasitic, and anti-microbial properties.

In this chapter, we are going to describe the botany, local distribution, the phyto-chemicals, and finally the potential uses of *Annona muricata* in the current COVID 19 pandemic.

2. Origin and geographical distribution of African medicinal plants namely *A. muricata*

Annonaceae plant species are native to south tropical America and south Mexico [1].

Its center of geographic diversity is in the north of South America and it is distributed in different tropical regions of the world (Love and Paull, 2011).

Soursop is used in food, beverages, and other preparations [2].

The most of African annonaceae are observed mostly in lowland or mountainous rain forests in Africa and Madagascar. However, a limited diversity of plants has adjusted to slightly more arid conditions and can be found in thickets or savanna vegetation [3].

Africa is a botanical continent which corresponds to its geographic distribution.

Although its origin is unknown, *Annona muricata* is believed to be native to tropical America, especially the West Indies. It was one of very first fruit trees to be introduced to the East after Columbus' expedition to America; Spaniards introduced it to the Philippines early on, and it today develops in nearly any tropical country. Before World War II, this species was introduced to the most of the Pacific Islands. In tropical America and west Africa, it is widely planted and naturalized [4].

The morphological characteristics of these plant species are depicted in **Figures 1–3.**

Its geographic distribution is well documented on the agroforestry species database.

Annona muricata is native from Antigua and Barbuda, Argentina, Bahamas, Barbados, Bolivia, Brazil, Chile, Colombia, Cuba, Dominica, Dominican Republic, Ecuador, French Guiana, Grenada, Guadeloupe, Guatemala, Guyana, Haiti, Honduras, Jamaica, Martinique, Mexico, Montserrat, Netherlands Antilles, Nicaragua, Panama, Paraguay, Peru, Puerto Rico, Sri Lanka, St Kitts and Nevis,

St Lucia, St Vincent and the Grenadines, Surinam, Trinidad and Tobago, Uruguay, Venezuela, Virgin Islands (US), Zanzibar [5].

There are some places where tree species have not been not planted but yet introduced as exotic Fruit species like Benin, Cambodia, China, Cote d'Ivoire, Eritrea, Ethiopia, Ghana, Guinea, India, Indonesia, Laos, Liberia, Mauritania, Nigeria, Papua New Guinea, Philippines, Reunion, Senegal, Sierra Leone, Tanzania, Thailand, Togo, Uganda, US, Vietnam.

Below is a map showing countries where these plant species have been planted. (**Figure 4**).

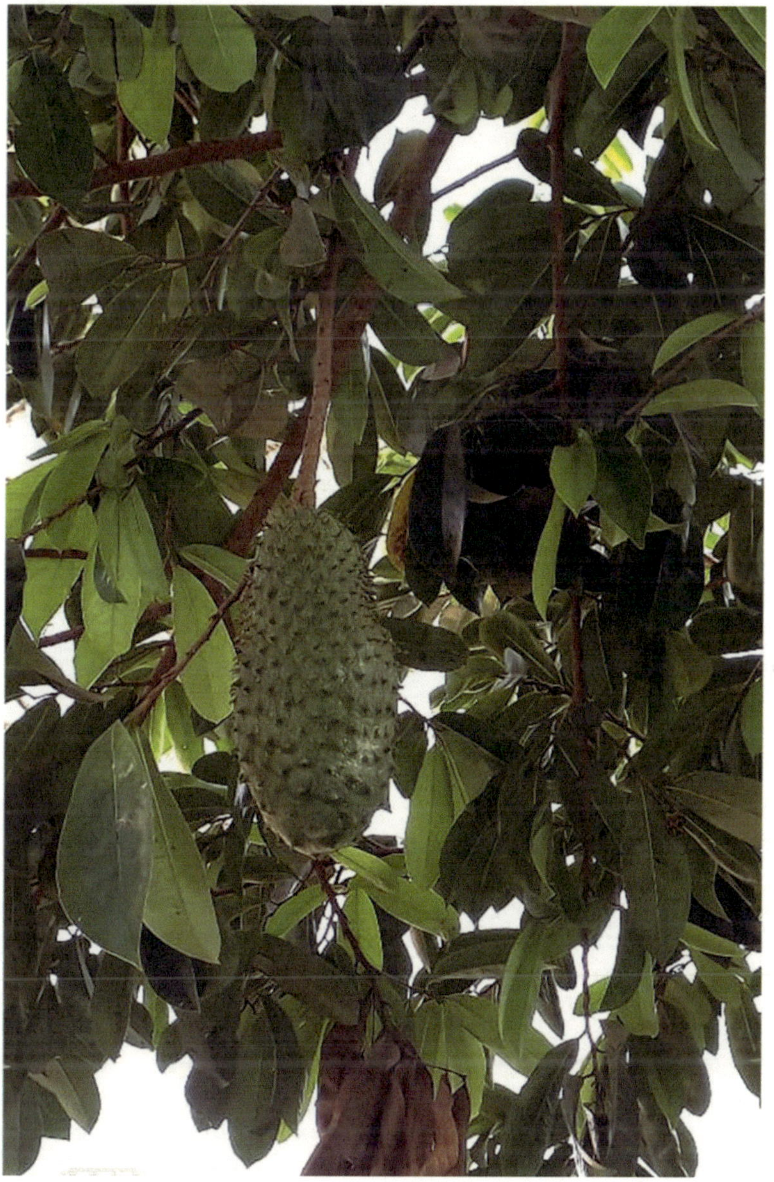

Figure 1.
Soursop tree and leaves (own image).

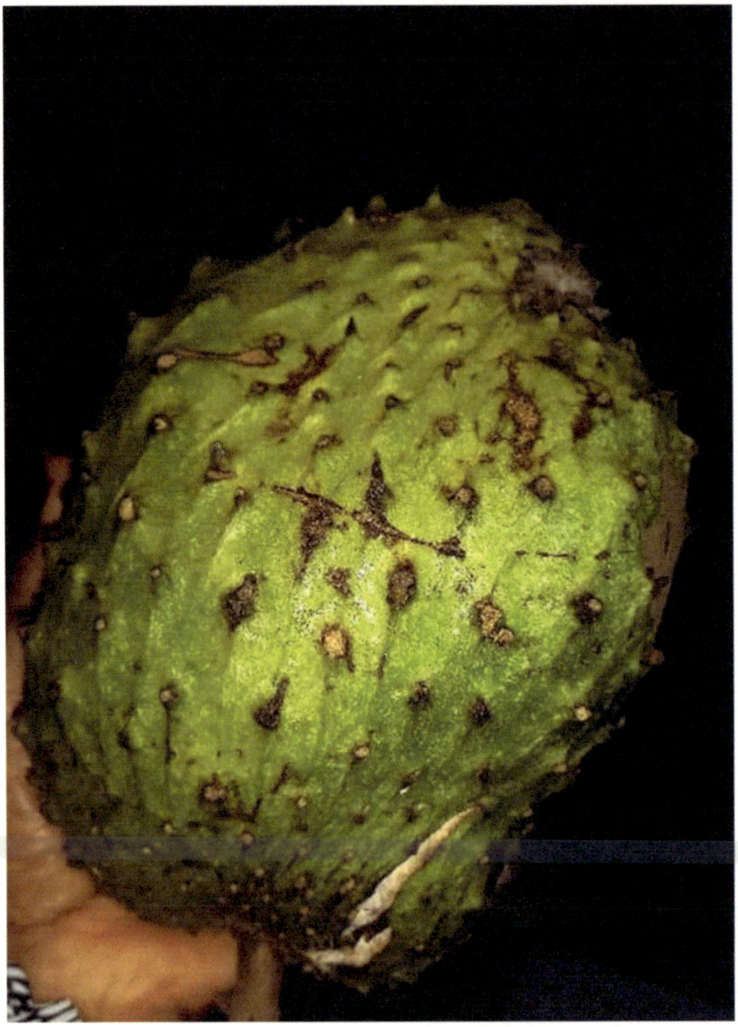

Figure 2.
Soursop fruit skin (own image).

2.1 Botanical description

Annona muricata is a lowland tropical, fruit-bearing tree of the annonaceae family found in African, South American, and Southeast Asian rainforests. *A. muricata*, as well known as soursop, guanabana, or Brazilian pawpaw, has large, glossy, dark green leaves but also edible, green heart-shaped fruits [6, 7]. The leathery skin of the fruits is made of a soft, curved spines, and each fruit may contain 55–170 black seeds distributed in a creamy white flesh with a clearly different aroma and flavor [8].

Coria-Téllez et al., have reported 212 bioactive compounds in *A. muricata* extracts [8]. Reports in the literature indicate that 74 of these bioactive compounds exhibit a variety of anticancer effects in preclinical cell culture and animal model systems.

The genus name "annona" is from the Latin word "anon", meaning "yearly produce", referring to the fruit production habits of the various species in this genus [9].

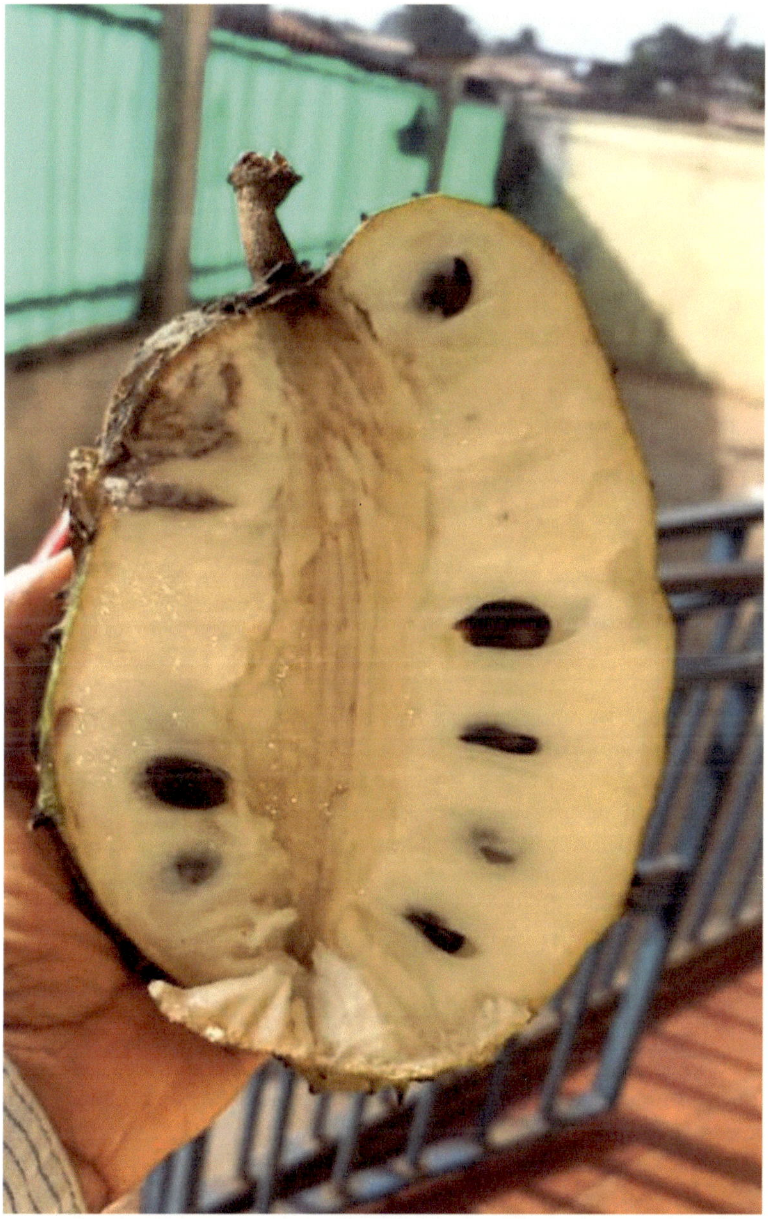

Figure 3.
Soursop fruit white pulp and seeds (own image).

2.2 Chemical constituents

There are 212 bioactive chemicals found in *A. muricata*, per the studies. Acetogenins are the most common chemicals, followed by alkaloids, phenols, and other active ingredients. The leaves and seeds are the most frequently investigated plant parts, probably because they are the most often used.

More than 200 bioactive compounds have been isolated from *A. muricata*, including six types of acetogenins, various alkaloids (mostly isoquinolines,

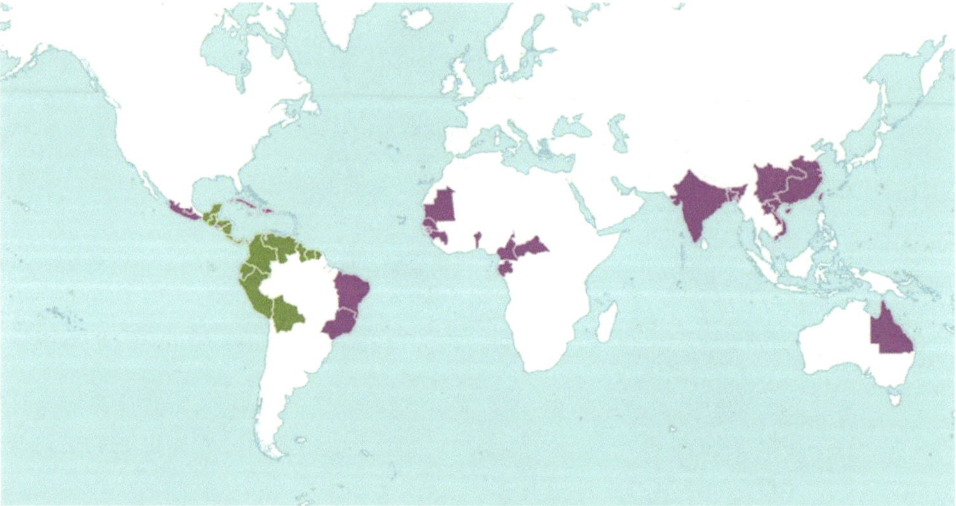

Figure 4.
Geographical distribution of A. muricata [1]. ■ *native,* ■ *introduced. Note:* ■ *South American native plant species,* ■ *west, central Africa, and south Asia introduced plant species.*

aporphines, and protoberberines, notably reticuline and coreximine), phenols (e.g., quercetin and gallic acids), and other compounds, including sesquite rpene derivatives. At least 50 pharmacological studies have already been conducted, with two-thirds in vitro and one-third in vivo studies involving mice models. Coria-Tellez et al., 2017 have recently published extensive studies of the above.

There are six prominent phytochemicals which have been isolated from *A. muricata* plant species as alkaloid, annonaceous acetogenin, megastigmane, flavonol triglycoside, phenolic, cyclopeptide.

Annonaceous acetogenins are one class of phytochemicals exclusive to the annonacae plant species [10].

2.3 Medicinal uses

A number of medicinal uses have been reported across the globe ranging from the use of leaves, bark, roots, fruits to seeds of *A. muricata* [11].

The most widely used preparation in traditional medicine is the decoction of bark, root, seed or leaf but applications are varied. In a number of tropical sub-Saharan countries such as Uganda, all parts are used to treat malaria, stomachache, parasitic infections, diabetes [12], and cancer [13].

The use of graviola leaves extract can cure malaria in tropical countries like Cameroon, Togo, and Vietnam [14–16]. In Ghana, *A. muricata* and some other plants are decocted into a mixture and used in bath for pregnant mothers prior to birth [17].

In west Africa, *Annona muricata* is mostly used as food as fruit because of its anti-oxidant properties which have been evaluated in fresh or frozen pulp, juice, and fresh or dried leaves [12].

Lately, the medicinal uses of *A. muricata* leaves included treatments for hypertension [11–19], diabetes and cancer.

According to Linn Churchill et al., (1980) *Annona muricata* Fruit and fruit juice are taken for worms and parasites, to cool fevers, to increase mother's milk after childbirth, as an astringent for diarrhea and dysentery. The crushed seeds are used against internal and external parasites, head lice. The bark, leaves, and roots are considered as sedative, ulcer treatment, hypotensive, and nervine, and a tea is made for various disorders towards those effects.

Coria-Téllez et al., (2018) explained that in fruits and roots of *annona murricata* contains acetogenins proved to have anticarcinogenic effect.

Acetogenins have been reported to show significant antiviral activities against herpes simplex virus-I (HSV-I) (Padma et al., 1998), herpes simplex virus-II (HSV-II) (Betancur-Galvis et al., 1999), human papillomavirus (HPV) (Donne et al., 2017), hepatitis C virus (HCV) (Apriyanto et al., 2018), dengue virus type 2 (DENV-2), human immunodeficiency virus-I (HIV-I) (van de Venter et al., 2014; [12]).

3. Plant based drug for the management of COVID 19: reality or hope?

At the end of 2019, a novel coronavirus was identified as the cause of a cluster of pneumonia cases in Wuhan, a city in the Hubei Province of China. It rapidly spread, resulting in a global pandemic. The disease is designated COVID-19, which stands for coronavirus disease 2019 [20].

Corona disease caused by the acute respiratory syndrome coronavirus 2 (SARS-CoV-2) is a major threat to global health.

Disinfection is one of the trending public health measure implemented in community settings to help in reducing the transmission of the disease by the elimination of the viral agent.

The long term use of these disinfectants can cause skin damage or hypersensitivity [21].

According to A. Taghizadehghalehjoughi et al., graviola has a strong protective effect on PH changes damage induction. Therefore, we recommend the use of graviola after hand disinfections.

In Cameroon, the first case was reported on the 06th March 2020, a traveler who arrived there on the 24th February 2020 from France [22].

The socio-economic and health situations of indigenous people allow them with no alternative to the less expensive readily available traditional concoctions [23].

Cameroon is located in central Africa with a population of over 25 million of young people with a median age of 18.7 years and 41.25% of the population being between zero and 14 years old [24].

In Cameroon, access to health care services is challenging. One out of every 1000 patients is able to see a specialist and 3 out of 20 patients are able to buy prescribed drugs in hospitals [25].

According to E. Fongnzossie Fedoung et al., since the first case was reported in our country, several herbal recipes have been popularized in social media, as alleged solutions to manage COVID 19. According to a recent release from the Cameroon Radio and Television Corporation, the Archbishop of Douala, His grace Samuel Kleda, has made public an attempt at treating symptoms of COVID-19 with an herbal remedy, free of charge and the Ministry of Public Health is showing commitment to support the process of development and homologation of this treatment (CRTV, 2020).

Nowadays, the COVID 19 care in Cameroon relies mostly on vaccination and trending public health interventions like wearing a mask in public spaces, the use of hand sanitizers and/or social distancing.

During the pandemic, people were afraid to attend health facilities to get tested for COVID 19 and isolated in specialized treatment centers, also personnel was not well prepared to handle this type of public health emergency.

Confirmed cases were admitted to various hospitals for treatment regimens that included oral chloroquine, azithromycin, immune system support vitamins such as vit C and zinc, and other treatment options for moderate to severe conditions.

Most people experienced mild form of COVID 19 and were admitted in a treatment center in Yaoundé according to Fouda Mbarga et al., [22].

The Ministry of Health encourages people to get the full COVID 19 vaccine, but people prefer to get herbal medicine from the informal sector.

According to World Health Organization (WHO) coronavirus dashboard, from January 3, 2020 to February 21, 2022, in Cameroon, there have been 118,933 confirmed cases of COVID-19 with 1918 deaths, reported to the organization. As of February 15, 2022, a total of 1,024,333 vaccine doses have been administered [26]. Since the start of the global pandemic, the number of confirmed cases and deaths has increased, according to this situation report.

4. *Annona muricata* as an antiviral agent for the management of SARS-CoV-2?

According to WHO, the current management of COVID 19 at home of patients or confirmed cases consists mainly of antipyretics for fever and headache, as well as good diet and hydration [27].

Cameroon is among the highest species diversity in Africa, yet herbal medicines is not yet completely acknowledged by the country's healthcare system, and herbal drug development is limited despite numerous ethnopharmacological surveys on various African plant species.

According to Matshidiso Moeti, the WHO regional director for Africa, interest in African traditional medicine is growing as a potential treatment for COVID 19 [28].

Malagasy is the only African country to already have succeeded in producing a potential cure for COVID 19.

Madagascar is the only African country to have previously succeeded in developing a COVID 19 treatment.

Researchers from Madagascar's Malagasy Institute for Applied Research recently developed COVID Organics, a novel coronavirus antidote (IMRA). According to the country's president, Rajoelina, it has anti-coronavirus potential [29].

There was no specific antiviral agent or vaccine ready for healthy people at the beginning of the epidemic.

Nowadays, there are many antiviral agents for the treatment of COVID 19 including such hydroxychloroquine (HCQ), chloroquine (CQ), and ivermectine (IVM) that are not yet approved by the FDA and are not recommended for use in the treatment of COVID 19 [30].

Graviola's bioactive compounds give it a potential antiviral agent, however it's not optimal.

5. Conclusions

Graviola is not only a medicinal plant but also a food supplement that has been used for decades by indigenous people to face health challenges.

Cameroon is a country with a large biodiversity but has not integrate herbal medicine in the public health system.

The Institute of Medical Research and Medicinal Plants Study of Cameroon should investigate *Annona muricata*'s potential antiviral effect further in order to support the state response strategy in the current global pandemic.

Acknowledgements

The author would like to thank Dr. Dongmo Michel for providing resources and his precious contribution to the development of this chapter.

Conflict of interest

Lysiane Marese Atcham Amougou declares no conflict of interest regarding the submission and the publication of this book chapter.

Acronyms and abbreviations

A. muricata	*Annona muricata.*
WAHO	West African Health Organization
CRTV	Cameroon Radio Television
SARS CoV 2	severe acute respiratory syndrome coronavirus 2
WHO	World Health Organization
IMRA	Malagasy Institute of Applied Research
HCQ	hydroxychloroquine
CQ	chloroquine
IVM	ivermectine

Author details

Lysiane Marèse Atcham Amougou
Yaounde University Teaching Hospital, Accredited Treatment Center for HIV-Positive People, Yaoundé, Cameroon

*Address all correspondence to: atcham4lysie@yahoo.fr

References

[1] Available from: https://powo.science.kew.org/taxon/14308-2#distribution-map [Accessed: January 29, 2022]

[2] Peter SS, Palmer VS. Chapter nine—Food plant chemicals linked with neurological and neurodegenerative disease. Advances in Neurotoxicology. 2017;**1**:247-278. DOI: 10.1016/bs.ant.2017.07.009

[3] Available from: https://afroannons.myspecies.info/content/african-annonaceae-diversity-and-beauty#overlay-context=category/african-annonaceae/annonaceae [Accessed: January 31, 2022]

[4] Neffati M et al., editors. Medicinal and Aromatic Plants of the World—Africa. Vol. 3. Netherlands: ©Springer Science+Business Media B.V, Springer Nature; 2017. DOI: 10.1007/978-94-024-1120-1_1

[5] Available from: https://www.prota4u.org/database/protav8.asp?h=M1,M11,M15,M18,M25,M26,M27,M34,M36,M4,M5,M7&t=Annona,muricata&p=Annona+muricata#Protologue [Accessed: February 18, 2022]

[6] Moghadamtousi S, Fadaeinasab M, Nikzad S, Mohan G, Ali H, Kadir H. *Annona muricata* (Annonaceae): A review of its traditional uses, isolated acetogenins and biological activities. International Journal of Molecular Sciences. 2015;**16**(7):15625-15658

[7] Ribeiro de Souza EB, da Silva RR, Afonso S, Scarminio IS. Enhanced extraction yields and mobile phase separations by solvent mixtures for the analysis of metabolites in *Annona muricata* L. leaves. Journal of Separation Science. 2009;**32**(23-24):4176-4185

[8] Coria-Téllez AV, Montalvo-Gónzalez E, Yahia EM, Obledo-Vázquez EN. *Annona muricata*: A comprehensive review on its traditional medicinal uses, phytochemicals, pharmacological activities, mechanisms of action and toxicity. Arabian Journal of Chemistry. 2016;**30**:8-11

[9] Orwa C, Mutua A, Kindt R, Jamnadass R, Simons A. Agroforestree Database:a tree reference and selection guide version 4.0. 2009. Available from: http://www.worldagroforestry.org/af/treedb/ [Accessed: February 07, 2022]

[10] Prasad SK, Pradeep S, Shimavallu C, Kollur SP, Syed A, Marraiki N, et al. Evaluation of *Annona muricata* acetogenins as potential anti-SARS-CoV-2 agents through computational approaches. Frontiers in Chemistry. 2021;**8**:624716. DOI: 10.3389/fchem.2020.624716

[11] N. Badrie, A. Schauss Soursop (*Annona muricata* L.): Composition, nutritional value, medicinal uses, and toxicology R. Watson, V. Preedy, Bioactive Foods in Promoting Health, Academic Press, Oxford (2010), pp. 621-643

[12] Gavamukulya Y, Wamunyokoli F, El-Shemy HA. Annona muricata: Is the natural therapy to most disease conditions including cancer growing in our backyard? A systematic review of its research history and future prospects. Asian Pacific Journal of Tropical Medicine. 2017;**10**(9):835-848. DOI: 10.1016/j.apjtm.2017.08.009. ISSN 1995-7645

[13] Gavamukulya Y, Abou-Elella F, Wamunyokoli F, El-Shemy H. Phytochemical screening, anti-oxidant

activity and in vitro anticancer potential of ethanolic and water leaves extracts of *Annona muricata* (Graviola). Asian Pacific Journal of Tropical Medicine. 2014;**7**(1):S355-S363

[14] Boyom FF, Fokou PVT, Yamthe LRT, Mfopa AN, Kemgne EM, Mbacham WF, et al. Potent antiplasmodial extracts from Cameroonian Annonaceae. Journal of Ethnopharmacology. 2011;**134**(3):717-724

[15] Nguyen-Pouplin J, Tran H, Tran H, Phan TA, Dolecek C, Farrar J, et al. Antimalarial and cytotoxic activities of ethnopharmacologically selected medicinal plants from South Vietnam. Journal of Ethnopharmacology. 2007;**109**(3):417-427

[16] Ross IA. Medicinal Plants of the World: Chemical Constituents, Traditional and Modern Medicinal Uses. Vol. 2. New Jersey: Humana Press; 2001

[17] Asase A, Hesse DN, Simmonds MSJ. Uses of multiple plants prescriptions for treatment of malaria by some communities in southern Ghana. Journal of Ethnopharmacology. 2012;**144**(2):448-452. DOI: 10.1016/j.jep.2012.09.028. ISSN 0378-8741

[18] Hajdu Z, Hohmann J. An ethnopharmacological survey of the traditional medicine utilized in the community of Porvenir, Bajo Paraguá Indian Reservation. Bolivia Journal of Ethnopharmacology. 2012;**139**(3):838-857

[19] Ezuruike U, Prieto J. The use of plants in the traditional management of diabetes in Nigeria: Pharmacological and toxicological considerations. Journal of Ethnopharmacology. 2014;**155**(2):857-924

[20] World Health Organization. Director-General's remarks at the media briefing on 2019-nCoV on 11 February 2020. Available from: http://www.who.int/dg/speeches/detail/who-director-general-s-remarks-at-the-media-briefing-on-2019-ncov-on-11-february-2020 [Accessed: February 15, 2022]

[21] Taghizadehghalehjoughi A et al. Investigation of protective effects of Graviola (*Annona muricata*) plant against disinfectants used in different pHs in Covid-19 process. Acta Scientific Pharmaceutical Sciences. 2021;**5**(5):45-50

[22] Fouda Mbarga N, Epee E, Mbarga M, Ouamba P, Nanda H, Nkengni A, et al. Clinical profile and factors associated with COVID-19 in Yaounde, Cameroon: A prospective cohort study. PLoS One. 2021;**16**(5):e0251504. DOI: 10.1371/journal.pone.0251504

[23] Abia WE, Fonchang GN, Kaoke MD, Fomboh R, Ageh MT, Abia EA, et al. Interest and perceptions on traditional medicines in Cameroon. IJR. 2015;**2**(5):377. Available from: https://www.researchgate.net/publication/319312281_Interest_and_perceptions_on_traditional_medicines_in_Cameroon

[24] Available from: https://worldpopulationreview.com/countries/cameroon-population [Accessed: February 15, 2022]

[25] Fongnzossie Fedoung E, Biwole AB, Nyangono Biyegue CF, Ngansop Tounkam M, Akono Ntonga P, Nguiamba VP, et al. A review of Cameroonian medicinal plants with potentials for the management of the COVID-19 pandemic. Advances in Traditional Medicine (ADTM). 2021:1-26. DOI: 10.1007/s13596-021-00567-6. Epub ahead of print

[26] Available from: https://covid19.who.int/region/afro/country/cm [Accessed: February 22, 2022]

[27] World Health Organization. Clinical Management of COVID-19: Interim Guidance. Geneva: World Health Organization; 2020 Available from: https://apps.who.int/iris/handle/10665/332196

[28] WHO to Study Madagascar's Drug to Treat COVID-19. WHO Gets in Touch with Madagascar, after Country's President Slammed Global Health Body for Not Endorsing its Drug. Available from: https://www.aa.com.tr/en/africa/who-to-study-madagascars-drug-to-treat-covid-19-/1840971 [Accessed: February 23, 2022]

[29] Covid-Organics: WHO Sets Rules for Phase 3 Clinical Trials of African Herbal Medicine to Treat Coronavirus. Available from: https://www.timesnownews.com/health/article/covid-organics-who-sets-rules-for-phase-3-clinical-trials-of-african-herbal-medicine-to-treat-coronavirus/656173 [Accessed: February 23, 2022]

[30] Table 2f: Characteristics of Antiviral Agents. Available from: https://www.covid19treatmentguidelines.nih.gov/tables/antiviral-characteristics/ [Accessed: February 23, 2022]

Chapter 8

Carissa spinarum L.: A Case Study in Ethnobotany and Bioprospecting Research

Ciara Smyth and Helen Sheridan

Abstract

This study explores ethnobiological and bioprospecting research through the lens of *Carissa spinarum* L., using it as a case study to examine wider trends in such research. Hunn's Phasing in Ethnobiology is used as a framework, analysing the extensive research of a species used in healing, diet and other domains. Most reported studies are illustrative of Phase I Ethnobiological research based on the lack of basic context, emic or ecological detail, or a sense of collaboration with participants or across disciplines. Elements of Phases II, III and IV are evident in some studies highlighting ethnographic context, ecological issues or indigenous knowledge and rights. The extractive character of Phase I research, usually used for bioprospecting purposes, decontextualises plant use and may contribute to the historically poor results from ethno-directed bioprospecting. The widespread marginalisation of the social sciences in bioprospecting research can invalidate the whole research project and in turn ethnomedical plant use itself. A species such as *Carissa spinarum* L., emerging from Phase I research, can become a mere collection of its phytochemical parts, invalidated if those parts do not meet scientific measures of value. The collaborative character of Phase IV and V Ethnobiology would reward with more ethical and effective research with healing plants.

Keywords: Hunn phases of ethnobiology, ethnopharmacology, traditional medicine, medicinal plants, bioprospecting, emic, research ethics

1. Introduction

In August 2010, Reverend Ambilikile Mwasupile, a retired pastor in the Loliondo area of northern Tanzania began to treat people for a range of chronic ailments including diabetes, cancer, epilepsy, herpes, HIV/AIDS, liver disorders and asthma. A report on the phenomenon by Malebo and Mbwambo [1] describes how he was instructed in dreams to use a decoction of the root of the *Mugariga* tree to heal people with chronic illnesses. He would pray over the root before preparing the decoction, and pray again before personally administering it to the patient using Babu's own "miraculous cup" known as *kikombe cha Babu* [2]. He was, for a brief period, a media sensation throughout East Africa and was known as Babu wa Loliondo providing what was known as the "miracle cure". People travelled long distances by road and helicopter in order to get the once-off treatment. The flocks of people making their way to the remote village caused great disruption locally (**Figure 1**). The Loliondo cure was reported in local, national and international media including in the BBC [3] and the New York Times [4].

After initial scepticism, the Tanzanian government, local health officials and the national research hospital endorsed Babu wa Loliondo [2]. Popularity waned after 10 months, at least in part because the pastor called for a break due to the chaos caused locally. It was also reported that some elderly people died as they waited in queues for days [4] and that some HIV positive patients died, having stopped their anti-retroviral treatment subsequent to treatment with *Mugariga* [2]. Vähäkangas [2] describes how Babu wa Loliondo was, during that brief time, able to bridge the gap for people in the region between the scientific, traditional and Christian worldviews and between physical and spiritual healing.

Mugariga was identified as *Carissa spinarum* L. (*C. spinarum*), a plant known among several local ethnic groups as having healing properties [1]. In fact, prior to this, KEMRI (Kenya Medical Research Institute) was already investigating *C. spinarum* for its antiviral properties and in 2014 produced *Zedupex*™ containing *C. spinarum* [5]. Interest in the Loliondo "miracle cure" has re-emerged recently in relation to COVID-19. It was reported in the media that KEMRI was investigating *Zedupex*™ for efficacy against SARS-CoV-2 [6, 7].

C. spinarum, a member of the Apocynaceae family, is a complex and varied species that is widely distributed geographically throughout Sub-Saharan Africa, Australia, and parts of Asia [8]. This research will show that it has a large body of associated ethnobiological data, spanning its geographical range, dating from 1886 through to the present. This study aims to analyse this data through the lens of changes in ethnobiological research since its inception as a discipline, in the late nineteenth century, to the present.

Ethnobiology as a discipline is defined by the Society of Ethnobiology [9] as "the scientific study of dynamic relationships among peoples, biota, and environments"

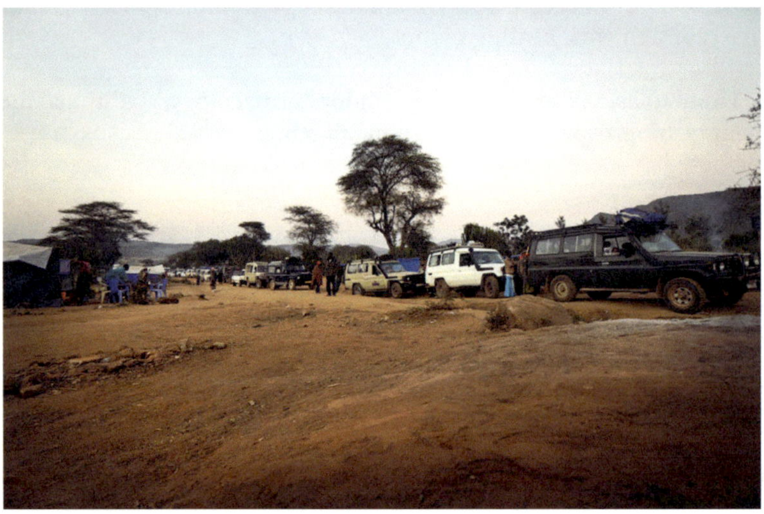

Figure 1.
Queues of traffic as people make their way to Loliondo (photo with permission from Jonathan Kalan).

with ethnobotany a major subdiscipline of ethnobiology. Ethnobiology is concerned with the material and symbolic aspects of interactions between humans and their environments, having multidisciplinary foundations and outlooks. It has undergone many changes since its academic beginnings in the late 1800s. Hunn describes four phases in the development of ethnobiology, although the characteristics of each phase are not limited to the defined time periods (see **Table 1**) [10]. Hunn's Phase I, characteristic of the later nineteenth century to the 1950s, is primarily descriptive presenting lists of plant species and their medicinal and other uses [11]. Phase II, dating from the 1950s to the 1970s, examined the role of cognition in human relationships with their environments researching folk classification, linguistics and symbolic aspects, representing the perspective of the person whose culture is being studied. It is described as the emic phase [12]. Phase III developed from the 1970s through to the 1990s examining indigenous knowledge and the broader ecological context which resulted in the formation of the ISE Code of Ethics [13]. Phase IV from the 1990s onwards is characterised by the rise to prominence of concerns around the rights of local communities, specifically: the exploitation of indigenous knowledge and intellectual property rights of indigenous knowledge holders. The indigenous voice is heard in this phase as a research collaborator rather than as a participant. A developing Phase V involves deeper networking and collaborative work between researchers across geographies and disciplines to address pressing issues of ecological and cultural crises [11]. D'Ambrosio identifies the same broad phasing as illustrated in **Table 1** [12]. In Phase IV, he identifies both biocultural and ethical components in the focus and conduct of research.

Ethnobiology has, thus, historically had a significant focus on ethnomedicine (EM). The main emphasis within EM research from its inception has been on finding new drug leads in what Reyes-García [14] called the "romance of ethnopharmacology" as a route to this end. The interest in mining medicinal plants for economic purposes dates back to the colonial period [15]. This search for new drugs has resulted in the prominence of Phase I-type research in Hunn's classification where medicinal species and their therapeutic uses are documented [11, 16].

C. spinarum is a species with a wealth of associated biocultural knowledge including practical and ritual uses across its range, with its use in health and healing

Time period	Hunn Phases	Character of era—D'Ambrosio	Some Academic Fields
Late 19th C–1940s	I	Ethnography Cultural Anthropology Uses of biota	Ethnography Economic Botany
1950s–1970s	II	Cognitive and emic classification Secondary metabolites	Ethnoscience Linguistics Ethnopharmacology Phytochemistry
1970s–1991	III	Ethnoecology Ethnopharmacology	Ecology and conservation Traditional Ecological Knowledge Bioprospecting
1992–present	IV	Indigenous Ethnobiology Bioculture Ethics Reflexivity	Indigenous rights Biocultural Diversity Research Ethics Global Change

Table 1.
Elements of history of ethnobiology (adapted from D'Ambrosio 2014).

being the most widely reported in the literature. Despite its widespread usage, it is not well-known outside the oral and folk traditions of Africa, South Asia and Australia as evidenced by a Google search. Using the Google Trends search function, as used in an analysis of global and regional interest of Açai berries [17], there is a low level of interest in *C. spinarum* relative to other medicinal species of global and regional importance such as *Azadirachta indica* A. Juss, *Withania somnifera* (L.) Dunal, *Argemone mexicana* L., and *Echinacea purpurea* (L.) Moench. Written records began during the colonial era and there has been recent media interest in its medical potential in East Africa [1]. There is limited recorded usage in the ancient texts of Traditional Chinese Medicine (TCM) and Ayurvedic and Siddha medicines although a similar species, *C. carandas* L., is listed in Ayurvedic databases [18]. The focus on healing properties may be a function of the studies that have been conducted where the emphasis is often on ethnomedicine (EM) and the ultimate potential for bioprospecting. Broad ethnobotanical studies and anthropological research would help to situate this healing focus in the context of the wider value of biodiversity as integral to existence in communities of the Global South [19].

Previous articles reviewing *C. spinarum* have examined the phytochemistry and pharmacology of the species with limited attention to the wider ethnobiology of this species [20–26]. The scope of this chapter is to:

- analyse the available indigenous knowledge regarding the cultural role of *C. spinarum* across the multiple reported domains with an in-depth analysis of the ethnomedical domain

- analyse the presentation of emic or insider's perspectives on the role of *C. spinarum* and other species in the study communities

- analyse the data through the framework of Hunn's phases of ethnobiology, using *C. spinarum* as a case study of wider trends in ethnobiology research of medicinal species

- question whether this analysis informs future research on *C. spinarum* and other species with substantial associated biocultural knowledge?

2. Botany of *Carissa spinarum L.*

2.1 Description and distribution

The species *Carissa spinarum* L. (*C. spinarum*) (Apocynaceae) grows as a thorny highly branched evergreen shrub or small tree of up to 6 m tall with evergreen leaves and masses of fragrant white flowers tinged with pink/purple. Fruits are green, then red ripening to purplish black and are edible when ripe (see **Figure 2**) [27].

C. spinarum is among the most widely distributed of all Apocynaceae species [28]. It occupies a wide range of habitats from wet or dry forest, to thickets and savannahs, at altitudes of 0–2450 m though it is not found in very wet climates or in equatorial rainforests [28]. Its wide ecological tolerance is reflected in the geographic distribution of botanical and ethnobotanical samples. *C. spinarum* is found in 74 countries and territories across 3 continents: Australia, throughout Sub-Saharan Africa and the Indian Ocean islands, the Arabian Peninsula; and in countries of South, East and Southeast Asia (see **Figure 3**) [8].

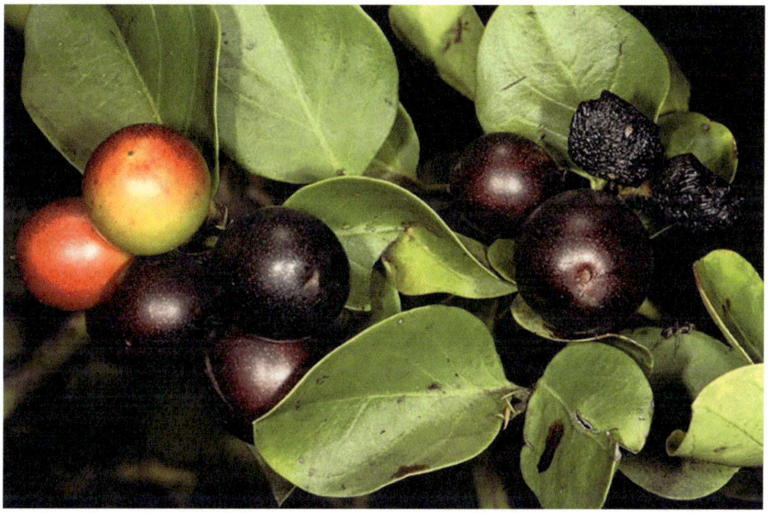

Figure 2.
C. spinarum *L., by SAplants, CC BY-SA 4.0 via Wikimedia Commons.*

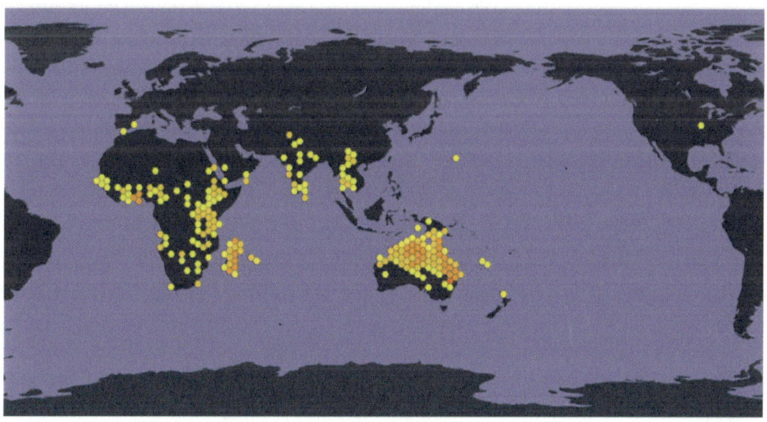

Figure 3.
C. spinarum *L. in GBIF Secretariat (2019). GBIF Backbone Taxonomy. Checklist dataset https://doi.org/10.15468/39omei accessed via GBIF.org on 2020-10-11.*

2.2 Botanical nomenclature and synonymy

C. spinarum is the currently accepted name of the species. It is listed in World Flora Online [29] as having 98 synonymic botanical names. The genus *Carissa* is described as having significant inter- and intra-species variation [30] and this, along with its wide geographic distribution, may contribute to its numerous botanical synonyms. The key synonyms that appear in the ethnobotanical literature are *C. spinarum* L. (accepted name), *C. edulis* (Forssk. Vahl.) (Sub-Saharan Africa), *C. opaca* Stapf ex Haines (India and Pakistan), *C. congesta* Wight (India), *C. xylopicron* Thouars (Mauritius) and *C. lanceolata* R.Br. (Australia). As a heterogeneous species, there are disagreements around plant identification, naming and synonymy with the added problem of misspellings. The complexities in the naming of *C. spinarum* carry through in all subsequent study findings as described in best-practice documents [31–33].

3. Ethnobiology of *C. spinarum*

This section will analyse the available indigenous knowledge regarding the cultural role of *C. spinarum* across the multiple reported domains. It begins with the ethnobiological distribution and nomenclature of the species. It then examines how the relationship of people and plants has been explored through qualitative and quantitative means. Specific cultural domains of use are then examined, with a particular focus on ethnomedical—human and animal—use as the most common domain (80%). Inclusion in human and animal diet is the second most common domain of use reported (9%). It is also valued as an insect and snake repellent, for firewood and charcoal making, for fencing and live hedging and as a timber. The examination of broad ethnobotanical usage across multiple domains is most commonly found in research from Ethiopia and Australia. The body of data is then analysed with respect to the historical phases of ethnobiological research.

3.1 Ethnobiological distribution and nomenclature of *C. spinarum* L.

C. spinarum has a wide ethnobiological distribution. Overall, a total of 284 documents were reviewed for this study including medical and other ethnobotanical uses. There are ethnobotanical reports from 35 countries across 3 continents as illustrated in the map in **Figure 4**. This is less than the botanical distributions and could indicate that it is not considered a useful species in the remaining 29 countries, that such research has not been conducted or that the knowledge has been lost. For the purposes of our analysis, the geographical regions have been divided as follows: Eastern Africa (Kenya, Tanzania, Rwanda, Uganda, Ethiopia); Southern Africa (Angola, Botswana, Mauritius, Madagascar, Malawi, Mayotte, South Africa, Zimbabwe); Central Africa (Chad, "Congo Belge" and "Ruanda-Urundi", DRC, Burundi); West Africa (Benin, Côte d'Ivoire, 'French West Africa', Ghana, Guinea, Mali, Nigeria, Senegal, Togo); Northern Africa (Sudan); Arabian Peninsula (Saudi Arabia); Eastern Asia (China); Southeast Asia

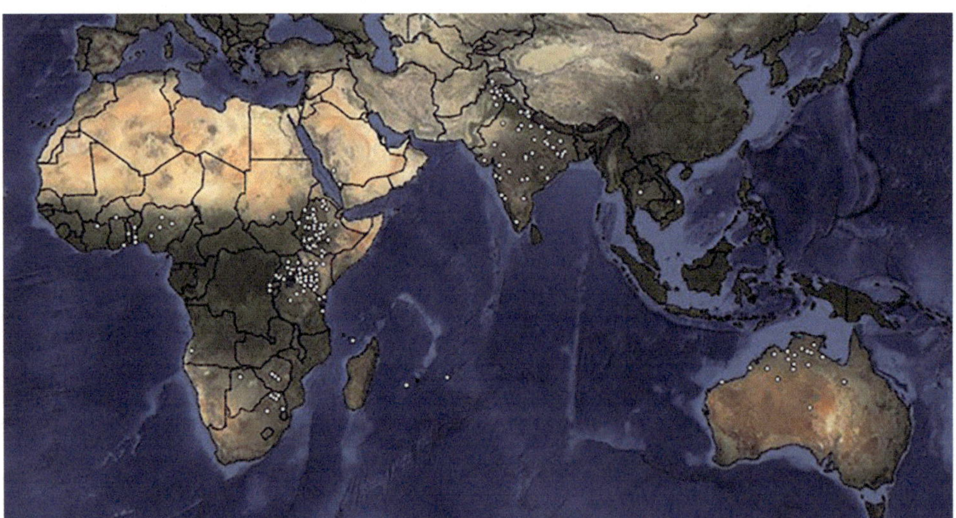

Figure 4.
Distribution of ethnobotanical reports on C. spinarum *(courtesy of Robbie Kelleher).*

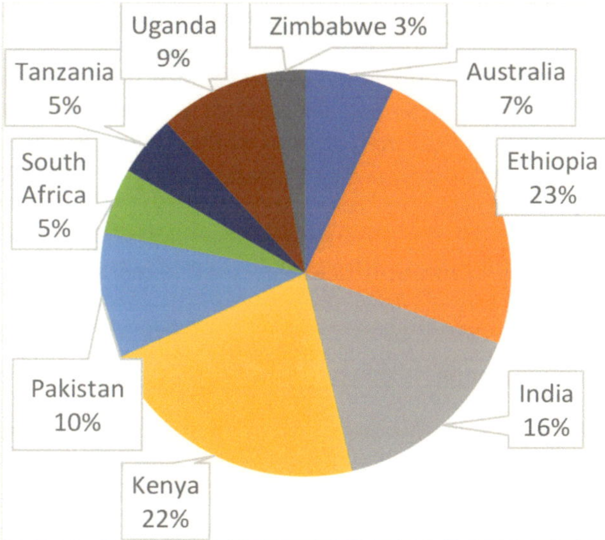

Figure 5.
Documents % per country (>6 = 80% total) citing ethnobotanical use of C. spinarum.

('Indo-China' i.e., Vietnam) and South Asia (India, Pakistan). The proportional geographical distribution of these studies is illustrated in the chart in **Figure 5** showing that most of the research has occurred in Kenya, Ethiopia and India with Uganda, Pakistan, South Africa, Tanzania and Australia being proportionally in a second tier of the data. The Kew Medicinal Plant Names Service [34] lists 162 common names. In this study, the most common vernacular names found are *Agam* (and variations—Ethiopia), *Muyonza* (and variations—Kenya), *Legetetwo* (and variations—Kenya), *Lamuriei* (and variations—East Africa), *Olamuriaki* (and variations—East Africa); *Bois drone* (Mauritius), *Konkerberry* (and variations—Australia), *Currant bush* (and variations—Australia), *Gara-asur* (India), *Karamarda* (and variations—India) and *Karaunda* (and variations—India and Pakistan).

3.2 Some emic perspectives on the ethnobiology of *C. spinarum*

Anthropology has historically been an integral part of ethnobotanical investigations dating to the colonial era. The emic approach in anthropology came to the fore in the 1960s whereby the researcher attempted to experience and interpret the culture from the insider's perspective. In ethnobiological research, techniques to gain the insider perspective are used in order to understand and interpret the relationship of people and plants. In ethnomedical research, this can take the form of understanding local illness aetiologies, concepts of health and healing, the meaning of different elements of the healing process and the meaning attached to different plants and habitats. In Hunn's four phases, the emic aspect becomes significant in Phase II from the 1950's through to the 1970's though Frazão-Moreira illustrates clearly the ongoing centrality of ethnographic research in ethnobiology [35]. An anthropological perspective in ethnobotanical and ethnomedical studies has been considered vital for decades [31, 32, 36, 37]. This view can give valuable context for the medicinal use of plants and can help direct further study and practice in many fields such as health care provision, sustainable plant use, environmental protection and bioprospecting. There is very little of the insider's understanding available in this analysis on *C. spinarum*. Of all primary ethnomedical studies involving *C. spinarum*, 75% have no contextual information at all including no information on local morbidity, mortality or availability of biomedical healthcare. Some 25% of studies, provide some emic information with short descriptions of selected aspects of local traditional medicine such as causation and diagnosis, specific illness understandings and descriptions, knowledge distribution and transmission, information on the place of plants in healing and biomedical health context [38–53]. However, a view on how this species has a role in health and healing in some communities is presented in research from Australia and Eastern Africa.

3.2.1 Australia: "Boonyja Bardag Gorna—All trees are good for something"

The phrase "*Boonyja Bardag Gorna*—All trees are good for something" is the title of the book authored by Esther and Sandy Paddy and Moya Smith [54] and is an illustration of the centrality of biocultural knowledge to life for the authors. Attempts to record that knowledge are ongoing in parts of Australia.

There are elements of Aboriginal biocultural knowledge that makes Australian ethnobiological research different to that conducted in other cultural contexts. These elements relate to the historical context and cultural norms relating to biocultural knowledge, knowledge transmission and plant usage. *C. spinarum* is a widely distributed species in northern Australia [55]. However, there is relatively little ethnobotanical data in comparison to the high level of botanical sampling. This might be explained by the fact that significant ethnobiological research in the area is relatively recent, being concentrated in the past 35 years with the greater part of that local ecological knowledge already lost (Glenn Wightmann, Ethnobiologist, Northern Territory Government pers. comm 2020). Most of the research analysed in relation to Australian Aboriginal ethnobiology is not published in online academic journals but is mostly in the form of Botanical Bulletins. The research is collaborative with community members as primary authors and is published for the purposes of transmission of biocultural knowledge, a cultural requirement for Aboriginal Elders [56]. Research with the Wik peoples in Queensland, has illustrated how ethnobotanical research methods need to be culturally appropriate [57]. They stated that for Aboriginal Communities with whom they have conducted research, widely used ethnobotanical methods such as those described by Cotton [58] and Martin [37] are not appropriate in this environment. Factors contributing to this include: categories of public and secret biocultural knowledge, inappropriate questions and inappropriate questioning. Researchers need to be aware that only selected people may speak on behalf of "country" by law. In this analysis of the ethnobotany of *C. spinarum*, the reality of public and secret knowledge is described by several authors [56, 59–62]. These studies highlight the fact there is a vast amount of knowledge of Aboriginal medicines including gendered knowledge, which is secret, culturally sensitive and cannot be shared in publications.

In a large study of Australian Aboriginal medicinal plant usage, Latz [63] found that, in contrast to western medicines, fewer than 10% are taken internally and that about 70% are used as a wash or an ointment. The use of fumes from heated plant parts is also common in Australia especially for children in a process known as "smoking" [63–65]. These general findings are reflected in the research on *C. spinarum* in Australia. The most common routes of administration are fumigation and external application. Latz stated that most important species have several uses. Connelly and Wallis [64] added that there is knowledge of all of the different elements of a plant

DOI: http://dx.doi.org/10.5772/intechopen.104665

and how they may each be used in different ways. In these Australian studies, *C. spinarum* is used medicinally and ritually but is also included in diet, as an insect repellent, for carving and for firewood. This multifunctionality of plant species is reflected across the global range of *C. spinarum*. The possibility of multifunctionality of species recorded in ethnobotanical research may be important to bear in mind when asking why a particular species may be chosen by local people. It's very multifunctionality may be a central reason for its choice as a medicinal species. While emic description of Australian aboriginal EM is provided in some documents, as elsewhere, detailed anthropological information in relation to *C. spinarum* in particular is limited. McDonald [66], in an anthropological study in the East Kimberley region researching concepts of health and illness, described the "smoking" process: Aboriginal peoples "smoke" the bodies of children and adults with medicinal plants in order to clear the body of "rubbish"—debris that can clog the flow of *birlirr*, the body's life-force. In the study community, *C. spinarum* is an excellent smoking medicine [60, 66]. Aromatic leaves are believed to be strong medicinally as the smoke can be felt entering the body through the senses and the skin:

> *You can feel the jiluwa working, feel the blood flowing [during a smoking treatment]. I was heavy before, just like sin. I'm fresh and light now. We can feel the medicine going into us. Feel cold coming through the body. When we take gardiya tablets, we don't feel anything. Gija woman, [66] p. 90. [Note: Jiluwa are body channels, gardiya tablets are whitefella medicine or pharmaceuticals. Coldness is a healthy state].*

For Aboriginal peoples, bush medicine is considered to have been in the ground from *ngarrangkarni*—the Dreaming time, placed there by the ancestors [66]. This elicits trust in users of bush medicine. *C. spinarum* is included in some Dreaming stories and thus is part of Aboriginal cosmology, which links plants, animals, humans, and places, past and present [67]. The inclusion of this and other aspects of the social and natural environment in these stories indicate a cultural importance that extends beyond the utilitarian realm.

The loss of biocultural knowledge is a well-established phenomenon in the ethnobotanical literature in general [68, 69]. Latz [63] and Wightmann (2020 pers. commun.) described the loss of many aspects of traditional Aboriginal knowledge due to changes in the way of life and the influx of new diseases. Other authors describe how many of the plant species and the practices involving them are still in use by many adults as "domestic" medicine and need to be documented [61]. The value of the publication of the Dalabon biocultural knowledge from North Australia was asserted in [56]. Given that traditional modes of transmission of knowledge relating to native species from elders to the next generation are being interrupted through the lack of access to sacred sites and ceremonial practices, some elders feel that the transmission of knowledge through publication is a way of fulfilling their duty.

3.2.2 Buda (Evil Eye) in Ethiopia

Spirit-Related Illness, usually *Buda* (Evil Eye) is commonly reported to be treated with *C. spinarum* in Ethiopian studies. Treatment often involves *C. spinarum* in combination with other species in the form of fumigation. Literature shows that there is a wide geographical and historical spread of Evil Eye. It is referenced in Classical Greek literature, the Bible, Islamic literature and is reported among some Asian peoples and in most European, African and American countries [70]. However, there is no description of the presentation of *Buda* or other spirit-related illness in any of the Ethiopian documents on *C. spinarum*. In other Ethiopian research with a sociological rather than ethnobiological focus, *Buda* has been studied. The ability to inflict Evil Eye/*Buda* is described as being innate and that the identity of people who can inflict *Buda* is secretly known within a community [71]. Abbink [72] wrote that the Amhara people of Ethiopia believe *Buda* to be held by people outside of the Amhara group, perhaps landless or with no permanent home or people of certain professions such as blacksmiths or potters. They have a hereditary, malevolent power which is used, perhaps involuntarily, to cause harm. He wrote that the victims of *Buda* become weakened with a sense of being drawn to their death. *Buda* is described as causing many animal and human health problems as well as damage to property and is commonly treated by ritual [71–74]. Jacobsson [75] wrote that it can cause any kind of illness including neuroses and psychosomatic illness, though it often manifests as gastrointestinal disorders. Jacobsson argues that there is no clear distinction between physical and mental disorders, and consequently there is none between associated healing methods. Thus, physical and spiritual means may be used as part of the healing process. The treatment with medicinal plants can have ritual and physical components, and the burning of *C. spinarum* in the treatment of *Buda* disorders could be interpreted in this light. The most common method of preparation of *C. spinarum* for treatment of *Buda* is the administration of root smoke by fumigation (for example see [51]). In a few cases, the root is mixed in water alone and inhaled or taken orally or the root may be tied around the neck as protection [76–78]. Ritual and physical effects may combine in the use of *C. spinarum* to treat *Buda*. In an examination of ritual plant use in Benin and Gabon from a biomedical (BM) (conventional medicine) perspective, Quiroz et al [79] illustrated that ritual use does not imply a lack of pharmacological activity. Pharmacological activity of the smoke of *C. spinarum* may augment the socio-cultural healing benefits of the ritual components of healing.

The example of spirit-related illnesses illustrates that an understanding of the context of healing, can help to situate the use of plants in the healing process and to interpret it from a cross cultural perspective.

3.2.3 Kenya: Pokot and Luo health-seeking behaviour

There are two anthropological studies from Kenya, whereby the context of *C. spinarum* use is provided through in-depth emic information in relation to health and illness in the study areas. These studies are conducted with the Pokot people in north western Kenya [80] and the Luo of Western Kenya [81] with some emic information from some other studies [41, 82–90].

The 1982 study of Pokot health-seeking behaviour illustrated the dynamic nature of this behaviour in the context of the availability of traditional and BM forms of health care [80]. The Pokot understanding of illness causation is detailed as having naturalistic/biological, interpersonal and/or spiritual basis. Treatment and prevention can involve addressing each of these planes of causation with the treatment for biological cause being more specific to the symptomatology and treatments for interpersonal and spiritual cause being more diffuse. Some ailments such as infertility and mental illness are considered to have an interpersonal or spiritual basis while others such as malaria are thought to have a more naturalistic causation. Treatments usually involve administration of medicinal plants, ritual and instructions on foods to eat or avoid. The use of purgatives and emetics by the Pokot in the study area to prevent and treat illness is understood in the context of illnesses residing in the gut. The process is thought to "clean up the system". The treatment for malaria, for instance, may involve the use of pharmaceuticals complemented by the subsequent use of purgatives and emetics to ensure the complete expulsion of the illness. The use of emetics and laxatives was likewise discussed elsewhere in the context of Pokot ethnobotany [89] and among the Luo [81].

Ethnobotanical research with Luo mothers was conducted with reference to the authors' earlier extensive anthropological research with the Luo of western Kenya [81]. It is an instance of rich emic understandings presented in this analysis of *C. spinarum*. As with the Australian example above, there is an amount of secret knowledge among the Luo mothers, especially in the treatment of more complex ailments resulting in lacunae in the recorded knowledge. Their research found that gastrointestinal illnesses are the most commonly treated with medicinal plants while fever and headache are rarely treated using plant medicines despite the high prevalence of malaria in the study area. The authors attribute this to the availability of pharmaceuticals in local shops to treat these symptoms. The extent of secret knowledge and the availability of effective pharmaceuticals could result in an overall skewing of the ethnobotanical findings towards gastrointestinal use. Illness itself is considered to be a constant element of life and plant remedies are used, not to eliminate illness but rather to find a balance in a constant process. In the case of helminth infections, worms are considered to live permanently in the gut and it is important to maintain worms in a healthy equilibrium in the gut for the health of the individual. Treatment of other illnesses, such as diarrhoea, require the illness to be removed from the body with purgatives. This concept of healing also finds the BM healing by suppression of illness to be unhealthy such that sometimes the use of BM is prohibited in the pursuit of health:

> *Luo medicine makes the illness come out; injections push it back inside. If you inject, it moves through the body and you swell and may die. (Luo mother [81] p. 44).*

Many illnesses including diarrhoea may be thought to be caused by *Yamo*, an overarching illness concept that can manifest in many ways but is treated through eliminating it from the body. The constant presence of illness in the body, even when it is healthy, requires that a child be constantly treated to make illness emerge from the body and as such keep the forces of *Yamo* and other forces of illness at bay:

> *'a (young) child ought to be ill regularly' (nyathi onego otuore) lest it would die, once the illness (i.e., Yamo) finally 'comes out'. (Luo saying, [81] p. 44).*

In their research with Luo mothers, the authors report the use of *C. spinarum* (*Ochuoga*) in the treatment of diarrhoea and *Ang'iew* (a childhood febrile illness with rash) [81]. While no individual species is singled out as culturally important, the presentation of in-depth emic understandings of health and illness described in brief here gives valuable context to the listing of 91 medicinal species. From a BM perspective such as researching health-seeking behaviour or bioprospecting, it is important to understand the socio-cultural understandings of health and illness as a backdrop to the choice of treatments. The use of *C. spinarum* as a purgative to treat malaria, for instance, does not imply that it is ineffective as an anti-malarial but the knowledge could modify the perspective of the bioprospecting ethnopharmacologists. For BM healthcare workers, the knowledge of local purgative and emetic practices is important in providing care to the communities served.

3.3 Ethnobotanical uses—*C. spinarum* in human and animal medicine

Ethnomedical (EM) analysis of *C. spinarum* took into consideration the following basic elements: plant parts used, methods of preparation, route of administration and ailments treated using *C. spinarum*, followed by analysis of the use of different plant parts for different ailments. Plant harvesting details were searched but were only reported on in three studies out of a total of 284 documents and 513 use reports (URs) analysed. Each of these aspects of EM plant use bears a relationship to the phytochemistry, bioactivity and toxicity of plant extracts which then have a bearing on the outcomes of ethno-directed bioprospecting studies. The global geographical variation in usage of *C. spinarum* and the ethnoveterinary use of *C. spinarum* were also examined.

The geographical distribution of the ethnobotanical data is illustrated in **Figure 6**. The key areas reporting the EM use of *C. spinarum* are Eastern Africa (mainly Kenya and Ethiopia) and South Asia (mainly India and Pakistan). *C. spinarum* is also used across the rest of Sub-Saharan Africa, Northern Africa and the Arabian Peninsula, East and South East Asia and Australia.

3.3.1 C. spinarum *in human ethnomedicine: plant parts used*

A summary of *C. spinarum* plant part used in medicinal preparations for human use across all regions is seen in **Figure 7**. It illustrates that, for *C. spinarum*, the primary plant part used is the root followed by leaf, fruit, rootbark, stem and bark while 9% of reports do not state what plant part is used (N/S).

The data was analysed across 5 key geographical regions: Eastern Africa, Western Africa, Southern Africa, South Asia and Australia. The summary of key plant parts used is illustrated in **Figure 8** and shows that, at regional level, the root is still the most commonly used plant part. However, in Eastern Africa, the predominance is more marked where the root and rootbark together account for three quarters of all URs. Fruit and leaf use are minimal by comparison. In Western Africa, the root and rootbark together account for most usage with leaf, fruit and stem used infrequently. In Southern Africa the root accounts for over half of usage with stem and other parts lower. In South Asia,

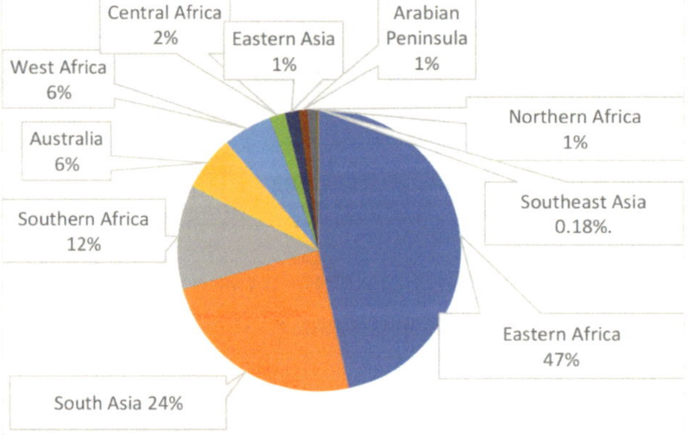

Figure 6.
Geographical distribution of human EM Use Reports (URs) for C. spinarum.

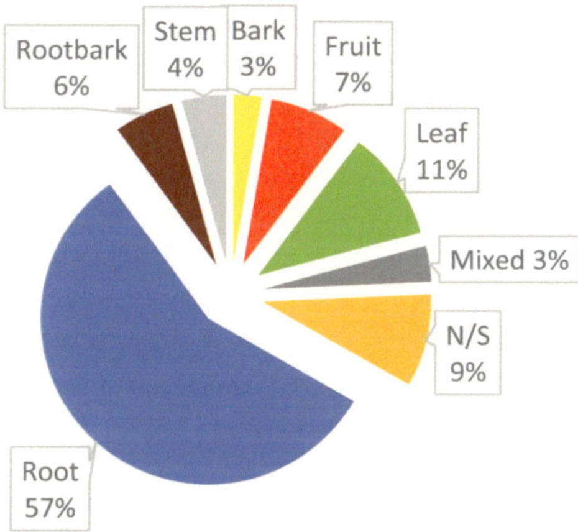

Figure 7.
C. spinarum *for human use: plant parts used in the preparation of EM.*

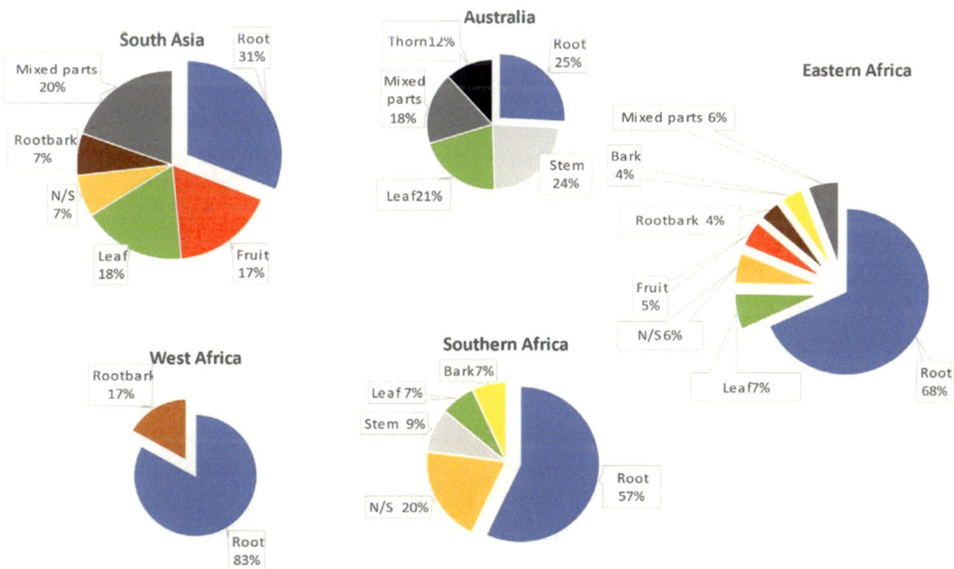

Figure 8.
C. spinarum *and variation in plant part usage across global regions (UR > 3, 85% of all URs; N/S = not stated; chart areas approximately reflect relative nos. of URs).*

root use is less dominant and followed by leaf and fruit. In Australia, the different plant parts are more evenly divided between root, stem and leaf. In most areas a proportion do not state what plant part is used, particularly so in Southern Africa.

More broadly in EM research, there are a number of reasons hypothesised for differences in the choice of plant and plant part such as availability and related cultural norms, the presence of bioactive metabolites, organoleptic qualities, appearance, time of year and location of a species.

A study of the most commonly used plant parts in East Africa stated that with trees and shrubs, the bark and root are more commonly used [91]. A study in a semi-arid region of Kenya found that most medicinal plants are trees and shrubs, and their bark and roots are the most commonly used parts [89]. Research in the Caatinga (semi-arid) region in North-eastern Brazil found that the species and plant parts that are available throughout the year are the most important medicinal species. Stem-bark was the most commonly used plant part [92]. The authors reported that herbaceous plants and leaves, which are only available for a few months of the year, are less commonly used in the same study. The authors examined tannin concentration in two medicinal species, assuming tannins to be responsible for much of the medicinal activity though they acknowledge that this may not be wholly correct. They found that both leaf and stem-bark contained significant quantities of tannins although the stem-bark is the part used medicinally. They postulated that the community develops a stronger relationship with the perennial woody plant parts regardless of the fact that the leaf may be as effective as the stem.

Organoleptic qualities of taste, smell, colour and texture are reported to be important to decision making around medicinal plants as described by Etkin [36] and are linked to explanatory models of illness. A study in Peru illustrated how sensation is at the centre of medicinal plant selection connecting culture and the environment [93]. A study in Brazil found that taste and smell are associated with therapeutic indications [94]. Studies in Mexico indicated a similar connection between taste, smell and therapeutic indication where, for instance, bitter and aromatic plants are valued in the treatment of gastrointestinal disorders [95]. Bitterness is a characteristic of aphrodisiac tonics in West Africa and the Caribbean [96]. Among the Pokot people in Kenya, bitter medicines were considered to be more effective at treating all illness [80]. Sensory attributes of plants were, likewise, seen, as an important indicator of healing power among the Suiei Dorobo of Northern Kenya [85]. The "doctrine of signatures" may be a contributor to the choice of plant or plant part such that, for instance, a root with a red extract may be considered to be useful in blood disorders [36, 97].

The choice of plant part in EM may be directly related to the presence of bioactive ingredients in different plant parts, an assumption often made in ethnodirected bioprospecting studies [98]. Secondary metabolites may benefit plants through action as pollinator attractants, as simple feeding repellents or as toxicants to prevent herbivory [99]. Voeks [99] states that this phenomenon, referencing a study on the presence of alkaloids, is more pronounced in low-latitude countries and is more likely in herbs and shrubs. Further studies in the Caatinga of Brazil reported that, in such semi-arid areas, plants invest more heavily in secondary metabolites based on phenolic compounds (such as tannins) providing quantitative defences against herbivory [98]. In comparison, in humid forest regions, plants are more likely to produce qualitative defences in the form of highly bioactive compounds such as alkaloids. Another consideration is that phenotypic plasticity is known to occur within a species across different habitats in response to different environmental stressors [98]. Plant defences are determined by the availability of resources such as light, water and nutrients in an ecosystem. The lack of resources such as water and nutrients in semi-arid habitats may result in a "metabolic specialisation" in quantitative defences such as phenolics [98]. The authors add that woody species growing in semi-arid areas could have lower concentrations of bioactive ingredients in the leaf than in perennial plant parts due to the short growth-period of the leaf, thus favouring the perennial parts as medicinal ingredients.

How do these general hypotheses and findings in relation to the choice of plant parts in EM relate to *C. spinarum*? While *C. spinarum* has a wide ecological tolerance, it can be seen from the map of ethnobotanical usage in **Figure 4** that many of the areas in which *C. spinarum* is used are semi-arid. This lends credence to the use of the perennial parts of this shrub, as these are available throughout the year. Organoleptic qualities may be a factor with choice of *C. spinarum* root. It is somewhat bitter in taste which, as described above, may lead to its being considered medicinal [89, 100, 101]. The root has an oily, volatile sap with a pleasant smell which lends itself to use as a rub for chest and muscle conditions and as an inhalant. *C. spinarum* is a member of the Apocynaceae family, a family which is known to produce toxic and medicinal metabolites such as the Vinca alkaloids. The choice of plant part may be related to the avoidance of toxic components in other plant parts. A review of the ethnobotany of Apocynaceae species in Kenya (25 in all), found that the root is the most commonly used plant part for medicinal use (63%) [102]. In contrast, a review of some medicinally important Apocynaceae species found that there is no particular preponderance of root use [103]. Rather, EM use in different species was found to be generally distributed across plant parts. This correlates with the finding in India and Pakistan where the plant part usage of *C. spinarum* is much more evenly distributed across plant parts than in Eastern Africa. This difference could point to factors such as availability of plant material, cultural norms around medicinal preparations or ecological differences across its range leading to different secondary metabolite patterns.

3.3.2 C. spinarum *in human ethnomedicine: methods of preparation*

The predominant methods of preparation of *C. spinarum* globally are summarised in **Figure 9**. In the data as a whole, where a method is given, it may be simply written as a single word such as decoction, infusion, paste, juice or raw. There is relatively little detailed description of the preparation of *C. spinarum* in the studies analysed. In the reviewed studies, over one third do not to include a method of preparation. The preparation of medicinal products by decoction i.e., boiling of the plant part in water for a length of time, is by far the most common method reported followed by use of the untreated plant, burning for smoke, cold water mixture, infusion, powder, juice, decoction with soup and mixing with alcohol (4 citations).

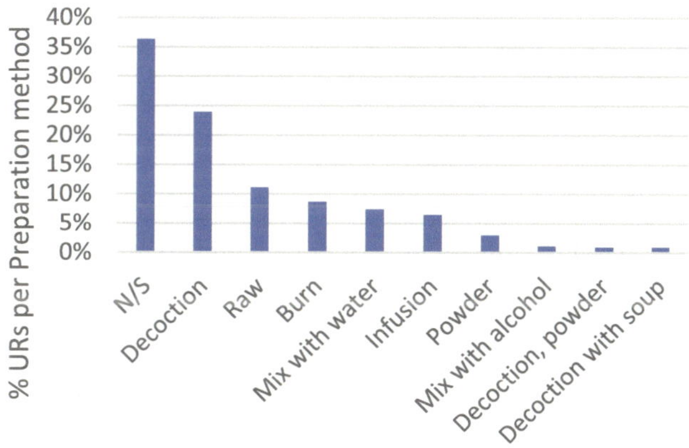

Figure 9.
Methods of preparation of human EM containing C. spinarum *(UR > 4) ("Decoction, powder" where unclear which method used per ailment).*

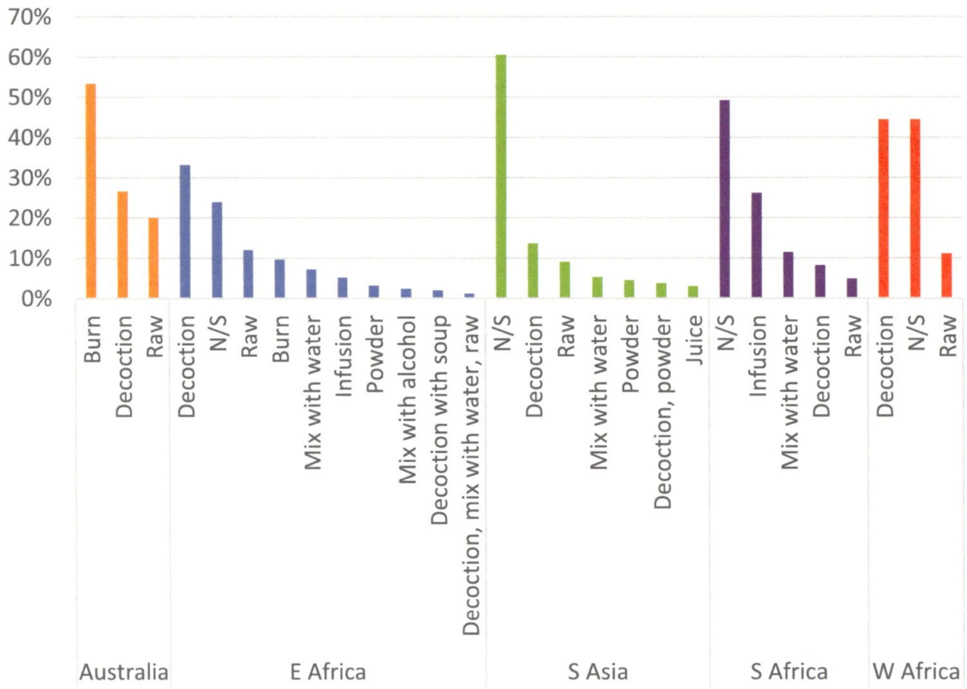

Figure 10.
Regional variation in method of preparation of C. spinarum *expressed as % URs per region (UR > 2). Methods with low occurrence are excluded.*

Methods of preparation vary across the geographical range represented in **Figure 10**. A significant proportion in each geographical area, except Australia, does not state the method of preparation. In South Asia, Eastern Africa and West Africa, decoction is the most common method used. In Southern Africa, infusion is the most popular method of preparation. In Australian studies the most common method is burning followed by decoction and untreated. Burning as a method of preparation globally is relatively high. When we examine the data in relation to burning, it is apparent that this is greatest in Australia and in Ethiopia with the emic context described above in Section 3.2. In Australia, burning is used in the main as a treatment to protect children by "smoking" while in Ethiopia, the primary illness category where burning is used is *Buda* (Evil Eye) (see Sections 3.2.1 and 3.2.2).

3.3.3 C. spinarum *in human ethnomedicine: methods of preparation x key plant parts*

It is useful to take a closer view of the methods of preparation that are used for each plant part. The chart in **Figure 11** presents an overview of the most common methods of preparation for each plant part. The chart shows that the fruit is most often used raw; the bark is most often prepared by infusion; the leaf, root and root-bark are each most commonly prepared by decoction and the stem by burning.

Where fruit is treated, the minimal treatment is illustrated as follows:

> *Fruits are crushed, dried, pounded into powder and sprayed on wound ([104] p. 6 Ethiopia).*

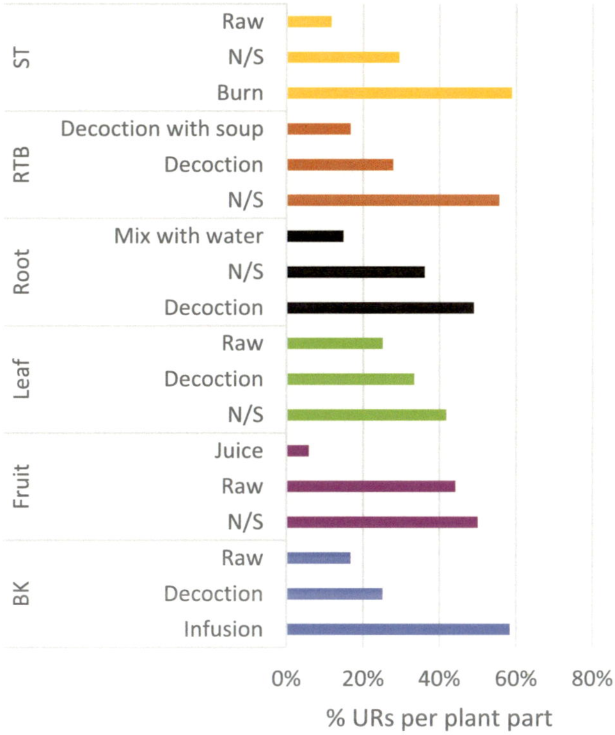

Figure 11.
Salient methods of preparation for each plant part (top 3, excludes combinations; 54% of total URs) (BK = Bark; ST = Stem; RTB = Rootbark).

and of leaf:

> *Leaves are crushed, squeezed and liquid taken (orally) with coffee (to treat febrile illness) ([104] p. 6 Ethiopia).*

Simple decoctions are prepared as follows:

> *Among the Mitakoodi, it [root] is scraped and soaked in water and then boiled. The resultant liquid is drunk as a tea to treat aches and pains and used as an eyewash ([64], p. 14, Australia).*

Leaves are boiled in water and liquor is used to treat jaundice [105] Pakistan. Some additional ingredients may be added as part of the treatment prescribed:

> *Rootbark is crushed and mixed with black pepper and given (for typhoid fever). [106] India.*
> *Fresh root of C. spinarum pounded mixed with cold water. One cup of tella [beer] is used as a drink for three days [to treat gonorrhoea] [49] Ethiopia*

The method of preparation of medicinal plants can have a significant influence on the extraction of active constituents. This can be seen in Chinese Herbal Medicine (CHM) whereby a variety of processing methods may be used to improve efficacy and/or to reduce toxic effects [107]. In a study on the preparation of CHM, a variety of extraction methods is described whereby special preparation instructions relate to different physical, chemical and pharmacological activities of active compounds [108]. The authors describe the preparation of the two-herb formula, Danggui Buxue Tang (DBT), illustrating the variability in yields of marker compounds with duration of boiling, the drug/solvent ratio, the number of extractions and co-extraction vs. individual extraction of each plant. In relation to *C. spinarum* preparation in the studies analysed, the level of detail seen in CHM research is not provided. However, the example of DBT illustrates the importance of accurate data recording in EM studies. The use of decoction or maceration for root preparation, as described with *C. spinarum*, can be seen to aid extraction of active compounds in harder plant materials such as roots, bark and stem [109]. It may also have a role in reducing the toxicity of phytochemicals or plant extracts given that *C. spinarum* belongs to the Apocynaceae family, known to produce toxic metabolites. In bioprospecting, detail on EM preparation can be a crucial guide for ethnopharmacologists in their investigations [108]. Detailed ethnographic descriptions on preparation give a clearer view of the elements of the healing process as a whole which has relevance across other research foci such as cultural record, health care provision and sustainable plant use [32].

3.3.4 C. spinarum *in human ethnomedicine: route of administration*

The most commonly used route of administration globally for *C. spinarum* is the oral route as seen in **Figure 12** with external application, fumigation and inhalation being the most commonly used routes otherwise. However, the route is not specified at all in 40% of URs. In **Table 2**, the primary methods of preparation and route of administration for each plant part are listed. The table illustrates that the root and rootbark are most commonly prepared by decoction and administered orally. The fruit usually undergoes no preparation and is administered orally. The stem is burned and used as a fumigant or inhalant. The leaf is most commonly burned as an inhalant and boiled as a decoction.

It can be seen from **Figure 13** that the predominance of the oral route is common to all geographical zones apart from Australia where it is more common to apply externally and to fumigate. The oral route of administration is common in EM as it is in BM [110, 111]. This may be explained by factors such as safety, convenience, cost and

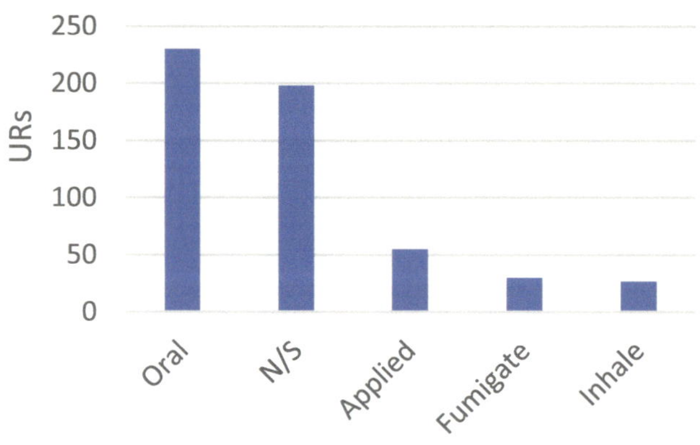

Figure 12.
Top 5 routes of administration of C. spinarum *globally.*

Plant part	Preparation	Route	URs
Root	Decoction	Oral	70
Root	Burn	Fumigate/inhale	21
Root	Mix with water	Oral	18
Root	Infusion	Oral	17
Fruit	Raw	Oral	15
Root	Decoction	Applied	9
Stem	Burn	Fumigate/inhale	9
Root	Mix with water	Applied	8
Root	Raw	Applied	8
Leaf	Burn	Inhale	8
Bark	Infusion	Oral	7
Leaf	Decoction	Oral	7
Root	Mix with alcohol	Oral	6
Root	Powder	Oral	6
Leaf	Raw	Oral	5
Root	Raw	Inhale	4
Leaf	Raw	Applied	3
Root	Powder	Applied	3
Root	Raw	Oral	3
Rootbark	Decoction	Oral	3
Rootbark	Decoction with soup	Oral	3
Leaf	Decoction	Applied	2
Leaf	Raw	Inhale	2

Table 2.
Most common route x preparation x plant part in C. spinarum *used in EM.*

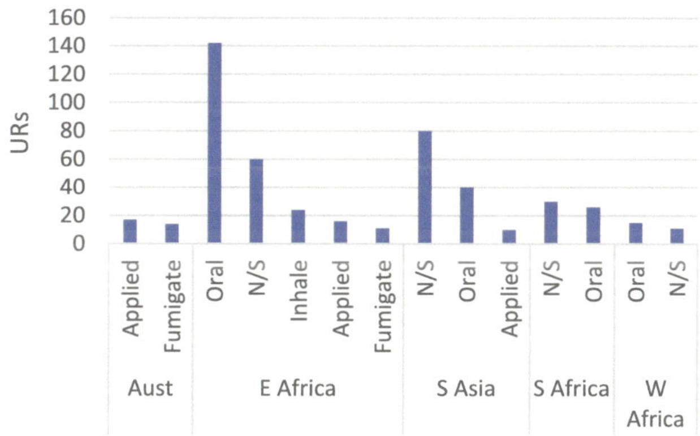

Figure 13.
Key routes of administration of C. spinarum *in different geographical regions (URs > 9).*

acceptability [111, 112]. Route of administration may also be related to the ailments treated. *C. spinarum* is commonly used to treat gastrointestinal ailments and oral administration would thus be logical. In addition, some theories of health and illness in the study areas necessitate the oral route of administration where emesis or purgation is required. In some cases, a mixture of routes is used for one treatment. In the following example oral and topical routes are combined for the treatment of syphilis:

> *Infusion (of root) drunk in malwa, sitz bath ([113] Uganda; malwa is local beer made from Eleusine coracana).*

In Tanzania, oral and topical use are combined for the treatment of unspecified chest conditions:

> *Root crushed and scraped and pulp is applied as a poultice for chest complaints. Root extract drunk at same time. Tanzania [114].*

In Uganda for the treatment of epilepsy, the root is used internally and externally as follows:

> *Powder drunk, bathed, smeared to body. Uganda [113].*

In a study in Uganda, where eight different species used to treat epilepsy, most are applied in some manner rather than taken orally [113]. This includes smearing, bathing, instilling into eye or nostril, fumigating, inhaling or licking. Use of non-oral routes could be a reflection of the practical difficulty of administering orally if a person is having a seizure, or may be a reflection of a ritual component of treatment of a complex illness, or both [79]. The choice of route could be related to the bioactive metabolites present. It is asserted by Le [111] that some phytochemicals such as alkaloids may be more active orally whereas terpenoids may be well absorbed through external or nasal administration.

3.3.5 Human ailments treated using C. spinarum

This section will first outline the form of classification used for this analysis on human ailments treated. The data is then analysed in relation to medicinal usage of *C. spinarum*. The WHO-ICPC system (International Classification of Primary Care) of illness classification was developed for the BM primary care setting as a patient-centred model of classification [115]. The ICPC template is promoted by some researchers to classify certain EM studies as they often lack precise BM diagnoses [32, 116]. This analysis of *C. spinarum* uses a modified ICPC classification system for cross-cultural comparison of EM usage. This is a bi-axial system of Body Systems and Ailment Categories. Modifications of the ICPC system are made to both axes to reflect salience in the *C. spinarum* data of particular body systems and ailments. A summary of the overall classification system is presented in **Table 3a and b**.

Some Body Systems listed in **Table 3a** are self-explanatory such as digestive, musculoskeletal etc. The General and Unspecified grouping is often used where the ailment relates to the whole body such as Malaria or other infectious diseases/symptoms. The *C. spinarum*-data-specific classifications of Spirit-Related and Ill-Defined are created to reflect their prevalence in the data, with the former including Evil Eye, bewitchment, sorcery and evil spirits. The classification of Ill-Defined is created to

(a)	
ICPC body system (plus)	**ICPC body system (plus)**
Blood, blood forming & immune	Psychological
Cardiovascular	Respiratory
Digestive	Skin
Endocrine/metabolic & nutrition	Spirit-related
Eye	**GU system sub-classification:**
General and unspecified	Andrology
Ill-defined	Genital (gender not specified)
Musculoskeletal	Women's Health
Neurological	Urology (gender not specified)

(b)	
ICPC ailment categories (selected)	**Added ailment categories**
Infection	Cough
Injury	Constipation
Neoplasm	Diarrhoea
Symptom/complaint	Evil Eye
Other/misc.	Fever
Added ailment categories	Jaundice
	Pain
Abdominal pain	Seizure
Asthma	Snakebite

Table 3.
Modified bi-axial ICPC classification for C. spinarum*: (a) body systems and (b) selected ailment categories (GU = Genito-urinary).*

reflect ambiguity or lack of descriptions of illness e.g., "Cold-sick" where it is not clear what this means from the text [117]. Genito-urinary (GU) ailments are frequently cited in EM systems as reflected in many global studies [118] and in African *C. spinarum* related studies [91, 119–124]. The ICPC Body System classifications of women's health, andrology and urology are modified in this analysis of *C. spinarum* such that the Genito-Urinary ailments are grouped under four Body System classifications: Women's Health, Genital (not gender specific), Urology (not gender specific) and Andrology. Women's Health includes the ICPC "Female Genital" and "Pregnancy, Childbearing, Family Planning and Female Reproductive System"; Genital includes ailments which are not gender specific and this mainly refers to Sexually Transmitted Infections (STIs); Urology refers mainly to urinary tract infections and Andrology refers mainly to virility. The ICPC modification is made so that the true prevalence of women's' health issues can be evaluated rather than splitting the data into smaller categories. The original ICPC Ailment Categories of Infection, Injury, Symptom/Complaint, Neoplasm and Other are retained while some symptoms, diagnoses and injuries are added as Ailment Categories to aid the analysis. These occur frequently in the data and would otherwise be subsumed under a broad generic Category such as

Symptom/Complaint (**Table 3b**). The added Ailment Categories are Abdominal Pain, Asthma, Cough, Diarrhoea, Evil Eye, Fever, Jaundice, Pain, Seizure and Snakebite. Examples of the bi-axial classification include: amoebiasis classified as Digestion (Body System) and Infection (Ailment Category); gonorrhoea classified as Genital and Infection; post-partum haemorrhage classified as Women's Health and Symptom/ Complaint. This is a means of analytical cross-referencing of the data.

The key Ailment Categories treated with *C. spinarum* are Infection, Pain, Evil Eye, Abdominal Pain, Fever, Diarrhoea and Symptom/Complaint, with a more complete list of 15 Categories presented in **Table 4**. These Key Ailment Categories are cross-referenced with the key ailments within those Categories. It illustrates that while.

Ailment category and ailment	URs
Infection	**94**
Malaria	24
Genital Infection	22
Worms/other parasites	14
Infectious disease other	11
Gastrointestinal infection	10
Upper respiratory infection	7
Pain	**47**
Teeth/gum symptom/complaint	15
Headache	14
Joint symptom/complaint	12
Pain general/multiple sites	6
Evil eye	**27**
Abdominal pain	**26**
Fever	**22**
Diarrhoea	**21**
Symptom/complaint	**20**
Impotence/sexual function—male	7
Digestive symptom/complaint other	7
Lymph gland(s) enlarged/painful	6
Constipation	**17**
Ill-defined	**14**
Jaundice	**10**
Cough	**13**
Snakebite	**13**
Injuries	**11**
Asthma	**8**

Table 4.
Key ailment categories with key ailments treated using C. spinarum *(ailment category UR > 5; ailment UR > 4) (61% of URs).*

Infection is the most common Category treated, Evil Eye is the most common specific Ailment treated followed by Abdominal pain, Malaria, Fever and Genital Infection.

C. spinarum is used across multiple Body Systems with the Digestive system predominant (**Table 5**). The other key Systems treated are General/Unspecified, Spirit-Related and Genital. The breakdown of key ailments treated within the Body Systems is illustrated showing that in the Digestive System, the key ailments treated are Abdominal pain, Diarrhoea and Constipation. The main ailments of the General/ Unspecified Body System are Malaria and Fever. Spirit-related illnesses are Evil Eye for the most part. STIs are the most common ailment treated in the Genital System, joint symptoms in the Musculoskeletal System, cough in the Respiratory System, headache in the Neurological System and snakebite is the most common ailment treated affecting the Skin.

Body system (plus) and ailment	**URs**
Digestive	**116**
Abdominal pain epigastric	26
Diarrhoea	24
Constipation	17
Teeth/gum symptom/complaint	15
Worms/other parasites	14
Gastrointestinal infection	10
Jaundice	10
General and unspecified	**58**
Malaria	24
Fever	22
Infectious disease other	12
Spirit-related	**32**
Evil Eye	32
Genital (gender not specified)	**22**
Genital Infection	22
Musculoskeletal	**14**
Joint symptom/complaint	14
Respiratory	**13**
Cough	13
Neurological	**14**
Headache	14
Skin	**24**
Snake bite	13
Laceration/cut	11

Table 5.
Main body system with key ailments treated with C. spinarum *(UR > 9; 54% of total URs).*

The four dominant geographical zones with EM data for the use of *C. spinarum* in humans are Eastern Africa and South Asia—having the most data—and Southern Africa and Australia. The top 4 ailments in each of these four regions are listed in **Table 6**, which illustrates a diversity in ailments treated across the regions. Spirit-related illness is the most reported ailment, mainly from Ethiopia. Eastern and Southern Africa both list Abdominal Pain and Genital Infection among the most commonly treated ailments. Southern Africa and South Asia both register Fever, Constipation and Diarrhoea among the top 4 ailments treated. Southern Africa and Australia alone list respiratory symptoms among the top individual ailments treated. The treatment of malaria is high in Eastern Africa relative to South Asia corresponding to current and historical relative incidence of malaria [125, 126]. The relatively low level of treatment of fever with *C. spinarum* in Eastern Africa could

Top 4 ailments in highest use global regions	URs
Australia	**17**
Upper respiratory infection	3
Teeth/gum symptom	3
Ill-defined	3
Breast/lactation symptom	2
Health maintenance/prevention	2
Eye symptom	2
Respiratory symptom	2
Eastern Africa	**85**
Spirit-related	30
Malaria	20
Genital infection	19
Abdominal pain epigastric	16
South Asia	**43**
Fever	16
Constipation	10
Jaundice	9
Diarrhoea	8
Southern Africa	**19**
Diarrhoea	5
Abdominal pain epigastric	4
Worms/other parasites	3
Cough	3
Genital infection	3
Fever	3
Constipation	3

Table 6.
Key ailments in each of the top 4 global regions (31% of URs).

reflect the choice of alternative treatments such as other plant species or pharmaceuticals as suggested in Section 3.2.3 or the overdiagnosis of fever as malaria, a recognised phenomenon [127]. Jaundice and hepatic complaints are mainly reported in South Asia. Given the prevalence in Sub-Saharan Africa of malaria and other contributors to liver ailments such as hepatitis, typhoid fever, dengue and leptospirosis this is unusual [128]. Possible explanations may be that jaundice may not be common in study areas other than South Asia, it may not be treated as a symptom *per se* in those regions or *C. spinarum* may not be a chosen treatment outside of South Asia.

Examining the Body Systems classifications illustrates more inter-regional similarity in the top 5 Systems treated (**Table 7**). The Digestive and Respiratory Systems are commonly treated in each region. The Digestive System is the most commonly treated System in all regions except Australia though to varying degrees. Likewise,

Region and body system	URs	% Total regional URs
Australia	**18**	**50% (total 36)**
Respiratory	6	17%
Skin	4	11%
General and unspecified	4	11%
Digestive	4	11%
Eastern Africa	**154**	**56% (total UR 274)**
Digestive	52	19%
General and unspecified	50	19%
Spirit related	30	12%
Neurological	22	8%
Respiratory	21	8%
South Asia	**97**	**72% (total UR 135)**
Digestive	48	36%
General and unspecified	24	17%
Skin	14	10%
Respiratory	11	8%
Cardiovascular	9	6%
Southern Africa	**41**	**60% (total UR 68)**
Digestive	19	28%
General and unspecified	9	13%
Skin	6	9%
Respiratory	6	9%
Neurological	4	6%
Genital	4	6%
Total	**347**	**513**

Table 7.
Top 5 ICPC body systems treated by CS across 4 geographical zones (68% of total URs).

the General and Unspecified Body System is commonly treated in each region, mainly accounted for by malaria in Eastern Africa and fever in South Asia.

The Skin has a high relative importance in all zones except Eastern Africa. The Musculoskeletal System is a key System treated with *C. spinarum* in Eastern Africa whereas the Cardiovascular System is commonly treated in South Asia. In Australia, the Body Systems treated are comparable to the other regions. Study aims and objectives contribute to variability in reports of ailments treated across different regions.

The Body Systems and Ailments treated by *C. spinarum* may be a true reflection of disease prevalence in the study areas. However, in the main there is no reporting of morbidity and mortality data in the ethnobotanical research analysed which makes it difficult to interpret the research results. Some studies have a particular disease focus such as malaria, respiratory disorders, HIV/AIDS, parasitic disease and others. However, the majority of EM information included is from general studies without focusing on a particular ailment. The most common specific research focus is malaria-related from Eastern Africa [82, 83, 129–136]. This could account for the relatively high ranking of malaria in this analysis. A study with the Luo community in Kenya found that abdominal complaints are most commonly treated with traditional medicine in the study area. The authors relate this to the availability of pharmaceuticals for the treatment of other common ailments [81]. An alternative explanation is presented in early research with the Kamba people in Kenya. The author found an organ hierarchy whereby the abdominal and reproductive symptoms were the most important [137]. This hierarchy may be relevant more broadly throughout the Eastern Africa region and could contribute to the prevalence of digestive disorders and treatment of genitourinary ailments with *C. spinarum*. The prevalence of treatment of genitourinary conditions is a common finding in EM studies and may be related as much to cultural treatment norms as to disease prevalence [118]. Its absence from Australian studies may relate to "secret business" not suitable for discussion with a researcher [57].

3.3.6 C. spinarum *in ethnoveterinary medicine (EVM)*

Plant species used for human EM are commonly used for animal healthcare as well, a subject explored in a study of traditional veterinary knowledge in the Algerian steppe [138]. The authors suggested that human use may stem from the observation of animal self-treatment, a behaviour known as zoopharmacognosy. In the case of *C. spinarum*, this may be an element in therapeutic choice. Animals are known to browse on the leaves of *C. spinarum* and it is used in EVM for the treatment of helminthoses and other digestive disorders in animals as in humans. In this analysis of *C. spinarum*, there are 39 documents citing its use in EVM. The geographical spread of documents includes Sub-Saharan Africa—mainly Ethiopia and Kenya and South Asia—mainly India and Pakistan.

The plant part used follows that for human use and is predominantly the root, followed by the bark, leaf, fruit and leaf in **Figure 14a**. Comparing the plant parts used in South Asia to Eastern Africa, **Figure 14b** indicates that while the root predominates in both regions, there is greater variation in Eastern Africa. Here, the root accounts for almost half of URs but the bark is also used a good deal. This contrasts with human use where in Eastern Africa, the root/rootbark far outstrips other plant parts used. This may imply that, in Eastern Africa, the root is considered to be less toxic to humans than other plant parts given the likelihood that greater care is taken with human than animal treatments. In EVM in South Asia, the root accounts for two-thirds of URs and the leaf is used in a minority of cases. This is at variance with the plant parts used for human

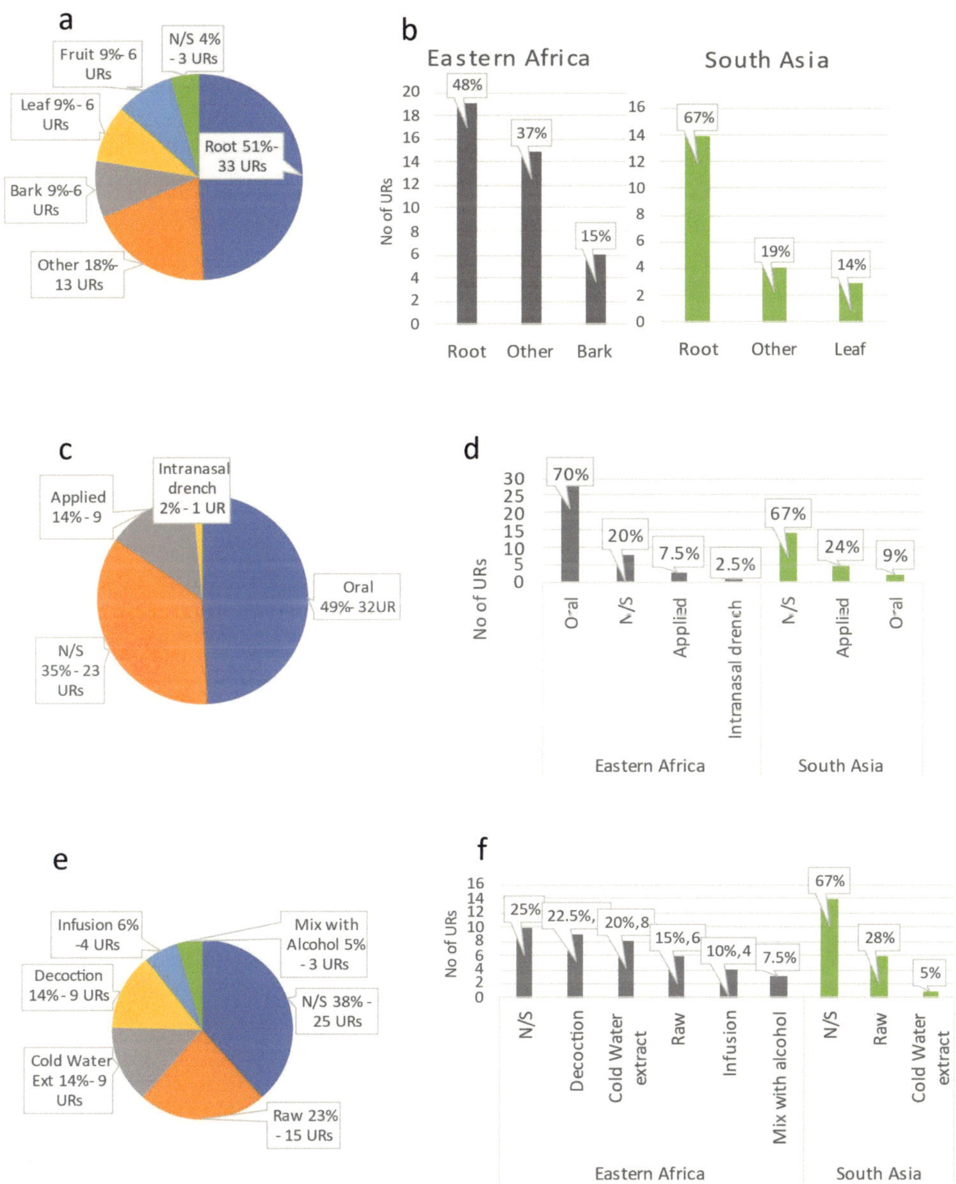

Figure 14.
EVM of CS: (a) key plant parts used globally; (b) key parts used in Eastern Africa and South Asia; (c) key routes of administration; (d) key routes in Eastern Africa and South Asia; (e) key methods of preparation; (f) key methods in Eastern Africa and South Asia.

treatment in South Asia where there is a more even spread between root, leaf and fruit. This could be explained by a number of factors such as the narrower range of diseases treated in EVM, cultural norms, perceived toxicity or acceptability. Similar to human EM of *C. spinarum*, globally the route of administration of EVM is predominantly oral (**Figure 14c**). However, the external route is more common than oral in South Asia whereas in Eastern Africa, the oral route predominates (**Figure 14d**). This may be due to the predominance of skin diseases in animal ailments treated in South Asian studies (see below). In Ethiopia, Tanzania and India it is applied in a similar way to treat worm-infested wounds in cattle whereby the root is ground and applied directly to the wounds [139–141]. The general methods of preparation are much more varied for EVM use. The method is divided more evenly across decoction, cold water extract and raw preparation (**Figure 14e**) though in South Asia the plant is more likely to be used in a raw state relative to the variety of preparations seen in Eastern Africa (**Figure 14f**).

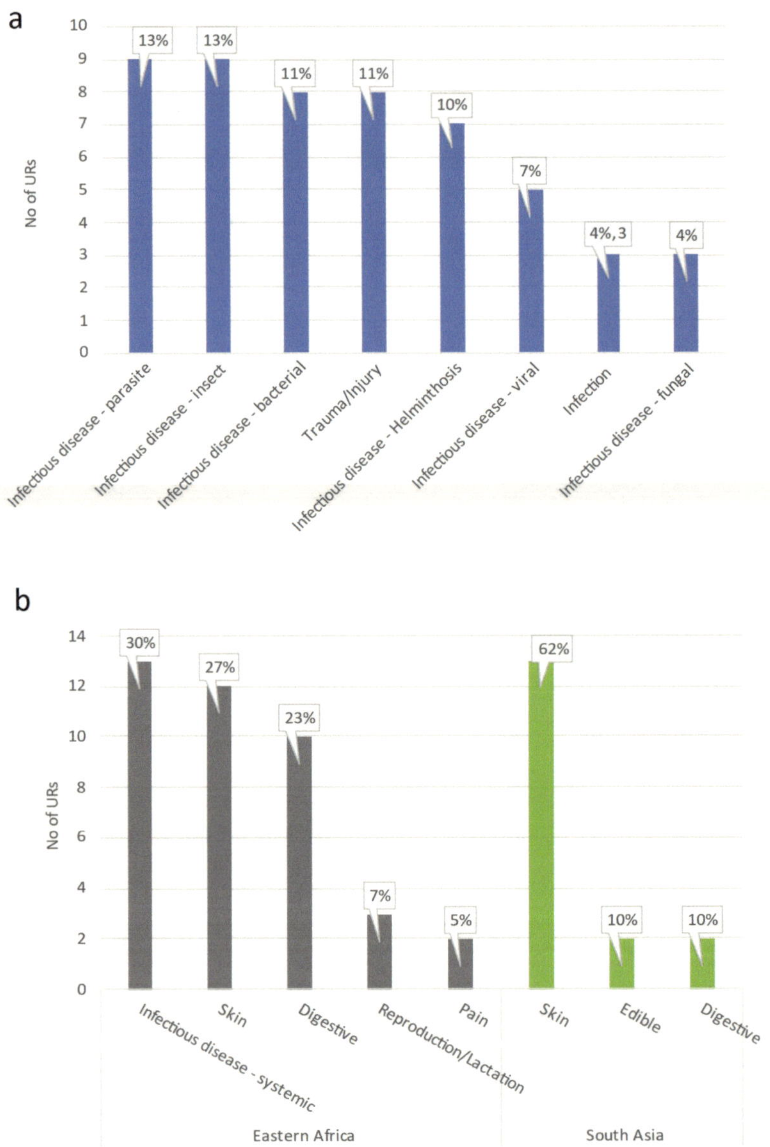

Figure 15.
EVM of CS: (a) key ailments treated globally; (b) key body systems treated in Eastern Africa and South Asia.

In examining the presenting ailments, they can be seen to be primarily related to infection (see **Figure 15a**) with some infections affecting the skin such as ringworm (fungal), lice, ticks, scabies and maggot infested wounds (ectoparasites—all insect related), digestive system (endoparasites—helminthosis), respiratory system in pleuropneumonia (bacterial) or more systemic infections such as theileriosis (endoparasites—protozoa), heartwater, anaplasmosis and salmonellosis (all bacterial), foot and mouth disease, chicken pox, rinderpest and lumpy skin disease (all viral). In a few of the studies, the research teams included members with BM veterinary knowledge and this explains the extent of BM diagnoses provided. Several studies from Eastern Africa have BM veterinary expertise on the research teams which set them apart from the human EM studies where it is rare to have BM diagnoses available [49, 142–149].

The majority of EVM ailments treated using *C. spinarum* are infections affecting the Skin, Digestive system and whole-body System. There is a marked difference in the classifications treated in Eastern Africa relative to South Asia. In the former, Skin infections, Digestive system and Systemic Infectious diseases are the most commonly treated Body System whereas in South Asia, Skin far outweighs any other System treated (**Figure 15b**). This is quite different to the BM systems treated with *C. spinarum* in human EM in South Asia (**Table 7**) where the digestive system is the predominant system treated. Other EVM research in South Asia shows that many body systems are commonly treated [150], which may indicate that *C. spinarum* is particularly effective in treating skin infections.

3.4 *C. spinarum:* structured ethnobotanical methods and cultural importance

The relationship between people and plants can be examined through qualitative and quantitative means. The results of qualitative research are described in Section 3.2. Structured quantitative methods provide an additional means of examining plant use in study communities [32].

The use of statistical methods in ethnopharmacological research dates back to the 1970s [151, 152]. A number of quantitative measures are employed that have been developed and modified over the years [153–155]. The most basic unit to measure is the Use Report (UR). Other measures used are Informant Consensus Factor (ICF), Fidelity level (FL) Relative Importance (RI) and Use Value (UV). The value ranges for these measures vary by study and method of calculation, making it difficult to compare studies [32].

3.4.1 Relative importance of C. spinarum*: primary use reports (URs)*

Given the number of primary studies that are reviewed here, there is relatively little statistical detail on the ethnobotanical use of *C. spinarum*. While there is commonly accurate detail on the number of participants in the studies, few studies provide accurate detail on URs for individual use categories as recommended in best practice documents [31, 32]. Of the Primary studies reviewed, three quarters stated the overall number of participants. Where the number of participants is stated, this could be given as a single number or as a combination of categories of participant: e.g., Focus Group plus Key Informant. One quarter of reviewed studies report the number of URs (number of participants reporting any use of a species) with one third of these being aggregated URs rather than UR per single use category or ailment. One fifth of studies present the primary data as the number of URs per use category. Thus, in 80% of primary studies, including recent ones, there is no indication of relative specific usage of any species. In overviewing the importance of *C. spinarum* where possible from UR data, it is of low to medium importance in most studies when compared to the use of other more frequently used species. This finding corresponds with a common finding in EM research whereby there are only a few species that are known by a large number of participants and many species that are known by just one or two participants [156]. The studies that indicate high importance of *C. spinarum* using the measure of URs include studies from Kenya, Sudan, Ethiopia, Angola, South Africa and Pakistan [43, 49, 157–163]. There are very few Asian studies presenting information on URs and most Australian studies involve participant-authors rather than large-scale surveys. Thus, the better assessments of value measured by UR are from African studies.

3.4.2 Relative importance of C. spinarum*: statistical calculations*

Primary research that includes statistical calculations on the relative importance of *C. spinarum* comes from Africa and Asia. Overall, where such research includes *C. spinarum* in its evaluations of importance, it is found to have a low-moderate relative importance. In parts of Uganda and Ethiopia, *C. spinarum* has a high relative importance as an edible species [164, 165]. In Zimbabwe, it has low relative importance for the treatment of schistosomiasis [166]. It is used in the treatment of Non-Communicable Diseases in a study conducted in Rodrigues Island where it has a low-moderate fidelity level for the treatment of diabetes mellitus [167]. In a study of species versatility in Saudi Arabia, *C. spinarum* has a low relative importance in the study area [120]. *C. spinarum* is used to treat malaria in a study in Pakistan but has low importance relative to the well-known *Azadirachta indica* A. Juss. (Neem tree) [168]. A study from southern India found that *C. spinarum* has a low UV and is reported for the treatment of cough alone [169].

The majority of studies that include *C. spinarum* have no measure of the cultural importance, contrary to current best practice recommendations [31, 32]. Where cultural importance is measured in Ethiopian studies, it is found in the main to have a relatively high importance over a broad range of ethnobotanical uses. In other areas, where reported, *C. spinarum* is of moderate or low cultural importance. Some early documents and the Australian studies included in this analysis contain no statistical information. The ethnobotanical information is often detailed but may involve very few participants. This would not be considered adequate according to current best practice guidelines but these studies are a valuable addition to ethnobotanical literature [80, 86, 89, 117, 170].

3.4.3 Relative importance of C. spinarum *in Ethiopia: participatory ranking*

Anthropological participatory Ranking exercises have been developed as central tools in ethnobotanical research [37, 58]. They are a feature of several Ethiopian studies examined for usage of *C. spinarum* and are a semi-quantitative method of measuring the relative frequency of use of species. Ranking exercises create a more in-depth examination of species use in the study area and follow from more general earlier explorations with participants, which can select out key species to include in comparison exercises. Inclusion in a ranking exercise for specific or general utility of itself indicates a high relative importance among participants. Participatory exercises involve the selection of a small number of key participants, 5–10 people, and a selected number of key plant species, usually 5–7 species, identified during the research as having importance for broad or narrow purposes. The exercises examine a range of ethnobotanical uses through one of a number of methods: direct matrix ranking (DMR), pairwise ranking, preference ranking or simply by number of uses.

A total of 25 Ethiopian ethnobotanical participatory ranking studies were identified including *C. spinarum* among the ethnobotanically known species of the area and 16 of these included *C. spinarum* in ranking exercises. There was a total of 170 species included in these exercises. It is evident that *C. spinarum* has a high relative importance in the study areas given its selection from a large pool of species.

3.4.4 Participatory general ethnobotanical rankings of C. spinarum *in Ethiopia*

Several Ethiopian studies examined the non-medical ethnobotanical importance of species using participatory ranking exercises. The range of ethnobotanical categories of importance in ranking exercises included medicine, firewood, furniture, construction, fencing, charcoal, forage, fodder and food.

There are 16 studies listed in **Table 8** that included *C. spinarum* in their ethnobotanical species list, with 7 exercises from these studies listing *C. spinarum* as having significant general ethnobotanical importance. The study areas exhibiting above the median ethnobotanical relative importance for *C. spinarum* are distributed throughout the country. This analysis indicates a high relative importance for *C. spinarum*, which is also evident in the statistical ranking analyses such as UV and RFC in the previous section.

Rank CS (total #) (1 is best)	Study authors
4 (8)	Amenu [49]
2 (6)	Amsalu, Bezie [172]
N/R	Araya, Abera [104]
N/R	Ashagre, Asfaw [165]
5 (6)	Jima and Megersa [173]
5 (11)	Kebebew and Leta [174]
1 (7)	Kebebew [175]
N/R	Kefalew, Asfaw [176]
N/R (uses)	Kidane [171]
11(46)	Kidane [171]
N/R	Lulekal, Kelbessa [43]
N/R	Lulekal, Asfaw [177]
N/R	Megersa, Asfaw [178]
N/R	Mekonen, Giday [179]
1 (6)	Meragiaw, Asfaw [180]
N/R	Tefera and Kim [181]
N/R	Teklay, Abera [182]

Table 8.
Ethiopian rankings of C. spinarum *use through participatory ranking for general ethnobotanical use (N/R = Not ranked) (all DMR except [171] species with >2 uses).*

Ranking exercise	Ranking method	CS rank (total #) 1 best	Study
General EM	Preference	N/R	[184]
Gonorrhoea	Pairwise	1 (6)	
Malaria	Preference	N/R	
Gonorrhoea	Preference	1 (5)	[49]
Evil Eye	Pairwise	2 (6)	
General EM	DMR	2 (6)	
Snakebite	Preference	N/R	[104]
Malaria	Preference	N/R	[185]
Cough	Pairwise	N/R	[186]
Stomach ache	Pairwise	N/R	[187]
Wound	Preference	N/R	
Stop bleeding	Preference	N/R	[188]
Stomach ache	Preference	4 (5)	[173]
General EM	DMR	1 (5)	
General EM	DMR	3 (11)	[174]
Diarrhoea	Preference	N/R	[175]
General EM	DMR	2 (7)	
Gonorrhoea	Pairwise	1 (5)	
Blackleg	Preference	N/R	[176]
Ascariasis	Preference	N/R	[189]
Gonorrhoea	Preference	N/R	[43]
General EM	URs	2 (10)	
Atopic eczema	Preference	N/R	[177]
Diarrhoea in livestock	Preference	N/R	[190]
Blackleg in cattle	Pairwise	N/R	[178]
General EM	DMR	N/R	
General EM	DMR	N/R	[179]
Febrile illness	Preference	N/R	[180]
Stomach ache	Preference	N/R	
General EM	DMR	1 (6)	
Mich	Preference	N/R	[183]
Cancer in humans and livestock	Preference	N/R	[181]
Stomach ache	Preference	N/R	
Wounds in livestock	Preference	N/R	
Abdominal pain	Preference	N/R	[182]
General EM	DMR	N/R	
General EM	Preference	N/R	[191]

Table 9.
*Ethiopian EM participatory ranking exercises in study locations listing CS. **Mich** is described as a febrile illness with headache and sore lips [183].*

3.4.5 Ethnomedical participatory rankings of C. spinarum *in Ethiopia*

Several ranking studies specifically examine EM importance both for broad utility and for particular medical purposes. An overview of these rankings is shown in **Table 9** and consists of 22 studies with a total of 37 ranking exercises. *C. spinarum* (CS) appears in 11 exercises using a variety of ranking methods: Preference Ranking, Pair-wise ranking and Direct Matrix Ranking (DMR). In most exercises that include *C. spinarum*, it is ranked above the median value. The study areas where it exhibits importance in the general EM category are distributed throughout the central regions of Ethiopia, north to south along the Rift Valley. The most common medical ranking exercises other than the general ranking are for gastrointestinal complaints and gonorrhoea. *C. spinarum* is ranked as the best for treating gonorrhoea in three studies, it is ranked in one gastrointestinal ranking exercise and in rankings for malaria and febrile illness, *C. spinarum* is not ranked [49, 173, 175, 180, 184, 185]. From these participatory exercises, *C. spinarum* appears to be highly ranked for the treatment of gonorrhoea and not for other specific ailments. It ranks high in several areas for general ethnomedical use.

3.4.6 C. spinarum*: a comparison of cultural value based on statistical measures vs. participatory ranking exercises in Ethiopia*

Interpretation of cultural importance by participatory ranking exercises and UR yields, sometimes, conflicting information. Ethnomedical participatory ranking exercises found that *C. spinarum* did not rank high in the treatment of gastrointestinal complaints. This is in contrast to the finding in **Table 7** whereby, in the ICPC classification, the Digestive system is the most treated Body System with *C. spinarum* in Eastern Africa. In Ethiopia specifically, it is second to Spirit-related illness in being the most commonly treated Body System. This indicates a potential discrepancy between the two forms of analysis. However, in ranking for treatment of gonorrhoea, *C. spinarum* is ranked best in three out of four exercises. This corresponds with that found in **Tables 4** and **6** which indicate its importance in treating genital infection globally and in Eastern Africa. That *C. spinarum* is not ranked in exercises for the treatment of malaria and for febrile illness is at odds with the findings in **Tables 4** and **6**, where malaria and fever are among the ailments most commonly treated with *C. spinarum* globally and in Eastern Africa. There are other sources of variability between statistical and participatory research. In participatory rankings, as in all research, there is a randomness to the choice of participant and all participants have necessarily a different knowledge base. There is also variability in the choice of species to include in the ranking exercises and it is not clarified how particular species are selected for analysis. The choice of a particular ranking subject is a function of the study design and researcher priorities and may not reflect the key ailments treated with traditional medicine in the study areas. This could lead to another layer of bias in the results.

The potential variability of outcomes, depending on research methods and study design should be borne in mind in any interpretation of the results or implementation of the research outcomes.

3.5 Phases in *C. spinarum* research

The framework of Hunn's phases of ethnobiology is applied to the ethnobiological documents analysed relating to *C. spinarum* research following a method employed in a study of Southeast Asian ethnobiology [11]. There were 219 primary ethnobiological research documents analysed. Of these, 85% are EM only, while the remainder relate to mainly to diet and general ethnobotany. Within these studies, in whatever phase they are classified, there is a general lack of detail on the practicalities of medicinal plant use. There is almost total silence on plant harvesting. In 9% of cases, there is no information on the plant part used. In over one third of cases, there is no method of preparation given and where a method is given, rarely is close detail provided. The route of administration is not given in 40% of cases. The lack of such basic detail on plant use devalues the research overall, whatever the research agenda, whether for cultural record, bioprospecting or other purposes. Added to these immediate aspects of medicinal plant use are the omissions on the fabric of local life. Culture is central to healing and plant use. However, cultural elements of EM are omitted in the majority of studies such as the meanings associated with plants, disease concepts, therapeutic indications, or what "healing" actually means in the local context as distinct from BM understandings of being healed [192]. Other aspects that are rarely addressed include, for instance, local healthcare provision, morbidity and mortality, environment and economy, which, among other things, contribute to healthcare choices and to the relationship of people with plants.

The majority of the studies that include *C. spinarum* fall into the Phase I classification, representing two thirds of the total and are, in the main, bioprospecting studies. They are largely descriptive in nature, containing lists of species and their uses, with sparse detail on how they are used, as described above. There is an implication built into this rudimentary data collection, that the "how" and "why" of ethnomedicine has little to do with science. In the bioscience laboratory, studies based on EM catalogues of species generally use organic solvents to extract single or multiple metabolites and test these extracts or compounds in *in-vitro* systems, none of which bears any resemblance to the use of traditional medicines in the field. In an unpublished review by these authors of 125 documents examined for phytochemistry and pharmacology of *C. spinarum*, nine (7%) test the pharmacology of aqueous plant extracts and six (5%) identify phytochemicals from aqueous or distilled extracts (data available on request[1]). This indicates the disjuncture between traditional medical practice and preclinical ethnopharmacological studies. There are some studies in the current analysis that have characteristics of each of Phases II to V even where they still contain catalogues of species and their uses. Those with some descriptions of local understandings of illness and healing are ascribed Phase II character. Descriptions such as of disease and causation of TB in a Ugandan community, liver dysfunction in a community in Togo or the meanings associated with plant names in a South African community add to the reader's understanding of EM in those communities [46, 47, 53]. Studies with some Phase II character represent a quarter of the total, with five studies having more detail. For instance, research with Luo mothers, already discussed in Section 3.2.3, situates the treatments of digestive disorders, worms and the use of pharmaceuticals in the study community. Two studies with the Marakwet of Kenya, from 1978 and 2014, give good descriptions of disease perceptions in the study communities. Studies with the Maasai and Samburu in Kenya, give good background descriptions of health in the communities and relationship to environment which allows a deeper understanding of plant usage. Each of these more detailed studies offer an emic perspective which better situates how people use plants for life [41, 81, 86, 87, 193].

[1] This data is part of a PhD dissertation by the first author which includes the phytochemistry and pharmacology of *Carissa spinarum* L.

Those using participatory ranking as described in Section 3.4.5 have Phase III character and represent 11% of the total. They give a sense of how plants form an integral part of life. The participatory studies allow researchers to understand how people think about plants in their immediate environment and how particular species may have cultural value across multiple practical and symbolic domains. Studies conducted in collaboration and co-authorship with community members have elements of Phase IV character such as several Australian publications as described in Section 3.2.1 and two Africa-based studies which mentioned benefit-sharing arrangements [41, 50, 54, 56, 59, 62, 194]. These represent 0.5% of the total. The Convention on Biodiversity (CBD) and related issues such as conservation, sustainable use of resources, prior informed consent and equitable benefit sharing relate to later phases in ethnobiology from the 1970s and Phase III onwards. They are rarely discussed in any of the documents. Consent in any form is reported in 40% of studies though there is no description of the process in any instance. Ethics is referred to where ethical approval of the research has been granted in 16% of studies though the process is not discussed nor the ethical issues examined. The International Society of Ethnobiology (ISE) code of ethics is referred to in six studies (3%) which may imply a greater attention to ethical standards in the research process. Research permits are cited in 15% of studies though the process is not elaborated upon. Intellectual property rights (IPRs) or benefit sharing arrangements are mentioned in eight studies (4%) [59, 62, 132, 157, 194–197]. Half of all studies have no mention of consent, ethics, permits, IPR or other research ethics related issues.

4. Discussion on ethnobiology of *C. spinarum*

C. spinarum (Apocynaceae) is a species that is varied and widely distributed across the globe covering many diverse habitats. There is a volume of ethnobiological knowledge recorded in many of the regions where it is found, particularly in Eastern Africa and South Asia. Across most of its range it is found to be part of the local culture, being valued in ritual, health and healing, diet and a range of other applications.

The predominant role of *C. spinarum*, in the studies examined in this analysis, is in healing and diet, reflecting the research focus in the analysed studies. All parts of the plant are eaten though eating of ripe berries is most commonly reported. The most common EM use of *C. spinarum* in humans across all geographical areas is in the treatment of digestive system, while other body systems such as respiratory and skin are represented to a lesser extent. An analysis of geographic variation reveals a different picture. In Eastern Africa, malaria, STIs and spirit-related illness such as Evil Eye, are the most commonly treated while in South Asia, fever and digestive complaints predominate. Though the particulars of treatment vary across geographical regions, the dominant documented pattern is that the root is prepared by decoction and administered orally. The exception to this is in Australia where use of *C. spinarum* matches trends in local EM practices more broadly and is mainly administered by fumigation or application.

Ethnobiology is a wide and varied discipline with research agendas covering the natural and social sciences including such diverse subjects as indigenous rights, migration, biocultural diversity, health, research ethics and reflexivity [12]. When conducting research on medicinal species, the research focus could involve, for instance, cultural record, health care provision, sustainable plant use, environmental protection or bioprospecting. The ongoing preponderance of Phase I research, lacking cultural contextualisation and theoretical focus, is continually critiqued within ethnobiology and ethnopharmacology [32, 36, 198]. This holds true whatever the research focus.

The phenomenon is reflected here in the studies containing *C. spinarum* with the majority falling into the Phase I category. Two-thirds of studies analysed are Phase I, lacking even minimal information on the context of plant use or examination of therapeutic indications. They also lack detail on the many aspects of plant remedy preparation and administration. As Phase I research usually represents a bioprospecting agenda, the findings show significant lacunae in the information available on *C. spinarum* for guiding further scientific study. One quarter of studies have Phase II character with some emic detail, providing cultural context to EM practices. The studies ascribed to Phase III involves participatory research and accounts for 11% of studies while 0.5% of studies have Phase IV or V character.

Phase I may be dominant in this analysis due to the nature of this analysis itself. Searching for an individual species may be biased towards cataloguing studies. *C. spinarum* is a medicinal and dietary species and this fact may self-select for Phase I studies with decontextualised catalogues of species and their therapeutic and dietary indications favoured in bioprospecting studies. Another reason for the lack of later phases in this analysis of the ethnobiology of *C. spinarum* could be the nature of ethnobiological research itself. In ethnobiology in general, there has been a shift recognised in Hunn's Phases towards an ecology and action-focused research agenda and away from its roots in anthropology [199]. These research agendas do not necessarily require the naming of particular species, which may explain the relative absence of later ethnobiological phases in this species analysis.

The absence of ethnographic content in this analysis places this body of *C. spinarum* data largely in the Phase I category. The emic perspective, limited in this research, is vital to an improved understanding of plant use and is an essential component of all ethnobiological research, whatever the phase. Frazão-Moreira illustrates the ongoing centrality of ethnographic research in ethnobiology [35]. However, in ethnopharmacological research, the socio-cultural focus has been in decline over the past three decades [200]. The relative lack of ethnographic content in ethno-directed bioprospecting has been criticised by numerous authors. Etkin's early critique of ethnopharmacology as generating lists of species that extract them from their cultural contexts has been reiterated more recently [14, 36]. In the bioprospecting process, the subsequent extraction of active metabolites can then diminish indigenous knowledge, even where it is validated by laboratory science [14]. In either case, indigenous use of medicinal species is reduced to its chemical components in what has been called its "molecularisation", disregarding the wider cultural contexts of use and perceptions of efficacy [15, 16]. With regard to medicinal uses, there has been criticism of the poor description and development of therapeutic indications leading to biased data and poor outcomes [16]. Weiskopf illustrated that there is an assumption that traditional ecological knowledge can be "plugged" in to "academic ecological knowledge" unchanged and that there is an assumed category and explanatory overlap between both as is the case, he argues, in the validation process in medical bioprospecting [201]. Taking the current analysis of *C. spinarum*, a local diagnosis of malaria is assumed in some studies to equate to the BM category malaria or "typhoid" to typhoid [202]. The use of an emetic or a laxative might be assumed to be used for the same purposes as an emetic or laxative in BM which may not be the case [89]. Category overlap thus cannot be assumed but must be underpinned by qualitative research exploring cognition among local participants. A hierarchy of convergence was prevalent in early ethnobiology research on folk classification between local and scientific categories whereby ethnotaxa that fit into the scientific categories were given priority and ethnotaxa that did not converge were marginalised

[199]. Such ethnotaxa could be names of plants, birds or of therapeutic indications in EM. One can interpret the analysis of *Buda* (Evil Eye) in Ethiopian studies in Section 3.2.2 in light of hierarchies of convergence. While it is included as a therapeutic indication, there is no examination of this ethnotaxon in any of the Ethiopian studies analysed here. The local importance of this category is clear, but why is it not explored? Is it thought to be self-explanatory as other therapeutic indications are? Is it being marginalised as described above, a desire to ignore that which did not fit? Is there a lack of anthropological expertise in a natural science focused research team? Is it beyond the scope of the research agenda? Is it due to secrecy among research participants as described in Australian research? Whatever the reason, the lack of exploration of *Buda* in these EM studies is a missed opportunity to document local understandings of health and healing and perhaps illuminate the wider use of *C. spinarum* and other species.

The detailed ethnography needed for a substantial emic perspective in ethnopharmacological research requires collaboration between the natural and social sciences. There are documented barriers to such collaboration which can militate against conducting ethnobiological research beyond Phase I. These include inadequate funding and time and a range of academic issues.

All ethnobiology research touches on material and symbolic aspects of interactions between humans and their environments and as such requires a multidisciplinary approach to research, but this is not common in practice [12, 14, 203, 204]. In the current analysis, some explicitly ethnobotanical studies have multidisciplinary teams however with some exceptions [81, 89], the team members belong to a natural science discipline [134, 205, 206]. D'Ambrosio [12] attributed this to the normal association of ethnobiology research with either anthropology or biology departments with few dedicated ethnobiology schools. He argued that the ethnobiology researcher, rather, takes the disciplinary approach of their primary discipline with either a natural science or a social science/humanities perspective, carrying through their disciplinary origins in their research questions. The natural sciences perspective is largely objective, quantitative and etic in its approach, while a social scientific outlook is more often subjective, qualitative and emic. The natural sciences perspective predominating in the Phase I character of *C. spinarum* studies analysed [12]. Significant roadblocks exist to cross-disciplinary collaboration including in ethnobiology. These barriers revolve around the interrelated aspects of status, funding, time and complexity. An analysis of research collaborations between social and natural sciences found that collaborative research has a lower academic status than natural sciences research [207]. Funding across disciplines is difficult as funding streams generally follow single disciplines [12, 208]. Added to this, it is argued that social science research is chronically underfunded [209]. Within ethnopharmacology, there is a demonstrable lack of funding for ethnographically directed research compared with that for laboratory-based screening for bioactive metabolites [210]. Where social science and humanities research is conducted in collaboration with natural sciences, the latter tends to be the dominant partner in such research. The social science element may be tagged on with no true commitment of time and funding necessary for the incorporation of the social science discipline into the project [209, 211]. Similarly, the time required for communication across disciplines, for creating relationships and mutual understandings among research team members and for integrating research findings is rarely considered in project timelines [209]. Frequently the social science elements of collaborative research are more difficult to translate into action rather than the faster, more reductive natural sciences research [209]. These limits on time and funding can hamper ethno-directed studies and result in poor outcomes in ethnopharmacological research [16].

Collaboration with study communities is a central feature of progressive ethnobiological research, with community voices heard rather than interpreted by academics [181]. However, in this analysis, there is near-total anonymity of the research participants themselves. This is the norm in earlier phases of ethnobiological research as described in recent works [15, 212]. The collaborative approach suffers from some of the same barriers as cross-disciplinary collaborations including skills, funding, time constraints and academic norms. The marginalisation of social sciences in interdisciplinary collaborative research means that the social science skills needed for in-depth community collaboration may not be available. Likewise, the time and associated funding requirements may be lacking making it more difficult to establish the necessary relationships of trust. Academically, research design varies whereby the social sciences often have a flexible approach to research design [213]. Where ethnobiology studies originate in natural sciences departments, academic structures may not permit this fluidity nor the processual approach needed in collaborative work. Collaboration and co-authorship are integral to Phase IV and V research and is considered to be essential to the future of ethnobiology [198]. If ethno-directed bioprospecting is to be conducted within an ethical and collaborative framework, then these barriers need to be addressed. All of these elements - disciplinary silos, funding, status and time-militate against the collaboration with communities and across disciplines necessary for high quality ethnobiological research that can capture the interpenetrative nature of the relationships of humans and their environments in an ethical manner.

Research design and methods used in ethnobiology may produce results which do not properly represent the relationships of people and plants. Shortcomings in quantitative studies, in choice of participants and questionnaire design, in use of common ethnobotanical methods and the interview itself, may each contribute to an ethnobiology that is not representative of the local voice. Quantitative analysis in ethnobiology has become a common component of ethnobiological research especially since the 1990's [214]. It can be a component of a progressive ethnobiology when used judiciously. However, its inclusion has also been critiqued by several authors. The indiscriminate use of statistical methods without a basis in theory or hypothesis is challenged, proposing a better fit of method with the research question [215]. The variability in the use and interpretation of statistics produces research that cannot be compared or synthesised across studies and geographies [32, 214]. In this analysis, the wide variation in sample sizes, the difference in formulae and terms used, different interpretations of use categories make comparisons and syntheses of data difficult or inaccurate. The varying application of statistical measures has led to the recommendation that primary data (URs) are reported to allow for comparison between studies and meta-analysis [32]. In health and medicine directed ethnobiology, there are pitfalls with statistical methods. The equation of the most popular species with the "best" could be misapplied since popularity may have more to do with ease of access or symbolic value than efficacy in BM terms [16]. The format of many ethnobiological studies which result in catalogues of plant knowledge does not necessarily translate into real-world plant use such that what is known is not necessarily what is used [204].

It has been argued at a more fundamental level, that study design including choice of participants and questionnaire design lead to more variability in results than the choices around statistical indices or the grouping of use categories [216]. Sampling bias may emerge when indigenous knowledge is not homogenously distributed across a community or region [217]. The recording and classification of ethnobotanical knowledge may focus mainly on practical utility of species and can ignore other elements of importance to local communities. Elements that may not be categories of interest in study protocols, such as the sacred or aesthetic, may be relevant to community members [218]. Common ethnobotanical methods may not be culturally appropriate in Australian aboriginal research and this necessitates the development of alternative culturally sensitive study designs [37, 57, 58]. The use of tools such as free-listing were found to produce variable outcomes, even within a single participant (in separate interviews), or relating to age or the presence of a third party at the interview [219]. Similarly, a Bolivian study found that even subtle changes in the use of methods of free-listing and semi-structured interviews can produce markedly different results [220]. The core method of the interview itself is a challenged process when the recorded portion, the verbal, is only a fraction of the whole communication. The interviewer changes the outcome of the interaction through their very presence and the questions they ask, bringing their own etic category biases and resulting in an inaccurate representation of indigenous knowledge [221].

As the discipline of Ethnobiology has progressed, the ethics of research has become increasingly central to its conduct. Vandebroek [204] has argued that the normal method of documenting traditional medicinal knowledge and subsequent laboratory research on pharmacological activities has limited if any health benefits for study communities. There are clear ethical implications to such research. There are increasing calls to develop action-focused research protocols, which ask questions that directly address public health problems and make ethnobiological research more relevant to study communities [14, 204]. Vandebroek [204] refers to ethnobiological research in Mali whereby research results were directly returned to the study community through a refinement of local knowledge on an anti-malarial traditional medicine and only secondarily directed towards the development of a phytopharmaceutical [222]. The area of researching traditional knowledge and genetic resources raises ethical issues including of intellectual property rights, benefit sharing and protection of biodiversity. However, in the *C. spinarum* documents, there is little stated attention to ethics. Where ethics is mentioned, it is usually perfunctory. It is true that the lack of discussion of ethics does not mean that the research was conducted unethically. Some journals may require evidence of ethical research conduct as a condition of publication such as the *Journal of Ethnopharmacology*, even though ethical issues are not discussed in the research paper as such. This may not be the case for all journals. Where ethical issues are discussed as in Australian research such as [61], there is a greater sense of the ethical conduct of the research. Likewise, benefit sharing and IPRs may be a component of some research permits. However, the mention or discussion of them within the research paper such as in those listed in Section 3.5 raises the reader's awareness of these essential aspects of ethical research which has a value in itself.

5. Conclusions

This analysis using *C. spinarum* as a case study of a medicinal species illustrates that it has been identified in ethnodirected bioprospecting studies and other forms of ethnobiological research across three continents. Most of the research is categorised as Phase I in Hunn's classification of ethnobiology with little contextual or ethnographic content. Where emic perspectives on the use of this species are reported, it is seen to profoundly alter the perspective of the reader on the use of this and other species within the study community. However, even a minimal "thin description" is lacking in most of the ethnobotanical research, where lists of EM species may be recorded without information on the plant part used, or on the preparation or administration of the plant remedy. The omission of such essential data can invalidate the documentation of ethnobotanical data whatever the purpose, whether cultural record, health care provision, sustainable plant use, environmental protection or bioprospecting.

There is more to be learned about this species and the many other species of broad biocultural value through the design and funding of research which allows local meanings and values to emerge. A more nuanced understanding of its meaning for indigenous people and local communities may be illuminated through study designs that incorporate a blending of qualitative and quantitative research methodologies as proposed in best practice documents in ethnobiology and in ethnopharmacology. A partnership approach with local communities can make for more ethical as well as more fruitful research. Allied to this, is the aim of trans-disciplinarity in ethnobiological research. Such a research process could reveal local ways of knowing biodiversity and environment beyond the categories of utility commonly captured in natural science-directed ethnobotanical research.

The evidence of the current analysis of the ethnobotany of *C. spinarum* illustrates that such an approach is essential to ethical, sustainable, and effective ethnobiological research of this and other culturally valued species. A move beyond the current obstacles to collaborative research is needed to examine in meaningful and effective ways how people interact with plants and the wider environment in response to health challenges with dynamism and creativity.

Acknowledgements

The authors acknowledge Trinity College Dublin 1252 scholarship and NatPro for co-funding of Ciara Smyth's postgraduate research.

Conflict of interest

The authors declare no conflict of interest.

Appendices and nomenclature

Additional information available on request from corresponding author.

Author details

Ciara Smyth* and Helen Sheridan
The NatPro Centre, School of Pharmacy and Pharmaceutical Sciences, Trinity College Dublin, Ireland

*Address all correspondence to: csmyth6@tcd.ie

References

[1] Malebo HM, Mbwambo ZH. Technical Report on Miracle Cure Prescribed by Rev. Ambilikile Mwasupile in Samunge Village, Loliondo, Arusha. Dar es Salaam. Tanzania: Institute of Traditional Medicine, Muhimbili University of Health and Allied Sciences; 2011

[2] Vähäkangas M. Babu Wa Loliondo - healing the tensions between Tanzanian worlds. Journal of Religion in Africa. 2015;**45**(1):3-36. DOI: 10.1163/15700666-12340029

[3] BBC News. Tanzanian 'miracle' pastor Mwasapile calls for a break: bbc.co.uk/news; 2011. Available from: https://www.bbc.com/news/world-africa-12878811

[4] Gettleman J. Crowds come over roads and by helicopters for Tanzanian's cure-all potion. New York Times. 2011. Available from: https://www.nytimes.com/2011/03/29/world/africa/29potion.html

[5] Tolo FM, Muthaura CN. Natural products research: A potential source of innovative new drug discovery and development. Journal of Infectious Diseases and Therapy. 2019;7:17. DOI: 10.4172/2332-0877-C2-062

[6] Siele M. Kenya turns to herbal 'Loliondo medicine' in search for Covid-19 cure. 2020. Available from: https://www.kenyans.co.ke/news/54317-kenya-turns-herbal-medicine-search-covid-19-cure-video

[7] Kenya CitizenTV. Coronavirus pandemic: Hope in herbs. Tolo: Zedupex shows anti-viral potential aginst herpes virus Kenya: YouTube; 2020. Available from: https://www.youtube.com/watch?v=yQQldlVL5Pw

[8] GBIF Occurrence Download [Internet]. 2022. Available from: https://www.gbif.org/occurrence/download/0191989-210914110416597

[9] Society of Ethnobiology. What is Ethnobiology?: ethnobiology.org; 2021. Available from: https://ethnobiology.org/about-ethnobiology/what-is-ethnobiology

[10] Hunn E. Ethnobiology in four phases. Journal of Ethnobiology. 2007;**27**(1):1-10

[11] Hidayati S, Franco FM, Bussmann RW. Ready for phase 5 - current status of ethnobiology in Southeast Asia. Journal of Ethnobiology and Ethnomedicine. 2015;**11**(17):1-8. DOI: 10.1186/s13002-015-0005-7

[12] D'Ambrosio U. Theoretical reflections on ethnobiology in the third millennium. Contributions to Science. 2014;**10**:49-64. DOI: 10.2436/20.7010.01.188

[13] International Society of Ethnobiology. ISE code of ethics (with 2008 additions). 11th International Congress of Ethnobiology. 2008. Available from: http://ethnobiology.net/code-of-ethics/

[14] Reyes-García V. The relevance of traditional knowledge systems for ethnopharmacological research: Theoretical and methodological contributions. Journal of Ethnobiology and Ethnomedicine. 2010;**6**(32):1-12. DOI: 10.1186/1746-4269-6-32

[15] Osseo-Asare AD. Bitter Roots: The Search for Healing Plants in Africa. Berkeley: University of California Press; 2014. p. 300

[16] Albuquerque UP, Medeiros PM, Ramos MA, Júnior WSF,

Nascimento ALB, Avilez WMT, et al. Are ethnopharmacological surveys useful for the discovery and development of drugs from medicinal plants? Revista Brasileira de Farmacognosia. 2014;**24**(2):110-115. DOI: 10.1016/j.bjp.2014.04.003

[17] Heinrich M, Dhanji T, Casselman I. Açai (*Euterpe oleracea* Mart.)—A phytochemical and pharmacological assessment of the species' health claims. Phytochemistry Letters. 2011;**4**(1):10-21. DOI: 10.1016/j.phytol.2010.11.005

[18] Sharma PC, Yelne MB, Dennis TJ, Joshi A, Ayurveda CCfRi, Siddha. Database on Medicinal Plants Used in Ayurveda: Central Council for Research in Ayurveda & Siddha. Deptt. of ISM & H, Min. of Health & Family Welfare, Government of India; 2001

[19] Kaphengst TM, Davis C, Gerstetter K, Klaas K, McGlade K, Naumann S. Quality of life, wellbeing and biodiversity. The role of biodiversity in future development. In: Final Report Submitted to Deutsche Gesellschaft für Internationale Zusammenarbeit (GIZ) GmbH. Berlin: Ecologic Institute Berlin; 2014

[20] Fatima A, Singh PP, Agarwal P, Irchhaiya R, Alok S, Verma A. Treatment of various diseases by *Carissa spinarum* L.—A promising shrub. International Journal of Pharmaceutical Sciences and Research. 2013;**4**(7):2489-2495. DOI: 10.13040/ijpsr.0975-8232.4(7).2489-95

[21] Ansari I, Patil DT. A brief review on phytochemical and pharmacological profile of *Carissa spinarum* L. Asian Journal of Pharmaceutical and Clinical Research. 2018;**11**(9):12-18. DOI: 10.22159/ajpcr.2018.v11i9.26316

[22] Al-Youssef HM, Hassan WHB. Phytochemical and pharmacological aspects of *Carissa edulis* Vahl: A review. International Journal of Current Research in Chemistry and Pharmaceutical Sciences. 2014;**1**(9):12-24

[23] Izhar S, Ahmed D. *Carissa opaca*: A plant with great potential for future drugs for degenerative and infectious diseases. ChemistrySelect. 2016;**1**:3005-3011. DOI: 10.1002/slct.201600462

[24] Devmurari V, Shivanand P, Goyani MB, Vaghani S, Jivani NP. A review: *Carissa congesta*: Phytochemical constituents, traditional use and pharmacological properties. Pharmacognosy Review. 2009;**3**(6):375-377

[25] Kaunda JS, Zhang YJ. The genus *Carissa*: An ethnopharmacological, phytochemical and pharmacological review. Natural Products and Bioprospecting. 2017;**7**(2):181-199. DOI: 10.1007/s13659-017-0123-0

[26] Dhatwalia J, Kumari A, Verma R, Upadhyay N, Guleria I, Lal S, et al. Phytochemistry, pharmacology, and nutraceutical profile of *Carissa* species: An updated review. Molecules. 2021;**26**(22):7010

[27] *Carissa spinarum* Linnaeus, Mant. Pl. 2: 559. 1771. [Internet]. www.efloras.org. n.d [cited 23 Feb 2021]. Available from: http://efloras.org/florataxon.aspx?flora_id=2&taxon_id=200018364

[28] Leeuwenberg AJM, Dilst FJH. Series of Revisions of Apocynaceae XLIX, *Carissa* L. Backhuys: Leiden; 2001. p.126

[29] WFO. *Carissa spinarum* L. Published on the Internet 2021. Available from: http://www.worldfloraonline.org/taxon/wfo-0000803913

[30] Salunke RJ, Ghate VS. Comparative pharmacognosy of medicinally important species of genus *Carissa*.

International Journal of Pharmacy and Life Sciences. 2013;**4**(8):2890-2904

[31] Heinrich M, Lardos A, Leonti M, Weckerle C, Willcox M, Applequist W, et al. Best practice in research: Consensus statement on ethnopharmacological field studies—ConSEFS. Journal of Ethnopharmacology. 2018;**211**:329-339. DOI: 10.1016/j.jep.2017.08.015

[32] Weckerle C, de Boer HJ, Puri RK, van Andel T, Bussmann RW, Leonti M. Recommended standards for conducting and reporting ethnopharmacological field studies. Journal of Ethnopharmacology. 2018;**210**:125-132. DOI: 10.1016/j.jep.2017.08.018

[33] Rivera D, Allkin R, Obón C, Alcaraz F, Verpoorte R, Heinrich M. What is in a name? The need for accurate scientific nomenclature for plants. Journal of Ethnopharmacology. 2014;**152**(3):393-402. DOI: 10.1016/j.jep.2013.12.022

[34] *Carissa spinarum* L. [Apocynaceae] [Internet]. Royal Botanic Gardens, Kew. 2020. Available from: https://mpns.science.kew.org/mpns-portal/plantDetail?plantId=34226&query=carissa+spinarum&filter=&fuzzy=false&nameType=all&dbs=wcs

[35] Frazão-Moreira A. Ethnobiological research and ethnographic challenges in the "ecological era". Etnografica. 2015;**19**(3):605-624. DOI: 10.4000/etnografica.4141

[36] Etkin NL. Ethnopharmacology: Biobehavioral approaches in the anthropological study of indigenous medicines. Annual Review of Anthropology. 1988;**17**:23-42

[37] Martin GJ. Ethnobotany: A Methods Manual. 1st ed. London; New York: Chapman & Hall; 1995. p. 268

[38] Paulos B, Fenta TG, Bisrat D, Asres K. Health seeking behavior and use of medicinal plants among the Hamer ethnic group, South Omo zone, southwestern Ethiopia. Journal of Ethnobiology and Ethnomedicine. 2016;**12**(44):1-13. DOI: 10.1186/s13002-016-0107-x

[39] Hermans M, Akoègninou A, Van Der Maesen LJG. Medicinal plants used to treat malaria in southern Benin. Economic Botany. 2004;**58**:S239-S252

[40] Mabano GO, Kakudidi EKZ, editors. Medicinal plant uses in Nyabushozi County, Mbarara District, western Uganda. In: Taxonomy and ecology of African plants, their conservation and sustainable use: Proceedings of the 17th AETFAT congress Addis Ababa, Ethiopia. Addis Ababa, Ethiopia: Royal Botanic Gardens, Kew; 2006. p. 505-518

[41] Bussmann RW, Gilbreath GG, Solio J, Lutura M, Lutuluo R, Kunguru K, et al. Plant use of the Maasai of Sekenani valley, Maasai Mara, Kenya. Journal of Ethnobiology and Ethnomedicine. 2006;**2**(27):1-7. DOI: 10.1186/1746-4269-2-22

[42] Abbasi AM. Medicinal Plant Biodiversity of Lesser Himalayas-Pakistan. New York; London: Springer; 2012. p. 220

[43] Lulekal E, Kelbessa E, Bekele T, Yineger H. An ethnobotanical study of medicinal plants in Mana Angetu District, southeastern Ethiopia. Journal of Ethnobiology and Ethnomedicine. 2008;**4**(10):1-10. DOI: 10.1186/1746-4269-4-10

[44] Maroyi A. An ethnobotanical survey of medicinal plants used by the people in Nhema communal area, Zimbabwe. Journal of Ethnopharmacology. 2011;**136**(2):347-354. DOI: 10.1016/j.jep.2011.05.003

[45] Malik S, Ahmad S, Sadiq A, Alam K, Wariss HM, Ahmad I, et al. A comparative ethno-botanical study of Cholistan (an arid area) and Pothwar (a semi-arid area) of Pakistan for traditional medicines. Journal of Ethnobiology and Ethnomedicine. 2015;**11**(31):1-20. DOI: 10.1186/s13002-015-0018-2

[46] Tabuti JRS, Kukunda CB, Waako PJ. Medicinal plants used by traditional medicine practitioners in the treatment of tuberculosis and related ailments in Uganda. Journal of Ethnopharmacology. 2010;**127**(1):130-136. DOI: 10.1016/j.jep.2009.09.035

[47] Kpodar MS, Karou SD, Katawa G, Anani K, Gbekley HE, Adjrah Y, et al. An ethnobotanical study of plants used to treat liver diseases in the Maritime Region of Togo. Journal of Ethnopharmacology. 2016;**181**:263-273. DOI: 10.1016/j.jep.2015.12.051

[48] Kristensen M, Balslev H. Perceptions, use and availability of woody plants among the Gourounsi in Burkina Faso. Biodiversity and Conservation. 2003;**12**(8):203-217

[49] Amenu E. Use and management of medicinal plants by indigenous people of Ejaji Area (Chelya Woreda) West Shoa, Ethiopia: An ethnobotanical approach [MSc]. Addis Ababa: Addis Ababa University; 2007

[50] Mchangama M, Salaün P. Recueil d'une pharmacopée à Mayotte Etud Océan Indien. 2012;**48**:1-42. DOI: 10.4000/oceanindien.1770

[51] Teklehaymanot T, Giday M, Medhin G, Mekonnen Y. Knowledge and use of medicinal plants by people around Debre Libanos monastery in Ethiopia. Journal of Ethnopharmacology. 2007;**111**(2):271-283. DOI: 10.1016/j.jep.2006.11.019

[52] Abbink J. Medicinal and ritual plants of the Ethiopian southwest: An account of recent research. Indigenous Knowledge and Development Monitor. 1995;**3**(2):6-8

[53] Mongalo NI, Makhafola TJ. Ethnobotanical knowledge of the lay people of Blouberg area (Pedi tribe), Limpopo Province, South Africa. Journal of Ethnobiology and Ethnomedicine. 2018;**14**(46):1-23. DOI: 10.1186/s13002-018-0245-4

[54] Paddy E, Paddy S, Smith M. Boonyja Bardag Gorna: All Trees Are Good for Something. Anthropology Department, Western Australian Museum: Perth; 1993. p. 33

[55] GBIF Secretariat. *Carissa spinarum* L. in GBIF Backbone Taxonomy. Checklist dataset: GBIF.org; 2019. Available from: https://doi.org/10.15468/39omei

[56] Bordulk D, Nikipini D, Tukumba M, Bennett L, Bordro Tingey R, Katherine M, et al. Dalabon (Ngalkbon/Dangbon) Plants and Animals: Aboriginal Biocultural Knowledge from Southern Arnhem Land, North Australia. Palmerston; Katherine: Department of Land Resource Management Diwurruwurru-Jaru Aboriginal Corp./Mimi Aboriginal Art & Craft; 2012. p. 256

[57] Edwards S, Nebel S, Heinrich M. Questionnaire surveys: Methodological and epistemological problems for field-based ethnopharmacologists. Journal of Ethnopharmacology. 2005;**100**(1):30-36. DOI: 10.1016/j.jep.2005.05.026

[58] Cotton CM. Ethnobotany: Principles and Applications. New York: John Wiley and Sons Ltd.; 1996. p. 434

[59] Jones JM, Bardbariya D, Raymond E, Roberts D, McDonald D, McDonald D,

et al. Jaminjung, Ngaliwurru and Nungali Plants and Animals: Aboriginal Knowledge of Flora and Fauna from the Bradshaw and Judbarra/Gregory National Park Area, North Australia. Darwin: Jawoyn Association,Nortern Territory Department of Natural Resources, Environment, Arts & Sport, Diwurruwurru-Jaru Aboriginal Corporation, Mimi Aboriginal Art and Craft; 2011. p. 188

[60] Wightman GM, Jungurra Kalabidi G, Nungari ND, Topsy, Nawurla Dujngari Frith R, Nampin Jiwitjiwitj M, et al. Gurindji Ethnobotany: Aboriginal Plant Use from Daguragu, Northern Australia. Conservation Commission of the Northern Territory: Darwin; 1994. p. 76

[61] Aboriginal Communities of the Northern Territory of Australia. Traditional Aboriginal Medicines in the Northern Territory of Australia. Darwin: Conservation Commission of the Northern Territory of Australia; 1993. p. 651

[62] Doonday B, Wightman GM, Samuels C, Clancy M, Milner J, Chungulla R, et al. Walmajarri Plants and Animals: Aboriginal Biocultural Knowledge from the Paruku IPA, southern Kimberley, Australia. Halls Creek, WA; Sydney, NSW; Palmerston, N.T.: Paruku IPA; WWF-Australia: Department of Land Resource Management; 2013. p. 240

[63] Latz P. Bushfires and Bushtucker : Aboriginal Plant Use in Central Australia. Alice Springs, Australia: Iad Press; 1995. p. 415

[64] Connelly P, Wallis L. Kar-Kar: Mitakoodi Traditional Medicinal Plant Uses of the Cloncurry Region. Southern Gulf Catchments: Mount Isa, Queensland; 2013. p. 74

[65] PAKAM—Pilbara and Kimberley Aboriginal Media. Gija bush food and medicine [Video]. Australia: www.ictv.com.au; 2009 [00:22:7]. Available from: https://ictv.com.au/video/item/890?lp=1

[66] McDonald H. East Kimberley concepts of health and illness: A contribution to intercultural health programs in northern Australia. Australian Aboriginal Studies. 2006;**2006**(2):86-97

[67] Central Art Aboriginal art store. Conkerberry dreaming Alice Springs: https://www.aboriginalartstore.com.au/; 2021. Available from: https://www.aboriginalartstore.com.au/artists/roxella-napangardi-marshall/conkerberry-dreaming-(326-18)

[68] Cox P. Will tribal knowledge survive the millennium? Science. 2000;**287**:44-45. DOI: 10.1126/science.287.5450.44

[69] Swiderska K, Argumedo A, Pant R, Vedavathy S, Nellithanam J, Munyi P, et al. Protecting Community Rights over Traditional Knowledge: Implications of Customary Laws and Practices. London: IIED; 2006. p. 21

[70] Pagani E, Santos JFL, Rodrigues E. Culture-bound syndromes of a Brazilian Amazon riverine population: Tentative correspondence between traditional and conventional medicine terms and possible ethnopharmacological implications. Journal of Ethnopharmacology. 2017;**203**: 80-89 DOI: 10.1016/j.jep.2017.03.024

[71] Amenu K, Szonyi B, Grace D, Wieland B. Important knowledge gaps among pastoralists on causes and treatment of udder health problems in livestock in southern Ethiopia: Results of qualitative investigation. BMC Veterinary Research. 2017;**13**:1-13. DOI: 10.1186/s12917-017-1222-1

[72] Abbink J. A socio-structural analysis of the Beta Esra'el as an "infamous group"

in traditional Ethiopia. Sociologus. 1987;**37**(2):140-154

[73] Tareke KG, Lemu YK, Yidenekal SA, Feyissa GT. Community's perception, experiences and health seeking behavior towards newborn illnesses in Debre Libanos District, North Shoa, Oromia, Ethiopia: Qualitative study. PLoS One. 2020;**15**(1): 1-19. DOI: 10.1371/journal.pone.0227542

[74] Kahissay MH, Fenta TG, Boon H. Beliefs and perception of ill-health causation: A socio-cultural qualitative study in rural North-Eastern Ethiopia. BMC Public Health. 2017;**17**(1):1-10. DOI: 10.1186/s12889-017-4052-y

[75] Jacobsson L. Traditional treatment of mental and psychosomatic disorders in Ethiopia. International Congress Series. 2002;**1241**:265-269. DOI: 10.1016/S0531-5131(02)00678-7

[76] Abebe W. A survey of prescriptions used in traditional medicine in Gondar region, northwestern Ethiopia: General pharmaceutical practice. Journal of Ethnopharmacology. 1986;**18**(2):147-165

[77] Mengesha GG. Ethnobotanical survey of medicinal plants used in treating human and livestock health problems in Mandura Woreda of Benishangul Gumuz, Ethiopia. Advancement in Medicinal Plant Research. 2016;**4**(1):11-26

[78] Giday M, Teklehaymanot T, Animut A, Mekonnen Y. Medicinal plants of the Shinasha, Agew-awi and Amhara peoples in Northwest Ethiopia. Journal of Ethnopharmacology. 2007;**110**(3):516-525. DOI: 10.1016/j.jep.2006.10.011

[79] Quiroz D, Sosef M, van Andel T. Why ritual plant use has ethnopharmacological relevance. Journal of Ethnopharmacology. 2016;**188**:48-56. DOI: 10.1016/j.jep.2016.05.006

[80] Nyamwaya DO. The Management of Illness in an East African Society : A Study of Choice and Constraint in Health Care among the Pokot. Cambridge: Cambridge; 1982. p. 274

[81] Geissler PW, Harris SA, Prince RJ, Olsen A, Odhiambo RA, Oketch-Rabah H, et al. Medicinal plants used by Luo mothers and children in Bondo District, Kenya. Journal of Ethnopharmacology. 2002;**83**(1-2):39-54. DOI: 10.1016/S0378-8741(02)00191-5

[82] Muthaura CN, Keriko JM, Mutai C, Yenesew A, Gathirwa JW, Irungu BN, et al. Antiplasmodial potential of traditional antimalarial phytotherapy remedies used by the Kwale community of the Kenyan coast. Journal of Ethnopharmacology. 2015;**170**:148-157. DOI: 10.1016/j.jep.2015.05.024

[83] Orwa JA, Mwitari PG, Matu EN, Rukunga GM. Traditional healers and the management of malaria in Kisumu District, Kenya. East African Medical Journal. 2007;**84**(2):51-55

[84] Johns T, Kokwaro JO, Kimanani EK. Herbal remedies of the Luo of Siaya District, Kenya—Establishing quantitative criteria for consensus. Economic Botany. 1990;**44**(3):369-381

[85] Ichikawa M. A preliminary report on the ethnobotany of the Suiei Dorobo in northern Kenya. African Study Monographs. 1987;7(suppl):1-52. DOI: 10.14989/68347

[86] Lindsay RS. In: Hepper FN, editor. Medicinal Plants of Marakwet, Kenya. Kew, England: Royal Botanic Gardens, Kew; 1978. p. 1-49

[87] Kipkore W, Wanjohi B, Rono H, Kigen G. A study of the medicinal plants used by the Marakwet community in Kenya. Journal of Ethnobiology and

Ethnomedicine. 2014;**10**(1):24-58. DOI: 10.1186/1746-4269-10-24

[88] Bussmann RW. Ethnobotany of the Samburu of Mt. Nyiru, South Turkana, Kenya. Journal of Ethnobiology and Ethnomedicine. 2006;**2**(35):1-10. DOI: 10.1186/1746-4269-2-35

[89] Timberlake JR. Ethnobotany of the Pokot of Northern Kenya. London: Royal Botanic Gardens, Kew; 1987. p. 105

[90] Nagata JM, Jew AR, Kimeu JM, Salmen CR, Bukusi EA, Cohen CR. Medical pluralism on Mfangano Island: Use of medicinal plants among persons living with HIV/AIDS in Suba District, Kenya. Journal of Ethnopharmacology. 2011;**135**(2):501-509. DOI: 10.1016/j.jep.2011.03.051

[91] Kokwaro JO. Medicinal Plants of East Africa. 3rd ed. University of Nairobi Press; 2009. p. 478

[92] Monteiro JM, de Albuquerque UP, Lins-Neto EM, de Araujo EL, de Amorim EL. Use patterns and knowledge of medicinal species among two rural communities in Brazil's semi-arid northeastern region. Journal of Ethnopharmacology. 2006;**105**(1-2):173-186. DOI: 10.1016/j.jep.2005.10.016

[93] Shepard GH. A sensory ecology of medicinal plant therapy in two Amazonian societies. American Anthropologist. 2004;**106**(2):252-266

[94] Medeiros PM, Santos Pinto BL, do Nascimento VT. Can organoleptic properties explain the differential use of medicinal plants? Evidence from Northeastern Brazil. Journal of Ethnopharmacology. 2015;**159**:43-48. DOI: 10.1016/j.jep.2014.11.001

[95] Heinrich M. Ethnobotany and natural products: The search for new molecules, new treatments of old diseases or a better understanding of indigenous cultures? Current Topics in Medicinal Chemistry. 2003;**3**(2):141-154. DOI: 10.2174/1568026033392570

[96] van Andel T, Mitchell S, Volpato G, Vandebroek I, Swier J, Ruysschaert S, et al. In search of the perfect aphrodisiac: Parallel use of bitter tonics in West Africa and the Caribbean. Journal of Ethnopharmacology. 2012;**143**(3):840-850. DOI: 10.1016/j.jep.2012.08.008

[97] Mabogo DEN. The ethnobotany of the Vhavenda [MSc]. Pretoria: University of Pretoria; 1990

[98] Albuquerque UP, Ramos MA, Melo JG. New strategies for drug discovery in tropical forests based on ethnobotanical and chemical ecological studies. Journal of Ethnopharmacology. 2012;**140**(1):197-201. DOI: 10.1016/j.jep.2011.12.042

[99] Voeks RA. Disturbance pharmacopoeias: Medicine and myth from the humid tropics. Annals of the Association of American Geographers. 2004;**94**(4):868-888

[100] Doshi GM, Chaskar PK, Zine S, Une HD. Cold extraction of *Carissa congesta* Wight monitored by a comparative revision of HPLC and HPTLC. Pharmacognosy Communication. 2014;**4**(2):29-33. DOI: 10.5530/pc.2014.2.6

[101] Joshi D, Boyce S. Notes—Chemical investigation of roots of *Carissa congesta*, Santapau. I. Isolation of Carissone and D-glucoside of β-Sitosterol. The Journal of Organic Chemistry. 1957;**22**(1):95-97. DOI: 10.1021/jo01352a617

[102] Omino EA, Kokwaro JO. Ethnobotany of Apocynaceae species in

Kenya. Journal of Ethnopharmacology. 1993;**40**(3):167-180. DOI: 10.1016/0378-8741(93)90065-d

[103] Bhadane BS, Patil MP, Maheshwari VL, Patil RH. Ethnopharmacology, phytochemistry, and biotechnological advances of family Apocynaceae: A review. Phytotherapy Research. 2018;**32**(7):1181-1210. DOI: 10.1002/ptr.6066

[104] Araya S, Abera B, Giday M. Study of plants traditionally used in public and animal health management in Seharti Samre district, southern Tigray, Ethiopia, Journal of Ethnobiology and Ethnomedicine 2015;**11**(22):1-25. doi:10.1186/s13002-015-0015-5

[105] Mahmood A, Qureshi R, Mahmood A, Sangi Y, Shaheen H, Ahmad I, et al. Ethnobotanical survey of common medicinal plants used by people of District Mirpur, AJK. Pakistan Journal of Medicinal Plant Research. 2011;**5**(18):4493-4498

[106] Singh VK, Anwar AZ. Folk medicines in primary health care: Common plants used for the treatment of fevers in India. Fitoterapia. 1994;**65**(1):68-74

[107] Guo P, Brand E, Zhao Z. Chinese medicinal processing: A characteristic aspect of the ethnopharmacology of Traditional Chinese Medicine. In: Heinrich M, Jäger AK, editors. Ethnopharmacology. Chichester: John Wiley & Sons Inc. 2015. p. 303-316

[108] Sheridan H, Krenn L, Jiang R, Sutherland I, Ignatova S, Marmann A, et al. The potential of metabolic fingerprinting as a tool for the modernisation of TCM preparations. Journal of Ethnopharmacology. 2012;**140**(3):482-491. DOI: 10.1016/j.jep.2012.01.050

[109] Nagalingam A. Drug delivery aspects of herbal medicines. In: Arumugam S, Watanabe K, editors. Japanese Kampo Medicines for the Treatment of Common Diseases. Japan: Academic Press; 2017. pp. 143-164

[110] Shepherd M, Shepherd E. Medicines administration 1: Understanding routes of administration. Nursing Times. 2020;**116**(6):42-44

[111] Le J. Drug administration: MSD; 2020. Available from: https://www.msdmanuals.com/en-gb/home/drugs/administration-and-kinetics-of-drugs/drug-administration

[112] Boadu AA, Asase A. Documentation of herbal medicines used for the treatment and management of human diseases by some communities in southern Ghana. Evidence-based Complementary and Alternative Medicine. 2017;1-12. DOI: 10.1155/2017/3043061

[113] Tabuti JRS, Lye KA, Dhillion SS. Traditional herbal drugs of Bulamogi, Uganda: Plants, use and administration. Journal of Ethnopharmacology. 2003;**88**(1):19-44. DOI: 10.1016/s0378-8741(03)00161-2

[114] von Koenen E. Medicinal, poisonous and edible plants in Namibia. Göttingen: Klaus Hess Verlag; 2001

[115] Wonca International Classification Committee (WICC). ICPC-2—English—international classification of primary care—2nd edition. 2012. Available from: https://www.globalfamilydoctor.com/groups/WorkingParties/wicc.aspx

[116] Staub PO, Geck MS, Weckerle CS, Casu L, Leonti M. Ethnopharmacological communication: Classifying diseases and remedies in ethnomedicine and ethnopharmacology. Journal of Ethnopharmacology. 2015;**174**:514-519. DOI: 10.1016/j.jep.2015.08.051

[117] Reid EJ, Betts TJ. Records of Western Australian plants used by aboriginals as medicinal agents. Planta Medica. 1979;**36**(2):164-173. DOI: 10.1055/s-0028-1097257

[118] van Andel T, de Boer HJ, Towns A. Gynaecological, andrological and urological problems: An ethnopharmacological perspective. In: Heinrich M, Jäger AK, editors. Ethnopharmacology. Chichester: John Wiley & Sons Inc. 2015. p. 199-212

[119] Tabuti JRS, Dhillion SS, Lye KA. Traditional medicine in Bulamogi County, Uganda: Its practitioners, users and viability. Journal of Ethnopharmacology. 2003;**85**(1):119-129. DOI: 10.1016/S0378-8741(02)00378-1

[120] Tounekti T, Mahdhi M, Khemira H. Ethnobotanical study of indigenous medicinal plants of Jazan region, Saudi Arabia. Evidence-Based Complementary and Alternative Medicine. 2019;1-45. DOI: 10.1155/2019/3190670

[121] Delbanco A-S, Burgess N, Cuni-Sanchez A. Medicinal plant trade in northern Kenya: Economic importance, uses and origin. Economic Botany. 2017;**71**(1):13-31. DOI: 10.1007/s12231-017-9368-0

[122] Nanyingi MO, Mbaria JM, Lanyasunya AL, Wagate CG, Koros KB, Kaburia HF, et al. Ethnopharmacological survey of Samburu District, Kenya. Journal of Ethnobiology and Ethnomedicine. 2008;**4**(14):1-12. DOI: 10.1186/1746-4269-4-14

[123] Muthee JK, Gakuya DW, Mbaria JM, Kareru PG, Mulei CM, Njonge FK. Ethnobotanical study of anthelmintic and other medicinal plants traditionally used in Loitoktok District of Kenya. Journal of Ethnopharmacology. 2011;**135**(1):15-21. DOI: 10.1016/j.jep.2011.02.005

[124] Kaingu CK, Oduma JA, Kanui TI. Practices of traditional birth attendants in Machakos District, Kenya. Journal of Ethnopharmacology. 2011;**137**(1):495-502. DOI: 10.1016/j.jep.2011.05.044

[125] WHO. World malaria situation in 1990. Bulletin of the World Health Organization. 1992;**70**(6):801-807

[126] Roser M, Ritchie H. Death rate from malaria, 2017: OurWorldInData.org; 2019. Available from: https://ourworldindata.org/malaria#malaria-incidence

[127] Gwer S, Newton CRJC, Berkley JA. Over-diagnosis and co-morbidity of severe malaria in African children: A guide for clinicians. American Journal of Tropical Medicine and Hygiene. 2007;77:6-13

[128] Beeching N, Gill G. Tropical Medicine. 7th ed. Chichester: Wiley-Blackwell. 2014. p.408

[129] Koch A, Tamez P, Pezzuto J, Soejarto D. Evaluation of plants used for antimalarial treatment by the Maasai of Kenya. Journal of Ethnopharmacology. 2005;**101**(1):95-99. DOI: 10.1016/j.jep.2005.03.011

[130] Muthaura CN, Rukunga GM, Chhabra SC, Mungai GM, Njagi ENM. Traditional antimalarial phytotherapy remedies used by the Kwale community of the Kenyan coast. Journal of Ethnopharmacology. 2007;**114**(3):377-386. DOI: 10.1016/j.jep.2007.08.033

[131] Muthaura CN, Rukunga GM, Chhabra SC, Mungai GM, Njagi ENM. Traditional phytotherapy of some remedies used in treatment of malaria in Meru District of Kenya. South African Journal of Botany. 2007;**73**(3):402-411. DOI: 10.1016/j.sajb.2007.03.004

[132] Njoroge GN, Bussmann RW. Diversity and utilization of antimalarial

ethnophytotherapeutic remedies among the Kikuyus (Central Kenya). Journal of Ethnobiology and Ethnomedicine. 2006;**2**(8):1-7. DOI: 10.1186/1746-4269-2-8

[133] Tabuti JRS. Herbal medicines used in the treatment of malaria in Budiope County, Uganda. Journal of Ethnopharmacology. 2008;**116**(1):33-42. DOI: 10.1016/j.jep.2007.10.036

[134] Stangeland T, Alele PE, Katuura E, Lye KA. Plants used to treat malaria in Nyakayojo sub-county, western Uganda. Journal of Ethnopharmacology. 2011;**137**(1):154-166. DOI: 10.1016/j.jep.2011.05.002

[135] Ayuko TA, Njau RN, Wanjala C, Nyangasi L, Ndiege IO. *In vitro* antiplasmodial activity and toxicity assessment of plant extracts used in traditional malaria therapy in the Lake Victoria region. Memórias do Instituto Oswaldo Cruz. 2009;**104**(5):689-694. DOI: 10.1590/s0074-02762009000500004

[136] Kirira PG, Rukunga GM, Wanyonyi AW, Muregi FM, Gathirwa JW, Muthaura CN, et al. Anti-plasmodial activity and toxicity of extracts of plants used in traditional malaria therapy in Meru and Kilifi districts of Kenya. Journal of Ethnopharmacology. 2006;**106**(3):403-407. DOI: 10.1016/j.jep.2006.01.017

[137] Good CM. Ethnomedical Systems in Africa: Patterns of Traditional Medicine in Rural and Urban. Kenya: Guilford Publications; 1987. p. 343

[138] Miara MD, Bendif H, Ouabed A, Rebbas K, Ait Hammou M, Amirat M, et al. Ethnoveterinary remedies used in the Algerian steppe: Exploring the relationship with traditional human herbal medicine. Journal of Ethnopharmacology. 2019;**244**:1-13. DOI: 10.1016/j.jep.2019.112164

[139] Teklehaymanot T. Ethnobotanical study of knowledge and medicinal plants use by the people in Dek Island in Ethiopia. Journal of Ethnopharmacology. 2009;**124**(1):69-78. DOI: 10.1016/j.jep.2009.04.005

[140] Rimbach L. Traditional methods of treating cattle diseases. Report for ASA (Studienaufenthalte in Afrika, Asien und Latein-Amerika). Berlin: ASA Programme. 1977. p.19

[141] Singh VK, Khan AM, Govil JN. Medicinal Plants and Folklores: A Strategy towards Conquest of Human Ailments. New Delhi: Today & Tomorrow's Printers and Publishers; 1990.p. 250

[142] Gradé JT, Tabuti JRS, Van Damme P. Ethnoveterinary knowledge in pastoral Karamoja, Uganda. Journal of Ethnopharmacology. 2009;**122**(2):273-293. DOI: 10.1016/j.jep.2009.01.005

[143] ITDG, IIRR. Ethnoveterinary Medicine in Kenya: A Field Manual of Traditional Animal Health Care Practices. Nairobi, Kenya: Intermediate Technology Development Group and International Institute of Rural Reconstruction; 1996. p. 226

[144] Tabuti JRS, Dhillion SS, Lye KA. Ethnoveterinary medicines for cattle (*Bos indicus*) in Bulamogi County, Uganda: Plant species and mode of use. Journal of Ethnopharmacology. 2003;**88**(2-3):279-286. DOI: 10.1016/s0378-8741(03)00265-4

[145] Ejobi F, Mosha R, Ndege S, Kamoga D. Ethno-veterinary medicinal plants of the Lake Victoria basin: A bioprospection. Journal of Animal and Veterinary Advances. 2007;**6**(2):257-261

[146] Gakuubi MM, Wanzala W. A survey of plants and plant products traditionally used in livestock health

management in Buuri District, Meru County, Kenya. Journal of Ethnobiology and Ethnomedicine. 2012;**8**(39):1-19. DOI: 10.1186/1746-4269-8-39

[147] Teshale S, Bekana M, Adugna G, Kelbessa E. Medicinal plants in the ethnoveterinary practices of Borana pastoralists, southern Ethiopia. International Journal of Applied Research in Veterinary Medicine. 2004;**2**(3):220-225

[148] Birhanu T, Abera D. Survey of ethno-veterinary medicinal plants at selected Horro Gudurru districts, Western Ethiopia. African Journal of Plant Science. 2015;**9**(3):185-192. DOI: 10.5897/AJPS2014.1229

[149] Ndizihiwe D, Nkuuhe D, Ahishakiye E, Sunday B, Tumwesigye W. Utilization of medicinal plants in treating livestock diseases around Queen Elizabeth national park, western Uganda. International Journal of Herbal Medicine. 2019;**7**(2):4-07

[150] Shrivastava S, Jain AK. Ethno-veterinary practices in India: A review. In: Jain AK, editor. Indian Ethnobotany: Emerging Trends. Jodhpur: Scientific Publishers (India); 2016. p. 276-285

[151] Moerman DE. Symbols and selectivity: A statistical analysis of native American medical ethnobotany. Journal of Ethnopharmacology. 1979;**1**(2):111-119. DOI: 10.1016/0378-8741(79)90002-3

[152] Adu-Tutu M, Afful Y, Asante-Appiah K, Lieberman D, Hall JB, Elvin-Lewis M. Chewing stick usage in southern Ghana. Economic Botany. 1979;**33**(3):320-328. DOI: 10.1007/BF02858262

[153] Trotter R, Logan M. Informant consensus: A new approach for identifying potentially effective medicinal plants. In: Etkin N, editor. Plants in Indigenous Medicine and Diet: Biobehavioral Approaches. New York: Redgrave Publishing Company. 1986. pp. 91-112

[154] Phillips O, Gentry AH, Reynel C, Wilkin P, Galvez-Durand B C. Quantitative ethnobotany and Amazonian conservation. Conservation Biology. 1994;**8**(1):225-248

[155] Heinrich M, Ankli A, Frei B, Weimann C, Sticher O. Medicinal plants in Mexico: Healers' consensus and cultural importance. Social Science and Medicine. 1998;**47**(11):1859-1871. DOI: 10.1016/S0277-9536(98)00181-6

[156] Thomas E, Vandebroek I, Sanca S, Van Damme P. Cultural significance of medicinal plant families and species among Quechua farmers in Apillapampa, Bolivia. Journal of Ethnopharmacology. 2009;**122**(1):60-67. DOI: 10.1016/j.jep.2008.11.021

[157] Wambugu SN, Mathiu PM, Gakuya DW, Kanui TI, Kabasa JD, Kiama SG. Medicinal plants used in the management of chronic joint pains in Machakos and Makueni counties, Kenya. Journal of Ethnopharmacology. 2011;**137**(2):945-955. DOI: 10.1016/j.jep.2011.06.038

[158] Njoroge GN, Kaibui IM, Njenga PK, Odhiambo PO. Utilisation of priority traditional medicinal plants and local people's knowledge on their conservation status in arid lands of Kenya (Mwingi District). Journal of Ethnobiology and Ethnomedicine. 2010;**6**(22):1-8. DOI: 10.1186/1746-4269-6-22

[159] Kama-Kama F, Midiwo J, Nganga J, Maina N, Schiek E, Omosa LK, et al. Selected ethno-medicinal plants from Kenya with *in vitro* activity against major African livestock pathogens

belonging to the "*Mycoplasma mycoides* cluster". Journal of Ethnopharmacology. 2016;**192**:524-534. DOI: 10.1016/j.jep.2016.09.034

[160] Issa TO, Mohamed YS, Yagi S, Ahmed RH, Najeeb TM, Makhawi AM, et al. Ethnobotanical investigation on medicinal plants in Algoz area (South Kordofan), Sudan. Journal of Ethnobiology and Ethnomedicine. 2018;**14**(31):1-22. DOI: 10.1186/s13002-018-0230-y

[161] Urso V, Signorini MA, Tonini M, Bruschi P. Wild medicinal and food plants used by communities living in Mopane woodlands of southern Angola: Results of an ethnobotanical field investigation. Journal of Ethnopharmacology. 2016;**177**:126-139. DOI: 10.1016/j.jep.2015.11.041

[162] Mashile SP, Tshisikhawe MP, Masevhe NA. Indigenous fruit plants species of the Mapulana of Ehlanzeni District in Mpumalanga province, South Africa. South African Journal of Botany. 2019;**122**:180-183. DOI: 10.1016/j.sajb.2018.09.031

[163] Saqib Z, Mahmood A, Naseem Malik R, Mahmood A, Hussian Syed J, Ahmad T. Indigenous knowledge of medicinal plants in Kotli Sattian, Rawalpindi District, Pakistan. Journal of Ethnopharmacology. 2014;**151**(2):820-828. DOI: 10.1016/j.jep.2013.11.034

[164] Ojelel S, Mucunguzi P, Katuura E, Kakudidi EK, Namaganda M, Kalema J. Wild edible plants used by communities in and around selected forest reserves of Teso-Karamoja region, Uganda. Journal of Ethnobiology and Ethnomedicine. 2019;**15**(3):1-14. DOI: 10.1186/s13002-018-0278-8

[165] Ashagre M, Asfaw Z, Kelbessa E. Ethnobotanical study of wild edible plants in Burji district, Segan area Zone of Southern Nations, Nationalities and Peoples Region (SNNPR), Ethiopia. Journal of Ethnobiology and Ethnomedicine. 2016;**12**(32):1-15. DOI: 10.1186/s13002-016-0103-1

[166] Ndamba J, Nyazema N, Makaza N, Anderson C, Kaondera KC. Traditional herbal remedies used for the treatment of urinary schistosomiasis in Zimbabwe. Journal of Ethnopharmacology. 1994;**42**(2):125-132

[167] Samoisy Anne K, Mahomoodally MF. Ethnopharmacological analysis of medicinal plants used against non-communicable diseases in Rodrigues Island, Indian Ocean. Journal of Ethnopharmacology. 2015;**173**:20-38. DOI: 10.1016/j.jep.2015.06.036

[168] Mujtaba Shah G, Abbasi AM, Khan N, Guo X, Ajab Khan M, Hussain M, et al. Traditional uses of medicinal plants against malarial disease by the tribal communities of lesser Himalayas–Pakistan. Journal of Ethnopharmacology. 2014;**155**(1):450-462. DOI: 10.1016/j.jep.2014.05.047

[169] Venkatachalapathi A, Sangeeth T, Ali MA, Tamilselvi SS, Paulsamy S, Al-Hemaidc FMA. Ethnomedicinal assessment of Irula tribes of Walayar valley of southern Western Ghats, India. Saudi Journal of Biological Sciences. 2018;**25**(4):760-775. DOI: 10.1016/j.sjbs.2016.10.011

[170] Dalziel JM. The Useful Plants of West Tropical Africa (being an Appendix to "The flora of West Tropical Africa"). London: Crown Agents for the Colonies; 1937. p. 612

[171] Kidane L, Gebremedhin G, Beyene T. Ethnobotanical study of medicinal plants in Ganta Afeshum District, eastern zone of Tigray, northern Ethiopia. Journal

of Ethnobiology and Ethnomedicine. 2018;**14**(64):1-19. DOI: 10.1186/s13002-018-0266-z

[172] Amsalu N, Bezie Y, Fentahun M, Alemayehu A, Amsalu G. Use and conservation of medicinal plants by indigenous people of Gozamin Wereda, east Gojjam zone of Amhara region, Ethiopia: An ethnobotanical approach. Evidence-Based Complementary and Alternative Medicine. 2018;**2018**:1-23. DOI: 10.1155/2018/2973513

[173] Jima TT, Megersa M. Ethnobotanical study of medicinal plants used to treat human diseases in Berbere District, Bale Zone of Oromia regional state, south East Ethiopia. Evidence-based Complementary and Alternative Medicine. 2018;**2018**:1-16. DOI: 10.1155/2018/8602945

[174] Kebebew M, Leta G. Wild edible plant bio-diversity and utilization system in Nech Sar National park, Ethiopia. International Journal of Bio-resource and Stress Management. 2016;7(4):885-896. DOI: 10.5958/0976-4038.2016.00143.3

[175] Kebebew M. Diversity, knowledge and use of medicinal plants in Abay Chomen District, Horo Guduru Wollega Zone, Oromia Region of Ethiopia. Journal of Medicinal Plants Research. 2017;**11**(31):480-500. DOI: 10.5897/jmpr2016.6274

[176] Kefalew A, Asfaw Z, Kelbessa E. Ethnobotany of medicinal plants in Ada'a District, East Shewa Zone of Oromia regional state, Ethiopia. Journal of Ethnobiology and Ethnomedicine. 2015;**11**(25):1-28. DOI: 10.1186/s13002-015-0014-6

[177] Lulekal E, Asfaw Z, Kelbessa E, Van Damme P. Ethnomedicinal study of plants used for human ailments in Ankober District, North Shewa Zone, Amhara Region, Ethiopia. Journal of Ethnobiology and Ethnomedicine. 2013;**9**(63):1-13. DOI: 10.1186/1746-4269-9-63

[178] Megersa M, Asfaw Z, Kelbessa E, Beyene A, Woldeab B. An ethnobotanical study of medicinal plants in Wayu Tuka District, East Welega Zone of Oromia regional state, west Ethiopia. Journal of Ethnobiology and Ethnomedicine. 2013;**9**(68):1-18. DOI: 10.1186/1746-4269-9-68

[179] Mekonen T, Giday M, Kelbessa E. Ethnobotanical study of homegarden plants in Sebeta-Awas District of the Oromia Region of Ethiopia to assess use, species diversity and management practices. Journal of Ethnobiology and Ethnomedicine. 2015;**11**(64):1-13. DOI: 10.1186/s13002-015-0049-8

[180] Meragiaw M, Asfaw Z, Argaw M. The status of ethnobotanical knowledge of medicinal plants and the impacts of resettlement in Delanta, northwestern Wello, northern Ethiopia. Evidence-based Complementary and Alternative Medicine. 2016;**2016**:1-24. DOI: 10.1155/2016/5060247

[181] Tefera BN, Kim Y-D. Ethnobotanical study of medicinal plants in the Hawassa Zuria District, Sidama Zone, southern Ethiopia. Journal of Ethnobiology and Ethnomedicine. 2019;**15**(25):1-21. DOI: 10.1186/s13002-019-0302-7

[182] Teklay A, Abera B, Giday M. An ethnobotanical study of medicinal plants used in Kilte Awulaelo District, Tigray Region of Ethiopia. Journal of Ethnobiology and Ethnomedicine. 2013;**9**(65):1-23. DOI: 10.1186/1746-4269-9-65

[183] Osman A, Sbhatu DB, Giday M. Medicinal plants used to manage human

and livestock ailments in Raya Kobo District of Amhara regional state, Ethiopia. Evidence-Based Complementary and Alternative Medicine. 2020;**2020**:1-19. DOI: 10.1155/2020/1329170

[184] Abera B. Medicinal plants used in traditional medicine by Oromo people, Ghimbi District, Southwest Ethiopia. Journal of Ethnobiology and Ethnomedicine. 2014;**10**(40):1-15. DOI: 10.1186/1746-4269-10-40

[185] Asnake S, Teklehaymanot T, Hymete A, Erko B, Giday M. Survey of medicinal plants used to treat malaria by Sidama people of Boricha district, Sidama Zone, south region of Ethiopia. Evidence-based Complementary and Alternative Medicine. 2016;**2016**:1-9. DOI: 10.1155/2016/9690164

[186] Bekalo TH, Woodmatas SD, Woldemariam ZA. An ethnobotanical study of medicinal plants used by local people in the lowlands of Konta Special Woreda, Southern Nations, Nationalities and Peoples' regional state, Ethiopia. Journal of Ethnobiology and Ethnomedicine. 2009;**5**(26):1-15. DOI: 10.1186/1746-4269-5-26

[187] Chekole G, Asfaw Z, Kelbessa E. Ethnobotanical study of medicinal plants in the environs of Tara-gedam and Amba remnant forests of Libo Kemkem District, Northwest Ethiopia. Journal of Ethnobiology and Ethnomedicine. 2015;**11**(4):1-38. DOI: 10.1186/1746-4269-11-4

[188] Chekole G. Ethnobotanical study of medicinal plants used against human ailments in Gubalafto District, northern Ethiopia. Journal of Ethnobiology and Ethnomedicine. 2017;**13**(55):1-29. DOI: 10.1186/s13002-017-0182-7

[189] Kidane B, van Andel T, van der Maesen LJG, Asfaw Z. Use and management of traditional medicinal plants by Maale and Ari ethnic communities in southern Ethiopia. Journal of Ethnobiology and Ethnomedicine. 2014;**10**(46):1-15. DOI: 10.1186/1746-4269-10-46

[190] Lulekal E, Asfaw Z, Kelbessa E, Van Damme P. Ethnoveterinary plants of Ankober District, North Shewa Zone, Amhara Region, Ethiopia. Journal of Ethnobiology and Ethnomedicine. 2014;**10**(21):1-19. DOI: 10.1186/1746-4269-10-21

[191] Teklehaymanot T. An ethnobotanical survey of medicinal and edible plants of Yalo Woreda in Afar regional state, Ethiopia. Journal of Ethnobiology and Ethnomedicine. 2017;**13**(40):1-25. DOI: 10.1186/s13002-017-0166-7

[192] Vandebroek I, Moerman DE. The Anthropology of Ethnopharmacology. Ethnopharmacology. 2015. Chichester: John Wiley & Sons Inc. 2015. p. 17-28

[193] Bussmann RW. Ethnobotany of the Samburu of Mt. Nyiru, south Turkana, Kenya additional file. Journal of Ethnobiology and Ethnomedicine. 2006;**2**(35):1-10

[194] Raymond E, Blutja J, Gingina L, Raymond M, Raymond L, Raymond O, et al. Wardaman ethnobiology: Aboriginal plant and animal knowledge from the Flora river and south-west Katherine region, north Australia. Darwin: Centre for Indigenous Natural and Cultural Resource Management, Northern Territory University and Parks and Wildlife Commission of the Northern Territory; 1999. p. 191

[195] Nyahangare ET, Mvumi BM, Mutibvu T. Ethnoveterinary plants and

practices used for ecto-parasite control in semi-arid smallholder farming areas of Zimbabwe. Journal of Ethnobiology and Ethnomedicine. 2015;**11**(30):1-16. DOI: 10.1186/s13002-015-0006-6

[196] Arshad M, Ahmad M, Ahmed E, Saboor A, Abbas A, Sadiq S. An ethnobiological study in Kala Chitta hills of Pothwar region, Pakistan: Multinomial logit specification. Journal of Ethnobiology and Ethnomedicine. 2014;**10**(13):1-17. DOI: 10.1186/1746-4269-10-13

[197] Saidulu P, Suthari S, Kandagatla R, Ajmeera R, Vatsavaya R. Ethnobotanical knowledge studied in Pocharam wildlife sanctuary, Telangana, India. Notulae Scientia Biologicae. 2015;7(2): 164-170

[198] Vandebroek I, Pieroni A, Stepp JR, Hanazaki N, Ladio A, Alves RRN, et al. Reshaping the future of ethnobiology research after the COVID-19 pandemic. Nature Plants. 2020;**6**(7):723-730. DOI: 10.1038/s41477-020-0691-6

[199] Ludwig D. Revamping the metaphysics of ethnobiological classification. Current Anthropology. 2018;**59**(4):415-438. DOI: 10.1086/698958

[200] Yeung AWK, Heinrich M, Kijjoa A, Tzvetkov NT, Atanasov AG. The ethnopharmacological literature: An analysis of the scientific landscape. Journal of Ethnopharmacology. 2020;**250**:1-21. DOI: 10.1016/j.jep.2019.112414

[201] Weiskopf DA. Representing and coordinating ethnobiological knowledge. Studies in History and Philosophy of Biological and Biomedical Sciences. 2020;**84**:1-11. DOI: 10.1016/j.shpsc.2020.101328

[202] Carrière S, Andrianotahiananahary H, Ranaivoarivelo N, Randriamalala J. Savoirs et Usages des Recrus Post-agricoles du Pays Betsileo : Valorisation d'une Biodiversité Oubliée à Madagascar. VertigO. 2005;**6**(1):1-14. DOI: 10.4000/vertigo.3047

[203] Etkin NL, Elisabetsky E. Seeking a transdisciplinary and culturally germane science: The future of ethnopharmacology. Journal of Ethnopharmacology. 2005;**100**(1-2):23-26. DOI: 10.1016/j.jep.2005.05.025

[204] Vandebroek I. Intercultural health and ethnobotany: How to improve healthcare for underserved and minority communities? Journal of Ethnopharmacology. 2013;**148**(3):746-754. DOI: 10.1016/j.jep.2013.05.039

[205] Kigen G, Kipkore W, Wanjohi B, Haruki B, Kembol J. Medicinal plants used by traditional healers in Sangurur, Elgeyo Marakwet County, Kenya. Pharmacognosy Research. 2017;**9**(4):333-347. DOI: 10.4103/pr.pr_42_17

[206] Kigen G, Kamuren Z, Njiru E, Wanjohi B, Kipkore W. Ethnomedical survey of the plants used by traditional healers in Narok County, Kenya. Evidence-based Complementary & Alternative Medicine (eCAM). 2019;**2019**:1-8. DOI: 10.1155/2019/8976937

[207] Barthel R, Seidl R. Interdisciplinary collaboration between natural and social sciences—Status and trends exemplified in groundwater research. PLoS One. 2017;**12**(1):1-27. DOI: 10.1371/journal.pone.0170754

[208] Jahn T, Bergmann M, Keil F. Transdisciplinarity: Between mainstreaming and marginalization. Ecological Economics. 2012;**79**:1-10. DOI: 10.1016/j.ecolecon.2012.04.017

[209] Strang V. Integrating the social and natural sciences in environmental research: A discussion paper. Environment, Development and Sustainability. 2009;**11**(1):1-18. DOI: 10.1007/s10668-007-9095-2

[210] Albuquerque UP, Melo JG, Medeiros MF, Menezes IR, Moura GJ, Asfora El-Deir AC, et al. Natural products from ethnodirected studies: Revisiting the ethnobiology of the zombie poison. Evidence-based Complementary and Alternative Medicine. 2012;**2012**:1-19. DOI: 10.1155/2012/202508

[211] Ledford H. Team science. Nature. 2015;**525**(7569):308-311. DOI: 10.1038/525308a

[212] Langwick SA. Healers and scientists: The epistemological politics of research about medicinal plants in Tanzania, or 'moving away from traditional medicine'. In: Geissler W, Molyneux C, editors. Evidence, Ethos and Experiment: The Anthropology and History of Medical Research in Africa. Oxford: Berghahn Books; 2011. p. 263-295

[213] Robson C, McCartan K. Real World Research: A Resource for Users of Social Research Methods in Applied Settings. 4th ed. Chichester: John Wiley & Sons, Inc; 2016. p. 560

[214] Albuquerque UP, Hanazaki N. Five problems in current ethnobotanical research—And some suggestions for strengthening them. Human Ecology. 2009;**37**(5):653-661. DOI: 10.1007/s10745-009-9259-9

[215] Ferreira Júnior WS. Reflections on the theoretical advance in ethnobiology: Are we pointing to the wrong direction? Ethnobiology and Conservation. 2020; **9**(20):1-8. DOI: 10.15451/ec2020-05-9.20-1-8

[216] Dudney K, Warren S, Sills E, Jacka J. How study design influences the ranking of medicinal plant importance: A case study from Ghana, West Africa. Economic Botany. 2015;**69**(4):306-317. DOI: 10.1007/s12231-015-9322-y

[217] Tardío J, Pardo-de-Santayana M. Cultural importance indices: A comparative analysis based on the useful wild plants of southern Cantabria (northern Spain). Economic Botany. 2008;**62**(1):24-39. DOI: 10.1007/s12231-007-9004-5

[218] Turnhout E, Bloomfield B, Hulme M, Vogel J, Wynne B. Conservation policy: Listen to the voices of experience. Nature. 2012;**488**(7412):454-455. DOI: 10.1038/488454a

[219] Meireles MPA, Albuquerque UP, Medeiros PM. What interferes with conducting free lists? A comparative ethnobotanical experiment. Journal of Ethnobiology and Ethnomedicine. 2021;**17**(4):1-11. DOI: 10.1186/s13002-021-00432-5

[220] Paniagua Zambrana NY, Bussmann RW, Hart RE, Huanca ALM, Soria GO, Vaca MO, et al. To list or not to list? The value and detriment of freelisting in ethnobotanical studies. Nature Plants. 2018;**4**(4):201-204. DOI: 10.1038/s41477-018-0128-7

[221] Albuquerque UP, Nascimento ALB, Soldati GT, Feitosa IS, Campos JLA, Hurrell JA, et al. Ten important questions/issues for ethnobotanical research. Acta Botanica Brasilica. 2019;**33**(2):376-385. DOI: 10.1590/0102-33062018abb0331

[222] Graz B, Willcox ML, Diakite C, Falquet J, Dackuo F, Sidibe O, et al. *Argemone mexicana* decoction versus

artesunate-amodiaquine for the management of malaria in Mali: Policy and public-health implications. Transactions of the Royal Society of Tropical Medicine and Hygiene. 2010;**104**(1):33-41. DOI: https://doi.org/10.1016/j.trstmh.2009.07.005

Chapter 9

Ethnomedicinal Appraisal of Traditionally Used Wild Edible Plants of District Bagh, Azad Jammu & Kashmir, Pakistan

Sadia Shabbir and Muhammad Shoaib Amjad

Abstract

The present study was aim to document the traditional knowledge about medicinal uses of wild edible plants in District Bagh Azad Kashmir. Ethnomedicinal data was gathered from 80 informants using open ended and semi structured interview, field observation and group discussion. A total of 51 wild edible plant species mentioned by informants' as medicinal belonging to 42 botanical genera and 32 botanical families with Legumenaceae (6 spp.) and Rosaceae (5 spp.) being most frequently used. Herbs (45.09%) were most commonly used for prepration of herbal recipies. The preferably used plant part for herbal preparation are leaves (64.7%). The plant species with highest relative frequency of citation are *Morus nigra* (0.9) and *Melia azedarach* (0.9). The highest UV values was recorded for *M. nigra* (1) and *Berberis lycium* (1). The highest RI value was calculated for *Urginea indica* (90). *Berberis lycium* had 100% fidelity level. Wild edible plants species are under high anthropogenic pressure and need immediate conservation through community base management, public awareness and germplasm collection. There is dire need for reappraisal of traditionally knowledge on wild edible plants which not only conserve this traditional heritage but may also contribute in future drug discovery.

Keywords: wild edible plants, Bagh, UV, RFC, ICF

1. Introduction

Humans have quite complex relationship with plants extending far back from the beging of human civilization on the earth. Plants are intially used for food, medicine and shelter. However various other uses ared discover by human beging with the passage of time and the dependence of human being on plant incresaed many fold, and in this manner support various other aspects of human proseperity and walfare [1, 2]. Ethnobotany paly key role in understaning the past and present dynamic interrelationship between socioculture system and phytodiversity [3]. The term Ethonotany was first coined by John W. Harsberge in 1896 [4]. However Ford (1978) developed the ethnobotanical discipline which descirbed the collection, identifcation and uses of plants by the people [5]. In borader aspect, ethnobotany referes to the discipline which use various anthropolgical approaches to understand the knowledge systems. During the current era, the ethnobotany emerge as mutidisplinay subject which focus on people plant relationship not only by collection and documentation of plants and their potential uses but also invovle economy, anthorpology, botany, pharmacology, public heatlh and vaious other fields. Thus people palnt interaction is quite broader aspect encompassing religious, social, artistic, commerical and symbolic relationship.

Ethnobotanical survey play pivotal role in highlighing the important plant species of the particular area. These species may be quite significant in pharmaceutical, farming, medicine and nuraceutical industry. The documentation of tradiational knowledge provide the basis for development of various modern drugs. It has been estimated that about 25% of modern medicine are plant based and majority of allopatheic medicine are synthetic analogue to the natural compound isolated from various plant species [6]. About 70–80% population of developing countries still depend upon herbal remedies for curing various ailments. This may due their cost effectivness, less side effect, cultural acceptibility and lack of modern health facilites. Herbal remedies are even extensivly used in various developed countries e.g. 40–50% population in Germany, 30–50% in China, 42% in the USA, 49% in France and 48% in Australia used plant based medicine as supplementary health care [7–9].

Wild plants species grows in natural or semi natural ecosystem spontaneously and exist independently without any human intervention. In contrast cultivated or domesticated plants have grown under human intervention, such as collection or breeding, and rely on management for their continuing survival. Wild edibel plant are gathered throughout the world using tradiational practice from different habitats such as forests, wetlands cultivateable fields and roadside. Since ancient times, wild plants have played a pivotal role in survival and livlehood of number of ethnic communities across the world by providing medicine, food, colors, shelter, poisons, textiles and also used in cultruarl and religious cermonies [10]. They are preffered by the people because of their aromatic and fresh taste, growing in pollutant free envirnoment, rich mineral nutrients, strong vitality and number of health and medicinal benefits [11].

According to estimate there are about 20,000 wild plant species across the world [12, 13]. In the past, more than 7000 wild edible plant species have been used by the humans [14]. Out of total, only 3000 speccies have been ued as agricultural crop and 150 species are commercially cultivated. However 90% of our food is obtained from only 20 species [12, 15, 16]. The usage of wild edible plant as food occur both in the time of food shortage and surplus and this usage has not completely disappeared even in the agricultural socities where people primarly depends upon crop plant [17, 18]. Throughout the contemporary world, about 200 million people full fill their food and livilehood requirments from frorest [12]. Previous reports also documented the theraputic potential and nturional value of wild edible plants [15, 16, 19].

The wild edible plants (WEPs) are an integral component of biodiversity and there in situ conservation offers various sociocultural, economic and agriculture benefits [10, 20]. The role of wild edible plants in folk tradiations is quite significant. However the most relevant and consistent reason for better management of wild edible plants are there use as food and medicine. Therefore, the ethnobotanical research is important in identifying new source for food and providing raw material for drug discovery. The presence of high amount of various micrnonutrients, minerals and vitamin increase the nutritional quality of wild edible as compared to domesticated varieties and hence prefered by ethnic communities [21]. Some areas of the world have particular diversity of plants and animals [15, 16]. District Bagh, is one of such area located in western Himalayan region of Azad Jammu & Kashmir. The area harbored number of wild edible plants, which are use by local in variety of ways. Large numbers of wild edible plants are widely distributed throughout the District and consumed in various ways. Nutritionally, most of these plants are highly important because of presence of fiber contents, minerals and vitamins. Root, nut, tubers, fruit and bark are commonly consumed parts, which were analyzed for carbohydrate, protein, fats and minerals.

Previous epidemiological reports confirmed that diet have key role in curing various chronic ailments. This evidence suggest that change in behavior of diet such as high consumption of grains, fruits and vegetable is a practical strategy in minimizing or controlling the incidence of various chronic ailments. High consumption of wild fruits and vegetables have strong link with low risk of cancer, cardiovascular and inflammatory diseases, Alzheimer's disease, diabetes, Aging, cataracts. The connection between food and health is becoming highly significant as people now demand tasty, healthy and natural functional foods which grow in uncontaminated environment. In different regions of the world the knowledge about such wild edible plants as medicine and food is disappearing. This is because it mainly transferred orally and vertically from generation to generation as a part of traditional knowledge. Hence it is very crucial to document the data about popular uses of such plants before this knowledge become extinct. Therefore, current study is design to (a) document ethnomedicinal knowledge about wild edible plants (b) quantitatively analyze the data by using various indices such as frequency of citation, use value, informant consent factor, relative importance and fidelity level.

2. Material and methods

2.1 Study area

District Bagh is one of the diversity rich area lies in western Himalayan region of Azad Kashmir. Its geographical coordinates are between latitude 33°53′–4°07′ N and longitude 73°30′ to 74° E. The altitude of the area varies between 600 and 3300 m. The total land area is 770 m^2 and total population is 0.397 illion. Map of the study area is given in **Figure 1**. The climate of the area is of Mediterranean type with annual precipitation of 1500 mm. January is coldest month with average minimum temperature fall below −2°C and June is warmest month where average maximum temperature remains close to 40°C.

The local inhabitant of the area belongs to diverse ethnic group mainly Maldial, Abbasi, Khawa, Rajpoot, Gujar and Sadaat. The whole population is Muslim. Commonly spoken languages include Hinko, Pahari, Kashmiri and Gojri. The vegetation of the area varies from subtropical to temperate type comprises a wide variety herbs, shrubs, trees and climbers. The people residing at higher altitude have poor socioeconomic condition and have a long abundant and tradition practices of eating wild plants. Due very limited access to modern health facilities, they still use these plants to

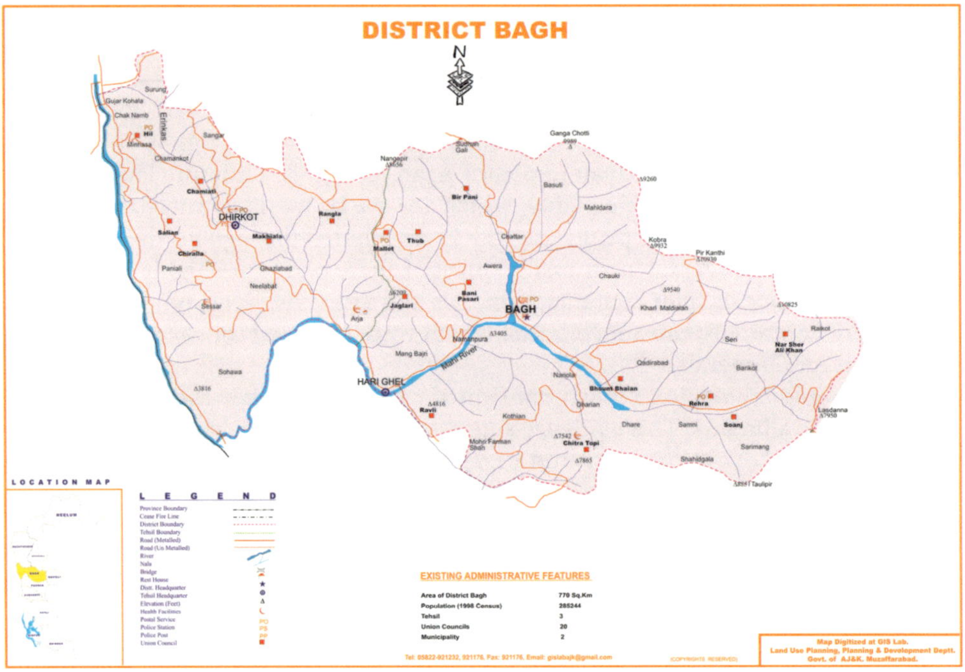

Figure 1.
Map of study area.

cure various ailments. However, knowledge about medicinal and other use of plants are mainly confine to elder peoples and health Practionaire (hakims).

2.2 Ethnobotanical data collection

Ethnomedicinal data about wild edible plants was obtained from 80 informants (35 males; females) open ended and semi structured interviews, field observation and group discussion. The consent was verbally obtained from the participant before starting interview. Ethical codes of American society of Ethnobiology was followed strictly during survey. Ethical permission to conduct survey was obtained from ethical committee of university, while legal permission was obtained from members of municipality. Complete information about wild edible plants such as local name, medicinal usage, part used in herbal recipie, cooking recipe, mode of consumption, disease treated were carefully recorded.

2.3 Plant collection and identification

Field survey was conducted during March 2020 to February 2021. The wild edible plants specimens were collected in triplicate during different season throughout year. The specimens were properly dried, pressed and pasted on herbarium sheets. By using flora of Pakistan (https://http://www.efloras.org) the specimens were identified. APG IV (2016) system was adopted for taxonomical verification of families while the correct botanical nomenclature was given by using The Plant List (2013). The identified specimens were further confirmed at Pakistan Agriculture and

DOI: http://dx.doi.org/10.5772/intechopen.104492

Research Council (PARC), Islamabad. The finally idenetified speciemen were submitted finally in herbarium of Botany Department of Women University.

2.4 Quantitative ethnobotanical indices

The collected ethno medicinal data of wild edible plants was quantitatively analyzed by using following indices:

2.4.1 *Relative frequency of citation (RFC)*

The local significance of particular plant species as cited by the informants was determined by using relative Frequency of Citation. It was figured out after Vijayakumar et al. [22] by given formula:

$$\text{RFC} = \text{FC}/\text{N} \tag{1}$$

whereas, FC is informant who reported specific wild edible plant species and N is total informants. Its value range between 0 and 1.0 when no informant cited use of species as useful and 1 when all the infsormant cited the species as useful.

2.4.2 *Use value index*

The relative importance of particular specie in region is reflected by use value (UV) and determined by following Vijayakumar et al. [22] by given formula:

$$\text{UV} = \frac{\sum Ui}{N} \tag{2}$$

Where, UV are use reports cited by each informant for given wild edible plant species and N are total informants.

2.4.3 *Relative importance*

It was figured out after Khan et al. [23] by given formula:

$$\text{RI} = (\text{Rel PH} + \text{Rel BS}) \times 100/2 \tag{3}$$

$$\text{Rel PH} = \frac{\text{PH of a given plant}}{\text{maximum PH of all reported species}} \tag{4}$$

Where PH is the pharmacological attribute of the selected plant, Rel PH = relative pharmacological attributes of a given plant.

$$\text{Rel BS} = \frac{\text{BS of a given plant}}{\text{maximum BS of all reported species}} \tag{5}$$

Where BS is body systems healed by given species and Rel BS is relative body systems healed by that species.

2.4.4 Informant consensus factor (ICF)

The consensus among the informants about usage of wild edible plants for treating different disease categories will check by using ICF. It was determined after Heinrich et al. [24] using given formula:

$$\mathrm{ICF} = \frac{\mathrm{Nur} - \mathrm{Nt}}{(\mathrm{Nur} - 1)} \tag{6}$$

Where, Nur is use reports in given diseases category, Nt are species numbers used for curing various diseases of that category.

2.4.5 Fidelity level (FL)

It reflect weigtage of particular plant species by informants to heal given ailment and was figured out after Alexiades and Sheldon [25] using given formula

$$FL\% = Np/N \times 100. \tag{7}$$

Where Np are informants citing use of specific wild plant species for a particular ailment and N are the total informants mentioning uses for a particular wild plant species for all disease category.

3. Results and discussion

3.1 Demography and knowledge variation

A total of 80 informants (35 males; 45 females) were selected to gathered knowledge about usage of wild edible plants from District Bagh. The informants were divided into four groups i.e. gender, age, education and profession (**Table 1**). The informants were first classified on the base of gender. Women informants were more in number as compared to men because the interviewee was female and women do not hesitate to share information with her. Besides, the women had high traditional knowledge (average cited species 3.90; average cited uses 5.15) about usage of wild edible plants as compared to male (average cited species 4.56; average cited uses 6.73) This may because the women generally mange the indoor and domestic activities while the males mostly engage in earning and field works. The other reason may be strongly connected network among the women and greater knowledge sharing with high number of central individual. These findings are strongly supported by Kayani et al., Aziz et al., Shaheen et al., Farooq et al. and Amjad et al.

Age was second criteria used for classification of informants. Base on age the informants were categorized into three categories i. e. 20–40, 41–60 and 60–80. The older age people (between 60 and 80) had more knowledge (average cited species 11.32; average cited uses 12.91) about wild edible followed by elder (average cited species 8.16; average cited uses 7.31) and younger (average cited species 3.44; average cited uses 3.67). The older age people had vast experience of practicing wild plants. While the younger had limited interest in learning and practicing traditional

DOI: http://dx.doi.org/10.5772/intechopen.104492

Variables	Informants category	Numbers	Percentage	ANSCI	ANUCI
Gender	Male	35	43.75	3.90	5.15
	Female	45	56.25	4.56	6.73
	Total	80			
Age class	20–40	21	26.25	3.44	3.67
	41–60	46	57.5	8.16	7.31
	60–80	13	16.25	11.32	12.91
Education	Illiterate	26	32.5	7.46	5.35
	Elementary education	19	23.75	10.56	9.67
	Secondary education	16	20	6.33	7.23
	Bachelors degree	11	13.75	5.34	3.42
	Higher education	8	10	3.94	2.37
Profession	Traditional health practionaires	9	11.25	20.48	13.98
	House wives	23	28.75	5.95	7.56
	Teachers	12	15	4.22	4.95
	Farmers	3	3.75	5.25	4.75
	Mid wives	10	12.5	8.15	8.67
	Herders	5	6.25	5.95	7.10
	Doctor	1	1.25	3.34	4.15
	Student	6	7.5	2.30	2.77
	Others	11	13.75	4.58	3.45

Key: ANSCI, average species cited by each informant; ANUCI, average N use cited by each informant.

Table 1.
Demographic characteristic of informants.

knowledge due to change in lifestyle and modernization. Similar trend were also observed by Qaseem et al. in Kotli, Shaheen et al. in Pearl valley and Umair et al. [26] in Hafizabad.

The third significant factor was education. Educated peoples had less knowledge about wild edible plants as compared to educated people. This is due to frequent utilization and direct attachment of uneducated informants with wild edible plants species. Beside they mostly contact with traditional healers during illness. The modern education and culture mostly detach the people from nature. Likewise, the traditional health practitioner (hakim) had more knowledge about wild plants because they remain in touch with them. They have strong academic knowledge about usage of herbs for curing various ailments. Previous reports from other areas of Pakistan and other world also report similar findings.

3.2 Taxonomic diversity of wild edible plants

A total of 51 wild edible plant species distributed among 42 genera and 32 families were documented from District Bagh. Maximum plant species were herbs (24 spp.; 45.09%) followed by shrubs (14 spp.; 27.45%) trees (12 spp.; 23.52%) and climber

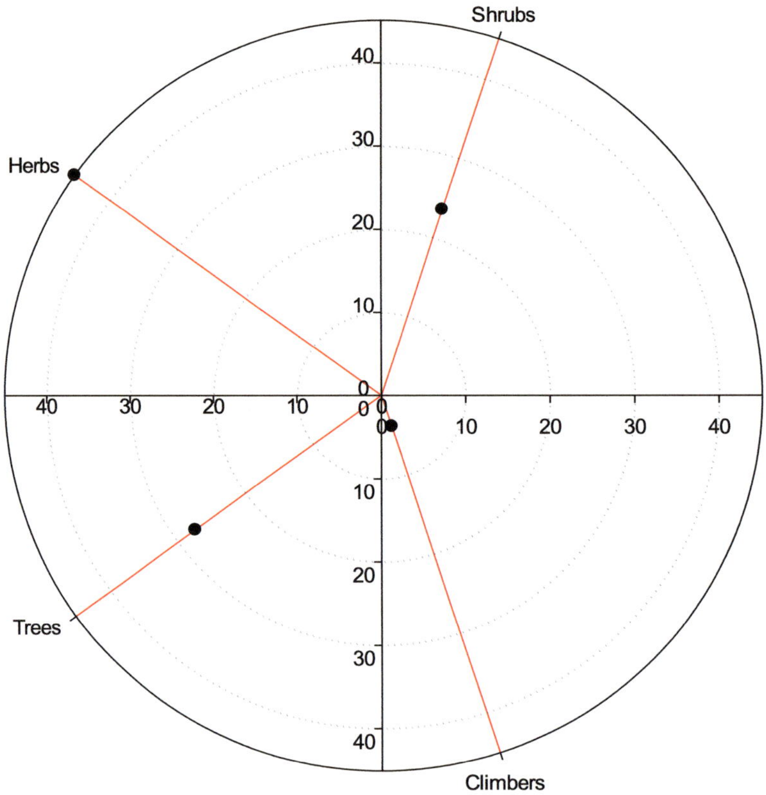

Figure 2.
Life form distribution of wild edible plants.

(2 spp.; 3.92%) (**Figure 2**). The dominance of herbaceous flora is due to location of study area in dense forest at higher altitude where there is high rainfall and moisture content.

Legumenaceae is a dominant family in the area having 6 species followed by Rosaceae (5 spp.) and Moraceae (4 spp.) (**Figure 3**). The dominance of these families in the study area might because the habitat and environmental conditions of the area are favorable for the member of these families. The local inhabitants of the area had great familiarity to the member of these families. The presence of high amount of active ingredients in its members might be another reason for their dominance. Previous reports from other areas of Pakistan and world support our findings [7, 27, 28].

3.2.1 Plants parts used

Local inhabitant of study area used various plants part to prepare different herbal recipes. Leaves were most frequently used plant part (64.7%) for herbal preparation followed by whole plants (5.88%) root (9.8), fruit (27.4), seed (19.6), flowers (7.8) bark (11.7%) bulb (3.92%) bark gal (1.96%)and petals (1.96%) as shown in (**Figure 4**). The high efficacy of leaves in phytotherapy might be due to presence of extractable crude drugs, phytochemicals and many other mixtures. This studies conducted with different regions of Pakistan Bano et al. and Ahmad et al.

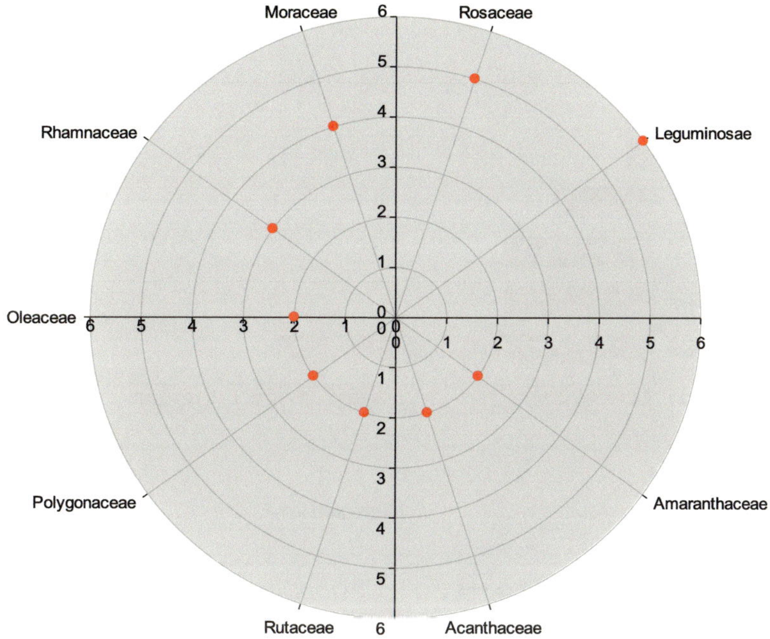

Figure 3.
Top ranked families of wild edible plant species.

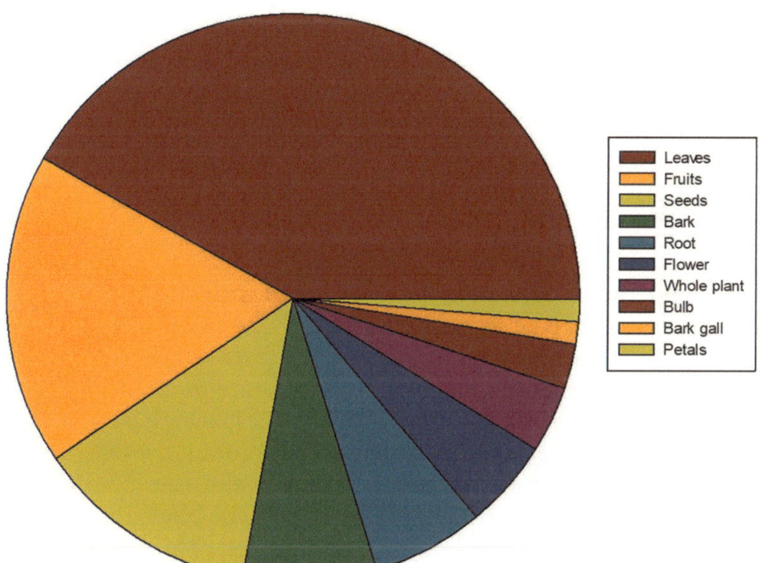

Figure 4.
Plant used in prepation of herbal recipes.

3.2.2 Mode of consumption

Wild edible plants were consumed in different ways by local inhbatiant to cure various ailments. Maximum species (species; 41.1%) were used in cooked form, followed by raw (15 species; 29.4), extract (6 species; 11.7%), soup (6 species; 11.7%)

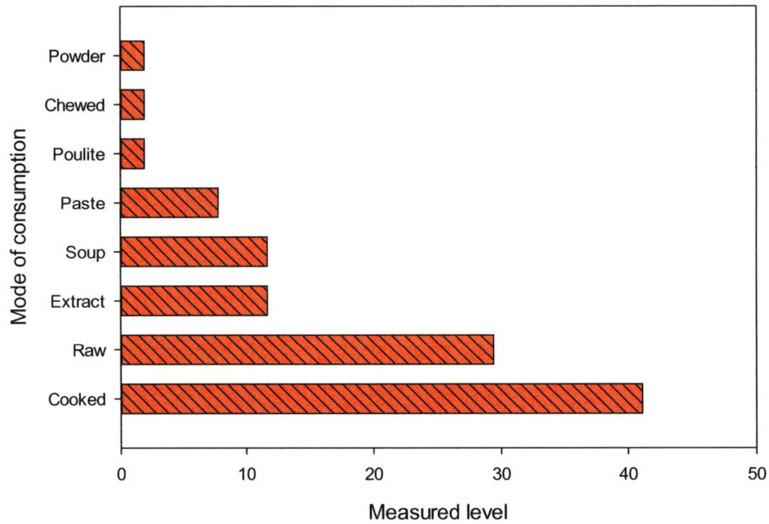

Figure 5.
Mode of consumption of wild edible plant species.

paste (4 species; 7.8%), powder (1 species; 1.9%) chewed (1 species; 1.9%) and poulite (1 species; 1.9) as shown in (**Figure 5**). Our findings are supported by previous documentation [7, 29–31]). Cooking and eating raw snakes are common practice in food anthropoglogy as descibed in various previous reports. The specific parts of wild edible plants are diectly cooked as a vegetable by mixing with water, soup and milk friuts are eat in raw form. Paste and poulite are apply on skin for various diseases treatment like scabies, skin worms.

3.2.3 Quantitative etnobotanical indices

3.2.3.1 Use value (UV)

The relative importance of plant species associated with the use of particular species reported by the informants is reflected by use value. The use value of document species ranges from 0.1 to 1. The maximum UV values was reported for *Berberis lycium Royle* (1) and *Morus nigra* (1). Other species with high use value are *Melia azedarach* (0.9), *Ficus palmata* (0.9) and *Dryopertis racemose* (0.8) (**Table 2**). The high usage of the reported species indicates a strong association and dependence of local communities on surrounding flora, specifically for the treatment of various diseases [32]. Moreover, the plant species which are used excessively are assumed to be biologically more active; therefore, these should be subjected to phytochemical and pharmacological screening to increase sustainable utilization and conservation of plant resources [33].

3.2.3.2 Relative importance (RI)

Relative importance reflect diversity of particular species for curing various ailments in area. The relative importance of the documented species ranges between 12.14 and 90.00. The highest RI value was calculated for *Urginea indica* (90.00) followed by *Elaeagnus umbellata* (77.86), *Pimpinella diversifolia* (73.57) and *Oxalis corniculata* (68.57) [34] (**Table 2**). The speies having high relative importance are

Sr. no.	Botanical name/Voucher number	UI	UV	FC	RFC	PH	BS	Rel PH	Rel BS	RI
1.	*Berberis lycium*	80	1	68	0.9	4	3	0.4	0.43	21.43
2.	*Ficus carica*	60	0.75	50	0.6	1	2	0.1	0.29	14.29
3.	*Olea ferruginea*	52	0.65	32	0.4	7	3	0.7	0.43	21.43
4.	*Oxalis corniculata*	44	0.55	22	0.2	6	4	0.6	0.57	28.57
5.	*Phyllanthus emblica*	32	0.4	20	0.2	2	3	0.2	0.43	21.43
6.	*Pimpinella diversifolia*	64	0.8	54	0.6	3	3	0.3	0.43	21.43
7.	*Pistacia chinensis*	12	0.15	6	0.1	7	2	0.7	0.29	14.29
8.	*Rosa abietina*	36	0.45	28	0.3	2	1	0.2	0.14	7.14
9.	*Rumex hastatus*	56	0.7	16	0.2	3	2	0.3	0.29	14.29
10.	*Solanum americanum*	40	0.5	20	0.2	2	5	0.2	0.71	35.71
11.	*Zanthoxylum armatum*	60	0.75	44	0.5	2	3	0.2	0.43	21.43
12.	*Ziziphus nummularia*	20	0.25	34	0.4	5	2	0.5	0.29	14.29
13.	*Ziziphus oxyphylla*	30	0.35	56	0.7	2	3	0.2	0.43	21.43
14.	*Rumex dentatus*	30	0.35	70	0.8	1	2	0.1	0.29	14.29
15.	*Taraxacum officinale F.H.Wigg./SS-15*	34	0.43	60	0.7	1	5	0.1	0.71	35.71
16.	*Dryopertis racemose*	71	0.88	67	0.8	5	2	0.5	0.29	14.29
17.	*Lathyrus aphaca*	66	0.82	50	0.6	1	5	0.1	0.71	35.71
18.	*Portulaca quadrifida*	46	0.58	23	0.2	4	2	0.4	0.29	14.29
19.	*Trigonella gracilis*	22	0.28	45	0.5	2	4	0.2	0.57	28.57
20.	*Vicia faba*	42	0.53	54	0.6	2	4	0.2	0.57	28.57
21.	*Pinus roxburghi*	68	0.85	67	0.8	10	3	1	0.43	21.43
22.	*Punica granatum*	26	0.33	54	0.6	6	4	0.6	0.57	28.57
23.	*Melia azedarach*	75	0.94	77	0.9	4	6	0.4	0.86	42.86
24.	*Morus alba*	66	0.83	53	0.6	3	7	0.3	1.00	50.00
25.	*Morus nigra*	80	1	78	0.9	4	5	0.4	0.71	35.71
26.	*Ficus palmata*	79	0.99	64	0.8	2	6	0.2	0.86	42.86
27.	*Urginea indica*	74	0.93	56	0.7	6	3	0.6	0.43	21.43
28.	*Rubus fruticocus*	56	0.7	45	0.5	8	2	0.8	0.29	14.29
29.	*Artemisia maritima*	48	0.6	58	0.7	2	2	0.2	0.29	14.29
30.	*Allium sativum*	63	0.79	46	0.5	5	1	0.5	0.14	7.14
31.	*Rosa rubiginosa*	61	0.76	58	0.7	3	3	0.3	0.43	21.43
32.	*Asystasia gangetica T.Anderson/SS-32*	79	0.99	21	0.2	11	1	1.1	0.14	7.14
33.	*Elaeagnus umbellata*	72	0.9	48	0.6	4	2	0.4	0.29	14.29
34.	*Robinia pseudoacacia*	65	0.81	33	0.4	5	3	0.5	0.43	21.43
35.	*Amaranthus caudatus*	50	0.63	25	0.3	8	2	0.8	0.29	14.29
36.	*Amaranthus viridis*	45	0.56	20	0.2	5	1	0.5	0.14	7.14
37.	*Urtica dioica*	49	0.61	54	0.6	3	3	0.3	0.43	21.43
38.	*Quercus incana*	33	0.41	49	0.6	2	2	0.2	0.29	14.29

Sr. no.	Botanical name/Voucher number	UI	UV	FC	RFC	PH	BS	Rel PH	Rel BS	RI
39.	*Diospyros lotus*	53	0.66	28	0.3	4	4	0.4	0.57	28.57
40.	*Zanthoxylum alatum*	23	0.29	70	0.8	5	3	0.5	0.43	21.43
41.	*Nasturtium officinale*	36	0.45	30	0.3	4	5	0.4	0.71	35.71
42.	*Canabis sativa*	67	0.84	56	0.7	4	1	0.4	0.14	7.14
43.	*Justicia adhatoda*	12	0.15	14	0.1	8	3	0.8	0.43	21.43
44.	*Capsella bursa-pastoris Medik./SS-44*	27	0.34	36	0.4	6	2	0.6	0.29	14.29
45.	*Melilotus albus*	39	0.49	21	0.4	6	1	0.6	0.14	7.14
46.	*Veronica arvensis*	40	0.5	13	0.1	2	3	0.2	0.43	21.43
47.	*Vicia sativa*	21	0.26	19	0.2	2	2	0.2	0.29	14.29
48.	*Medicago polymorpha*	37	0.46	20	0.2	1	1	0.1	0.14	7.14
49.	*Duchesnea indica*	26	0.33	60	0.7	1	6	0.1	0.86	42.86
50.	*Ziziphus sativa*	13	0.16	50	0.6	3	2	0.3	0.29	14.29
51.	*Prunus domestica*	37	0.46	34	0.4	1	3	0.1	0.43	21.43

Key: UV, use value; Ui, the number of uses that account for each species through every number of informants; FC, frequency of citation; RFC, relative frequency of citation; PH, relative number of pharmacological properties attributed to a single plant, BS, Number of body systems treated by a single species; Rel, relative number; RI, relative importance.

Table 2.
Quantitative ethnomedicinal data of wild edible plants.

used in excess by the native and have strong pharmacological potential [2] and their significance increases when used for curing number of ailments [35].

3.2.4 Informant consensus factor

The consensus of informants on wild edible plants to cure various diseases was determined by using ICF. To develop this consensus, all the treated aliments are categorized into 10 diseases groups. The value of ICF varied between 0.4 and 0.94. (**Figure 6**). The highest value of ICF (0.94) is digestive system and liver disease categoreis. The most frequently used plants for this category are *Berberis lycium*, *Dryopertis racemose*, *Ziziphus oxyphylla*, *Melia azedarach*, *Ficus palmata*, *Allium sativum*, *Zanthoxylum alatum*, *Medicago polymorpha*, *Ziziphus sativa*, *Prunus domestica*, *Taraxacum officinale*, *Rubus fruticocus*, *Amarantus caudatus*, *Elaeagnus umbellata*, *Morus nigra*. Previous reports from other study area also reflect high ICF for this disease category [2, 36–38]. The prevalance of diestive system disorder might be due to unavilabilty o clean drinking water and poor hygenic condition in the area. The secound highest ICF value was recorded for skin diseases.

3.2.5 Fidelity level

The fidelity level of wild edible plants species for curing different ailments in the study area varies between 30 and 100%. The fidelity level of only *Berberis lycium* was found 100 FL% which was used for the treatment of various diseases like diabetes, jaundice, diarrhea and stomach treatment. It was followed by *Rubus fruticocus* (83.3%) used to cure sore thorat, *Ziziphus oxyphylla* (83.3%) used to cure Jaundice and *Rumex dentatus* (80%) used to cure jaundice. Other species with high FL value are *Urginea*

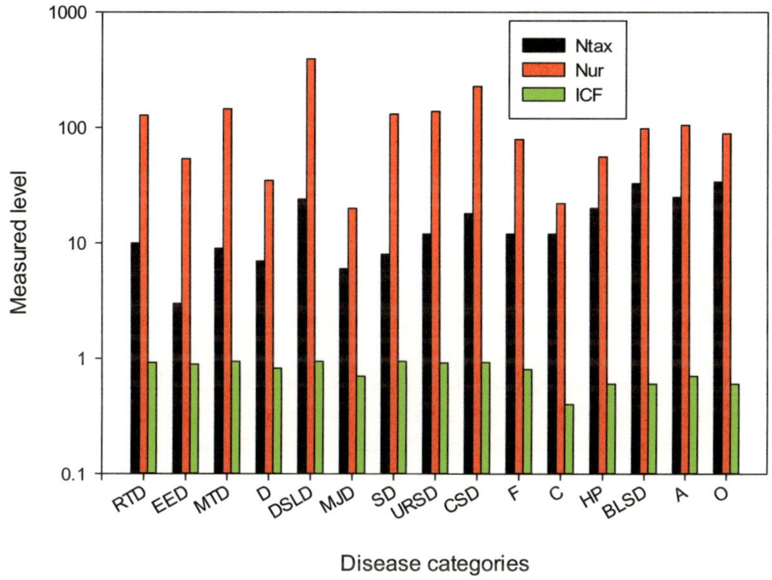

Figure 6.
Diseases categories treated by wild edible plant species in District Bagh. Key: RST, respiratory system diseases; EED, eye and ear diseases; MTD, mouth throat diseases; D, diabetes; DSLD, digestive system and liver diseases; MJD, muscular and joint diseases; SD, skin diseases; URSD, urinary and reproductive system diseases; CSD, circulatory system diseases; F, fever; C, cancer; HP, hair problems; BLSD, blood and lymphatic system diseases; A, antidote; O, others.

indica (76.7%), *Artemisia maritima* (76.5%), *Ziziphus nummularia* (76.0%), *Rosa abietina* (75%) and *Trigonella gracilis* (75%) (**Figure 7**). These spp. are mostly use to cure the digestive respiratory skin diseases like cold, dyscentery, diarrhea, fever and ulcer. Some other reserachers also recoded high fidelity level of these species in their

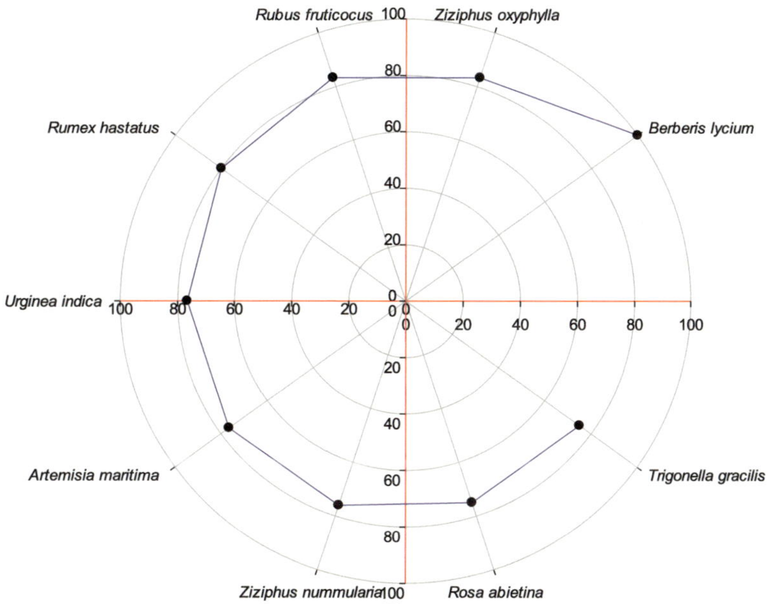

Figure 7.
Top ranked species with high fidelity level of wild edible plants.

investigated area [39]. These results reflect the dominance of particular disease in the investigated area, which are cured by using medicinal plant species with high fidelity level [7, 40]. The species with high FL are highly used in the investigated area as compared to the species with low FL value. The species having low FL values are not most important by the native of the study area [36]. The species with high FL value should be subject to further phytochemical and pharmacological investigation to validate the traditional knowledge.

4. Conclusion

The present study revealed that the rural communities of District Baghs still use wild edible plants for medicne, food and other purposes. But this indigenous knowledge on plant usage is disappearing rapidly due to moderanization, which should be conserved before it extinct. Ther use pattren of wild edible plants mainly infulenced by socio ecnomic factor instead of climatic factors. Study of the results showed that in the study area, most of the wild edible plants are used by poor families during difficult and normal time. However ther is rapid decline in use of several species which may lead to the extinction of this tradiational knowledge. The citation and use reports of wild vegetables verified that cultural heritage and cultural worth regarding collection of wild edible palnts is analogue because most of cited species are same. The majority of the plants were employed to treat digestive system and liver disorders, skin diseasess and respiratory tract diseases. The plant species with high RFC, UV, RI and FL should be subjecte to further pharmacological and phytochemical studies to verify this tradiational knowledge which can be used in future for novel drugh development. The current study also revlead that wild edible plants species are under high anthorpogenic pressure and need immidate conservation thorugh community base management, public awaness and germplasm collection. Besides, The conribution of ethnic communities for diversification of medicine and food sources should be recognize at the national and international level. There is dire need for reappraisal of tradiational knowledge on wilde edible palnts which not only conserve this tradiational heritage but may also contribute in furture drug discovery.

Appendix

Pictures of wild edible plants reported from study area.

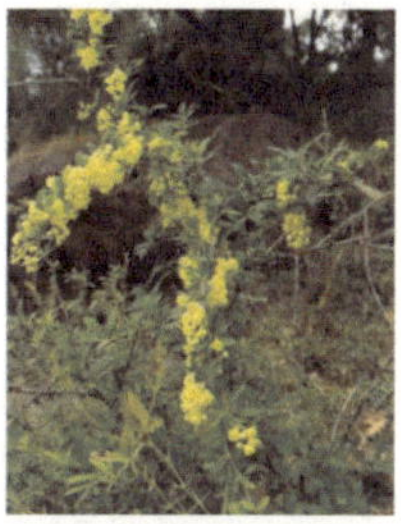

Berberis lycium

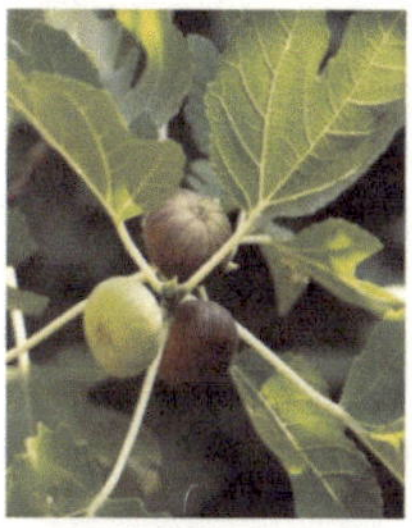

Ficus carica

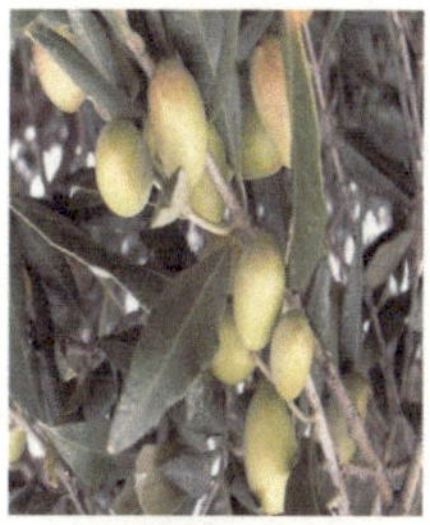

Olea ferruginea

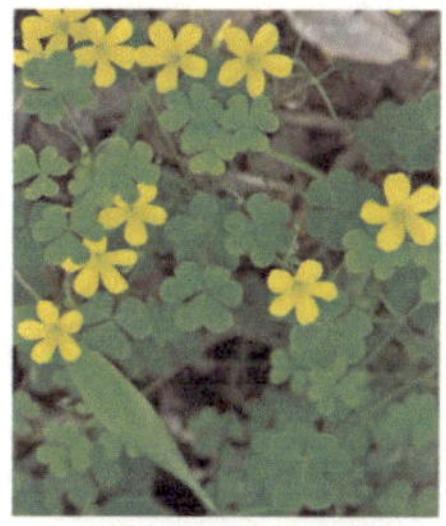

Oxalis corniculata

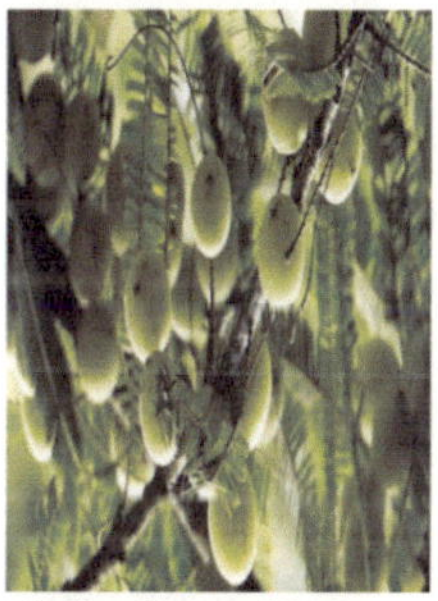

Phyllanthus emblica

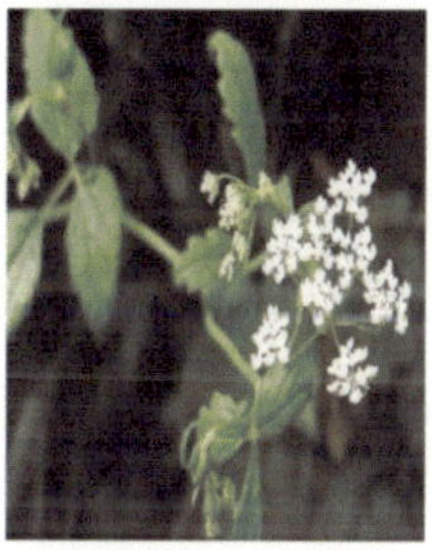

Pimpinella diversifolia

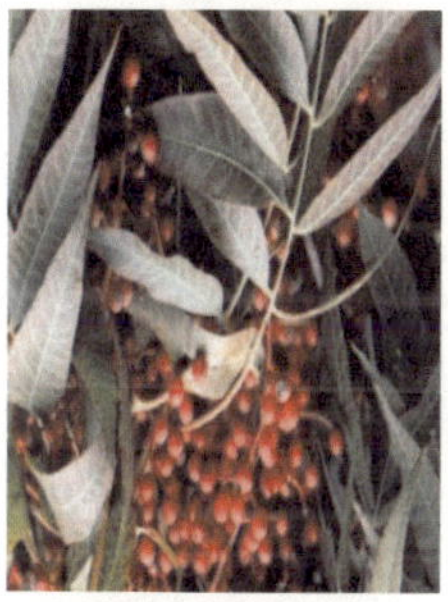

Pistacia chinensis

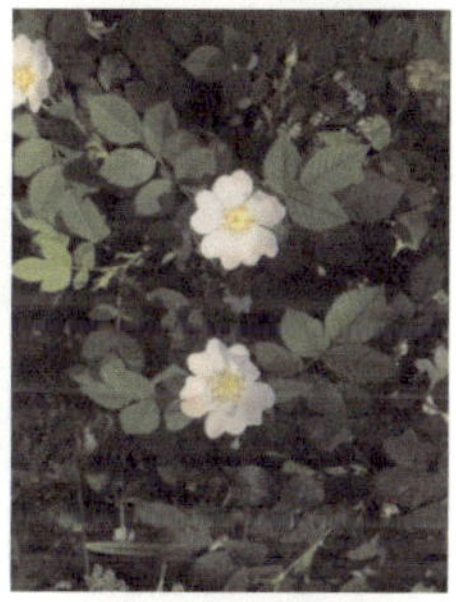

Rosa abietina

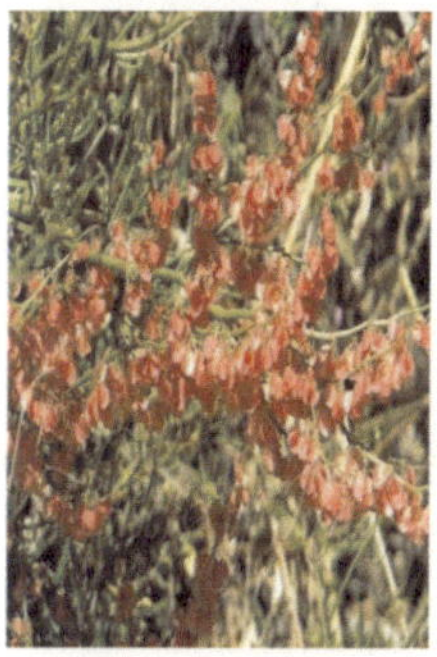

Rumex hastatus

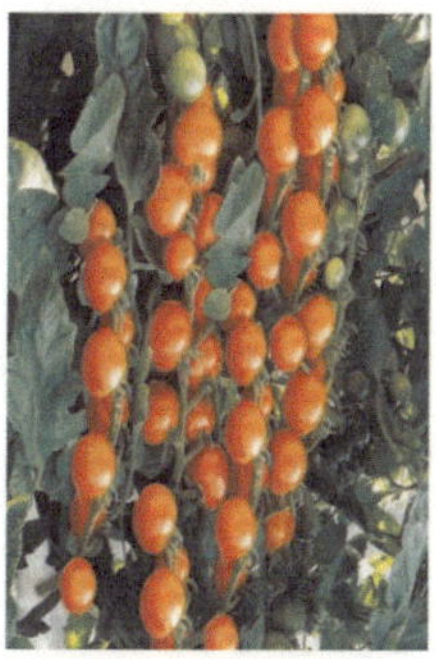

Solanum americanum

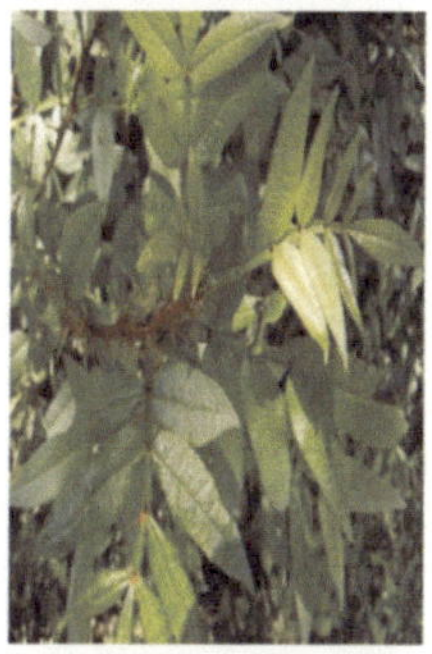

Zanthoxylum armatum

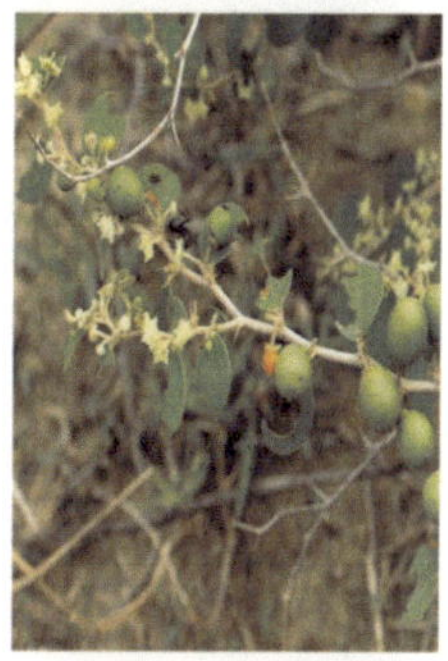

Ziziphus nummularia

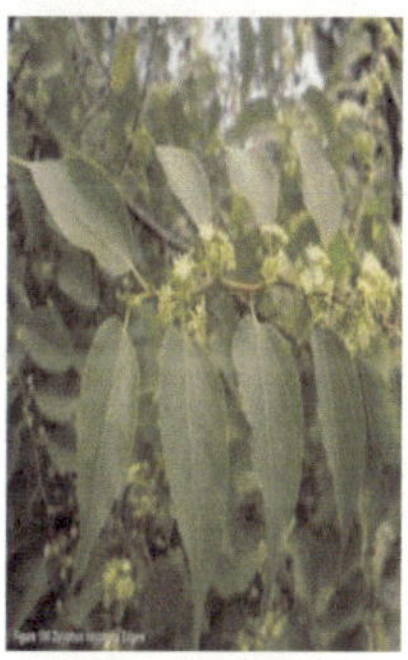

Ziziphus oxyphylla

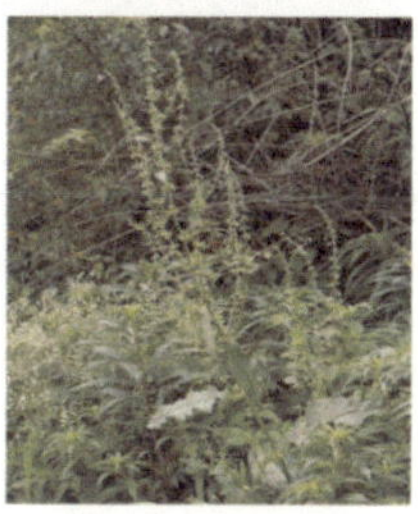

Rumex dentatus

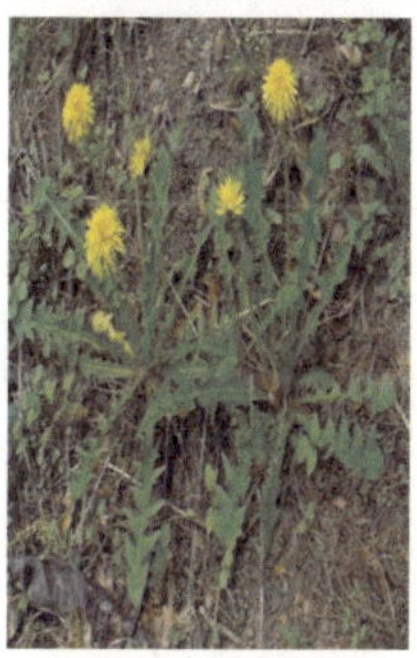

Taraxacum officinale

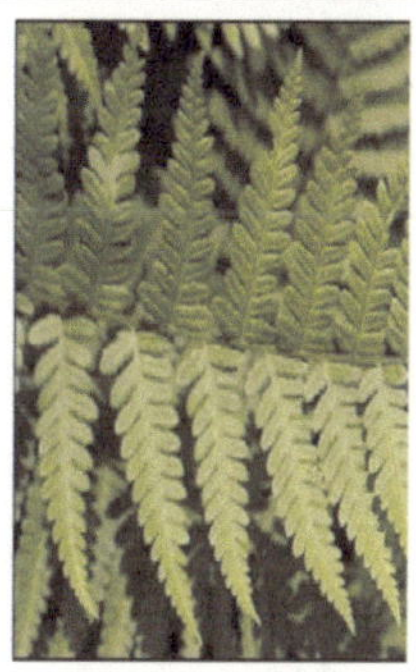

Dryopertis racemose

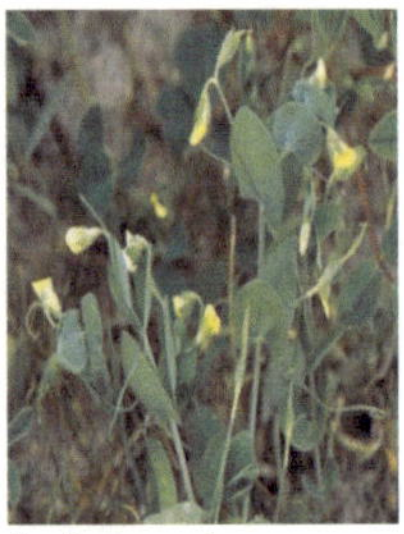
Lathyrus aphaca

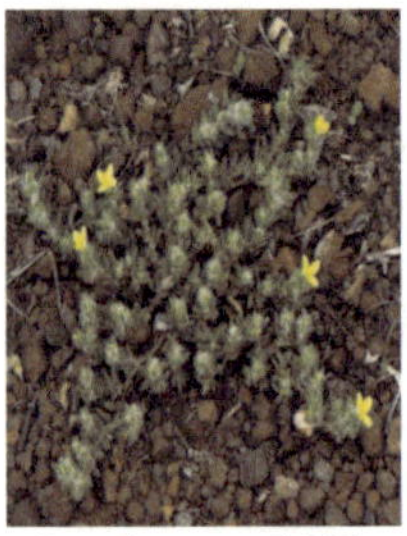
Portulaca quadrifida

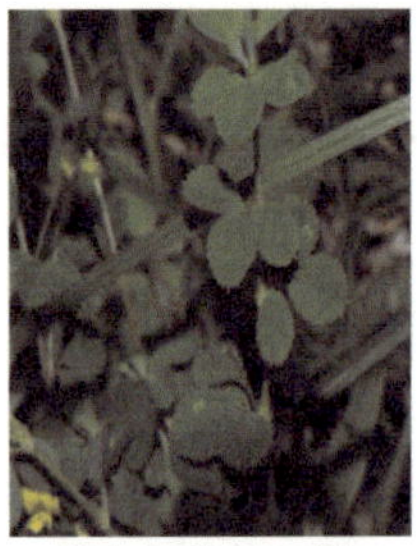
Trigonella gracilis

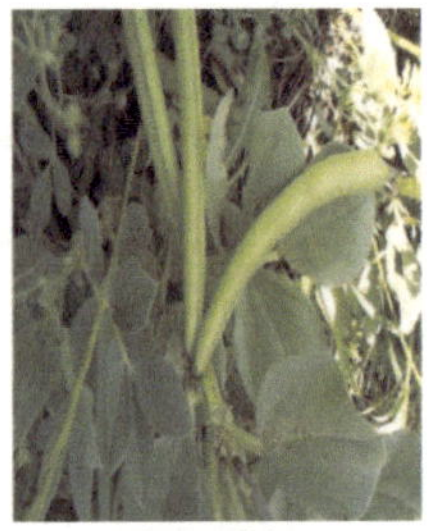
Vicia faba

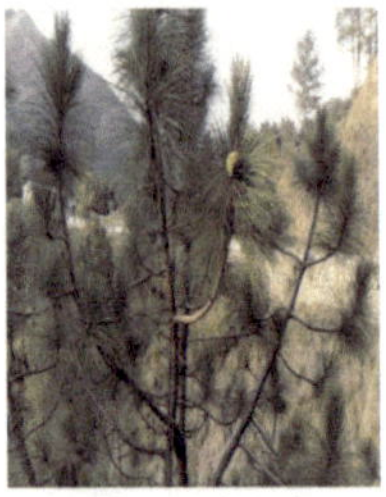
pinus roxburghi

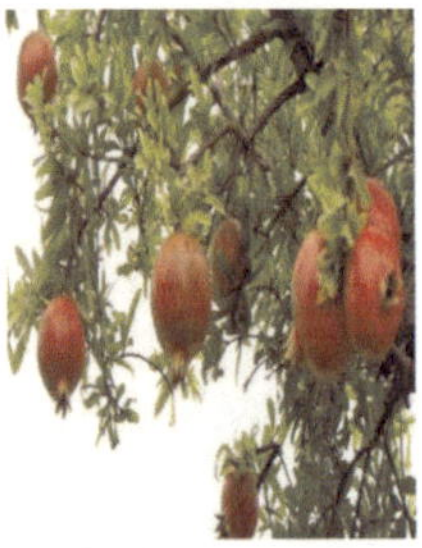
Punica granatum

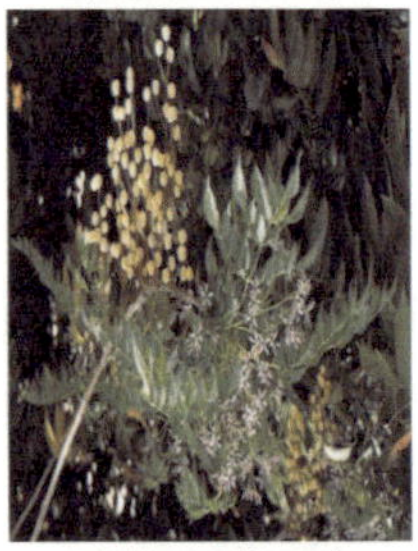
Melia azedarach

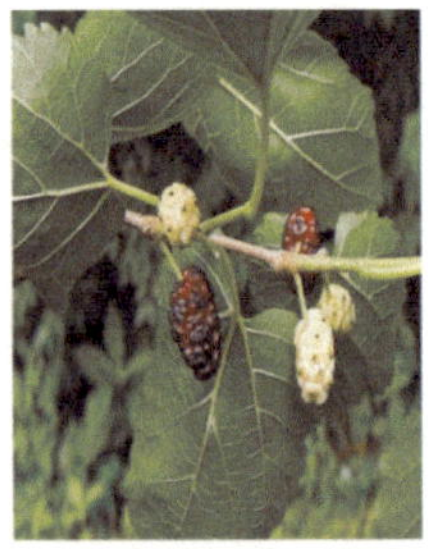
Morus alba

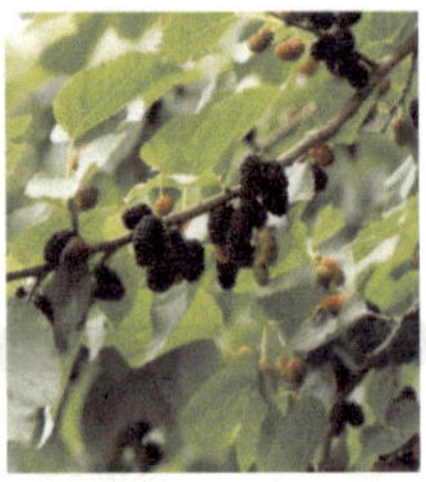
Morus nigra

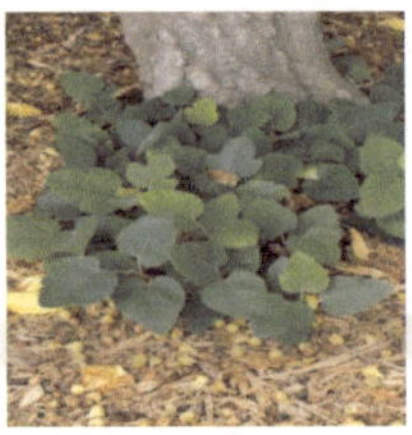
Ficus palmata

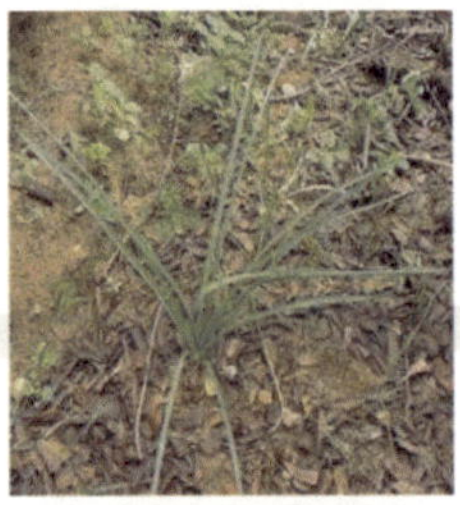
Urginea indica

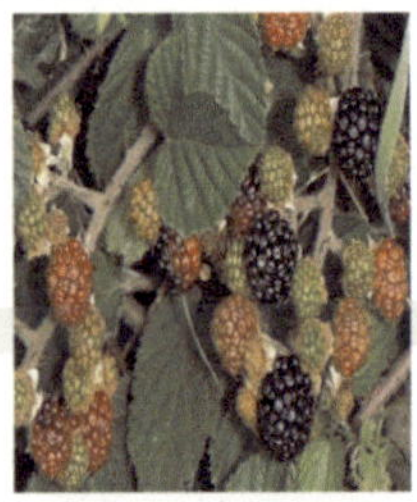
Rubus fruticocus

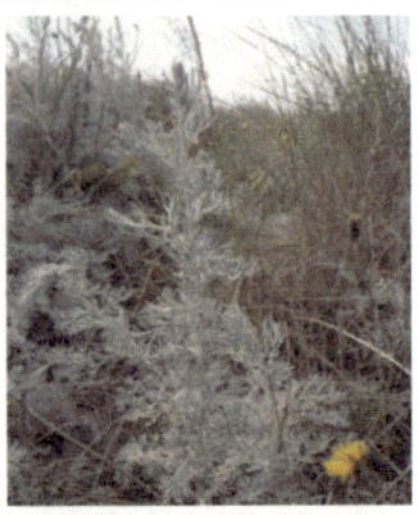
Artemisia maritima

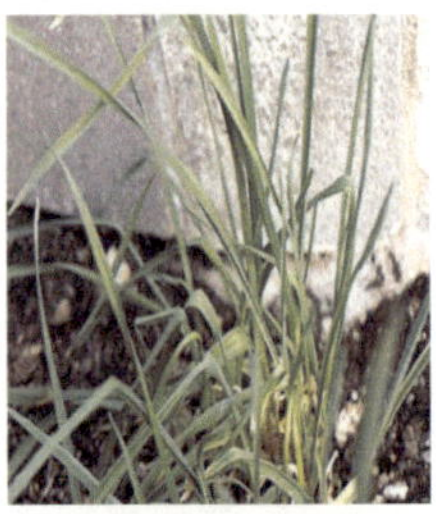
Allium sativum

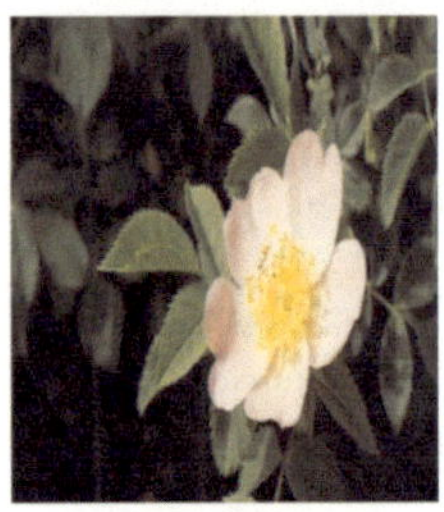
Rosa rubiginosa

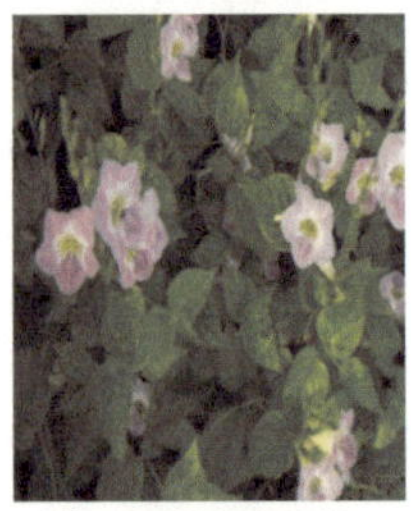
Asystasia gangetica

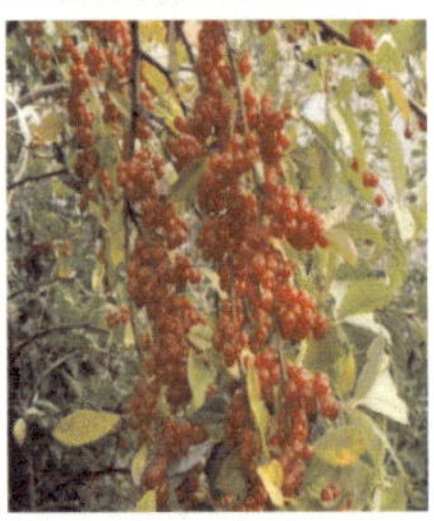
Elaeagnus umbellata

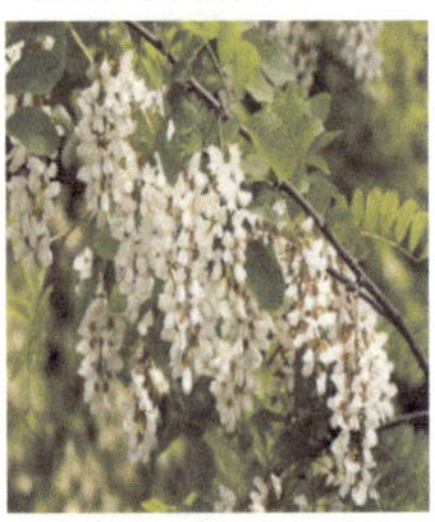
Robinia pseudoacacia

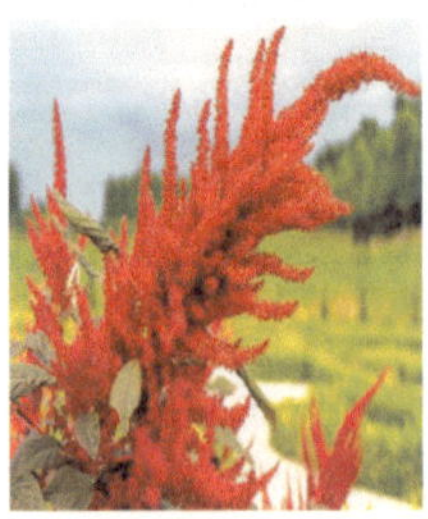
Amaranthus caudatus

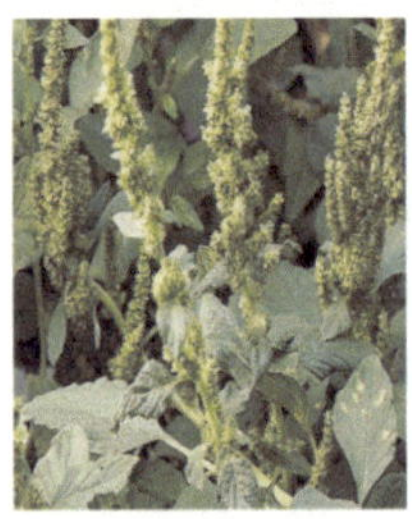
Amaranthus viridis

DOI: http://dx.doi.org/10.5772/intechopen.104492

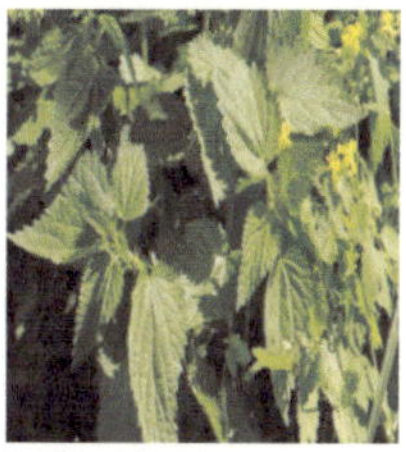

Urtica dioica

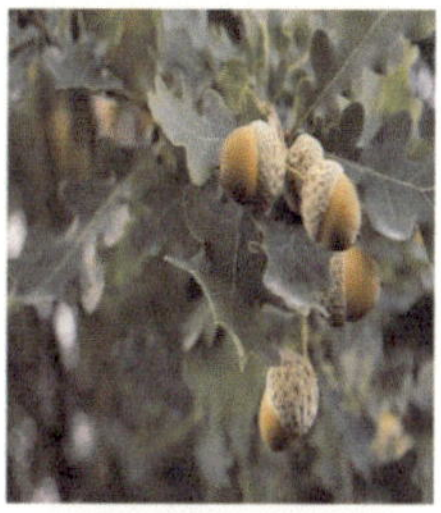

Quercus incana

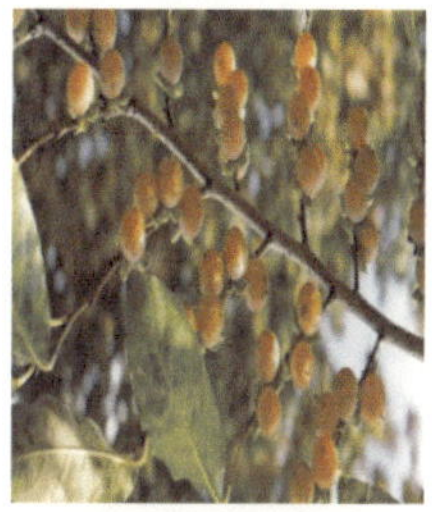

Diospyros lotus

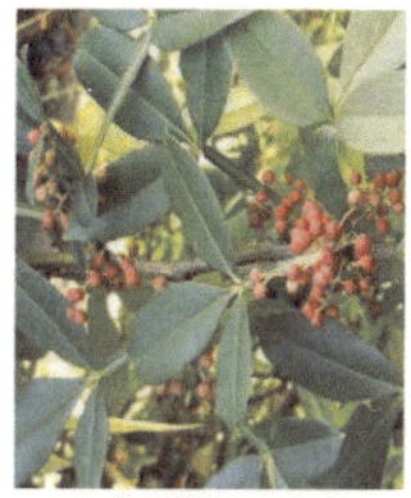

Zanthoxylum alatum

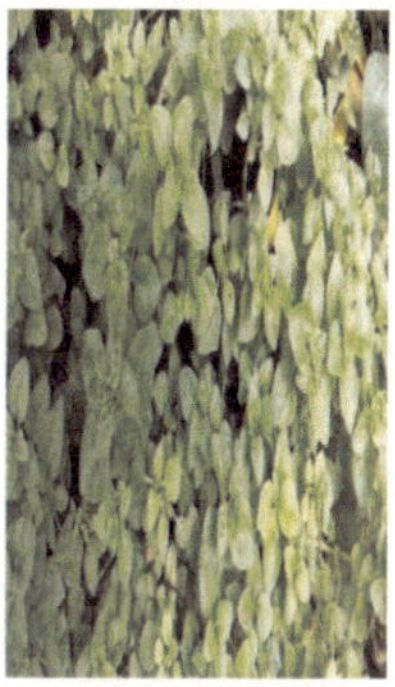

Nasturtium officinale

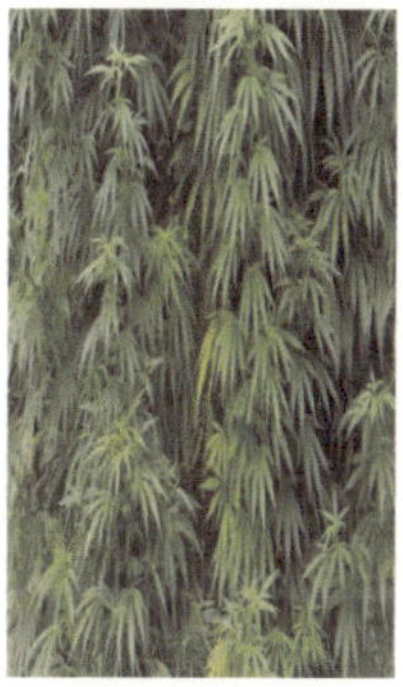

Canabis sativa

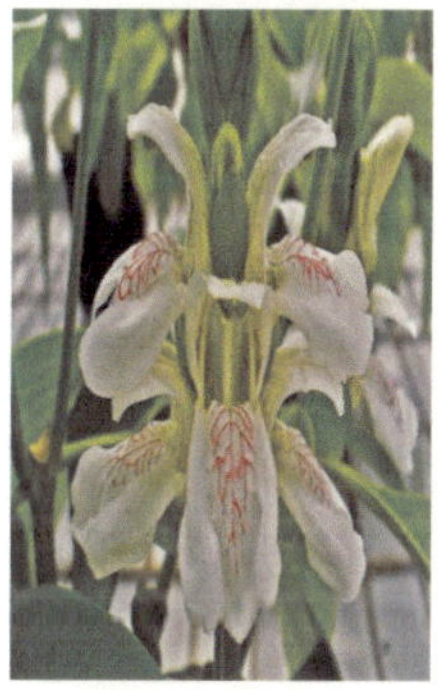

Justicia adhatoda

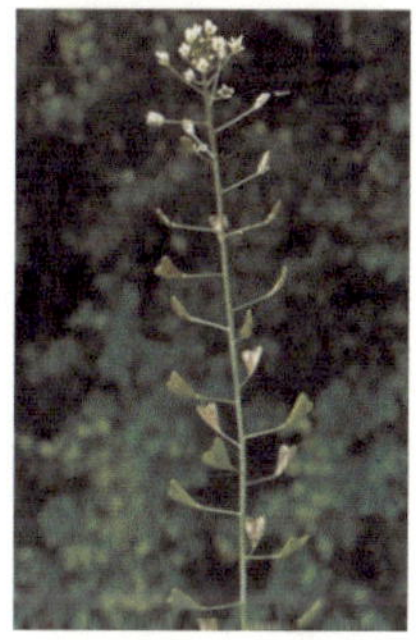

Capsella bursa-pastoris

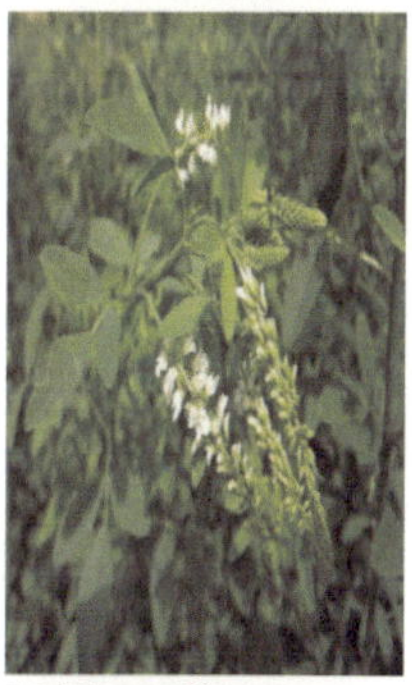

Melilotus albus

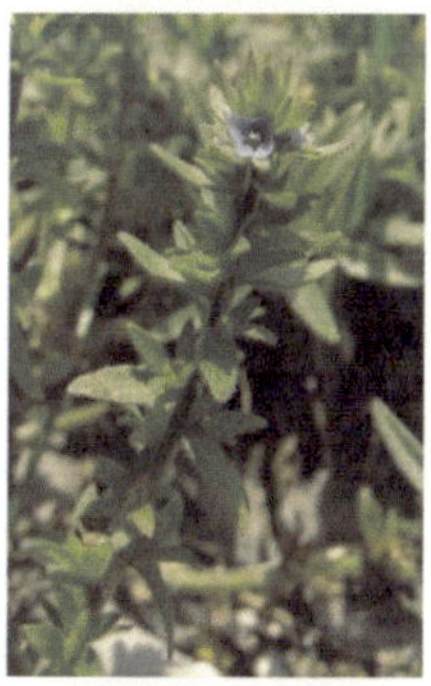

Veronica arvensis

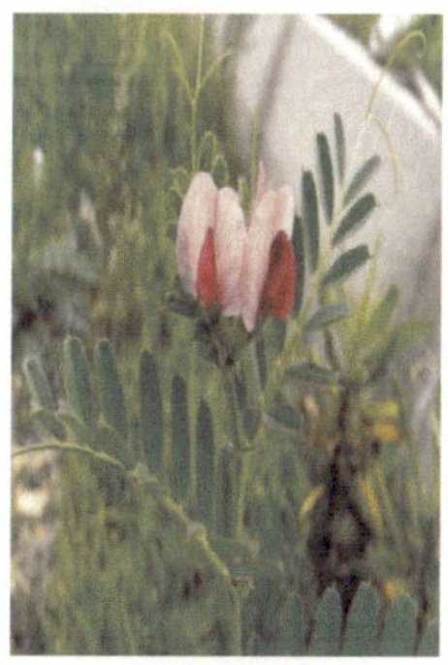

Vicia sativa

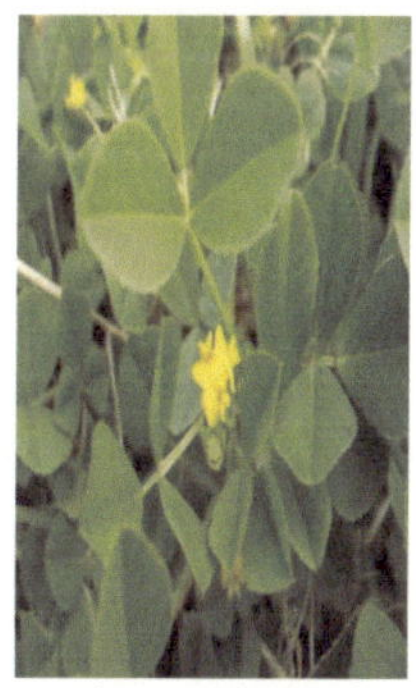

Medicago polymorpha

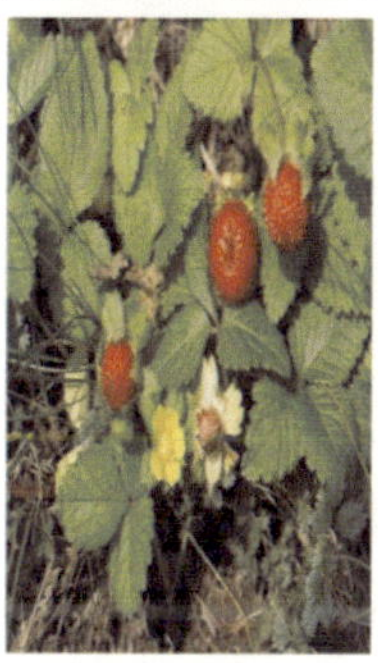

Duchesnea indica

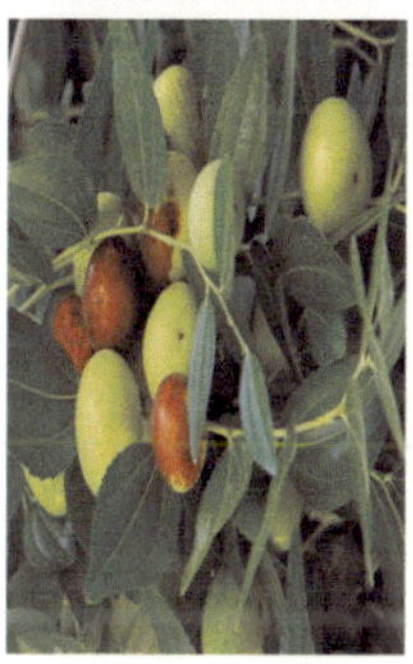

Ziziphus sativa

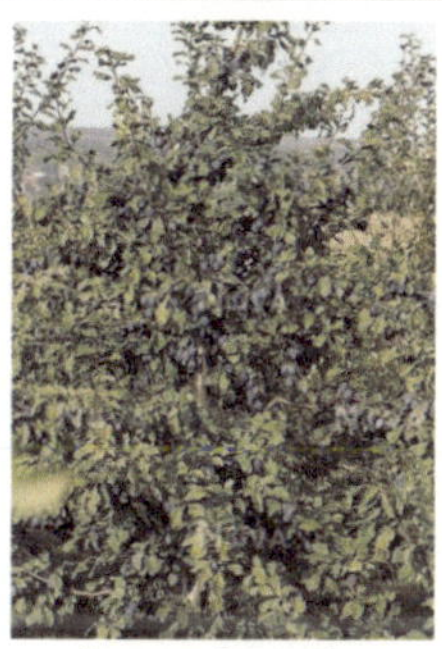

Prunus domestica

Ethnomedicinal uses of wild edible plants of District Bagh.

Sr no.	Botanical name/ voucher number	Vernacular name	Family	Habitat	Part used	Mode of consumption	Mode of administration	Diseases treatment
1.	*Berberis lycium* Royle/ SS-01	Sumbal	Berberdaceae	Shrub	Root	Extract	Internal	Jaundice
					Bark	Powder		Diabetes, stomach disorder
					Leaves	Raw		Diarrhea
2.	*Ficus carica* L./SS-02	Jangli ingeer	Moraceae	Tree	Leaves	Cooked	External	Throat
3.	*Olea ferruginea* Wall.ex Aitch/SS-03	Kao	Oleaceae	Tree	Seed	Extract	Internal	Toothache, Stomach disorder, diarrhea, heart diseases, High cholesterol, high blood pressure
4.	*Oxalis corniculata* L./SS-04	Khatti booti	Oxalidaceae	Herb	Leaves	Cooked	Internal	Influenza, fever
					Seed	Cooked	Internal	urinary tract infection, wash to rid children hookworms
					Bark	Paste	External	Insect bites
5.	*Phyllanthus emblica* L./ SS-05	Amala	Phyllanthaceae	Tree	Seed	Extract	External	Hair care, skin care
6.	*Pimpinella diversifolia* DC./SS-06	Sonf	Apiaceae	Herb	Seed	Soup	Internal	Respiratory tract diseases, urinary tract infection, kidney stone
7.	*Pistacia chinensis* Bunge/SS-07	Karkatshringi	Anacardiaceae	Tree	Fruit	Soup	Internal	Cough, asthma, dysentery, liver, disorders, snake bite
8.	*Rosa abietina* Gren. ex H. Christ/SS-08	Jangli gulab	Rosaceae	Shrub	Leaf	Extract	Internal	Blood purifier, wound healing
9.	*Rumex hastatus* D. Don/SS-09	Chukhare	Polygonaceae	Shrub	Fruit	Soup	Internal	Asthma, cough
					Root			Fever
10.	*Solanum americanum* Mill./SS10	Kachmach	Solanaceae	Herb	Whole plant	Paste	External	Scabies, skin worms
11.	*Zanthoxylum armatum* DC./SS-11	Timber	Rutaceae	Shrub	Leaves	Paste	Internal	Asthma
					Seed		External	Toothaches
12.	*Ziziphus nummularia* (Burm.f.) Wight & Arn./SS-12	Karken ber	Rhamnaceae	Shrub	Leaves	Soup	Internal	Cold, dysentery
					Seed			Diarrhea, Fever
					Bark			Ulcer
13.	*Ziziphus oxyphylla* Edgew./SS-13	Phitni	Rhamnaceae	Shrub	Fruit	Raw	Internal	Diabetes, jaundice

Sr no.	Botanical name/ voucher number	Vernacular name	Family	Habitat	Part used	Mode of consumption	Mode of administration	Diseases treatment
14.	*Rumex dentatus* L./ SS-14	Jungli palak, Hula	Polygonaceae	Herb	Fruit, Root	Cooked	External	Skin diseases
15.	*Taraxacum officinale* (L.) Weber ex F. H.Wigg./SS-15	Haund	Asteraceae	Herb	Leaves	Cooked	Internal	Diabetes
16.	*Dryopertis racemose*/SS-16	Kunji	Dryopteridaceae	Herb	Leaves	Cooked	Internal	Diarrhea, headache, heart diseases, respiratory disorder, uterus disorders
17.	*Lathyrus aphaca* L./ SS-17	Jungli matter	Leguminosae	Climber	Seed	Cooked	Internal	Toothache
18.	*Portulaca quadrifida* L./33-18	—	Portulacaceae	Herb	Whole plant	Extract	Internal	Diuretic, fever, urinary disorders, dysentery
19.	*Trigonella gracilis* Benth./SS-19	Not Known	Leguminosae	Herb	Leaves	Cooked	Internal	diabetes, decreasing blood, cholesterol.
20.	*Vicia faba* L./ SS-20	Faba bean	Leguminosae	Tree	Flowers	Cooked	Internal & External	Diuretic, removal of wards
21.	*pinus roxburghi*/ SS-21	Cheer	Pinaceace	Tree	Fruit	Poultice	External	TB
					Resin			Wound healing
22.	*Punica granatum* L./SS-22	Daru	Lythraceae	Shrub	Fruit	Raw	Internal	Sore throats, coughs, urinary infection, digestive disorders
							External	Skin disorder
23.	*Melia azedarach* L./SS-23	Darkh	Meliaceae	Tree	Fruit	Soup	Internal	Malarial fever, purify blood, diabetes
						Raw		Gas trouble
24.	*Morus alba* L./SS-24	Shatoot	Moraceae	Tree	Fruit	Raw	Internal	Dizziness, liver, kidney disorder
25.	*Morus nigra* L./SS-25	Khaa shattot	Moraceae	Tree	Fruit	Raw	Internal	Cough, bronchitis
					Leaves			Diuretic, Asthma
26.	*Ficus palmata* Forssk./SS-26	Pagwara	Moraceae	Tree	Fruits	Cooked	Internal	Constipation
					Leaves	Latex	External	Warts
27.	*Urginea indica* (Roxb.) Kunth/SS-27	Jungli piazz	Asparagaceae	Herb	Whole plant	Cooked	Internal	Diuretic, cough, asthma
28.	*Rubus fruticocus*/SS-28	Pahunay/ black berry	Rosaceae	Herb	Fruit	Raw	Internal	Anticancer, dysentery, diarrhea, whopping cough, toothache,

Sr no.	Botanical name/ voucher number	Vernacular name	Family	Habitat	Part used	Mode of consumption	Mode of administration	Diseases treatment
								sore throat, mouth ulcer, mouthwash
29.	*Artemisia maritima* L./SS-29	Chahu	Compositae	Herb	Leaves	Chewed	External	Toothache
						Cooked	Internal	Flavoring
30	*Allium* sativum L./SS-30	Jungli lashun	Amaryllidaceae	Herb	Whole plant	Cooked	Internal	Diabetes, fever, intestinal worms, dysentery, high blood pressure
31.	*Rosa rubiginosa*/ SS-31	Chal	Rosaceae	Shrub	Flowers	Cooked	Internal	Headaches, dizziness, blood purifier
32.	*Asystasia gangetica* (L.) T.Anderson/ SS-32	Aheer	Acanthaceae	Climber	Fruit	Extract	Internal	Hypertension, asthma, fever, epilepsy, stomach, heart pain, urethral discharge, nose bleeding, dry cough, irritated throat, chest infection
33.	*Elaeagnus umbellata* Thunb./SS-33	Kankoli	Elaeagnaceae	Shrub	Seed	Raw	Internal	Respiratory diseases, cough, pulmonary infection
34.	*Robinia pseudoacacia* L./SS-34	Kiker	Leguminosae	Tree	Fruit	Raw	Internal	Calms stomach, burns, eye aliment
35.	*Amaranthus caudatus* Linn./SS-35	Rata ganayar	Amaranthaceae	Herb	Leaves	Cooked	Internal	Eyes diseases, diuretic, diabetes, Malaria, ulcer,
					Seed			Diarrhea, swelling of the mouth, high cholesterol
36.	*Amaranthus viridis* L./SS-36	Chetta ganayar	Amaranthaceae	Herb	Leaves	Cooked	Internal	Ulcer, Throats, headaches, tumors
						Paste	External	Warts
37.	*Urtica dioica* L./SS-37	Kengi	Urticaceae	Herb	Leaves	Cooked	Internal	Diabetes, urinary, tract infection,
					Seed			Kidney stone
38.	*Quercus incana* Bartram/SS-38	Reeyun	Fagaceae	Tree	Leaves	Raw	Internal	Diuretic
					Seed			Diarrhea
39.	*Diospyros lotus* L./SS-39	Kala amlook	Ebenaceae	Tree	Fruit	Raw	Internal	Fever, diarrhea, constipation, dysentery
40.	*Zanthoxylum alatum*/ SS-40	Timber	Rutaceacae	Shrub	Fruit	Raw	Internal	Asthma, bronchitis, indigestion, diarrhea, cholera
41.	*Nasturtium officinale* R. Br./SS-41	Tara mera	Brassicaceae	Herb	Whole plant	Cooked	Internal	Urinary, tract infection, cough, bronchitis, muscular pain

Sr no.	Botanical name/ voucher number	Vernacular name	Family	Habitat	Part used	Mode of consumption	Mode of administration	Diseases treatment
42.	*Canabis sativa*/SS-42	Bang	Cannabaceae	Herb	Leaves	Extract	Internal	Control nausea, vomiting, Cancer, muscles spasms
43.	*Justicia adhatoda* L./SS-43	Bhikar	Acanthaceae	Herb	Leaves	Cooked	Internal	Bronchitis, asthma, TB, control bleeding from gums
					Flowers			Cough, diarrhea, dysentery, chest infection
44.	*Capsella bursa-pastoris* (L.) Medik./SS-44	Berg e bansa, bakar	Brassicaceae	Herb	Whole plant	Cooked	Internal	Nose bleeding, menstrual cycle, headache, heart problems, Diarrhea, urinary problems
45.	*Melilotus albus* Medik./SS-45	Sag	Leguminosae	Herb	Leaves	—	Internal	Inflammation joint pain, fever, cold, diuretic, wound healing
46.	*Veronica arvensis* L./SS-46	Honey colve	Plantaginaceae	Herb	Leaves	Cooked	Internal	Skin infection, blood purifier
47.	*Vicia sativa* L./SS-47	—	Leguminosae	Herb	Leaves	Cooked	Internal	Kidney pain, eye infection
48.	*Medicago polymorpha* L./SS-48	Jungli phali	Fabaceae	Shrub	Leaves& Fruit	Raw	Internal	Dysentery
49.	*Duchesnea indica* (Jacks.) Focke/SS-49	Sinjii	Rosaceae	Herb	Leaves	Cooked	External	Skin problems
50.	*Ziziphus sativa*/SS-50	Budi meva	Rhamnaceae	Herb	Fruit	Raw	Internal	Skin problems, liver disease, ulcer, weight loss
51.	*Prunus domestica* L./SS-51	Barr	Rosaceae	Shrub	Fruit	Raw	Internal	Constipation

Author details

Sadia Shabbir and Muhammad Shoaib Amjad*
Department of Botany, Women University of Azad Jammu & Kashmir, Bagh, Pakistan

*Address all correspondence to: malikshoaib1165@yahoo.com

References

[1] Ali H, Qaiser M. The ethnobotany of Chitral valley, Pakistan with particular reference to medicinal plants. Pakistan Journal of Botany. 2009;**41**(4):2009-2041

[2] Amjad MS, Qaeem MF, Ahmad I, Khan SU, Chaudhari SK, Zahid Malik N, et al. Descriptive study of plant resources in the context of the ethnomedicinal relevance of indigenous flora: A case study from Toli Peer National Park, Azad Jammu and Kashmir, Pakistan. PLoS One. 2017;**12**(2): e0171896

[3] Hussain W, Badshah L, Ullah M, Ali M, Ali A, Hussain F. Quantitative study of medicinal plants used by the communities residing in Koh-e-Safaid Range, northern Pakistani-Afghan borders. Journal of Ethnobiology and Ethnomedicine. 2018;**14**(1):1-18

[4] Campbell EA, Masuda S, Sun JL, Muzzin O, Olson CA, Wang S, et al. Crystal structure of the Bacillus stearothermophilus anti-σ factor SpoIIAB with the sporulation σ factor σF. Cell. 2002;**108**(6):795-807

[5] Asch DL, Asch NB. The economic potential of Iva annua and its prehistoric importance in the lower Illinois Valley. The Nature and Status of Ethnobotany. 1978:300-341

[6] Cox PA. Will tribal knowledge survive the millennium? Science. 2000; **287**(5450):44-45

[7] Bibi T, Ahmad M, Tareen RB, Tareen NM, Jabeen R, Rehman SU, et al. Ethnobotany of medicinal plants in district Mastung of Balochistan province-Pakistan. Journal of Ethnopharmacology. 2014;**157**: 79-89

[8] Heinrich M, Kufer J, Leonti M, Pardo-de-Santayana M. Ethnobotany and ethnopharmacology—Interdisciplinary links with the historical sciences. Journal of Ethnopharmacology. 2006;**107**(2): 157-160

[9] Kassaye KD, Amberbir A, Getachew B, Mussema Y. A historical overview of traditional medicine practices and policy in Ethiopia. Ethiopian Journal of Health Development. 2006;**20**(2):127-134

[10] Heywood V, Skoula M. The MEDUSA network: Conservation and sustainable use of wild plants of the Mediterranean region. In: Janick J, editor. Perspectives on New Crops and New Uses. Alexandria, VA: ASHS Press; 1999. pp. 148-151

[11] Alam MJ, Ahmed KS, Nahar MK, Akter S, Uddin MA. Effect of different sowing dates on the performance of maize. Journal of Krishi Vigyan. 2020; **8**(2):75-81

[12] Ladio AH, Lozada M. Patterns of use and knowledge of wild edible plants in distinct ecological environments: A case study of a Mapuche community from northwestern Patagonia. Biodiversity and Conservation. 2004;**13**(6):1153-1173

[13] Schaal B. Plants and people: Our shared history and future. Plants, People, Planet. 2019;**1**(1):14-19

[14] Grivetti LE, Ogle BM. Value of traditional foods in meeting macro-and micronutrient needs: The wild plant connection. Nutrition Research Reviews. 2000;**13**(1):31-46

[15] Abbasi AM, Khan MA, Zafar M. Ethno-medicinal assessment of some selected wild edible fruits and vegetables

of Lesser-Himalayas, Pakistan. Pakistan Journal of Botany. 2013;**45**(SI):215-222

[16] Abbasi AM, Khan MA, Shah MH, Shah MM, Pervez A, Ahmad M. Ethnobotanical appraisal and cultural values of medicinally important wild edible vegetables of Lesser Himalayas-Pakistan. Journal of Ethnobiology and Ethnomedicine. 2013;**9**(1):1-13

[17] Majeed M, Bhatti KH, Pieroni A, Sõukand R, Bussmann RW, Khan AM, et al. Gathered wild food plants among diverse religious groups in Jhelum District, Punjab, Pakistan. Foods. 2021; **10**(3):594

[18] Pimentel D, Nair MM, Buck L, Pimentel M, Kami J. The value of forests to world food security. Human Ecology. 1997;**25**:91-120

[19] Ansari D, Garcia N, Lucas E, Hamon K, Dhital B. Neural correlates of symbolic number processing in children and adults. Neuroreport. 2005;**16**(16): 1769-1773

[20] Ahmad K, Pieroni A. Folk knowledge of wild food plants among the tribal communities of Thakht-e-Sulaiman Hills, North-West Pakistan. Journal of Ethnobiology and Ethnomedicine. 2016;**12**(1):1-15

[21] Msuya TS, Kideghesho JR, Mosha TC. Availability, preference, and consumption of indigenous forest foods in the Eastern Arc Mountains, Tanzania. Ecology of Food and Nutrition. 2010; **49**(3):208-227

[22] Vijayakumar S, Yabesh JM, Prabhu S, Manikandan R, Muralidharan B. Quantitative ethnomedicinal study of plants used in the Nelliyampathy hills of Kerala, India. Journal of Ethnopharmacology. 2015;**161**: 238-254

[23] Khan MPZ, Ahmad M, Zafar M, Sultana S, Ali MI, Sun H. Ethnomedicinal uses of edible wild fruits (EWFs) in Swat Valley, Northern Pakistan. Journal of Ethnopharmacology. 2015;**173**:191-203

[24] Heinrich M, Ankli A, Frei B, Weimann C, Sticher O. Medicinal plants in Mexico: Healers' consensus and cultural importance. Social Science & Medicine. 1998;**47**(11):1859-1871

[25] Alexiades MN, Sheldon JW.. Selected guidelines for ethnobotanical research: A field manual (No. Sirsi i9780893274047). 1996

[26] Umair M, Altaf M, Abbasi AM. An ethnobotanical survey of indigenous medicinal plants in Hafizabad district, Punjab-Pakistan. PloS One. 2017;**12**(6): e0177912

[27] Arnold BC. Pareto Distribution. Wiley StatsRef: Statistics Reference Online; 2014. pp. 1-10

[28] Lulekal E, Asfaw Z, Kelbessa E, Van Damme P. Ethnomedicinal study of plants used for human ailments in Ankober District, North Shewa Zone, Amhara region, Ethiopia. Journal of Ethnobiology and Ethnomedicine. 2013; **9**(1):1-13

[29] Ahmad M, Sultana S, Fazl-i-Hadi S, Ben Hadda T, Rashid S, Zafar M, et al. An ethnobotanical study of medicinal plants in high mountainous region of Chail valley (district Swat-Pakistan). Journal of Ethnobiology and Ethnomedicine. 2014;**10**(1):1-18

[30] Inta A, Trisonthi P, Trisonthi C. Analysis of traditional knowledge in medicinal plants used by Yuan in Thailand. Journal of Ethnopharmacology. 2013;**149**(1): 344-351

[31] Kadir MF, Sayeed MSB, Setu NI, Mostafa A, Mia MMK. Ethnopharmacological survey of medicinal plants used by traditional health practitioners in Thanchi, Bandarban Hill Tracts, Bangladesh. Journal of Ethnopharmacology. 2014; **155**(1):495-508

[32] Kayani S, Ahmad M, Zafar M, Sultana S, Khan MPZ, Ashraf MA, et al. Ethnobotanical uses of medicinal plants for respiratory disorders among the inhabitants of Gallies–Abbottabad, Northern Pakistan. Journal of Ethnopharmacology. 2014;**156**: 47-60

[33] Trotter RT, Logan MH. Informant consensus: A new approach for identifying potentially effective medicinal plants. In: Plants in Indigenous Medicine & Diet. Routledge; 2019. pp. 91-112

[34] Faruque MO et al. Quantitative ethnobotany of medicinal plants used by indigenous communities in the Bandarban District of Bangladesh. Frontiers in Pharmacology. 2018;**9**:40

[35] Albuquerque UP, Lucena RF, Monteiro JM, Florentino AT, Cecília de Fátima CBR. Evaluating two quantitative ethnobotanical techniques. Ethnobotany Research and Applications. 2006;**4**: 051-060

[36] Ahmad KS, Hamid A, Nawaz F, Hameed M, Ahmad F, Deng J, et al. Ethnopharmacological studies of indigenous plants in Kel village, Neelum valley, Azad Kashmir, Pakistan. Journal of Ethnobiology and Ethnomedicine. 2017;**13**(1):1-16

[37] Schlage C, Mabula C, Mahunnah RLA, Heinrich AM. Medicinal plants of the Washambaa (Tanzania): Documentation and ethnopharmacological evaluation. Plant Biology. 2000;**2**(1):83-92

[38] Umair M, Altaf M, Bussmann RW, Abbasi AM. Ethnomedicinal uses of the local flora in Chenab riverine area, Punjab province Pakistan. Journal of Ethnobiology and Ethnomedicine. 2019; **15**(1):1-31

[39] Yineger H, Yewhalaw D, Teketay D. Ethnomedicinal plant knowledge and practice of the Oromo ethnic group in southwestern Ethiopia. Journal of Ethnobiology and Ethnomedicine. 2008; **4**(1):1-10

[40] Srithi K, Balslev H, Wangpakapattanawong P, Srisanga P, Trisonthi C. Medicinal plant knowledge and its erosion among the Mien (Yao) in northern Thailand. Journal of Ethnopharmacology. 2009;**123**(2): 335-342

Section 2

Secondary Metabolites of Medicinal Plants

Chapter 10

Phytochemicals from Solanaceae Family and Their Anticancer Properties

Sangilimuthu Alagar Yadav and Feba Sara Koshi

Abstract

Cancer is one of the most dreadful disease conditions all over the world. With the side effects and cost of conventional treatment, there is a demand for new therapies to prevent cancer. Research studies proved many plant products possess anticancer properties. Currently, a few plant-based drugs are used to treat it. The phytochemicals are investigated by in vitro and in vivo to assess their mechanism of action against cancer. This chapter is an overview of anticancer compounds extracted from plants of Solanaceae family with the potentials results. Many research has confirmed the anticancer efficiency of the biomolecules, such as solanine, solamargine, tomatidine, Withanolides, scopoletin, capsaicin found in Solanaceae, and their mode of action, such as cell cycle arrest, inhibiting signaling pathways, autophagy, suppression of enzymes in various human cancer cell lines of breast, pancreas, colorectal, liver, and cervical and also in animal models. This chapter seeks to provide an outline of key examples of anticancer activity of phytochemicals from the Solanaceae family, which offers a track for the development of novel medicines for cancer treatment as a single drug or in combinational drug. This chapter helps to identify the novel bioactive molecule for cancer treatment as lead molecule with less side effects in future.

Keywords: cancer, solanaceae, flavonoids, saponins, terpenes, anticancer properties, solanine, solamargine, tomatidine, withanolides apoptosis, cell cycle arrest

1. Introduction

Plants have been used for the treatment of diseases for centuries ago. Ancient manuscripts of different civilizations show evidence of using herbs as medicine. Now, this system is used in Unani, Ayurveda, and Siddha medicines also. According to WHO, 21,000 plant species have the potential to use as medicinal plants [1]. The plant is used as a whole or parts as medicine. The plant contains various chemicals called phytochemicals or phytonutrients, which are primary metabolites or secondary metabolites. These metabolites protect the plants from the attack of microbes, such as bacteria, fungi, and viruses. These chemicals are rich in fruits, vegetables, grains, and other plants. The intake of these plants decreases the risk of developing cancer, diabetes, and heart diseases. These chemicals may act as antioxidants or nutrient protectors [2].

Cancer, the abnormal growth of cells that can invade the nearby cells and even spread to other organs called metastasis, which can occur in any part of the body results due to various causes and factor is one of the most dreadful conditions in the world. Common cancer reported are breast, lung, colon, rectum, etc. Among those mentioned types high-mortality rate reported was because of lung cancer. The number of people affected is male [3]. The common treatment methods are radiation therapy, chemotherapy, and surgery. These treatments are quite expensive and also possess many side effects. These side effects can be reduced by using plant or plant-based drugs. Scientists prove that several plants and their components have the potential to fight against cancer and mechanism of action include cessation of the cell cycle, regulation of the transcription process, induction of autophagy, downregulation of proteins in biochemical pathways, and rupturing of the membrane. Also, it was reported that some chemicals are effective against more than one type of cancer [4].

There are different classes of phytochemicals derived anticancer drugs available on market. The drugs were used as tinctures, tea, powders, decoctions, etc. *In vitro* studies also prove that many plants in different parts of the world possess anticancer properties. Studies should be continued about the *in vivo* experimentation and clinical trials to integrate traditional medicine into modern treatment for the patients.

One among the family which possesses anticancer properties is the Solanaceae family. It is an angiosperm with 102 genera and more than 3000–4000 species of plants. Glycoalkaloids from Solanum species, such as solanine, solasonine, and solanidine, isolated from *Withania somnifera* L. have an anticancer property by arresting the cell cycle. David O Nwke et al. reviewed that Physapubescin B, a withanolide remoted from *Physalis pubescens* L. is used in the treatment of colorectal cancer. Extracts from *Datura metel* L. also show cell arrest in various studies [5]. The detailed evaluation of the mode of action of these chemicals in the Solanaceae members against cancer growth and multiplication opens a pathway for the future treatment of cancer.

2. Solanaceae family

Solanaceae family belongs to the order Solanales of angiosperms. Generally, they are called as potato family. This group is also called as nightshade family because of the poisonous alkaloids present in some members of the family. Most of the plants are economically important because of their food, ornamental or medicinal values. Some of the plants in this family are potato, tomato, all peppers, eggplant, etc. It also contains deadly toxic plants. These family members are found throughout the world but are widely distributed in the tropical regions of South America. Members of this family show different morphological and ecological characteristics [6]. Some of the medicinal plants are *Atropa, Hyosymus, Withania, Nicotiana,* and *Capsicum. Petunia, Datura,* and *Schizanthus* are used as ornamental plants [7] (**Table 1**), (**Figure 1**).

Afroz et al. reported, "Bioactive secondary metabolites reported from the members of the Solanaceae include AMPs, alkaloids, flavonoids, glycosides, lactones, lignans, steroids, simple phenols, sugars, and terpenoids" [7].

Genus name	Plant name	Uses
Solanum	*Solanum nigrum* L.	Used for dysentery, stomach complaints, antitumorigenic, and antioxidant.
	Solanum americanum L.	used for the treatment of rheumatic pains, eye diseases, heart pain
	Solanum melongena L.	lower blood cholesterol level, used in the treatment of internal bleeding, piles, and toothache
	Solanum surattense Burm. F.	Used against cough, sore throat, etc.
	Solanum lycopersicum L.	To prevent prostate cancer, breast cancer, and skin diseases
Atropa	*Atropa acuminate* Royle	Used as diuretics
	Atropa belladonna L.	Used in traditional medicine
Capsicum	*Capsicum annum* L.	Lowering blood pressure and Cholesterol.
	Caspsicum frutescens L.	Treatment of cancer
Datura	*Datura stramonium* L. *Datura metel* L.	antispasmodic and antiasthmatic diabetes, cancer, and viral infections
Withania	*Withania somnifera* L.	Used as a tranquilizer, Cancer treatment
	Withanaia coagulans L.	Is used to treat nervous prostration, sleeplessness, infertility, multiple sclerosis, etc.
Hyoscyamus	*Hyoscyamus niger* L. *Hyoscyamus pusillus* L.	Cerebral and spinal sedative Used as anesthetics
Nicotiana	*Nicotiana tobacum* L.	antispasmodics, diuretics, antioxidant activity along with other pharmacological effects
Physalis	*Physalissubglabrata* Mack & Bush	Used as a hallucinogen, used as a remedy for abscesses, coughs, fevers, and sore throats.
Scopolia	*Scopolia carniolica* Jacq.	Used as antispasmodic

Table 1.
Important plants of the Solanaceae family and their uses [8].

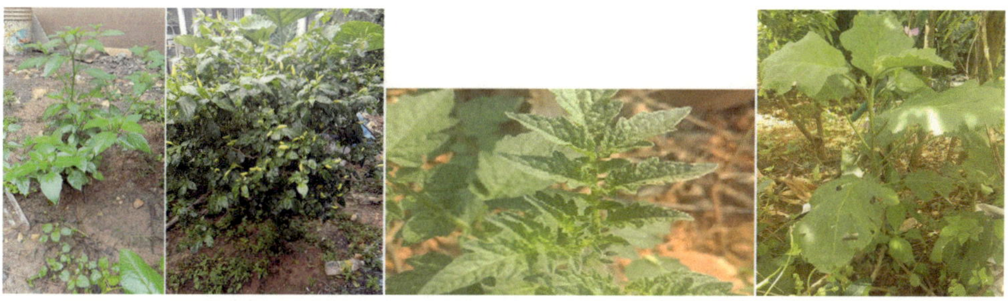

Figure 1.
Some members of the Solanaceae family plants: 1. Capsicum frutescens .L. 2. Solanum nigrum L. 3. Solanum lycopersicum L. 4. Solanum melongena L.

3. Phytochemicals

Phytochemicals or phytonutrients are produced by plants. These chemicals are the basic principle for the nutritive as well as pharmacological action of plants. These chemicals also provide a defense mechanism to the plants against plant pathogens.

The main pathogens belong to the class of bacteria, fungi, protozoa, and viruses [9]. The common vegetables and fruits, such as broccoli, berries, carrot, tomato, garlic, seeds, and onion, contain these chemicals in large quantities which increase the immune capacity of the body.

There are two types of metabolites in all living organisms including plants. They are primary metabolites, such as sugar, amino acids, nucleotides, and lipids, which are essential for their functioning. Plants also produce certain molecules which are not used directly in their life process such chemicals are called secondary metabolites synthesized by biochemical pathways, such as alkaloids, flavonoids, glycosides, phenolics, and terpenoids discovered with various properties, such as induction of flowering, protection from pathogens, protection from the external environment, attractant or repellant for pollination, antimicrobial, antioxidant, anti-inflammatory, and antitumor activity. These chemicals and their product are used in herbal medicine and modern medicines [10–12].

3.1 Types of phytochemicals in the Solanaceae family

The phytochemicals are classified on the basis of their biosynthetic origin, structure, and solubility properties. The different types of phytochemicals are alkaloids, glycosides, flavonoids, saponins, terpenes, steroids, etc. [13]. The Solanaceae family is rich in phytochemicals showing their effectiveness as medicinal plants (**Table 2**). The review studies show that most of these common plants in the selective family show anticancer properties (**Figure 2**) which can enlighten the treatment of cancer in the near future.

Genus name	Plant name	Phytochemical	Class
Solanum	*Solanum. nigrum* L.	Solasonine, Solamargine, Solanigroside P Solamargine	Steroidal glycoalkaloids
	Solanum anguivi Lam	Anguivioside A,B,C	Saponins
	Solanum incanum L.	Solamargine, Methylprotodioscin Indioside D	Steroidal glycoalkaloids
	Solanum lycopersicum L.	Lycopene. Diosgenin	Carotenoid Saponins
Atropa	*Atropa acuminata* Royle	Atropine	Alkaloids
	Atropa belladonna L.	Atropine, Apoatropine Scopolamine Kaempferol 3,7-diglycosides	Alkaloids Alkaloids Alkaloids Flavonoids
Capsicum	*Capsicum annum* L.	Caffeic acid, capsinoids Canusesnol kaempferol-3-O-glucoside	Phenolics sesquiterpenoids flavonols
	Capsicum frutescens L.	Capsaicin	capsaicinoids
Datura	*Datura stramonium* L. *Datura metal* L.	Apoatropine Tropine tropate Withanolides,	Nitrogen-containing polyhydroxylated heterocyclic compounds steroidal lactones

Genus name	Plant name	Phytochemical	Class
Withania	*Withania somnifera* L.	Withanolides, Withaferin A,, Physagulin D, Withanoside IV	Steroids steroidal lactone Glycoside Glycoside
	Withania coagulans L.	Withanolides	Steroidal lactone
Hyoscyamus	*Hyoscyamus niger* L.	Hyoscyamine, Apo atropine, hyoscine, skimmianine, scopolamine, belladonines	Alkaloids
Nicotiana	*Nicotiana tobacum* L.	Nicotine	Alkaloid

Table 2.
List of some phytochemicals and their classes in the Solanaceae family [14–17].

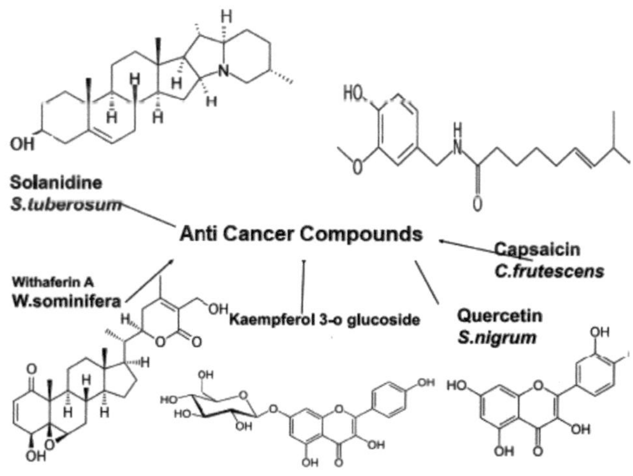

Figure 2.
Plants of Solanaceae family and their phytochemicals against cancer.

The use of phytochemicals in pharmaceutical and agrochemical industries is an ongoing process that requires continuous and elaborate study.

4. Alkaloids in Solanaceae

Alkaloids are cyclic nitrogenous secondary metabolites seen in many plants. They are synthesized during the biochemical synthesis of proteins and nucleic acid. These alkaloids have wide applications as drugs, narcotics, or poisons. Jerzykiewicz et al. reported, "Chenopodiaceae, Lauraceae, Magnoliaceae, Berberidaceae, Menispermaceae, Ranunculaceae, Papaveraceae, Fumariaceae, Papilionaceae, Rutaceae, Apocynaceae, Loganiaceae, Rubiaceae, Boraginaceae, Convolvulaceae, Solanaceae, and Campanulaceae are some of the families that rich in alkaloids which protect the plant from insects, pest and also give disease resistant capacity to plants" [18]. This property of alkaloids in Solanaceae can be utilized for anticancer medicine production.

Alkaloids are classified into different categories based the on nature of the precursor molecule for its biosynthesis, chemical structure, biological effect, and heterocyclic or non-heterocyclic types [19]. The biological effects of alkaloids include hallucinogens, antimalarial, tranquilizer, anticancer, CNS stimulant, insecticidal, antiviral, antihypertension, antimicrobial, antirheumatics, anti-inflammatory, antioxidant, and diuretics. The alkaloids are used in the drug industry because they are the precursor for medicines for cardiovascular disease, menopause, etc.

In vitro and *in vivo* synthesis and production of alkaloids from the Solanaceae family were studied and showed successful results. In different members of Solanaceae alkaloid, the composition is between 0.01 and 3% [20]. "Tropane, indole, pyridine, pyrrolidine, steroidal, and glycoalkaloids" are mostly seen as classes of alkaloids of the above-mentioned group of the plant [21] (**Table 3**).

Alkaloid	Type of Alkaloid	Source	Biological Action
Atropine	Tropane	*Atropa belladonna* L.	Para sympatholytic, Anticholinergic.
Hyoscyamine	Tropane	*Brugmansia candida* Pers	
Scopolamine	Tropane	*Hyoscyanus niger* L.	Antidepressant and Antinausea
Daturametelindoles A-D (1–4)	Indole Alkaloids	*Datura metel* L.	Anticancer Effect
Anabasine	Pyridine Alkaloids	*Nicotiana tabacum* L.	Insecticide
Nicotine	Pyridine Alkaloids	*N. tabacum* L.	Insecticidal
Chaconine	Glycoalkaloid	*Solanum tuberosum* L.	Fungicidal
Solanidane; Solanidine	Steroidal Alkaloid	*S. tuberosum* L.	Anticancer
Solamargine	Glycoalkaloid	*Solanum palinacanthum* Dunal *Solanum lycocarpum* L. *Solanum melongena* L.	anticancer
Solamarine	Glycoalkaloid	*Solanum dulcamara* L.	Antibacterial
Solanine	Saponins	*Solanum nigrum* L., *S. tuberosum* L.	Antifungal
Solanopubamine	Steroidal alkaloid	*Solanum schimperianum* Hochst.	Anticancer
Solasodine	glycoalkaloid	*Solanum leucocarpum* L. *Solanum trilobatum* L.	Antibacterial
Solasonine	glycoalkaloid	*S. lycocarpum* L. *Solanum asperum* Rich	substrate for the production of important steroids
Tomatidine	steroid glycosides	*Solanum arboretum* Humb. & Bonpl. *Solanum aculeastrum* Dunal	Anticancerous

Table 3.
List of some of the alkaloids and its source [22–24].

The review studies show that tomatidine, solanopubamine, solamargine, solanidane; solanidine, daturametelindoles A-D (1–4) chemicals show anticancer activity in in vitro conditions by activation of caspase-3 and regulation of cell cycle to induce apoptosis. The detailed mechanism of action of these chemicals and their clinical trials will be an asset for developments in cancer medicine.

5. Flavonoids in Solanaceae

Flavonoids have several potential effects in plants system such as attracting pollination, seed germination, aromatic flavors in defense mechanisms, stress tolerance, UV photoprotection, inducing root nodulation, and controlling transport of plant hormones [25–27]. Panche et al. reviewed that flavonoids have pharmaceutical, medicine, and cosmetic applications.

The different polyphenolic and glycosidic compounds had been reported from various members of the Solanaceae family (**Table 4**). Scopoletin (7-hydroxy-6-methoxycoumarin), a coumarin, was isolated from *Solanum lyratum* Thunb. showed hepatoprotective activity [28]. One of the most common flavonols in *Solanum nigrum* L. is Quercetin showed antiproliferation effect in different types of cancer models by apoptosis by inducing DNA methylation [29].

The flavonoids, such as apigenin, kaempferol, quercetin, and anthocyanin are some of the chemicals isolated from the respective family that possesses antiproliferation effects against cancer cell lines [30].

Sl	Flavonoids	Plant Source	Biological Action
1	Luteolin	*Solanum schimperianum* Hochst. *Capsicum annum* L.	Anticancer
2	Apigenin	*Solanum lycoparpum* L.	Antioxidant,antibacterial, cytotoxic
3	Kaempferol	*Solanum lycoparpum* L.	Anticancer
4	Quercetin	*Solanum nigrum* L.	Anticancer
5	Tangeretin	*Physalis angulate* L. *Physalis micranta* L.	Antioxidant, anti-inflamotory,antitumour
6	Mycicetin	*Solanum agrarium* Sendtn	Antispasmodic effect
7	Scopoletin	*Solanum lyratium* Thunb	Hepatoprotective activity
8	Anthocyanidins	*Solanum scabrum* Mill	
9	Anthocyanin	*Solanum. Tuberosum* L.	Inhibition of cell proliferation

Table 4.
List of flavonoid from Solanaceae [27–30].

6. Saponins in the Solanaceae family

More than 100 plant families, a few starfishes, and sea cucumber reported the presence of saponins. Dicot families, such as Leguminosae, Araliaceae, and Caryophyllaceae, are sources of triterpenoid saponins. Steroidal saponins are found in families, such as Agavaceae, Alliaceae, Asparagaceae, Dioscoreaceae, Liliaceae, Amaryllidaceae, Bromeliaceae, Palmae, and Scrophulariaceae. Solanaceae families contain steroidal glycoalkaloids [31]. Some of the biological activities of saponins are anti- cancer activity, reducing cholesterol levels, decreasing blood glucose, anti-inflammatory potentials, antibacterial, antifungal and antiviral activity [32, 33].

Figueiredo et al. isolated steroidal saponins from the roots of *Solanum sisymbriifolium* Lam. (Solanaceae)which showed a response against dengue virus and yellow fever virus [34]. Chlorogenone, (5α,25S)-Spirostan-3,6-dione are isolated from *Solanum torvum* Sw. Nuatigenosido isolated from *S. sisymbriifolium* Lam. root shows an antihypertensive effect. The antifungal property was exhibited by leaves of *Solanum chrysotrichum* Schltdl [35].

7. Terpenes in the Solanaceae family

Terpenes are used in herbal medicines because of their biological activities. Some of the activities include antiplasmodial, especially antimalarial, anticancer, antidiabetic, anti-inflammatory, antioxidant, etc. Curcumin is one of the terpenes used in folk medicine Terpenes are used as flavors and fragrances in food and cosmetics [36].

Diterpene phytol was isolated from Solanum schimperianum, and Betulinic acid was isolated from Solanum buddleifolium. 3β-Hydroxysolavetivone from the root of S. abutiloides showed antifungal activities. Solavetivone and Lubimin also showed antifungal activities isolated from *S. abutiloides.*

8. Anticancer effects of Solanaceae family and their mechanism

The common conventional treatment of cancer causes side effects and drug resistance in patients, so many plant species were attempted as anticancer drugs. α-chaconine a derivative of solanidine shows an antimetastatic effect individually also in combination with gallic acid by caspase-dependent apoptosis Reddivari et al. [37]. Solanine a glycoalkaloid present in *Solanum tuberosum* L. showed chemoprotective and chemotherapeutic effects. It also inhibited the proliferation of human pancreatic carcinoma cell lines, human melanoma cell lines, and human prostate cancer cells by apoptosis [38]. Solanidine a steroidal alkaloid from *S. tuberosum* L. and *Solanum americanuum* Mill. showed inhibition of cancer cells under laboratory conditions and also from the chemically derived compound of the same by the inhibition of DNA synthesis [39]. Tomatidine A steroid glycoside from *Solanum arboretum* Humb., *Solanum aculeastrum* Dunal. exhibited the suppression of cell invasion by inhibition of ERK and Akt signaling pathways in *in vitro* studies [40]. Tomatine spirosolane-type glycoalkaloids present in *Solanum cathayanum* Wu, *Lycopersicon esculentum* L. showed positive results against prostate cancer in mice when mixed with common drug for cancer by the induction of apoptosis mediated by P13K/Akt pro-signaling pathway [41].

Solamargine glycoalkaloid present in *Solanum palinacanthum, Solanum lycocarpum, Solanum melongena* reduced cell—viability by arresting cell cycle at the G2/M phase. Solasodine was evaluated by many workers for the induction of apoptosis [42]. Steroidal alkaloid soladulcidine, Beta-solamarine, and solanopubamine also show anticancer activity. Capsaicin, from *Capsicum frutescens* L., has anticancer effects on human cell lines of different origins [43]. The mechanism of action of the compound is apoptosis, cell-cycle arrest, and transcription factor regulation. Withanolides isolated from *D. metel* L. leaf extract inhibit tumor cell proliferation against human colorectal carcinoma [44]. Nicotine an alkaloid from *Nicotiana tabacuum* L. inhibits cancer cells by regulation of tumor necrosis factor [45]. Anthocyanins from *S. tuberosum* L. were found to cause inhibition of cell multiplication and apoptosis in different cancer cell models [30]. Degalactotigonin was isolated from *S. nigrum* L. showed cytotoxic effect for human tumor cell lines for pancreatic cancer cells induces apoptosis and cell cycle arrest by inhibiting signaling pathway [46].

Saponins from *Solanum trilobatum* L. leaf extract showed anticancer effect and initiation of apoptosis in human larynx cancer cell lines [47]. Saponins Torvosides M, Yamoscin, Indioside H, Borassoside E, Indioside I, and Dioscin isolated from *S. torvum, Solanum violaceum,* and *Solanum indicum* showed anticancer property [48]. Sesquiterpenoids from *S. lyratum*, named solajiangxin D and solajiangxins E, and 2-hydroxysolajiangxin E were isolated and were found to show significant cytotoxicity against three human cancer lines [49]. It has been reported that *W. somnifera* L. inhibits DMBA-induced carcinogenesis in mice [50]. Cycloeucalenone,24-oxo-31-norcycloartanone isolated from *Solanum cernuum*, Lyratol D, Solajiangxin B, Blumenol A, Dehydrovomifoliol from *S. lyratum*. Flavonoids rutin, Tiliroside from *Solanum anguvi*, *Solanum elaeagnifolium* exhibit anticancer activity. *Solanum betaceum* contains flavonoids, such as keracyanin, pelargonidin 3-rutinoside, tulipanin, delphinidin 3-O-α-L-rhamnosyl-(1–6)-β-D-glucoside-3′-O-β-D-glucoside show anticancer properties [35]. The ethanol extract from ripe fruits of *S. nigrum* L. showed anticancer activity by inhibiting the proliferation of human MCF-7 breast cancer cells and inducing cell death by apoptosis [51].

The above-mentioned plants exhibit anticancer mechanisms by cell cycle arrest: The cell cycle contains several proteins at the checkpoint. Cancer cells overcome this checkpoint leads to the multiplication of cells. So inducing cell cycle arrest can be an alternative method in the treatment of cancer. Various researches show that this is possible by phytochemicals. The phytochemicals, such as solanine, solanidine, solamargine, and α-chaconine, result in cell cycle arrest at the S phase of the cell cycle and thereby induce apoptosis based on various concentrations [52] (**Figure 3**).

Studies prove that these chemicals have anticancer properties against different types of cancer, such as breast cancer, colon cancer, cervical cancer, and liver cancer.

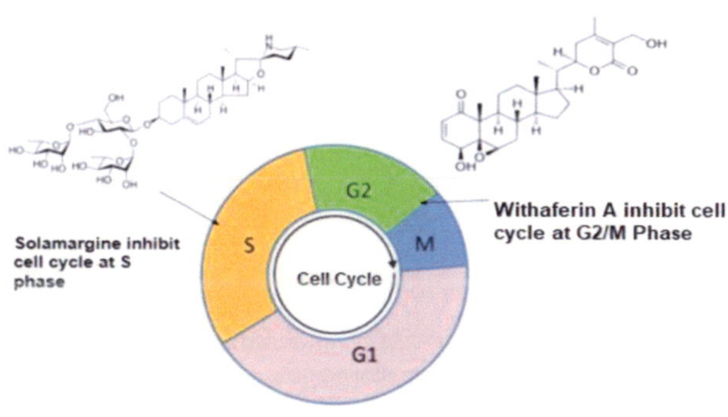

Figure 3.
Mechanism of cell cycle inhibition by phytochemicals of Solanaceae [50, 52].

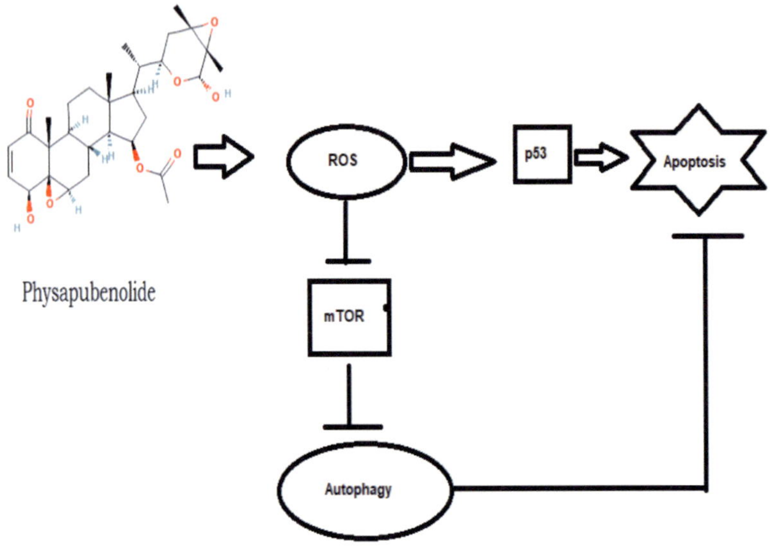

Figure 4.
Anticancer mechanism of physapubenolide [53].

Another mechanism involved in anticancer therapy is the regulation of transcription by inhibiting oncogenic transcription factors. Withaferin isolated from Withania sominifera shows antitumor activity by regulating transcription factors [5].

Physapubescin B and physapubenolide isolated from Physalis pubescens exhibit anticancer mechanisms by autophagy (**Figure 4**) and apoptosis in colorectal cancer cell lines [53].

Other mechanisms include the suppression of metabolic enzymes. Some plant molecules can cause apoptosis by breaking the mitochondrial membrane. Defensin isolated from Nicotiana alata induces necrotic-like cell death in a number of tumor cells [5]. The summary of the anticancer potential of selected plants that are economically useful to humans of the Solanaceae family with the mechanism of their action against different cancer cell lines which is reviewed in this literature from previous works by eminent workers is given in the table (**Table 5**).

The effective study of the mechanism of phytochemicals in the Solanaceae family will open a new approach to the treatment of cancer.

Plant Source	Phytochemical	Model	Mechanism of Action
Solanum tuberosum L.	Solanine	Human pancreatic cancer cell lines, human melanoma cell lines, human prostate cancer cells	Apoptosis
S. tuberosum L. *Solanum americanuum* L.	Solanidine	Human lung adenocarcinoma cell line (A549) A549 CAM xenograft BALB/c mouse model	Inhibition of DNA synthesis
Solanum arboretum Humb. *Solanum aculeastrum* Dunal.	Tomatidine	Human fibrosarcoma cells, human lung adenocarcinoma cell A549	Suppression of cell invasion by inhibition of ERK and Akt signaling pathways

Plant Source	Phytochemical	Model	Mechanism of Action
Solanum cathayanum C.Y.Wu. *Lycopersicum esculentum* L.	Tomatine	Prostate cancer in mice	Induction of apoptosis mediated by P13K/Akt pro-signaling pathway
Solanum palinacanthum Dunal *Solanum lycocarpum* Hil *Solanum melongena* L.	Solamargine	Human liver cancer cell lines, i.e., HepG2 and Huh-7 cells Human neuroblastoma cell line (SH-SY5Y)	By arresting the cell cycle at the G2/M phase
Solanum incanum L.	Solasodine	Human colorectal cancer cells	Suppression of the AKT/glycogen synthase kinase-3β/β-catenin pathway
Capsicum frutescens L.	Capsaicin	Human cell lines of different origins	Apoptosis, cell-cycle arrest, transcription factor regulation
Datura metel L.	Withanolides	Human colorectal carcinoma	Inhibit tumor cell proliferation
Nicotiana tabacuum L.	Nicotine	Human airway epithelial cells.	By regulation of tumor necrosis factor
S. tuberosum L.	Anthocyanins	Different cancer cell models	Inhibition of cell multiplication and apoptosis
Solanum nigrum L.	Degalactotigonin	Human Pancreatic cancer cell lines	Induces apoptosis and cell cycle arrest by inhibiting the signaling pathway
Solanum trilobatum L.	Saponins	Human larynx cancer cell lines	Initiation of apoptosis
Withania sominifera L.	Withaferin	Chicken myeloid cell lines (HD11-C3-GFP1 Myb reporter cell line) Human Myeloid leukemia cell line (HL60) Quail Japanese fibrosarcoma (QT6) Mouse preadipocyte cell line (3T3-L1)	By regulating transcription factors
Physalis pubescens L.	Physapubescin B and physapubenolide	Colorectal cancer cell lines.	Autophagy and apoptosis

Table 5.
Mechanism of action of phytochemicals in Solanaceae on different models of cell lines [30, 35, 40–54].

Many of these are commercially interesting because of their use as flavors and fragrances in foods and cosmetics.

Many of these are commercially interesting because of their use as flavors and fragrances in foods and cosmetics.

9. Conclusion

Cancer is one of the major public health problems across the world. The pandemic condition of the current world results in the delay of diagnosis and treatment that may lead to increased complications in the treatment of cancer. Phytochemicals from Solanaceae exhibit anticancer activity against various type of cancer.

These compounds proved their efficiency in the inhibition of cancer cell line proliferation by cell cycle arrest, regulation of transcription factors, blocking the signal pathways, initiation of apoptosis, and suppression of metastasis. Most of the compound shows positive results with a combination of other phytochemicals in cancer treatment. The effective study of these biomolecules as anticancer targets can lead to clinical trials and in the future, it opens an effective area for the treatment of cancer and prevention.

Acknowledgements

The author acknowledges and thanks to Karpagam Academy of Higher Education, Coimbatore providing the internet facility to complete this review process.

Author details

Sangilimuthu Alagar Yadav* and Feba Sara Koshi
Department of Biotechnology, Karpagam Academy of Higher Education, Coimbatore, Tamil Nadu, India

*Address all correspondence to: smuthu.al@gmail.com

References

[1] Kaliyaperumal Karunamoorthi MM. Traditional medicinal plants: A source of Phytotherapeutic modality in resource-constrained health care settings. Journal of Evidence-Based Complementary & Alternative Medicine. 2013;**18**(1):67-74. DOI: 10.1177/2156587212460241

[2] Lavecchia T, Rea G, Antonacci A, Giardi MT. Healthy and adverse effects of plant-derived functional metabolites: The need of revealing their content and bioactivity in a complex food matrix. Critical Reviews in Food Science and Nutrition. 2013;**53**(2):198-213. DOI: 10.1080/10408398.2010.520829

[3] Bray F, Ferlay J, Soerjomataram I, Siegel RL, Torre LA, Jemal A. Global cancer statistics 2018: GLOBOCAN estimates of incidence and mortality worldwide for 36 cancers in 185 countries. CA: A Cancer Journal for Clinicians. 2018;**68**(6):394-424

[4] Javed Iqbal BA. Plant-derived anticancer agents: A green anticancer approach. Asian Pacific Journal of Tropical Biomedicine. 2017;7(12):1129-1150. DOI: 10.1016/j.apjtb.2017.10.016

[5] David O, Nkwe BL. Anticancer mechanisms of bioactive compounds from Solanaceae: An update. Cancers. 2021;**13**(19):4989. DOI: 10.3390/cancers13194989

[6] Morris WL, Taylor MA. The solanaceous vegetable crops: Potato, tomato, pepper, and eggplant. In: Encyclopedia of Applied Plant Sciences. Second ed. Cambridge, Massachusetts, United States: Academic Press; 2017. pp. 55-58. DOI: 10.1016/B978-0-12-394807-6.00129-5

[7] Afroz M, Afroz M, Akter S, Ahmed A, Rouf R, Shilpi JA, et al. Ethnobotany and antimicrobial peptides from plants of the solanaceae family: An update and future prospects. Frontiers in Pharmacology. 2020;**11**:565. DOI: 10.3389/fphar.2020.00565

[8] Shah VV, Shah ND, Patrekar PV. Medicinal plants from Solanaceae family. Research Journal of Pharmacy and Technology. 2013;**6**(2):143-151

[9] Mendoza N, Silva EME. Introduction to Phytochemicals: Secondary Metabolites from Plants with Active Principles for Pharmacological Importance. London: IntechOpen; 2018, 2018. DOI: 10.5772/intechopen.78226

[10] Erb M, Kliebenstein DJ. Plant secondary metabolites as defenses, regulators, and primary metabolites: The blurred functional trichotomy. Plant Physiology. 2020;**184**(1):39-52. DOI: 10.1104/pp.20.00433

[11] Tijjani H, Egbuna C, Carrol LD. Biosynthesis of Phytochemicals. Oxfordshire United Kingdom: Apple Academic Press, Taylor and Francis; 2019. DOI: 10.1201/9780429426223

[12] Teoh ES. Secondary metabolites of plants. In: Medicinal Orchids of Asia. Cham: Springer; 2016. pp. 59-73. DOI: 10.1007/978-3-319-24274-3_5

[13] Koche D, Shirsat R, Kawale M. An overerview of major classes of phytochemicals: Their types and role in disease prevention. Hislopia Journal. 2016;**9**:1-11

[14] Ding X, Zhu F, Yang Y, Li M. Purification, antitumor activity in vitro of steroidal glycoalkaloids from black nightshade (Solanum nigrum L.). Food Chemistry. 2013;**141**(2):1181-1186

[15] Mannawar Hussain A, W. A. Ethnopharmacological investigations of phytochemical constituents isolated from the genus Atropa. International Journal of Scientific and Engineering Research. 2019;**10**:589

[16] Sinisgalli C, Faraone I, Vassallo A, Caddeo C, Bisaccia F, Armentano MF, et al. Phytochemical profile of Capsicum annuum L. cv Senise, incorporation into liposomes, and evaluation of cellular antioxidant activity. Antioxidants. 2020;**9**(5):428. DOI: 10.3390/antiox9050428

[17] Joshi DK. Pyto chemical and pharmacological profiles of Hyoscyamus niger Linn-A review. Pharma Science Monitor. 2015;**6**:153-159

[18] Jerzykiewicz J. Alkaloids of Solanacea. Postepy Biochemii. 2007;**53**(3):280-286

[19] Jayakumar K, Murugan K. Solanum alkaloids and their pharmaceutical roles: A review. Journal of Analytical & Pharmaceutical Research. 2016;**3**(6):00075. DOI: 10.15406/japlr.2016.03.00075

[20] Oksman-Caldentey KM, Arroo R. Regulation of tropane alkaloid metabolism in plants and plant cell cultures. In: Metabolic Engineering of Plant Secondary Metabolism. Dordrecht: Springer; 2000. pp. 253-281

[21] E, E. Solanaceae and Convolvulacea: Secondary Metabolities. Berlin: Springer; 2008

[22] Kukula-Koch WA, Widelski J. Alkaloids: Pharmacognosy: Fundamentals. Applications and Strategies. 2017:163-198. DOI: 10.1016/B978-0-12-802104-0.00009-3

[23] Bock JH, Norris DO. Introduction to forensic plant science. Forensic Plant Science. 2016;**2016**:1-22

[24] Liu Y, Jiang HB, Liu Y, Zhou YY. New indole alkaloids from the seeds of Datura metel L. Fitoterapia. 2020. DOI: 10.1016/j.fitote.2020.104726

[25] Kumar S, Pandey AK. Chemistry and biological activities of flavonoids: An overview. The Scientific World Journal. 2013;**2013**:162750. DOI: 10.1155/2013/162750

[26] Falcone Ferreyra ML, Rius S, Casati P. Flavonoids: biosynthesis, biological functions, and biotechnological applications. Frontiers in Plant Science. 2012;**3**:222. DOI: 10.3389/fpls.2012.00222

[27] Panche AN, Diwan AD, Chandra SR. Flavonoids: An overview. Journal of Nutritional Science. 2016;**5**:e47. DOI: 10.1017/jns.2016.41

[28] Kang SY, Sung SH, Park JH, Kim YC. Hepatoprotective activity of scopoletin, a constituent of Solanum lyratum. Archives of Pharmacal Research. 1998;**21**(6):718-722. DOI: 10.1007/BF02976764

[29] Jeong JH, An JY, Kwon YT, Rhee JG, Lee YJ. Effects of low dose quercetin: Cancer cell-specific inhibition of cell cycle progression. Journal of Cellular Biochemistry. 2009;**106**(1):73-82. DOI: 10.1002/jcb.21977

[30] Bontempo P, De Masi L, Carafa V, Rigano D, Scisciola L, Iside C, et al. Anticancer activities of anthocyanin extract from genotyped Solanum tuberosum L."Vitelotte". Journal of Functional Foods. 2015;**19**:584-593. DOI: 10.1016/j.jff.2015.09.063

[31] Kregiel D, Berlowska J, Witonska I, Antolak H, Proestos C, Babic M, et al. Saponin-based, biological-active surfactants from plants. Application and Characterization of Surfactants. 2017;**6**(1):184-205. DOI: 10.5772/68062

[32] El Aziz MMA, Ashour AS, Melad ASG. A review on saponins from medicinal plants: Chemistry, isolation, and determination. Journal of Nanomedicine Research. 2019;**8**(1):282-288. DOI: 10.15406/jnmr.2019.07.00199

[33] Shi J, Arunasalam K, Yeung D, Kakuda Y, Mittal G, Jiang Y. Saponins from edible legumes: Chemistry, processing, and health benefits. Journal of Medicinal Food. 2004;**7**(1):67-78. DOI: 10.1089/1096620041224111

[34] Figueiredo GG, Coronel OA, Trabuco AC, Bazán DE, Russo RR, Alvarenga NL, et al. Steroidal saponins from the roots of Solanum sisymbriifolium Lam. (Solanaceae) have inhibitory activity against dengue virus and yellow fever virus. Brazilian Journal of Medical and Biological Research. 2021;**54**(7):e10240. DOI: 10.1590/1414-431X2020e10240

[35] Kaunda JS, Zhang YJ. The genus solanum: An ethnopharmacological, phytochemical and biological properties review. Natural Products and Bioprospecting. 2019;**9**(2):77-137

[36] Cox-Georgian D, Ramadoss N, Dona C, Basu C. Therapeutic and medicinal uses of terpenes. In: Medicinal Plants. Cham: Springer; 2019. pp. 333-359. DOI: 10.1007/978-3-030-31269-5_15

[37] Reddivari L, Vanamala J, Safe SH, Miller JC Jr. The bioactive compounds alpha-chaconine and gallic acid in potato extracts decrease survival and induce apoptosis in LNCaP and PC3 prostate cancer cells. Nutrition and Cancer. 2010;**62**(5):601-610. DOI: 10.1080/01635580903532358

[38] Lv C, Kong H, Dong G, Liu L, Tong K, Sun H, et al. Antitumor efficacy of α-solanine against pancreatic cancer in vitro and in vivo. PLoS One. 2014;**9**(2):e87868

[39] Minorics R, Szekeres T, Krupitza G, Saiko P, Giessrigl B, Wölfling J, et al. Antiproliferative effects of some novel synthetic solanidine analogs on HL-60 human leukemia cells in vitro. Steroids. 2011;**76**(1-2):156-162. DOI: 10.1016/j.steroids.2010.10.006

[40] Yan K-H, Lee L-M, Yan S-H, Huang H-C, Li C-C, Lin H-T, et al. Tomatidine inhibits invasion of human lung adenocarcinoma cell A549 by reducing matrix metallo proteinases expression. Chemico-Biological Interactions. 2013;**203**(3):580-587. DOI: 10.1016/j.cbi.2013.03.016

[41] Lee ST, Wong PF, Hooper JD, Mustafa MR. Alpha-tomatine synergises with paclitaxel to enhance apoptosis of androgen-independent human prostate cancer PC-3 cells in vitro and in vivo. Phytomedicine. 2013;**20**(14):1297-1305. DOI: 10.1016/j.phymed.2013.07.002

[42] Akter R, U. S. A new cytotoxic steroidal glycoalkaloid from the methanol extract of Blumea lacera leaves. Journal of Pharmacy & Pharmaceutical Sciences. 2015;**18**(4):616-633

[43] Elkholi IE, Hazem NM, ElKashef WF, Sobh MA, Shaalan D, Sobh M, et al. Evaluation of anti-cancer potential of capsaicin-loaded trimethyl chitosan-based nanoparticles in HepG2 hepatocarcinoma cells. Journal of Nanomedicine & Nanotechnology. 2014;**5**(6):1-8. DOI: 10.4172/2157-7439.1000240

[44] Poddar S, Sarkar T, Choudhury S, Chatterjee S, Ghosh P. Indian traditional medicinal plants: A concise review. International Journal of Botany Studies. 2020;**5**(5):174-190 ISSN: 2320-0189 2015

[45] Madretsma GS, Donze GJ, van Dijk AP, Tak CJ, Wilson JH, Zijlstra FJ. Nicotine inhibits the in

vitro production of interleukin 2 and tumour necrosis factor-alpha by human mononuclear cells. Immunopharmacology. 1996;**35**(1):47-51. DOI: 10.1016/0162-3109(96)00122-1

[46] Zhou X, He X, Wang G, Gao H, Zhou G, Ye W, et al. Steroidal saponins from Solanum nigrum. Journal of Natural Products. 2006;**69**(8):1158-1163. DOI: 10.1021/np060091z

[47] Kanchana A, Balakrishna M. Anti-cancer effect of saponins isolated from Solanum trilobatum leaf extract and induction of apoptosis in human larynx cancer cell lines. International Journal of Pharmacy and Pharmaceutical Sciences. 2011;**3**(4):356-364

[48] Man S, Gao W, Zhang Y, Huang L, Liu C. Chemical study and medical application of saponins as anti-cancer agents. Fitoterapia. 2010;**81**:703-714. DOI: 10.1016/j.fitote.2010.06.004

[49] Yao F, Song Q-L, Zhang L, Li G-S, Dai S-J. Solajiangxins A–C, three new cytotoxic sesquiterpenoids from Solanum lyratum. Fitoterapia. 2013;**89**:200-204. DOI: 10.1016/j.fitote.2013.05.020

[50] Christina AJM, Joseph DG, Packialakshmi M, Kothai R, Robert SJH, Chidambaranathan N, et al. Anticarcinogenic activity of Withania somnifera Dunal against Dalton's ascitic lymphoma. Journal of Ethnopharmacology. 2004;**93**(2-3):359-361. DOI: 10.1016/j.jep.2004.04.004

[51] Son YO, Kim J, Lim JC, Chung Y, Chung GH, Lee JC. Ripe fruits of Solanum nigrum L. inhibits cell growth and induces apoptosis in MCF-7 cells. Food and Chemical Toxicology. 2003;**41**(10):1421-1428. DOI: 10.1016/s0278-6915(03)00161-3

[52] Fekry MI, Ezzat SM, Salama MM, Alshehri OY, Al-Abd AM. Bioactive glycoalkaloides isolated from Solanum melongena fruit peels with potential anticancer properties against hepatocellular carcinoma cells. Scientific Reports. 2019;**9**(1):1-11. DOI: 10.1038/s41598-018-36089-6

[53] Xu J, Wu Y, Lu G, Xie S, Ma Z, Chen Z, et al. Importance of ROS-mediated autophagy in determining apoptotic cell death induced by physapubescin B. Redox Biology. 2017;**12**:198-207

[54] Zhuang YW, Wu CE, Zhou JY, Chen X, Wu J, Jiang S, et al. Solasodine inhibits human colorectal cancer cells through suppression of the AKT/glycogen synthase kinase-3β/β-catenin pathway. Cancer Science. 2017;**108**(11):2248-2264. DOI: 10.1111/cas.13354

Chapter 11

Diversity of Natural Bioactive Compound in Plant Origin

Murshida Mollik and Hamidul Islam

Abstract

Recent studies have claimed that people are now greatly relying on synthetic drug without considering any side effect; however, all the synthetic drugs have been formulated commercially by following the invention of an authentic source of crude drug; hence, people are still directly or indirectly dependent on natural source of medicine. Recently, I have completed a research work on black pepper (*Piper nigrum*), and piperine (in a crystal form) was isolated as a mother bioactive compound from black pepper through a plenty of in vitro investigations. After that, I have experimented some in vitro analysis to evaluate the antioxidant power of that pure compound, and it was found that the crystal compound has strong antioxidant power. After doing some theoretical analysis, it has been identified that piperine may exist in other medicinal plants also, and many plants belonging to the same species can able to show multiple types of biological activities, which actually reflected the diversity of bioactive compounds in nature. People can benefit from different types of bioactive compounds, such as piperine, if we biosysthesize and use them commercially.

Keywords: bioactive compound, crystal compound, commercial purpose, diversity, in vitro test, piperine

1. Introduction

Medicinal plants or herbal medicine has been utilized to prevent and cure diseases since the ancient period of time, and it has played a significant role in drug discovery [1, 2]. The earlier evidences had been declared that the existing medicinal plants were consumed from 60,000 year ago. Recently, a 5000-year-old Sumerian clay slab was invented by utilization of medicinal plants for the manufacture of drug [3]; moreover, the current study is showing that more than 50% of marketed drugs have been derived from medicinal plants [4, 5].

The safety, efficacy, and quality of this active constituents greatly rely on the source, cross-contamination, and simultaneously the formulation procedure of finished products. The popularity of medicinal plants had been raised from fifteenth to seventeenth century, and the descriptions of herbal medicine had started to be available in various languages. In the eighteenth century, a scheme for classifying plant species had been initiated by Linnaeus [6].

Primarily, the medicinal plants were used in casual pharmaceutical preparations such as macerations, infusions, and decoctions; however, in between sixteenth and eighteenth centuries, the compounded drug was on demand. The early nineteenth century was a crucial point in the development of knowledge about the consumption of medicinal plants and the drug discovery, substantiation, and screening of alkaloids from the poppy as well as quinine, ipecacuanha, pomegranate also under trial. Scientific pharmacy was initiated followed by the isolation of glycosides from other medicinal plants, and the upgradation of chemical methodologies to isolate tannins, saponins, hormones, and vitamins was started [7, 8].

In the late nineteenth and early twentieth centuries, a steady fall in the therapeutic use of herbal medicines has been noticed. Many authors have claimed that drugs obtained from the medicinal plants may be possessed shortcomings due to degradative action of different types of enzymes. In the early twentieth century, stabilization method for the preparation and utilization of fresh medicinal plants had been proposed. After that, several steps has been taken to cultivate medicinal plants [9] as they have offered more authentic natural sources of active pharmacological ingredients [10].

1.1 Blessings of medicinal plants

Recently, due to the prominent side effects of updated synthetic drugs and escalating contraindications about their consumptions, a great attempt has been made to enhance the utilization of diverse medicinal plants [11]. Medicinal plants have played a vital and integral role in healthcare system from the earliest period of time, and some diverse types of instances of this blessing are described below [12].

Analgesic:

Opioids (morphine) can bind with cerebral opioid receptor and can modify the pain sensation by exerting receptor-mediated function and eventually will show analgesic effect [13, 14] and exert their analgesic effect. All the cannabis and cannabinoids had been consumed to relieve pain [15].

Anticancer:

Medicinal-plant-derived constituents such as vinblastine, vincristine from alkaloids *Vinca rosea* demonstrate anticancer activity [16].

Antihypertensive:

A plenty of medicinal plants were suggested by the ancient communities for the management of hypertension that may introduce a new area of research on the antihypertensive activity, [17, 18] such as reserpine from *Rauwolfia serpentine*.

Antidiabetic:

Medicinal plants such as *Acacia arabica*, *Eucalyptus globulus* may improve insulin secretion from pancreatic beta cell, thereby capable of exhibiting antidiabetic property [19].

Besides this overall pharmacological coverage, medicinal plants may have thousands of phytoconstituents, for instances, compound atropine from *Atropa belladonna* exhibits antispasmodic activity, ephidrine from *Ephedra vulgaris* might have bronchodialating effect.

Our present study is to represent the blessings of medicinal plants, which are readily available in our nature. I have already discussed a little bit about diversity of bioactive compounds in the above section, and it actually clarifies that nature may conserve every type of remedy related to the pathological state of human body. Actually, most of marketed drugs were being explored with the help of the concept of biodiversity of medicinal plants. As disease state does not consider any class of people such as rich, poor, middle-class, allergic people (to synthetic drug), suburb, or any city belonging people, so we should have developed our dependency on bioactive constituents containing medicinal plants, which will be economically affordable rather than synthetic drug. My research work was related to identifying the medicinal plant having great biological activity, which will be very cheap in source and obviously included to our daily food supplement. I have chosen black pepper (BP) (*Piper nigrum)* shown in **Figure 1** as my research topic where my prime concern was to identify bioactive compound (antioxidant activity containing) and correlate the biodiversity of that compound in nature.

1.2 Black pepper

1.2.1 Scientific name: Piper nigrum *Linn*

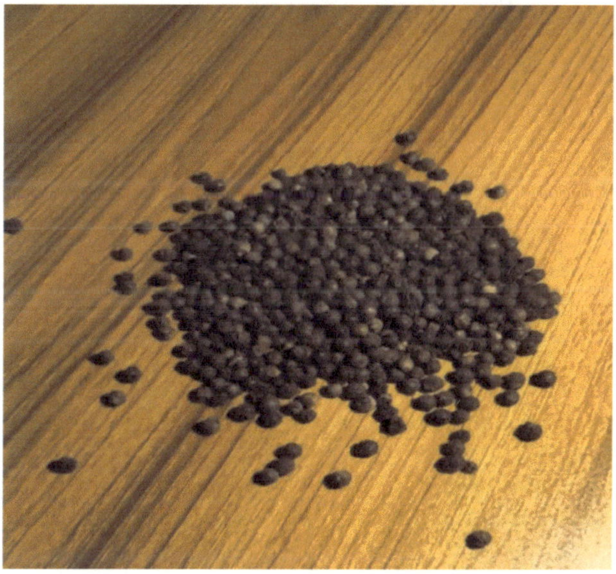

Figure 1.
*Black pepper (*Piper nigrum*) [20].*

1.2.2 Etymology of black pepper

The etymological background of black pepper was so complex, some believe that the word pepper has come from old English pipor, Latin pipor, and Sanskrit pippali for "long pepper." Besides this, people were using the word pepper to indicate the unrelated new word chili pepper (genous capsicum) during sixteenth century [21].

1.2.3 History of black pepper

Black peppercorns were explored stuffed in the nostril of Ramesses II, placed there as a part of the mummification rituals shortly after his death in 1213 BOE [22]. Someone has perceived that the black pepper was used in ancient Egypt, and it arrived in the Nile from south Asia. Black pepper is mainly popular in south Asia, southeast India, and is native to Kerala, a southwestern coast of India [23, 24].

1.2.4 Production and trade of black pepper (BP)

Ethiopia was the world's largest manufacturer and exporter of BP in 2019 producing 374,413 tonnes or 34 % of the world's total according to **Figure 2**. The rest of the major producers were Vietnam, Brazil, Indonesia, India, China, and Malaysia. Internationally pepper production has varied annually, which is dependent on the crop management, disease, and environmental impact [26, 27].

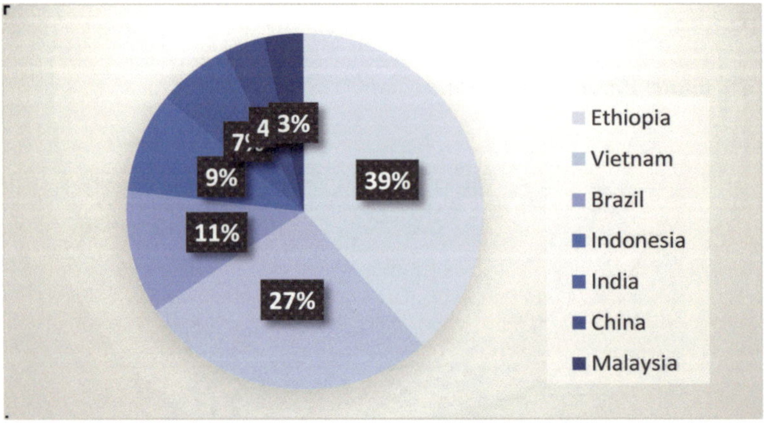

Figure 2.
Graphical representation of black pepper production, 2019 [25].

1.2.5 Perspective regarding antioxidant

I have tried my level best to isolate pure compound from black pepper and investigated a lot to identify antioxidant activity of that pure compound through a variety of in vitro evaluation processes.

The main target of any type of antioxidant or reductant is unpaired electron containing free radicals. Free radicals are a group of unstable chemicals, which can readily bind with biological components to be stable by gaining electrons resulting in destructive damage of cellular materials [28].

Typically, free radicals are formed inside the human body as a result of casual metabolic process, which can be both beneficial and harmful for human physiology; however, uncontrolled level of free radical production may initiate different types of diseases [29].

Antioxidant serves a prominent role in guarding our body from disease by neutralizing the series of oxidative stress produced by ROS [30]. During my research, my thought was to explore the free radical scavenging activity of sample and measure the extend of antioxidant power of that plant material as recent investigations have revealed that the plant-derived antioxidants with free-radical scavenging properties may have great therapeutic significance in diseases mediated by the free radicals such as neurodegenerative disease, autoimmune disorder, inflammatory disorder, cancer, and so on. To get relieved from these diseases, a variety of synthetic drugs are available in the market; however, these drugs may have some unavoidable side effects also. If people can put more concern on plant-based antioxidants, they will definitely get expected pharmacological effect with less or no side effects [31].

2. Experimental methodology with explaining physicochemical nature of that crystal compound

2.1 Extraction process

The extraction process has been completed based on the method described by Alam et al. [32]. About 500 g of sun and shade dried black pepper has been converted into powdered material by using a blender. Powdered black pepper was then transferred into an opaque bottle, and it has been filled with 1.5 L of methanol as a mother solvent for this experiment. The plant materials were kept in the bottle for 7 days with occasional shaking for better extraction (it can be called crude black pepper extract). The extracts of black pepper have been filtered through a fresh cotton plug and finally with Whatman No.1 filter papers. The filtrates found from the extraction process had been sent into the rotary evaporator (Bibby Sterlin Ltd, UK) to get a concentrated mass of sample under reduced pressure at 50 °C.

2.2 Fractionation (in between liquid-liquid solvent) process

The obtained concentrated mass of black pepper had been partitioned in between liquid solvent as described in **Figure 3**, where ultimately, a crystal seed fraction has been found.

2.3 Recrystallization process

Recrystallization is a process through which we can easily eradicate our desired compound from a mixture of undesired one by forming crystal of that compound in a favorable solvent, and simply it could be designated as an efficient method of purification [33]. As we have found a crystal seed fraction from black pepper, so we have utilized this recrystallization technique mentioned in **Figure 4** to purify crystal.

The flow diagram we have mentioned above had been followed to purify our crystal seed. The crystal seed was washed with KOH to remove resin-like compound or isomer of the crystal seed, and it was then filtered through filter paper for preliminary purification. Now it has been treated with petroleum ether for recrystallization and warmed up the combination to dissolve it at 50 °C. After that, the mixture was cooled to form crystal. The crystal is filtered for final purification.

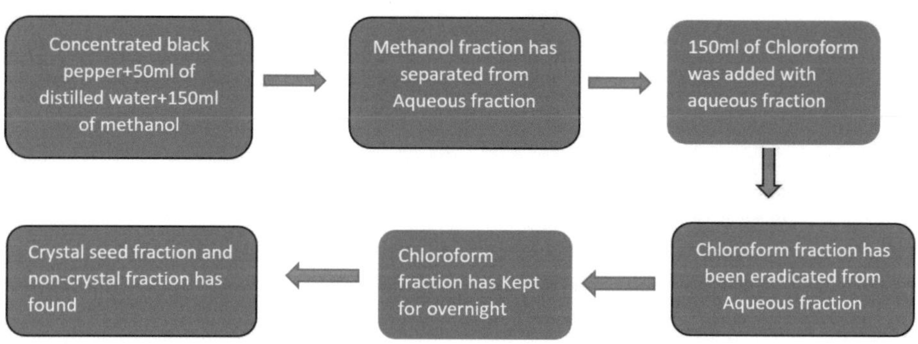

Figure 3.
Overall fractionation process of crude extract of black pepper in between liquid-liquid solvent.

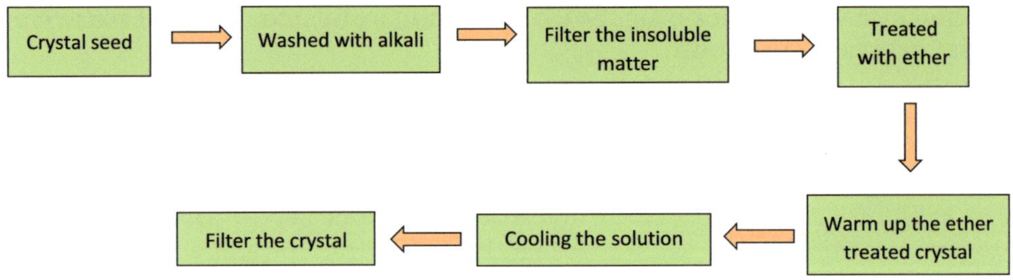

Figure 4.
Recrystallization technique for crystal seed produced from chloroform fraction.

2.4 Thin-layer chromatography (TLC)

It is the most convenient way to eradicate individual constituents from a mixture of compounds by using stationary phase and mobile phase, and the formation of a single spot actually indicates the presence of pure compound [34].

The spotted TLC paper was placed into the TLC chamber in such a way that the spot can stay just above the surface of the solvent system. After running of the solvent through a specified limit, then the operation was discontinued, and the TLC paper is dried in air. By treating with specified vanillin-sulfuric acid spray reagent, the paper was observed under UV light of different wavelengths to locate spots, so that can easily explore different types of medicinal constituents [35]. The paper was inserted into an iodine chamber to confirm about the spot is formed, and at last, I identified only single spot for the obtained crystal, which was examined under UV light and iodine chamber (**Figure 5**).

2.5 Calculating the R_f value of crystal

In TLC study, the retention factor has been utilized to screen and analyze the phytocompounds. The R_f value is a ratio of the distance moved by the compound and

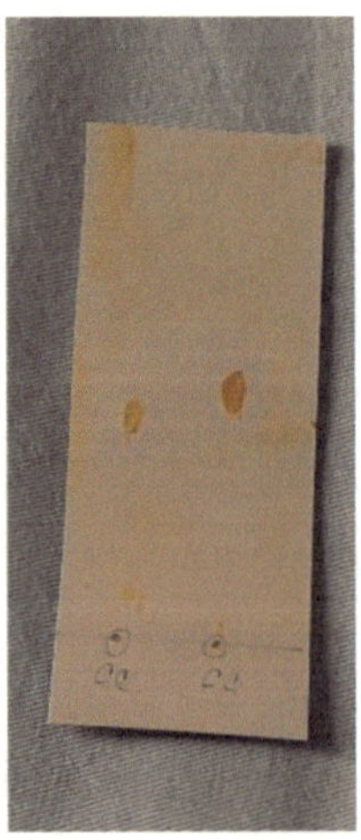

Figure 5.
TLC of crystal compound (CC) after spraying vanillin-sulfuric acid spray reagent.

the distance moved by the solvent. The obtained R_f value for crystal compound was found as 0.43.

2.6 Visual identification crystal

The crystal was light brown in color, and visually it was a needle-like structure, which has been shown in **Figure 6**.

2.7 Solubility of crystal compound

After doing a plethora of experiments, it has been found, as seen **Table 1** that the crystal compound was readily soluble in chloroform and likely insoluble in water.

2.8 Melting point

The melting point of that crystal was near 127°*C*.

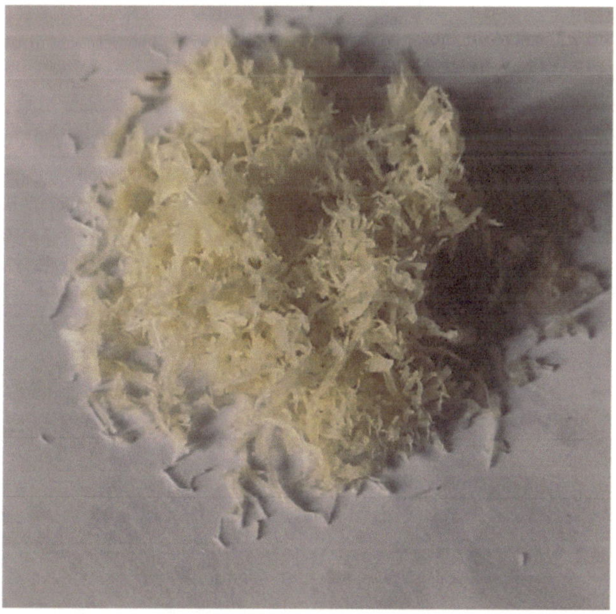

Figure 6.
Isolated crystal compound found in black pepper.

Solvent name	Solubility
Water	42 mg/L (likely insoluble)
Alcohol (ethanol)	1.5 gm/14.4 ml
Di-ethyl-ether	1 gm/35 ml
Chloroform	1 gm/1.5 ml

Table 1.
Solubility of crystal compound found through experimental method.

2.9 Boiling point

The crystal was so sensitive to increased level of heat, and it had been totally destructed during checking boiling point. So, the crystal material does not have any fixed boiling point.

2.10 Phytochemical contents

Alkaloid test for crystal (found from chloroform fraction of crude black pepper extract) had shown strong positive result according to **Table 2**, which clarifies that the crystal may have alkaloid compounds [36–38].

After comparing the physicochemical properties of crystal compound with standard one [39], it could be predicted that the crystal may be piperine.

3. In-vitro free radical scavenging assay with results interpretation

3.1 DPPH radical scavenging activity of different fractions of plant materials

Free radical scavenging ability of different fractions of sample had been evaluated by DPPH radical scavenging assay according to Blois and Desmarchelier et al. [40, 41]. The hydrogen atom donating capability of the plant extractives was estimated by identifying the color change of samples with 2,2-diphenyl-1-picrylhydrazyl (DPPH). DPPH exhibits made violet/purple color in samples having antioxidant property, and it was then faded into yellowish color. 2.4 ml of DPPH solution was mixed with 1.6 ml of sample solution at different concentration. The reaction mixture has been vortexed and left it for 30 min in a dark place at room temperature. The absorbance was taken for individual fractions at different concentration via spectrophotometer at 517 nm. Butylated hydroxy toluene had been used as standard. The percentage of DPPH radical scavenging activity was calculated by the following equation:

$$\%\text{DPPH radical scavenging activity} = \{(A0 - A1)/A0\} \times 100$$

where A_0 represents the absorbance of the control, and A_1 represents the absorbance of the sample materials. Then % of inhibition has been plotted against

Phytochemical test	Crystal compound (found from chloroform extract of black pepper)
Alkaloids	+++
Glycosides	−
Tannins	++
Steroids	−
Saponins	−
Carbohydrates	+
Terpenoids	+

Table 2.
Phytochemical contents explored in crystal (found from chloroform fraction of crude black pepper extract).

concentration, and the IC_{50} was calculated graphically. The same experiment was repeated for three times with every fraction at each concentration.

3.1.1 Data interpretation of DPPH radical scavenging assay

According to **Table 3**, it could be easily assumed that the crystal compound may have a great antioxidant power as the data for that compound had shown a nearly similar value of standard catechin. The IC_{50} value was so small, which was an indication for strong free radical scavenger.

3.2 Hydroxyl radical scavenging activity of different fraction of plant materials

Hydroxyl radical scavenging activity of samples has been evaluated according to the method of Halliwell et al. [42]. Hydroxyl radical has been generated by the Fe^{3+} -ascorbate-EDTA-H_2O_2 system, which is known as Fenton reaction. The overall reaction mixture was a combination of phosphate buffer solution, $FeCl_3$, EDTA, 2-deoxy-d-ribose, and sample extracts at different concentration. After that, it was placed into water bath at 36°C, and the reaction was initiated after addition of ascorbic acid and H_2O_2. The reaction had started, and it was sent for incubation at 36°C for maximum 1 hour, simultaneously thiobarbituric acid and HCl were added. The solution was heated for around 15 min at 100 °C followed by immediate cooling with water. The absorbance was taken at 532 nm, and it will reflect the free radical scavenging capability of samples by inhibiting the oxidation process in 2-deoxy-d-ribose in the presence of hydroxyl radical, and the ability was evaluated by using the following formula

Name of sample	Concentration (μg/ml)	% of scavenging (Mean±S.D)	IC_{50} (μg/ml)
Catechin (Standard)	0.78	19.09 ±0.01	3.2
	1.56	27.58±0.021	
	3.125	45.46±0.015	
	6.25	69.55±0.031	
	12.5	87.86 ±.02	
	25	94.39 ±0.0058	
	50	94.39±0.0058	
	100	94.39±0.0058	
Crystal compound (Pure)	1.56	27.67±2.006	4.1
	3.125	34.27 ±0.657	
	6.25	63.26 ±2.75	
	12.5	75.58±0.811	
	25	85.30±1.109	
	50	88.55 ±1.017	
	100	89.30±0.630	

Table 3.
DPPH radical scavenging data analysis for standard catechin and crystal compound.

Percentage of hydroxyl radical scavenging activity = [A0 − (A1 − A2] × 100/A0]

where A_0 represents the absorbance of control without any sample. A_1 represents the absorbance after incorporating the sample and 2-deoxy-D-ribose. A_2 represents the absorbance of the sample without adding 2-deoxy-d-ribose. IC_{50} was investigated graphically after plotting percentage of inhibition against concentration into the graph, and the test had been repeated for three times for individual concentration of samples.

3.2.1 Data interpretation of hydroxyl radical scavenging assay

The outcome of this assay was also close to standard one according to **Table 4**, where the IC_{50} for standard catechin was 31.77 (μg/ml), and for crystal, it was 35.01 (μg/ml).

3.3 Superoxide radical scavenging capability

This experiment had been completed based on the method mentioned in [43]. Superoxide radical scavenging assay actually estimated the scavenging efficiency of sample by reducing the nitro blue tetrazolium (NBT) by providing electron. The reaction mixture or solution was a combination of nonenzymatic phenazine methosulfate (PMS), nicotinamide adenine dinucleotide (NADH), phosphate buffer, and samples with various concentrations, and it was then incubated for 5 min at room temperature. The PMS-NADH system created free radical in the solution mixture. In the presence of sample solutions, the NBT was reduced into purple formazan. The overall activity has been evaluated by taking absorbance via spectrophotometer at 562 nm. All the tests had been operated for three times for better accuracy and blank has been determined to calculate the amount of formazan that has been produced, and quercetin has been taken as a standard for this experiment.

Name of sample	Concentration ($\mu g/ml$)	% of scavenging (Mean±S.D)	IC_{50} (μg/ml)
Catechin (Standard compound)	25	49.10±0.032	31.77
	50	55.14±0.14	
	75	58.38±0.87	
	100	68.44±1.21	
	125	73.51 ±1.01	
	150	80.69 ±1.09	
Crystal compound (Pure)	25	47.98 ± 0.45	35.01
	50	54.90 ± 1.22	
	75	57.11 ± 1.11	
	100	66.80±1.51	
	125	72.79 ± 0.53	
	150	78.95 ± 0.29	

Table 4.
Hydroxyl radical scavenging data analysis for standard catechin and crystal compound.

3.3.1 Data interpretation of superoxide radical scavenging assay

According to **Table 5**, the IC_{50} value for catechin was 26.79 (μg/ml), and crystal compound was 29.04 (μg/ml), which was satisfactory result for this in vitro test.

3.4 Graphical presentation of cumulative data obtained from in vitro antioxidant assay

From the above graph, it can easily assumed that the crystal compound may have great antioxidant activity. We know that lower the value of IC_{50} actually enhances the probability of having better antioxidant power of sample. When performing DPPH free radical scavenging activity, the sample had shown a very low value (4.1 $\mu g/ml$) of IC_{50} close to standard catechin (3.2 $\mu g/ml$), which ultimately provided a confirmation about the antioxidant capability of plant material.

Like DPPH test, the hydroxyl free radical scavenging assay and superoxide radical scavenging assay also convey messages regarding the free radical scavenging power and oxidant neutralizing potency of plant materials or samples. The IC_{50} value for hydroxyl radical scavenging assay of crystal compound was found as 35.01 ($\mu g/ml$), which was near the value of standard catechin of 31.77 ($\mu g/ml$); similarly the IC_{50} value was found as 29.04 and 26.79 for crystal compound and standard catechin, respectively, during super oxide radical scavenging assay (**Figure** 7).

3.5 Reducing power capacity assessment of crystal compound isolated from black pepper

The reducing power of plant material and standard material had been evaluated through the method of Oyaizu (1986) [44]. During this assay, the color of sample has

Name of sample	Concentration ($\mu g/ml$)	% of scavenging (Mean±S.D)	IC_{50} (μg/ml)
Catechin (Standard compound)	1.25	17.01±0.91	26.79
	2.50	19.25±0.53	
	5.00	24.27 ± 1.91	
	10	28.06 ±0.19	
	15	35.22 ±0.66	
	20	41.44 ±0.46	
Crystal compound (Pure)	1.25	15.29 ± 0.29	29.04
	2.50	19.01 ± 0.53	
	5.00	23.34 ± 0.26	
	10	26.51 ± 1.03	
	15	33.93 ± 1.13	
	20	39.32 ± 0.85	

Table 5.
Superoxide radical scavenging data analysis for standard catechin and crystal compound.

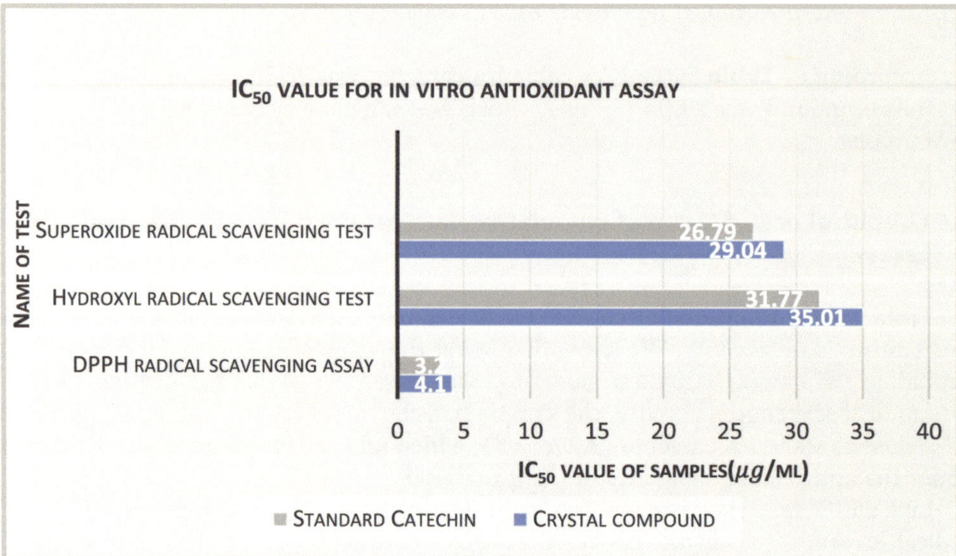

Figure 7.
Graphical representation for in vitro data analysis (DPPH radical scavenging test, hydroxyl radical scavenging test, superoxide radical scavenging test) regarding crystal compound found in black pepper and standard catechin.

altered to various shades of green and blue color based on the reducing capacity of the samples. The antioxidant compound actually served as reductant, and it induces reduction of the ferriccyanide to the ferrous form by releasing an electron. The overall reaction has been examined by monitoring the appearance of Perl's Prussian blue at 700 nm.

$$Fe^{3+} - \text{ferricyanide} + e \rightarrow Fe^{2+} - \text{ferrouscyanide}$$

Reducing power was investigated using the method developed by Oyaizu (1986). 2.5 ml of phosphate buffer (200Mm, p^H 6.6) and 2.5 ml 1% potassium ferricyanide had been incorporated into 2.5 ml of sample (crystal compound). The mixture was transferred into a water bath for maximum 20 min at 50°C followed by rapid cooling after warm-up. After that, 2.5 ml of 10% trichloro acetic acid was added, and it has centrifuged at 3000 rpm for 10 min. From the supernatant, 5 ml had been collected and being dispersed it into 5 ml of distilled water and 1 ml of ferric chloride, and absorbance has been taken, which reflects that higher the absorbance value, stronger the reducing capability. According to **Table 6**, the absorbance of crystal has increased with increasing concentration, which was close to similar with standard ascorbic acid.

3.5.1 Graphically presenting the data obtained from the reducing power assessment

It has been identified that the reducing power assay of crystal compound was slightly discriminable with standard ascorbic acid at low concentration; however, the difference between plant material and standard has diminished with escalating concentration with giving high absorbance value as shown in **Figure 8**.

Name of sample	Concentration ($\mu g/ml$)	Absorbance Mean±S.D
Ascorbic acid (Standard compound)	5	1.326 ±0.116
	10	2.119±0.116
	20	2.455±0.116
	40	2.5973 ±0.116
	80	2.756±0.1160
Crystal compound (Pure)	5	0.526 ±0.045
	10	0.842±0.127
	20	1.326±0.116
	40	2.119±0.1160
	80	2.59 ±0.106

Table 6.
Reducing power capacity assessment data analysis for standard ascorbic acid and crystal compound.

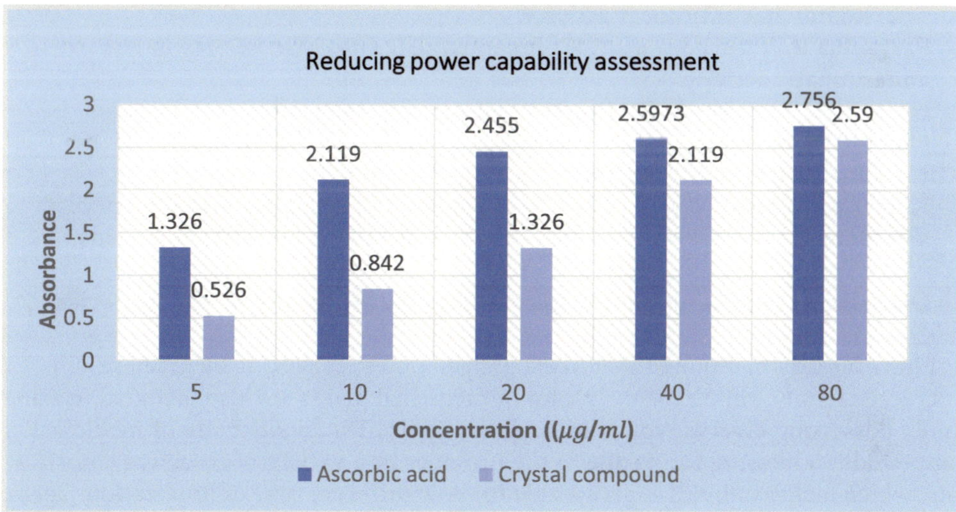

Figure 8.
Graphical representation of in vitro data analysis (reducing power capacity assessment) regarding standard ascorbic acid and crystal compound isolated from black pepper.

4. Discussions

4.1 Discussions regarding in vitro test

So, the overall in vitro antioxidant assay could be concluded that the obtained crystal compound (may be piperine) may have strong antioxidant power. By comparing with standard compound (catechin, ascorbic acid), the prediction could be extended that the black pepper is a great source of antioxidant compound with specifying the crystal constituent (may be piperine) as a prominent free radical scavenger.

4.2 Discussions regarding biodiversity of black pepper

The diversity of plant-derived medicinal constituents assists in a plenty of ways to enrich our research for instances in drug design and development. My current research was focused on merely to explore the free radical scavenger; however, my theoretical research through existing research article has claimed that piperine (crystal material) may exist in a lot of medicinal plants such as *Piper longum*, *Piper officinarum* rather than *Piper nigrum* (black pepper) also [45, 46].

Besides the antioxidant capability of piperine, the existing research has mentioned that it has a cluster of pharmacological implications also, which actually introduce the biodiversity of the piperine found in black pepper.

Li S, Wang C *et al.*, 2007 show that piperine could be effective against corticosterone-mediated depression.
Taqvi SI, Shah AJ *et al.*, 2008 have identified antihypertensive effect of piperine.
Bang JS, oh da H *et al.*, 2009 have observed that piperine found in black pepper may exhibit both antiarthritic and anti-inflammatory activity.
Manoharan S, Balakrishnan S *et al.*, 2009 have found that probably the piperine of *piper nigrum* has anticancer activity.
Parganiha R, Verma S *et al.*, 2011 invented that *Piper nigrum* may have in vitro antiasthmatic activity.
Hussain A, Naz S *et al.*, 2011 found that piperine may enhance saliva and pancreatic enzyme secretion, thereby accelerating the digestion process by reducing gastric emptying time.
Kumar KP, Vanaja M *et al.*, 2014 have explored that the leaf and stem of *piper nigrum* might possess antibacterial coverage against plant microorganisms.

4.3 Discussions regarding biodiversity of Piperaceae family or piper species

I have already mentioned that black pepper (*Piper nigrum*) is included in piperaceae family; simultaneously a lot of medicinal plants are also included in same family possessing diverse type of biological activity. The biodiversity of medicinal compound is a blessing for us due to the presence of a variety of bioactive constituents, which makes individual plants able to show different type of implications against several types of diseases or pathological conditions, and some of these are explained below.

Piper longum L. utilized as an antidote to snake bite, scorpion stings. Besides this, it can be applied in chronic bronchitis, cough, and cold [47].
Piper betle L. has a lot of implications such as in cuts, boils, scabies, mouth odor, cough remedy, bronchitis, and nosebleed [48].
Piper aduncum L. may have utilization in stomach aches, vaginitis, influenza, rheumatism, cough, fever, and general infections [49].
Piper aborescens Roxb. could be used in rheumatism, cytotoxic activity, and antiplatelet aggregation [50].
Piper capense L.F. might have application in renal disorder, gonorrhoea, syphilis, abdominal pain, enteritis, and asthma [51].
Piper ovatum Vahl possesses anti-inflammatory and analgesic activity [52].
Piper retrofractum Vahl can be consumed as digestive aid, stimulant, carminative, and in intestinal disorders, postpartum treatment (women) [53].

Piper tuberculatum Jacq. had been used as antidiuretic, analgesic, sedative, and antidote for snake bites [54].

5. Conclusions

Nowadays, we are suffering from several types of physiological abnormalities due to environmental impact or changes in lifestyle, which ultimately develop a lot of diseases that lead to acute or chronic effect on health. Now we are really blessed as nature has provided a plethora of medicinal plants in our surroundings, and we just need to identify them with their perfect implication. My overall research work was based on one type of plant with identifying bioactive compound with its pharmacological application; moreover, I have tried my best to explain how diversity of bioactive compound varies from one medicinal plant to another.

From the above analysis, it is clear that same type of plant may be applicable in different types of diseases, which is called biodiversity of medicinal plant. The invention of every type of synthetic drugs directly or indirectly relieson natural sources as the basis of production of synthetic drug comes from medicinal plants. With increasing diseases, the demand of synthetic drug has also proliferated, which may be life-threatening for humans as formulated drugs can cause damage of vital organs with frequent consumption. To diminish the side effects or dependency on synthetic drugs, we should raise awareness as early as possible.

Our future plan could be implemented by cultivating medicinal plants commercially and procuring the identified bioactive compound with maintaining all the precautions and after that it will be possible to mitigate the demand on synthetic drug. This is the ultimate way to get beneficial effect from medicinal plants and the adverse effect of marketed drug might be avoided.

Author details

Murshida Mollik[1*] and Hamidul Islam[2]

1 Department of Pharmacy, University of Rajshahi, Bangladesh

2 Department of Internal Medicine, Rajshahi Medical College, Bangladesh

*Address all correspondence to: m.mollik13@gmail.com

References

[1] Gu J, Gui Y, Chen L, Yuan G, Lu HZ, Xu X. Use of natural products as chemical library for drug discovery and network pharmacology. PLoS One. 2013; **8**:e62839

[2] Shinde VM, Dhalwal K, Potdar M, Mahadik KR. Application of quality control principles to herbal drugs. International Journal of Phytomedicine. 2009:**1**(1):4-8

[3] Sumner J. The Natural History of Medicinal Plants. London: Timber Press; 2000. p. 16

[4] Yarnell ND, Abascal JD. Dilemmas of traditional botanical research. Herbal Gram. 2002;**55**:46-54

[5] Fabricant DS, Farnsworth NR. The value of plants used in traditional medicine for drug discovery. Environmental Health Perspectives. 2001;**109**(Suppl 1):69-75

[6] Millie G. Reading medicine in the Codex De La Cruz Badiano. Journal of the History of Ideas. 2008;**69**(2): 169-192

[7] Swerdlow JL. Modern Science Embraces Medicinal Plants. Nature's Medicine: Plants that Heal. Washington, DC: National Geographic Society; 2000. pp. 110-157

[8] Brater D, Walter DJ. Clinical pharmacology in the middle ages: Principles that presage the 21st century. Clinical Pharmacology and Therapeutics. 2000;**67**:447-450

[9] Heidarian E, Rafieian-Kopaei M. Protective effect of artichoke (*Cynara scolymus*) leaf extract against lead toxicity in rat. Pharmaceutical Biology. 2013;**51**(9):1104-1109

[10] Nelson D, Cox M. Lehninger Principles of Biochemistry. 4th ed. New York: W.H. Freeman and Company; 2005. pp. 1-41

[11] Nasri H, Shirzad H. Toxicity and safety of medicinal plants. Journal of Herbal Medicine Plarmacology. 2013; **2**(2):21

[12] Sen S, Chakraborty R, Sridhar C, Reddy YSR, De B. Free radicals, antioxidants, diseases and phytomedicines: Current status and future prospect. International Journal of Pharmaceutical Sciences Review and Research. 2010;**3**:91-100

[13] Rauf A, Uddin G, Siddiqui BS, Khan A, Khan H, Arfan M, et al. In-vivo antino-ciceptive, anti-inflammatory and antipyretic activity of pistagremic acid isolated from Pistacia integerrima. Phytomedicine. 2014;**21**: 1509-1515

[14] Smith HS, Raffa RB, Pergolizzi JV, Taylor R, Tallarida RJ. Combining opioid and adrener-gic mechanisms for chronic pain. Postgraduate Medicine. 2014; **126**(4):98-114

[15] Jensen B, Chen J, Furnish T, Wallace M. Medical marijuana and chronic pain: A review of basic science and clinical evidence. Current Pain and Headache Reports. 2015;**19**(10):50-54

[16] Aggarwal BB, Harikumar KB. Potential therapeutic effects of curcumin, the anti-inflammatory agent, against neurodegenerative, cardiovascular, pulmonary, metabolic, autoimmune and neoplastic diseases. The International Journal of Biochemistry & Cell Biology. 2009;**41**: 40-59. DOI: 10.1016/j.biocel.2008. 06.010

[17] Ahmadi BB, Bahmani M, Tajeddini P, Kopaei RM, Naghdi N. An ethnobotanical study of medicinal plants administered for the treatment of hypertension. Journal of Renal Injury Prevention. 2016;**5**(3):123-128

[18] Lee SY, Hur SJ. Antihypertensive peptides from animal products, marine organisms, and plants. Food Chemistry. 2017;**228**:506-517

[19] Bhushan MS, Rao CHV, Ojha SK, Vijayakumar M, Verma A. An analytical review of plants for anti diabetic activity with their phytoconstituent & mechanism of action. International Journal of Pharmaceutical Sciences and Research. 2010;**1**(1):29-46

[20] *Piper nigrum*. Germplasm Resources Information Network (GRIN). Agricultural Research Service (ARS), United States Department of Agriculture (USDA). Retrieved 2 March 2008

[21] "Pepper (noun)". Online Etymology Dictionary, Douglas Harper. 2016. Retrieved 24 September 2016

[22] Fitzgerald S. Ramses II, Egyptian Pharaoh, Warrior, and Builder. Minneapolis, Minn: Compass Point Books; 2008. p. 88. ISBN 978-0-7565-3836-1. Retrieved 29 January 2008

[23] Harrison, Paul (2016). "What Are the Different Kinds of Peppercorns?." Food Republic. Retrieved 21 November 2019

[24] Sen CT. Food Culture in India: Food Culture around the World. Westport, Conn: Greenwood Publishing Group; 2004. p. 58. ISBN 9780313324871

[25] "Pepper (piper spp.), World regions/Production/Crops for 2019 (from pick list)." Food And Agriculture Organization of the United Nations: Statistical Division (FAOSTAT). 2019. Retrieved 25 March 2021

[26] "Karvy's special Reports — Seasonal Outlook Report Pepper" (PDF). Karvy Comtrade Limited. 15 May 2008. Retrieved 29 January 2008

[27] Krishnamuthry KS, Kandiannan K, Sibin C, Chempakam B, Ankegowda SJ. Trends in climate and productivity and relationship between climatic variables and productivity in black pepper (*Piper nigrum*). Indian Journal of Agricultural Sciences. 2011;**81**(8):729-733

[28] Leong CN, Tako M, Hanashiro I, Tamaki H. Antioxidant flavonoids glycosides from the leaves of *Ficus pumila* L. Food Chemistry. 2008;**109**: 415-420

[29] Valko M, Leibfritz D, Moncol J, Cronin MT, Mazur M, Telser J. Free radicals and antioxidants in normal physiological functions and human disease. The International Journal of Biochemistry & Cell Biology. 2007;**39**:44-84

[30] Huda AW, Munira MA, Fitrya SD, Salmah M. Antioxidant activity of *Aquilaria malaccensis* (Thymelaeaceae) leaves. Pharmaceutical Research. 2009;**1**: 270-273

[31] Nagulendran KR, Velavan S, Mahesh R, Begum VH. *In vitro* antioxidant activity and total polyphenolic content of *Cyperus rotundus* rhizomes. E-Journal of Chemistry. 2007; **4**:440-449

[32] Alam AHMK, Rahman MAA, Baki MA, Rashid MH, Bhuyan MSA, Sadik MG. Antidiarrhoeal principle of Achyranthes ferruginea Roxb. and their cytotoxic evaluation. Bangladesh Pharmacology Journal. 2002;**12**:1-4

[33] Harwood LM, Moody CJ. Experimental Organic Chemistry: Principles and Practice. Oxford, Boston, England: Blackwell Scientific Publications; 1990

[34] "Applications of Thin Layer Chromatography." News-Medical.net. 2018-09-18. Retrieved 2018-09-25

[35] Reich E, Schibli A. High-Performance Thin-layer Chromatography for the Analysis of Medicinal Plants. New York: Thieme; 2007

[36] Peach K, Tracey MV. Modern Methods of Plant Analysis,Vol. 4, p. 373

[37] Merck E. Dyeing reagents for Thin Layer Chromatography, 39, 1980

[38] Furniss BS et al. Vogels Text book of Practical Organic Chemistry. 4th ed. London: Longman; 1978. p. 934

[39] Barroso GM. Sistematica de angiosperms do Brazil. Sao Paulo: Epu Usp; 1978

[40] Blois MS. Antioxidant determinations by the use of a stable free radical. Nature. 1958;**181**:1199-1200

[41] Desmarchelier C, Bermudez MJN, Coussio J, Ciccia G, Boveris A. Antioxidant and prooxidant activities in aqueous extract of Argentine plants. International Journal of Pharmacognosy. 1997;**35**:116-120

[42] Halliwell B, Gutteridge JMC. Free radicals in biology and medicine. Clarendon Press. 1989;**3**:617-783

[43] Fontana M, Mosca L, Rosei MA. Interaction of enkephalines with oxyradicals. Biochemical Pharmacology. 2001;**61**:1253-1257

[44] Oyaizu M. Studies on products of browning reactions: antioxidant activities of products of browning reaction prepared from glucose amine. Japanese Journal of Nutrition. 1986;**44**: 307-315

[45] Oersted. Über das Piperin, einneuesPflanzenalkaloid [Onpiperine, new plant alkaloid]. JournalfürChemie und Physik. 1820;**29**(1):80-82

[46] Flueckiger FA, Hanbury D. Pharmacographia: London: Macmillan & Co; 1879. p. 534 584

[47] Chahal R, Ohlyan A, Kandale A, Walia SP. Introduction, phytochemistry, traditional uses and biological activity of genus *Piper*: A review. International Journal of Current Pharmaceutical Review and Research. 2011;**2**:131-144

[48] Ahmad GI. Medicinal plants used by Kadazandusun communities around rocker range. In: ASEAN Review of Biodiversity and Environmental Conservation (ARBEC), January, 1–10. 2003

[49] Martínez PT, Rosa LC, Ming MO, Marques M, Angela AM. Extraction of volatile oil from Piper aduncum leaves with supercritical carbon dioxide; 2003, pp. 65–70

[50] Tsai FP, Lee CC, Wu CY, Duh T, Ishikawa JJ, Chen YC, et al. New cytotoxic cyclobutanoid amides, a new furanoid lignan and anti-platelet aggregation constituents from *Piper arborescens*. Planta Medica. 2005;**71**: 535-542

[51] Tekwu T, Askun V, Kuete AE, Nkengfack B, Nyasse F, Etoa VPB. Antibacterial activity of selected Cameroonian dietary spices ethno-medically used against strains of

Mycobacterium tuberculosis. Journal of Ethnopharmacology. 2012;**142**:374-382

[52] Silva EH, Endo CV, Nakamura IE, Svidzinski A, De Souza MCM, Young T, Ueda-Nakamura DA. Chemical composition and antimicrobial properties of Piper ovatum Vahl., Molecules. 2009;**14**:1171-1182

[53] Muharini Z, Liu W, Lin P. New amides from the fruits of *Piper retrofractum*. Tetrahedron Letters. 2015; **56**:2521-2525

[54] Bezerra DP, Ferreira PMP, Machado CML, Aquino NC, Silveira ER, Chammas R, et al. Antitumour efficacy of *Piper tuberculatum* and piplartine based on the hollow fiber assay. Planta Medica. 2015;**81**:15-19

Section 3

Pharmacological Values of Medicinal Plants

Chapter 12

Detailed Pharmacognostical Standardization Studies on *Calotrophis Procera* (Aiton) Dryand Fruit

Devarakonda Ramadevi, Radha Rayi,
Subhash Chandra Mandal, Ganga Rao Battu, Babu Gajji
and Pachaiyappan Jayaram

Abstract

Calotropis procera (Aiton) Dryand (Asclepiadaceae) is very well-known latex wild plant, it is covered in tropical Asia and Africa, traditionally as well as medicinally the plant has been used for insecticidal, antimalarial, antiviral, antimicrobial, analgesic, antifertility, antitumor, antihyperglycemic, hepatoprotective, anti-inflammatory, antidiarrhoeal, anticonvulsant, oestrogenic, antidiabetic and anthelmintic activity. For this reason, the main theme of research work was carried out on detailed pharmacognistical studies for quality control and standardization and this study provides the basis for the herbal remedy and provide physiological information about plant species. This research is helpful to identify and estimate the purity of the drug and can also be used to screen for adulteration and gives a drug quality. This comprehensive research work is for identification, collection, authentication and it is easy to identify the adulterants. Detailed macroscopical, T.S, L.S, Powder microscopy, Physicochemical parameters, Extractive values, Fluorescence, Preliminary Phytochemical studies were performed as per the standard. It is a very important research work and the author had has been established the evaluation standards for a medicinal plant. This evaluation is for the authentication of a fruit plant of *Calotropis procera* and the fruit physiology is useful for both qualitative and quantitative estimation of the medicinal herbal drugs.

Keywords: *Calotropis procera* fruit, pharmacognostical standardization, quality control

1. Introduction

Calotropis procera (Aiton) Dryand has a powerful insecticidal, antimalarial, antiviral, antimicrobial, analgesic, antifertility, antitumor, antihyperglycemic, hepatoprotective, anti-inflammatory, antidiarrhoeal, anticonvulsant, oestrogenic, antidiabetic and anthelmintic activity. Actually where ever observe, the plant is available on road sides

[1]. *C. procera* is a flowering plant and it belongs to *Asclepiadaceae* family. The *C. procera* is native to Africa, Arabian Peninsula, Western Asia, the Indian Subcontinent and Indo-China. The plant is a most powerful latex plant, and it attracts insects. In this plant plenty of medicinally useful secondary metabolites are present, those are cardenolides, terpenoids and anthocyanins, for this reason, collected fresh fruit and coarse powder for detailed anatomy of T.S, L.S RLS, LRS, powder microscopy, Extractive, Fluorescence and Preliminary Phytochemical studies. Therefore, present work was carried out to study the Pharmacognostical studies on the fruit of *Calotropis procera* (Aiton) Dryand.

2. Methods

2.1 Material and methods for pharmacognostical studies

2.1.1 Collection of plant materials for authentication and for anatomical studies

The collected fruit of *Calotropis procera* from Titupathi, at the area of nalla malai forest, India. *C. procera* collected in the month of December, 2018. The *C. procera* fruit was authenticated by Prof. K. Madhavachetty, Department of botany, Srivenkateswara University, Andhra Pradesh, India. The given voucher for specimen number is 1221, deposited at College of Pharmaceutical Sciences, Andhra University.

2.1.2 Collection of specimens

The collected plant species are too healthy for the proposed study, specimens of organs are cutted and soaked into 70% of 90 ml ethyl alcohol, 5 ml of Formalin and 5 ml of acetic acid [2]. The organs of specimens are dehydrated with graded series of tertiary butyl alcohol as per the guidelines given by sass, 1940. Specimens of infiltration were carried by the addition of 58–60°C paraffin wax until TBA solution attained super saturation.

2.1.3 Morphological features

These plant species grow in all types of soil, collected fresh fruit from 2.8 mts height of the plant early in the morning at 6 am from red loamy soil land. The fruit is 10 cm long and 6 cm width outer and inner layer are green in color and in every fruit contains a plenty of brown-colored seeds more over every seed length is 5.5 to 6.0 mm length and 3.7 mm width many of white silky hairs are present and each silky hair length is 40 to 50 mm in long. Fruit color of the *Calotropis procera* is green in color, strong pungent odor, taste is characteristic/bitter and gummy in nature. Soluble in benzene, ethyl acetate, ethanol, methanol and hydroalcoholic.

2.1.4 Sectioning

The specimens of paraffin-embedded were sectioned with the help of a rotary microtome, the thickness of each section was 10–12 μm [3]. As per the standard method the obtained sections were stained in to toluidine blue [4] because toluidine blue is a polychromatic stain. The obtained strains are good because some phytochemical reactions were obtained. The obtained dye changed pink color to mucilage blue for the protein bodies, other sections are stained with safranin, fast green and iodine [5].

For studying the stomatal number, the pattern of venation and distribution of trichomes, sections of paradermal (sections taken parallel to the surface of leaf) as well as clearing of the leaf with 5% sodium hydroxide or epidermal peeling by partial maceration employing Jeffrey' s maceration fluid [5] were prepared. Glycerine mounted temporary preparations were made for macerated /cleared materials. Different parts of powdered materials were cleared with NaOH and mounted in glycerine medium after staining. Measurement of different cell components was studied.

2.1.5 Photomicrographs

Different magnifications of photographs are taken with the help of Nikon labphoto 2 microscopic unit, bright fields were used for normal observation. The polarized light was used for the identification of Different kinds of tissues, crystals, stone cells, starch grains, fibers, lignified and non-lignified cells. Since these obtained structures have fair finger print property, under polarized light they appear bright against the dark background. Magnifications of the figures are indicated by the scale –bars. Descriptive terms of the anatomical features are given in the standard anatomy books [6].

2.1.6 Instrumentation and technique

The obtained extracts and powder had examined under UV-light (254 nm, 354 nm) [7, 8]. The total ash value, Determination of Acid Insoluble Ash, Determination of Alcohol Soluble Extractive value, and Determination of Water-Soluble Extractive values in the obtained samples were performed, and in Loss on drying measured the amount of water and volatile oils, Swelling index, Foaming index were performed according to the standard procedure, for Extractive values, 2gms of an air-dried coarse powder of drug macerated with 40 ml of solvents (Hexane, Ethyl acetate, Chloroform, Acetone, Methanol and Distilled water) in a glass stoppered conical flask with frequent shaking for 6 hrs and then allowed to stand for 2 days, then filtered carefully, taking care against loss of solvent. The filtrate was evaporated in a silica crucible to dryness in the water bath and then dried 105° for 6 hrs, cooled in a desiccator for 30 min and weighed without delay [9]. Fluorescence Analysis of the drug was observed in UV light using various extracts of the drug. The drug powder was treated separately with different solutions [10, 11] and for Preliminary phytochemical studies. The prepared extracts were tested for the different types of chemical constituents present by known qualitative tests. The following tests were carried out on the extracts to detect various phytoconstituents present in them [12–14] were performed according to the official methods described in the Indian pharmacopeia (1996) and WHO guidelines on quality control methods -for medicinal plant materials.

3. Results and discussion

3.1 Anatomy of the fruit

The fruit of *Calotropis procera* is a double follicle that develops from bicarpellery apocarpous ovules. The mature fruit has fused stigma namely pentagonal stigma and the ovaries are free from each other. Later the stigma breaks and the two carpels become free from each other. The ovules develop into cylindrical, elongated fruits called follicles. The follicles are thick, soft and cylindrical. The ovules are many and attached to marginal placentum. When the follicles become fully matured they dehisce longitudinally along with the marginal layer of placental tissue.

3.2 Structure of the carpel

The carpel consists of the outer epicarp, middle mesocarp and inner endocarp (**Figure 1a**). The epicarp consists of an epidermal layer and inner thick compact parenchymatous tissue in which fairly prominent vascular strands are located (**Figures 2a** and **3a**). The inner pericarp is also thick with small circular, thin-walled compact.

Parenchymatous tissue (**Figures 2b** and **3b**) in the inner pericarp, the laticiferous canals are seen spreading in all directions. The middle part of the pericarp has wide air chambers and thin reticulate layers of parenchyma cells (**Figures 3a, b**) at certain places, thick horizontal layers of cells occur in between the outer and inner pericarp.

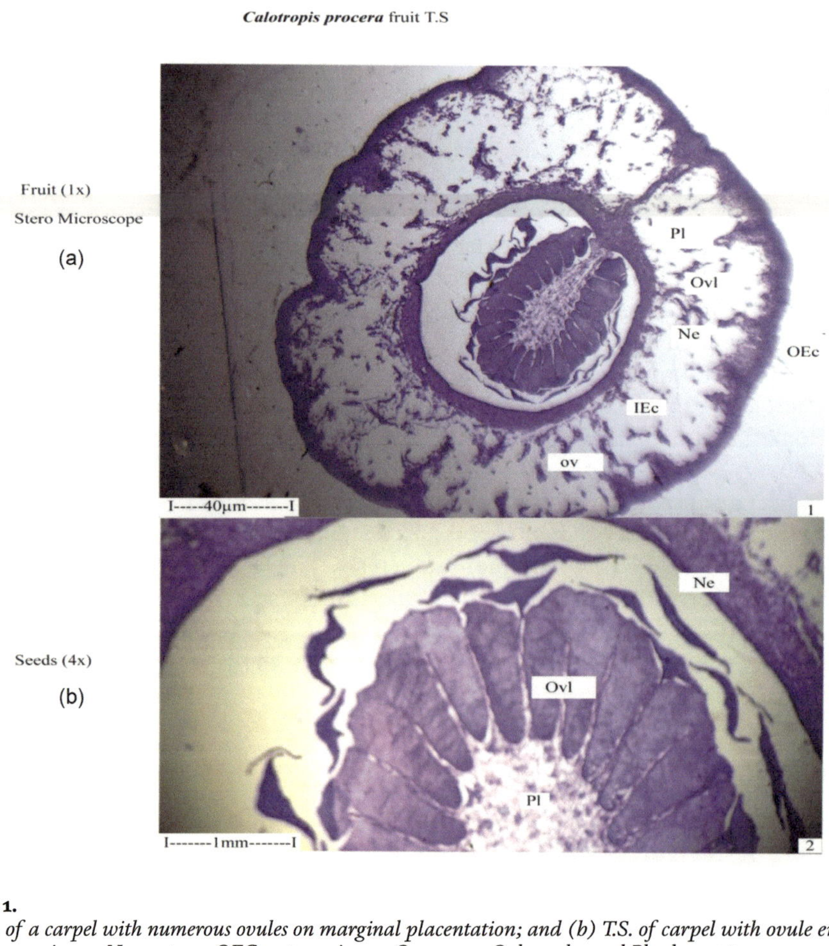

Figure 1.
(a) T.S. of a carpel with numerous ovules on marginal placentation; and (b) T.S. of carpel with ovule enlarged. IEP: inner epicarp; Ne: nectary; OEC: outer epicarp; Ov: ovary; Ovl: ovule; and Pl: plancenta.

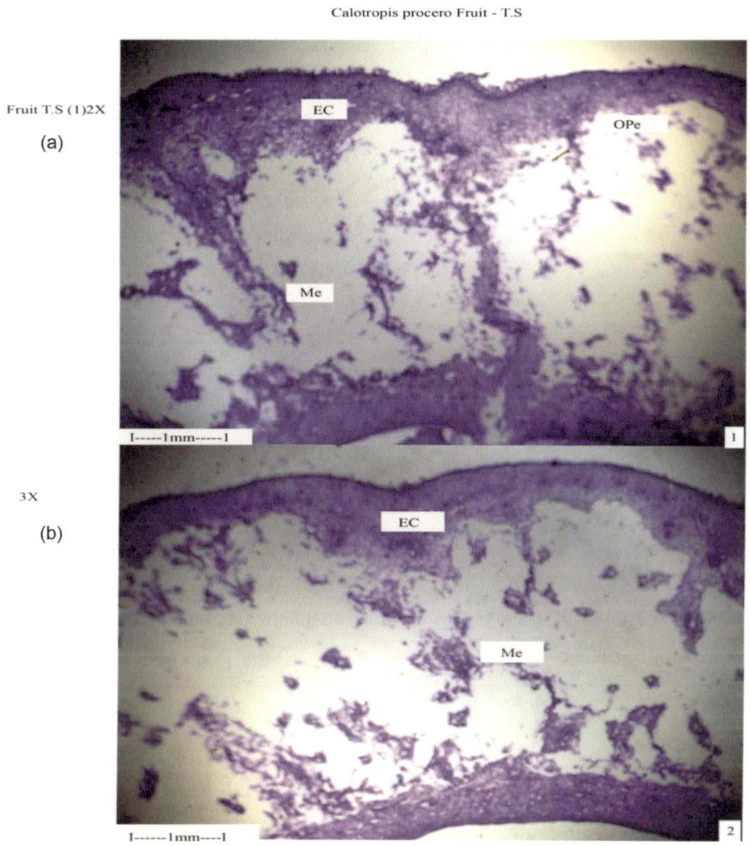

Figure 2.
(a) T.S. of pericarp: outer part; and (b) T.S. of pericarp: inner part. Ec: epicarp; IPe: inner pericarp; Ope: outer pericarp; and Me: mesocarp.

This horizontal plate of cells possesses small scattered vascular strands. In the outer pericarp also, there are numerous small vascular strands dispersed profusely in the parenchymatous ground tissue (**Figure 4a, b**).

3.3 Ovules and seeds

The ovules occur in marginal placentation a thick massive placental tissue occurs along one side of the carpel. On this elongated cylindrical placental tissue occurs, numerous club-shaped ovules (**Figures 1b**, 5, and **6a**).

The ovules are broad along the outer part and narrow towards the inner part (**Figure** 5). On the outer part of the carpel, there are numerous, curved elliptical, darkly stained appendages which are the nectarines (**Figures** 5 and **6a**, **b**).

3.4 Powder microscopy

In the powder preparation, fragments of tissues of the pericarp, seed coat and cell inclusions are seen. The inner surface of the pericarp consists of elongated, rectangular, thin-walled cells (**Figure 7a**). These cells have straight cell walls. The cells are parallel to each other forming a dense mat (**Figure 7a**). The outer surface of the pericarp

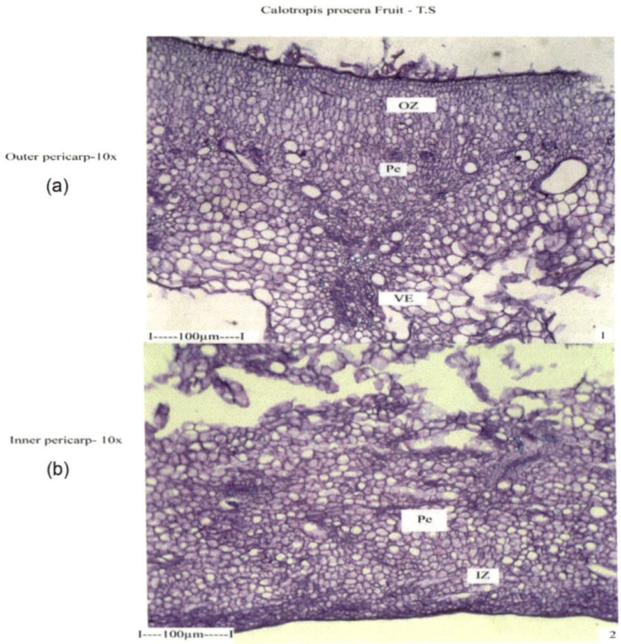

Figure 3.
(a) T.S. of pericarp outer part showing vascular elements; and (b) T.S. of pericarp inner part. IZ: inner zone; OZ: outer zone; Pe: pericarp; and Vs: Vascular strand.

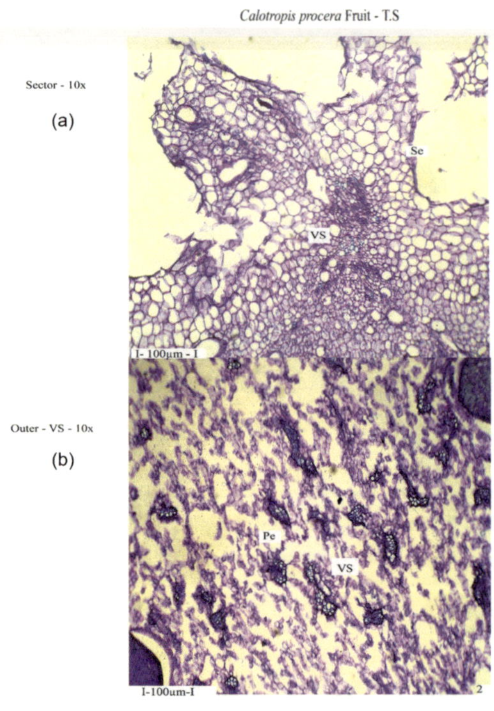

Figure 4.
(a and b) T.S. of pericarp with scattered vascular strands. Pe: pericarp; Se: segment of fruit wall; and Vs: vascular strand.

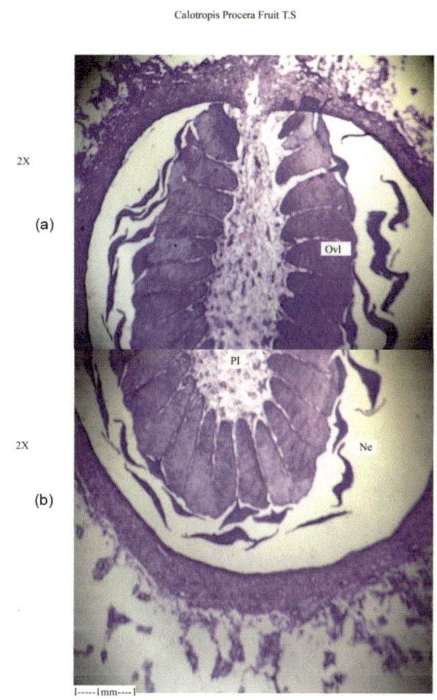

Figure 5.
T.S. of carpel enclosing a bundle of ovules in marginal placentation.Ne: nectary; ovl: ovule; Pl: placenta.

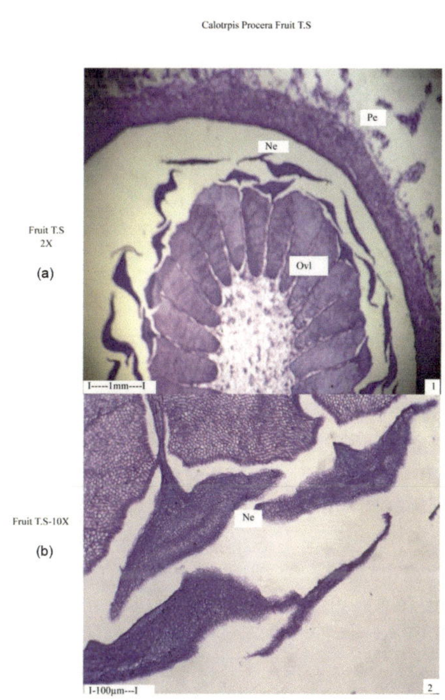

Figure 6.
(a) T.S. of carpel enclosing the ovules with peripheral nectarines; and (b) Nectaries enlarged. Ne: nectary; Ovl- ovule; and Pe: pericarp.

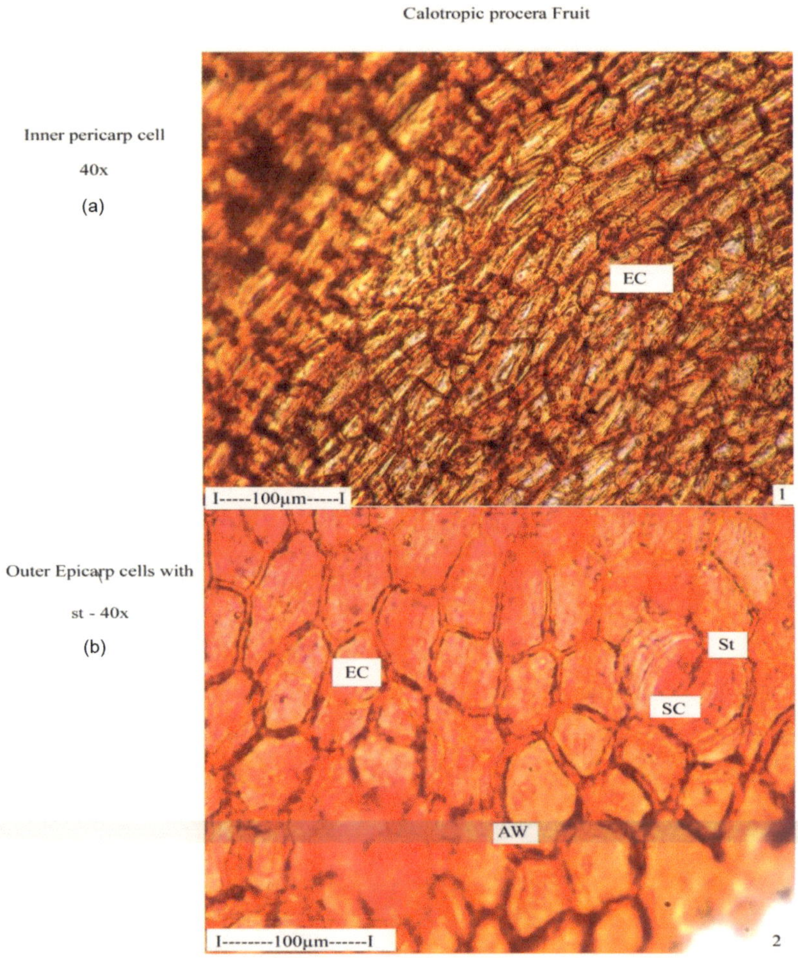

Figure 7.
(a) A piece of inner pericarp showing elongated compact parallel parenchyma cells; and (b) Surface view of the outer pericarp where the cells are polygonal with thick straight anticlinal walls and stomata. Aw: anti clinal wall; Ec: epidermal wall; Sc: subsidiary cell; and St: stomata.

consists of wide polygonal cells with thick, straight anticlinal walls. Stomata are also frequently seen on the outer epicarp. The stomata have narrow stomatal aperture and elliptical guard cells. The stomata appear to be paracytic type (**Figure 7b**).

Broken pieces of seed coats are frequently seen in the powder. The abundance of epidermal trichomes of non-gladular type are seen on the seed coat. The trichomes are thick at the base and become narrowly pointed at the tip. The cell walls of the trichome are thick and lignified and the cell lumen is narrow and canal like (**Figure 8a**, **b**). The trichomes are 130 μm long and 15 μm thick.

The epidermal cells of the seed coat are angular, polygonal and compact (**Figure 8a** and **9b**). Laticiferous canals are commonly present in the pericarp of the fruit. The laticiferous are long, canal-like, non-septate and unbranched. They contain dense white latex secreted from the laticifer (**Figure 9a**). The seeds have dense accumulation of different sizes of oil bodies. They appear white spherical bodies floating in water (**Figure 10a**). Prominent spherical or elliptical starch

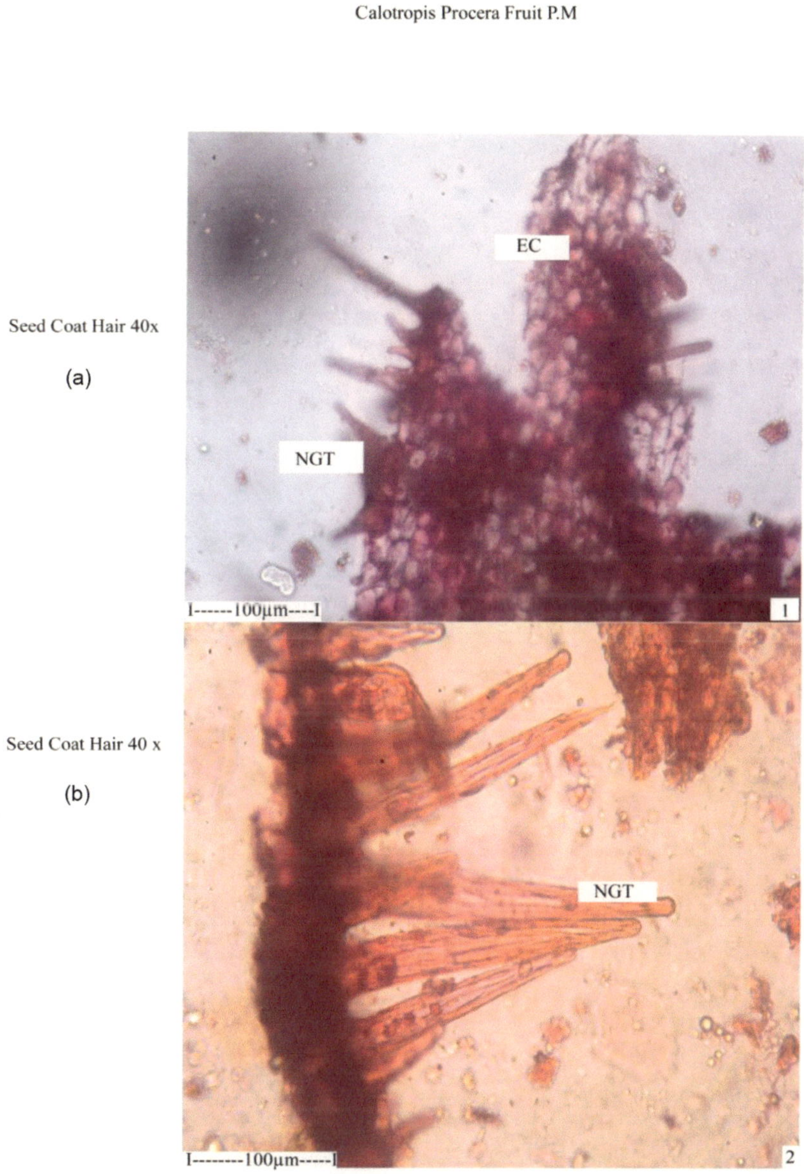

Figure 8.
(a) A broken piece of seed coat showing polygonal epidermal cells and non-glandular epidermal trichomes; and (b) Clusters of non-glandular trichomes seen in powder. Ec: epidermal cells; and NGT: non-gladular trichomes.

grains are common in the powder. When stained with IKI, the starch grains appear black or dark blue (**Figure 10b**). The seeds of *Calotropis* are flat, obovate and thin. One end of the seed is narrow and pointed. This pointed end of the seed bears a tuft of thin, white, soft trichomes. This tuft of trichomes is called coma. The trichomes of coma are also seen in the powder. These trichomes have thick walls and wide lumen. They are unicellular and unbranched. The trichomes are 30 µm thick (**Figure 10c**).

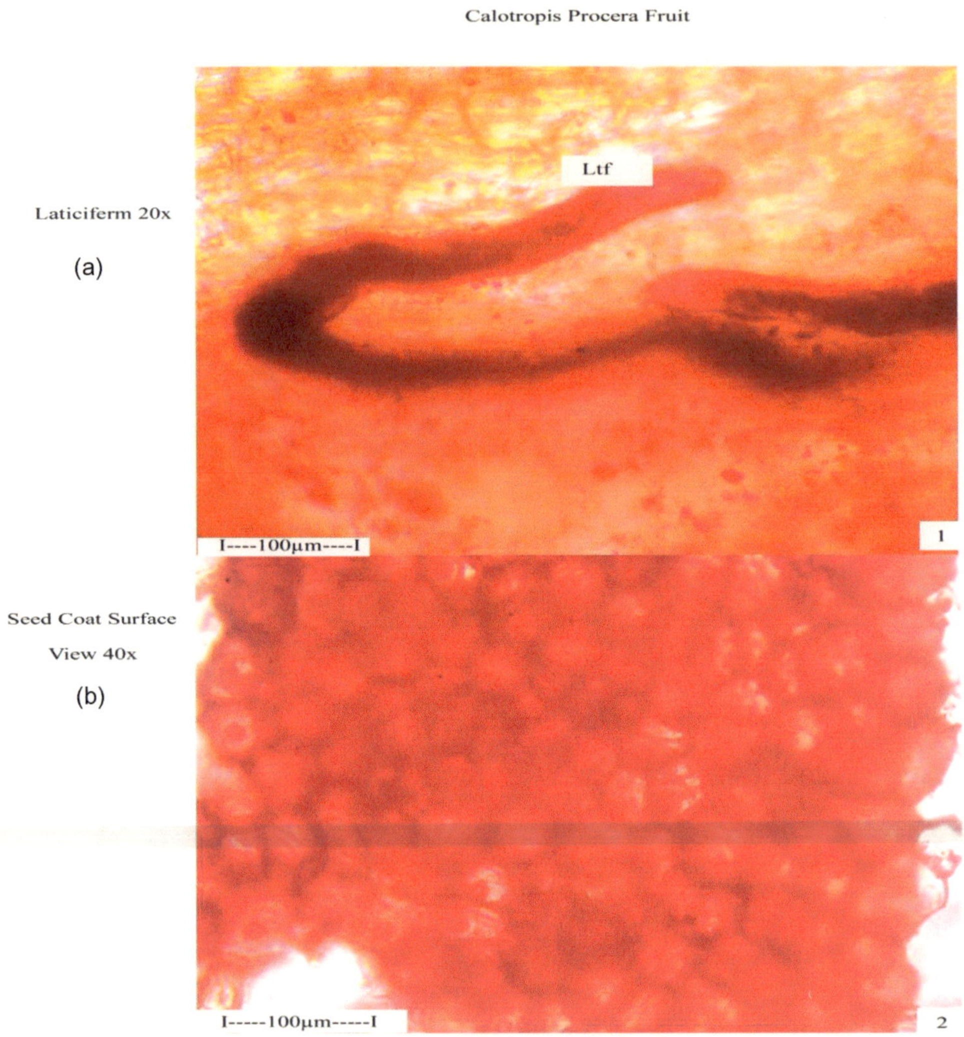

Figure 9.
(a) A piece of pericarp tissue with unicellular, unbranched laticiferous canal; and (b) Seed coat fragment showing thick-walled epidermal cells. Ec: epidermal cells; and LtF: laticifer.

The ash is mainly for the identification of carbonates, silicates, phosphates, sodium, potassium, calcium and magnesium without an organic matter. The obtained total ash value (11.4%), Water soluble ash (7.5), Acid insoluble ash (1.8), Foaming Index (<100), Swelling Index (52%), Loss on Drying (16.7%) And the extractive values are mainly for the estimation of primary and secondary metabolites in Petroleum ether (5.65%), it might be terpenoids, sterols, lipids and waxes and apart from Ethyl acetate extract (2.25%), Acetone extract (3.17%), Methanolic extract (4.53%) contains tepenoids, phenols, and glycoside containing components may be present. Distilled Water (10.11%) and Hydro-alcohol (6.05%) contains polyphenols, tannins and alkaloids present (**Tables 1–3**).

For herbal drugs, florescence analysis is very primary tool for the determination of constituents, this florescence analysis provides an informative data on nature of constituents [12]. The chemical reagents were used for the powdered drug analysis and

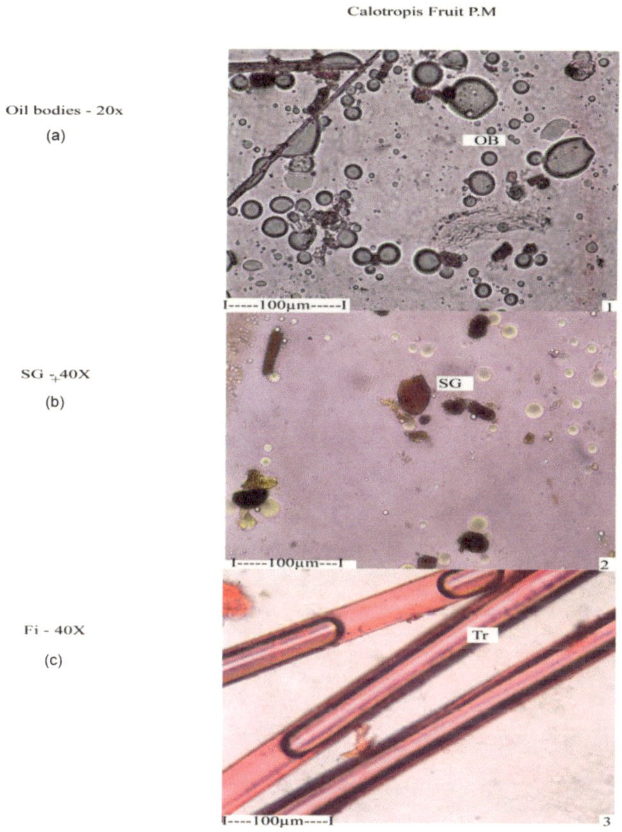

Figure 10.
Oil globules of different sizes found in the powder; (b) Starch grains stained with potassium iodide; and (c) Trichomes from coma of the seed. OB: oil bodies; SG: starch grains; and Tr: trichomes.

Parameters	Fruit
Color	Green
Shape	Been
Size	length10cm
Odor	Characteristic
Powdered drug study	
Color	Green
Odor	Characteristic
Taste	Strong Bitter
Filter paper test	

Table 1.
Morphological characters of Calotropis procera fruit.

observations are available in visible light and UV lights of Short and long wave lengths (**Table 4**).

The preliminary phytochemical screening on *Calotropis procera* was done by using hexane, n-butanol, ethanol, acetone, ethyl acetate, methanol and hydro alcoholic

Parameter	Percentage (%)
Total Ash	11.4
Water soluble ash	7.5
Acid insoluble ash	1.8
Foaming index	<100
Swelling index	52
Loss on drying	16.7

Table 2.
Results for physicochemical parameters.

Solvents	Percentage (%)
Petroleum ether	5.65
Ethyl acetate	2.25
Acetone	3.17
Methanol	4.53
Distilled water	9.11
Hydro-alcohol	6.05
± *Calculated as SEM of three reading.*	

Table 3.
Results of extractive values.

Chemical treatment	Day light	Fluorescence	UV longer (365 nm)	UVShort (254 nm)
Drug powder	Peanut Brownish green	Green	Dark green	Green
Hexane	Yellow	Yellowish green	Green	Green
Ethyl acetate	Yellowish green	Greenish yellow	Reddish green	Light reddish green
Methanol	Yellowish green	Yellow	yellow	light green
Water	Brown	Dark brown	Light green	Green
Drug powder+1 N NaOH in methanol	Yellowish green	Yellowish green	yellow	Light green
Drug powder+1 N NaOH in water	Brownish green	Brownish green	green	light green
5% NaOH	Light Yellowish	Yellowish	Yellowish	Yellowish
10% NaOH	Yellowish	Yellowish	Yellowish	Yellowish
Powder+1 N Hcl solution	Dark brown	brownish	Light green	Colorless
Powder+50% HNO3	Yellow	Reddish yellow	Dark green	Light green
Powder+50%H2SO4	Light green	Reddish yellow	Light green	Light green
Powder+50% HCl	Dark brown	brownish	Light green	Colorless
5% FeCl3	Greenish peanut	Brownish green	Darkish yellowish red green	yellowish red green
Powder + picric acid	Orange yellowish green	Yellowish green	Darkish yellowish red green	yellowish red green
Powder +Dil. NH4	Dark green	Greenish peanut	Greenish peanut	Greenish peanut
Powder + acetic acid	Dark yellowish green	yellowish green	Dark green	Light green

Table 4.
Fluorescence analysis on Calotrophis procera fruit.

DOI: http://dx.doi.org/10.5772/intechopen.104549

Phytochemical analysis	**Hexane**	**N- Butanol**	**Ethylacetate**	**Ethanol**	**Acetone**	**Methanol ic**	**Hydroalcoh olic**
1. Alkaloids							
(a) Mayer's test	–	–	+	+	+	++	+
(b) Hager's test	–	–	+	–	–	++	++
(c) Dragendroff's test	–	–	++	–	–	++	++
2.Carbohydrates							
(a) Molisch's test	+	+	++	++	++	++	++
(b) Fehling's test	+	++	+	+	+	+	+
(c) Barfoed's test	+	++	++	++	++	++	++
(d) Benedict's test	+	+	+	+	+	++	++
3. Glycosides							
(a) Borntrager's test	+	++	++	+	++	++	++
(b) Legal's test	+	+	++	++	++	++	++
(c) Keller-Kiliani test	+	+	++	++	++	++	++
4. Phenols and Tannins							
(a) Ferric chloride test	+	++	++	++	++	+	++
(b) Gelatin test	–	++	++	++	++	+	++
(c) Lead acetate test	+	++	++	++	++	+	++
5. Flavonoids							
(a) Alkaline reagent test	–	+	+	+	+	+	+
(b) Schinoda test	–	++	++	++	++	++	++
(c) Zn + HCl test	+	++	++	++	++	++	++
6. Test for fixed oils							
(a) Spot test	++	++	++	++	++	++	++

Phytochemical analysis	Hexane	N- Butanol	Ethylacetate	Ethanol	Acetone	Methanol ic	Hydroalcoh olic
7. Saponins							
(b) Foam test	++	+	++	++	++	++	++
8. Proteins and Aminoacids	+	+	++	++	++	++	++
(a) Millon's test	+	+	+	+	+	+	+
(b) Biurettes test	+	+	+	+	+		+
(c) Ninhydrin test	+	+	+	+	+	+	+
9. Terpenoids/ Phytosterols							
(a) Libermann-Burchard test	++	++	++	++	+	+	+
10. Test for triterpenoids							
(a) Salkowski test	++	++	++	++	+	+	+
11. Gum and Mucilages							
(a) Alcoholic precipitation test	++	++	++	++	++	++	+
12. Test for lignin	+	++	++	++	++	++	+
(a) Lignin test	+	++	++	++	++	++	+
(b) Labat test	+	++	++	++	++	++	+

"–" indicates absent; "+" indicates presence; and "++" indicates more intense.

Table 5.
Preliminary phytochemical tests for identification of the class of primary and secondary components in the extract of C. procera fruit.

extracts. N-butanol, ethyl acetate and acetone extracts gave positive tests for alkaloids, carbohydrates, proteins, glycosides and terpenoids. Hexane extract showed only for terpenoids. Hydro alcoholic extract showed the presence of Alkaloids, Carbohydrates, Tannins, and Glycosides. Methanolic extract showed the presence of Alkaloids, Carbohydrates, Phenols, Tannins, Flavonoids, Proteins and Glycosides (**Table 5**).

4. Conclusion

This plant species is available in overall tropical and subtropical countries, standardization of crude drug work is the primary reference to do further step. Herbal Drugs are useful for different ailments in different countries. Pharmacognostical, Preliminary Phytochemical evaluation studies provide us a basis to establish the quality protocols of any medicinal herbs. In the Introduction part, we described about the species of plant, macroscopical, microscopical, preliminary phytochemical, ash values, extractive values, fluorescence analysis are the main tools to identify the purity, presence and absence of certain chemical groups in a herbal drug. Pharmacognostic studies are mainly useful for quality of a herbal drugs [15]. Breakthroughs and Innovations of *Calotropis procera* is mainly useful for insecticidal, antimalarial antiviral, antimicrobial, analgesic, antifertility, antitumor, antihyperglycemic, hepatoprotective, anti-inflammatory, antidiarrhoeal, anticonvulsant, oestrogenic, antidiabetic and anthelmintic activity etc. reported. In Andhra Pradesh state in India no pharmacognostic research work was established. So, this work is a primary and important for further studies. *Calotropis procera* is helpful for establishing the correct identification of a plant and the plant will be main tool for standardization, characterization and identification of *Calotropis procera* fruit. The plant is also helpful for the other research studies.

Acknowledgements

I thank to Prof. P. Jayaraman (Plant Anatomy Research Centre (PARC), helped me a lot when I worked on microscopical study. Prof B. Ganga Rao was given me a permission to do my research in Pharmacognosy and Phytochemistry Laboratory, AU College of Pharmaceutical Sciences, Andhra University, Visakhapatnam, Andhra Pradesh. Prof. SC Mandal and Dr. Radha Rayi, reviewer for comments on before draft of the manuscript and they helped me a lot to do this work and I thank to Dr. Babu Gajji was given me a lot of support to carry out my research.

Funding

This research work is one of my part of P. D. F research work and was fully funded under the grant number File No: PDF-SS-2015 – AND – 2017 10498 by University Grants Commission, New Delhi.

Conflicts of interests

Conflicts of interest is none.

Availability of data and material

Availability of data and material is our own, based on the literature we have written ourselves.

Ethics approval and consent to participate

Not applicable.

Consent for publication

Not applicable.

Author details

Devarakonda Ramadevi[1*], Radha Rayi[2], Subhash Chandra Mandal[3], Ganga Rao Battu[4], Babu Gajji[5] and Pachaiyappan Jayaram[6]

1 AU College of Pharmaceutical Sciences, Pharmacognosy and Phytochemistry Division, Andhra University, Visakhapatnam, India

2 Institute of Pharmaceutical Technology, Sri Padmavathi Mahila Visvavidyalayam, Tirupathi, Andhra Pradesh, India

3 Division of Pharmacognosy, Faculty of Engineering and Technology, Department of Pharmaceutical Technology, Kolkata, India

4 Adikavi Nannaya University, Rajamandry, Andhra Pradesh, India

5 CCRAS (Central Council Research in Ayurvedic Sciences), Ministry of Ayush, Uttar Pradesh, India

6 Plant Anatomy Research Centre (PARC), Chennai, Tamil Nadu, India

*Address all correspondence to: ramapathi.addepalli@gmail.com

References

[1] Murti Y, Yogi B, Pathak D. Pharmacognostic standardization of leaves of *Calotropis procera* (Ait.) RBr. (Asclepiadaceae). International Journal of Ayurveda Research. 2010;**1**(1):14-17

[2] Ramadevi D, Jayaram P, Rao BG, Babu ND, Radha R. Detailed pharmacognostical studies on Apocyanaceae family root from wild of South India (Andhra Pradesh). Journal of Pharmacognosy and Phytochemistry. 2020;**9**(5):2229-2239

[3] Johansen DA. Plant Microtechnique. New York: McGraw Hill Book Co; 1940

[4] Brien O, Feder CPN, Cull ME. Polychromatic staining of plant cell walls by toluidine blue-O protoplasma. Protoplasma. 1964;**59**:364-373

[5] Sass JE. Elements of Botanical Microtechnique. New York: McGraw Hill Book Co; 1940

[6] Easu K. Plant Anatomy. New York: John Wiley & Sons; 1964. p. 767

[7] Vijaya P, Devarakonda R. Preliminary phytochemical tests, physicochemical parameters and anti bacterial activity of *Artocarpus heterophyllus*. Indian Journal of Research. 2017;**6**(4):624-626

[8] Fahn A. Plant Antomy. Oxford, England: Pergamous Press; 1974. p. 611

[9] The Indian Pharmacopoeia. 1996. New Delhi: Govt. of India Publication Anonymous

[10] Chase CR, Pratt R. Fluorescence of powdered vegetable drugs with particular reference to development of a system of identification. American Pharmaceutical Association. 1949;**38**:324-331

[11] Brindha P, Sasikala P, Purushothamam KK. Bulletin of the Medical Ethno Botany Research. 1981;**3**:84-86

[12] Corner EJH. The Seeds of Dicotyledons. London: Cambridge University Press; 1976

[13] Lala PK. Lab Manuals of Pharmacognosy. Calcutta: CSI Publishers and Distributors; 1993

[14] Kokate CK, Purohit AP, Gokhale SB. Pharmacognosy. CBS Publishers and Distributors; 2005. p. 169

[15] Majid N, Nissar S, Raja WY, Nawchoo IA, Bhat ZA. Pharmacognostic standardization of Aralia cachemirica: A comparative study. Future Journal of Pharmaceutical Sciences. 2021;7:33

Chapter 13

Effect in Human Gene Regulation of Food-Derived Plant miRNAs

Daniel Sanchez Romo, Benito Pereyra Alferez and Jorge Hugo Garcia Garcia

Abstract

MicroRNAs (miRNAs) are a class of non-protein-coding RNA molecules with the ability to regulate gene expression at the posttranscriptional level, abundant in plants and animals, showing a high level of similarity due to their mechanism of biogenesis and action; this led to the discovery of cross-kingdom interactions mediated by exogenous miRNAs, which has been one of the most important scientific advances in recent years. Because plant-derived miRNAs after ingestion can be resistant to diverse conditions such as crossing the gastrointestinal tract in mammals, entering the body fluid and regulating the expression of endogenous mRNAs. Suggesting that food-derived plant miRNAs may control genes in humans through cross-kingdom regulation. More importantly, plant miRNAs may be a new class of molecules with utility in future epigenetic regulatory therapy applications in a wide range of diseases, demonstrating a new and highly specific strategy for the regulation of gene expression.

Keywords: MicroRNA, cross-kingdom, mRNA, human, gene regulation

1. Introduction

In recent years, non-protein-coding RNA transcripts have been associated to regulatory functions in plants and animals, particularly micro RNAs (miRNAs), a class of endogenous single-stranded molecules of ~22 nucleotides, transcribed by polymerase II from MIR genes, involved in negative regulatory activities at the posttranscriptional level in plants and mammals [1–3]. The sophisticated mechanism used by miRNAs for the regulation of their targets is based on perfect or near-perfect complementarity binding of miRNAs at the ORF, 5'UTR and 3'UTR sites of mRNA, resulting in repression of translation or degradation of the messenger [4]. Since the identification of the first miRNA in *Caenorhabditis elegans* [5], until now according to the miRBase version 22.1 database (http://www.mirbase.org, accessed April 2021), a total of 38,589 hairpin precursors (pre-miRNAs) from 217 organisms have been recorded. In plants some crucial functions of miRNAs have been established such as response to developmental signals, auxin responsive factors (ARFs), pathogen infection, cell division, metabolism, etc. [6, 7]. In human, these small transcripts have been found to endogenously participate in some diseases such as diabetes, cancer, heart disease, tumors, atherosclerosis, or biomarkers in early stages of particular diseases [8, 9]. Recently, several studies have shown that plant miRNAs can enter the gastrointestinal tract through food in humans, be identified in various tissues and circulatory system, perceiving genes in humans as potential regulatory targets [10]. Because exogenous miRNAs and endogenous miRNAs have no distinguishing characteristics from each other, therefore, it will be recognized as an endogenous miRNA [11]. The cross-kingdom regulation by miRNAs has developed a series of investigations because it is important to determine the effects of miRNAs from plants on gene expression in humans when they enter the human body through food [11–13].

This chapter will provide a brief overview of the evidence about the impact of exogenous miRNAs and their direct influence on various biological processes in human, a cross-kingdom approach.

2. Biogenesis and mechanisms of miRNAs

miRNAs are single-stranded strands of approximately (18–24) base pairs evolutionarily conserved in diverse species [14], they are transcribed by RNA polymerase II (pol II) giving rise to a miRNA-primary, which possesses a stem-loop structure [3]. The first step occurs in the nucleus and is carried out by cleavage by the RNase III enzyme Drosha and the double-stranded RNA-binding protein (dsRNA) DGCR8, generating a product of approximately 60 nt called pre-miRNA that contains an overhang of 2–3 nt [15]. It is subsequently exported to the cytoplasm by the pre-miRNA/Exportin5/Ran-GTP complex, in the cytoplasm GTP is hydrolyzed to GDP inducing the release of the pre-miRNA [16], then processed by the Dicer RNaseIII protein producing an RNA duplex of approximately 22 nt [17]. The double strand is incorporated into the RNA-induced silencing complex (RISC), a protein nuclease complex, an Argonaute protein (Ago2), and a double-stranded RNA-binding protein, upon incorporation one strand of the duplex is degraded and the other remains as a mature miRNA, with the faculty to regulate the expression of a target mRNA [17, 18]. While, in plants, the pri-miRNA synthesized by pol II in the nucleus is processed by an enzyme of the RNase III family DICER-LIKE1 (DCL1), resulting in an miRNA/miRNA duplex chain. To stabilize and protect from degradation these duplexes are 2′-O-methylated at the 3′-ends by a Hua Enhancer 1 (HEN1) methyltransferase [19]. Finally, one strand of the duplex is incorporated into AGO1 in the cytoplasm to form the RISC complex [20]. One of the determining mechanisms in the interaction of miRNA and its target mRNA is the seed region (nt 2–8, [21]). The seed region appears to be the most important site for miRNA recognition of its target [22]. In addition to taking advantage of its utility to predict regulatory targets, in relation to the characteristics in the mRNA sites necessary for the effective recognition of the miRNA [23].

3. Endogenous function by plant and animal miRNAS

In recent years, a series of research studies have provided important advances in plant molecular biology by discovering that plants can regulate the expression of some target genes [11, 24, 25]. The first example was discovered in the nematode *C. elegans* by studying the lin-4 gene in 1993, which transcribes for a small RNA complementary to some segments of the 3'untranslated region of an mRNA encoding the LIN-14 protein, required for passage to the late larval stage [26]. However, up until 2000, it was reported that these small transcripts, due to their size, had gone unnoticed. But they were the perpetrators of gene silencing. Over time it has been evidenced that animals and plants produce a large amount of miRNAs [27]. In plants miRNAs generally participate in the process of growth, disease resistance, morphogenesis, leaf and fruit size, development of healthy plant characteristics, and the process of flowering regulation [6]. Some miRNA targets have been found to be involved in processes such as metabolism, transport, cell signaling, stress response [28]. In humans, it is estimated that approximately 60% of all protein-coding genes are miRNA targets, which could practically affect most physiological processes in the body [29]. The miRNAs are, therefore, important regulatory molecules of gene expression in different processes, such as neuronal development, differentiation, proliferation, and cell survival [2]. There is evidence that miRNAs offer potential targets for the diagnosis, prognosis, and treatment of a wide variety of diseases [21]. More importantly, miRNA profiles, especially in serum, plasma, and urine, have been reported to be closely related to various diseases and disease states, including cancer, diabetes, inflammation, infections, and tissue injury [8, 14, 30].

4. Resistance and stability of plant miRNAs to harsh conditions

In 2017, Luo et al. [31] revealed the abundance of miRNAs in *Zea mays* (maize), obtaining 18 highly represented miRNAs, fresh maize samples were subjected to different treatments (elevated temperature and pressure, starch dextrinization, and protein denaturation), observing that all miRNAs resisted the treatments with only decrease in their concentrations. Subsequently, the resistance of miRNAs from maize was analyzed in pigs, due to their attractive biomedical model and organ size similar to humans, they were fed for 7 days with fresh maize-based diet, and evaluated the presence of the 18 previously selected miRNAs, finding 16 in tissue and serum. They verified the crossing of the gastrointestinal barrier of synthetic miRNAs and evaluated by bioinformatic analysis the possible regulation of pig genes by miRNAs from maize, obtaining as a result that MIR164a-5p has CSPG4, OTX1, and PLAGL2 genes as a potential target, with a reduction in the gene activity compared with control. This suggests the likelihood that exogenous miRNAs regulate gene expression in endogenous mRNAs in a similar way to mammalian miRNAs.

4.1 Mechanisms of transport and absorption

Exogenous miRNAs are selectively packaged into small microvesicles (MVs). MVs are a mixture of microparticles, exosomes, and other vesicular structures found in human plasma [12]. They are shed from epithelial cells under normal or pathological conditions and can enter the circulatory system to be transported. They contain receptors and ligands on the surfaces of the cells of origin, giving them the ability to interact with target cells and mediate intercellular communication. Exogenous miRNAs take advantage of this ability to regulate host cell gene expression. MVs serve as stable signaling molecules, they protect exogenous miRNAs against serum RNAases and facilitate their transport to target genes [12, 32–34]. They are classified according to their origin, size, and formulation mechanism: exosomes, microvesicles, and apoptotic bodies [35].

5. Regulation in human given by exogenous miRNAs from plant cross-kingdoms

5.1 MIR168a of plants first evidence of cross-kingdom regulation

The paradigm that miRNAs originated exclusively for endogenous assimilation was changed in 2012 by Zhang et al. [12], when the first evidence of cross-kingdom interactions was demonstrated by sequencing serum from men and women in China and finding present human and other animal miRNAs from dietary plant miRNAs, identifying MIR168a from *Oriza sativa* (rice), analyzed through bioinformatics, finding as a regulatory target the gene encoding for the low-density lipoprotein receptor adapter protein 1 (LDLRAP1). Confirming their various hypotheses on the regulation of the LDLRAP1 gene, predicted target of exogenous MIR168a, through an in vivo assay where serum and tissues were collected from mice previously fed with rice and in vitro transfecting HepG2 cells with MIR168a MVs, finding a decrease in the levels of the protein in vitro and in vivo, thus interfering with the cholesterol transport mechanism.

5.2 Stability and survival of plant miRNAs to the gastrointestinal tract in mammals

In a second approach to cross-kingdom approach, as far as was known, there was no major evidence demonstrating the survival of exogenous miRNAs to the gastrointestinal (GI) system, blood, or organs in mammals. Plant-derived MIR172 was detected in a range of 2–72 hours and remained stable in organs, tissues, feces, and blood in mice after being fed total RNA from *Brassica oleracea* in amounts between 10 and 50 μg, administered orally, suggesting the survival of exogenous miRNAs to the GI system, organs, and blood in mammals [36]. Subsequently, in another study in humans [10], 16 miRNAs from plants were evaluated and detected after ingestion (ath-MIR156a, ath-MIR157a, ath-MIR162a, ath-MIR167a, ath-MIR168a, ath-MIR172a, ath-MIR172a, ath-MIR390a, osa-MIR528, ppt-MIR894, ath-MIR166a, ath-MIR158a, ath-MIR159a, ath-MIR160a, ath-MIR163a, ath-MIR169a, ath-MIR824). The concentrations of plant miRNAs were measured by qRT-PCR, in nine volunteers administered orally with 2.5 L of watermelon juice and 2.5 kg total mixture of other fruits, finding the presence of exogenous miRNAs (MIR156a, MIR157a, MIR162a, MIR167a, MIR168a, MIR172a, MIR390a, MIR528, MIR894, and MIR166a) in serum for up to 9 hours, demonstrating that a variety of exogenous plant miRNAs can be found in human plasma following ingestion.

5.3 Antiviral activity of miR2911 from plants

According to the authors Zhou et al. [37], the repercussions, given by exogenous miRNAs from plants, together with the mechanisms involved in absorption and transfer "remain largely unknown". In their study they sequenced the plant honeysuckle (HS, *Lonicera japonica*) used for thousands of years to treat influenza infection and were able to obtain a total of 148 miRNAs in their reads. Additionally, the plant was subjected to a decoction process, finding only the MIR2911 stable after treatment, remaining in high concentrations (0.2 g HS/ml), was 0.06 pmol/ml suggesting its stability due to its sequence and high GC content. Subsequently, mice administered with the 500 μl decoction product of the plant reached a peak in the concentrations of MIR2911 in plasma and lung 6 h post-administration and a decrease to a basal level after 12 h. A series of potential target genes for MIR2911 of different viruses such as H1N1, H3N2, H5N1, and H7N9 were found through bioinformatic analysis. In cell lines infected with H1N1 and transfected with synthetic MIR2911, they achieved a significant decrease in viral count due to the fact that the target genes, PB2 and NS1, are essential for its replication. The in vivo study demonstrated that miR2911 inhibited the replication of several IAV (influenza A viruses) including H1N1, H5N1, and H7N9, decreasing mortality in mice, being the first evidence of a natural product that directly targets and suppresses IAV. In addition, the authors in 2020 conducted an emerging investigation of MIR2911, now against the SARS-CoV-2 virus, the cause of COVID-19, severe acute respiratory syndrome, which spread rapidly around the world, causing an unprecedented pandemic. Among the results, the researchers were able to inhibit viral replication in vitro, using exosomes from serum of donors who consumed the plant decoction and exosomes of synthetic MIR2911, showing a very high antiviral activity of plant MIR2911 on SARS-CoV-2 virus replication, since bioinformatics results showed at least 179 putative binding sites for the miRNA on the SARS-CoV-2 genome, with 28 binding sites subsequently confirmed, indicating that the plant miRNA could inhibit the translation of almost all SARS-CoV-2 proteins [38].

5.4 Potential role of plant miRNAs in breast cancer

According to the potential function of plant miRNAs, the authors sought to clarify the influence of exogenous molecules on tissues outside the GI tract. By sequencing serum and tumor tissue samples from stage II and III breast cancer patients, plant miR159 was detected up to six times more frequently than plant miRNAs. The results showed a higher abundance of miRNA in healthy patients than in breast cancer (BC) patients and patients with metastasis. Therefore, it was proposed that miR159 might influence breast cancer progression. By transfecting cells containing miR159 isolated from patient serum, they had the ability to reduce proliferation in BC cells. To identify miR159 target genes they used three independent methods: computational prediction, RNA-induced silencing, and sequencing. All three methods identified three potential target genes: transcription factor 7 (TCF7), nuclear receptor coactivator 6 (NCOA6), and engrailed homeobox 2 (EN2). Of which the TCF7 gene belongs to a family of transcription factors of the Wnt signaling pathway, which is overexpressed in breast cancer. Finally, the authors report that mice fed with MIR159 showed a significant reduction of TCF7 and MYC expression in their tumors with decreased tumor cell proliferation, reduced tumor growth, and increased apoptosis, providing important information on kingdom interactions for the prevention and treatment of various human diseases [39].

5.5 Plant MIR167e-5p suppresses intestinal cell proliferation

A recent study has found plant-derived MIR167e-5p to regulate enterocyte proliferation in vitro in cancer cell lines. Plant MIR167e-5p decreased cell proliferation following treatment with 20 pmol of MIR167e-5p over a 72 h period. The tests included viability assays determined by MTT at different times. In this study, a bioinformatic program was employed to identify plant miRNA targets due to their involvement in auxin response factor processes in plants, resulting in a conserved putative site in β-catenin gene in human, key in the Wnt/ β-catenin pathway related to cell proliferation, differentiation, and maintenance. Demonstrating that the plant MIR167e-5p could decrease protein levels and inhibit cell proliferation [40].

6. Future approaches and applications of miRNAs

Identifying gene targets in human in a timely manner using plant miRNAs offers a reliable, effective, and economical way to determine the possible effects of interactions given by exogenous molecules, regardless of their origin, in human mRNA, studies have focused on providing information of importance for future projects or research, as in 2017, Kumar et al. [41] presented a cross-kingdom bioinformatics analysis, showing the importance of some plant miRNAs, coming from the plant *Camptotheca acuminata* commonly known as Happy Tree, with anticancer attributions, showing in their results, a strong association with several cancer pathways in human, and a possible important role in the regulation of complex disease networks for humans. Similarly, another plant *Ocimum bascilicum*, used for its therapeutic properties, underwent a bioinformatics analysis, by Patel et al. in 2019 [42], finding a close relationship of plant miRNAs with various genes involved in signaling pathways, various functional processes, and several organs in human. Not only have predictive studies been performed in plants that are used for their medicinal properties, there are also analyses where foods of daily consumption have shown interesting results as in the year 2020, the authors Rakhmetullina et al. [43] searched for target genes in human for 227 miRNAs of the Oryza sativa (rice) plant, finding 942 possible genes, which represent 5.4% of the total number of human genes studied, being this of major importance, due to the fact that four miRNAs present (osa-miR2102-5p, osa-miR5075-3p, osa-miR2097-5p, and osa-miR2919) were associated with a greater number of target genes, and since miRNAs can reach some tissues, and the circulatory system through ingestion, some targets were related to some biological processes involved in the development of cardiovascular and neurodegenerative diseases, the authors emphasize the importance of continuing to study them. Likewise, in 2022, Sánchez-Romo et al. [44] determined through bioinformatics analysis the possible mRNA targets in humans, resulting in 787 different genes for 84 miRNAs of the plant Triticum aestivum (wheat), showing some genes involved in cancer processes, risk of dementia and schizophrenia. In addition, functional enrichment analysis highlighted some pathways such as the Fanconi anemia pathway, circadian rhythm, and the dopaminergic synapse pathway, related to attention deficit hyperactivity disorder ADHD.

7. Conclusion

The impact of endogenous and exogenous miRNAs that directly influence various biological processes is an important current topic, as it opens the horizons of understanding gene regulation in organisms. Considering that plants and humans are different species, plant miRNAs and their interactions have been actively studied, which has contributed to the knowledge of the mechanisms of coevolution between plant miRNAs and human mRNAs. The information gathered in these articles could facilitate the approach and could open a number of opportunities for the development of new studies and therapies for various diseases based on miRNAs, as well as extensive molecular validation of predictions.

Author details

Daniel Sanchez Romo, Benito Pereyra Alferez and Jorge Hugo Garcia Garcia*
Universidad Autonoma de Nuevo Leon, San Nicolas de los Garza, Mexico

*Address all correspondence to: jorge.garciagr@uanl.edu.mx

References

[1] Ambros V. The functions of animal microRNAs. Nature. 16 Sep 2004;**431**(7006):350-5. DOI: 10.1038/nature02871

[2] Bartel DP. MicroRNAs: Genomics, biogenesis, mechanism, and function. Cell. 2004;**116**:281-297. DOI: 10.1016/S0092-8674(04)00045-5

[3] Lee Y, Kim M, Han J, Yeom K-H, Lee S, Baek SH, et al. MicroRNA genes are transcribed by RNA polymerase II. The EMBO Journal. 2004;**23**:4051-4060. DOI: 10.1038/sj.emboj.7600385

[4] Axtell MJ, Westholm JO, Lai EC. Distinct characteristics of miRNA pathways in plants and animals. Genome Biology. 2010;**12**:1-13

[5] Lee RC, Feinbaum RL, Ambrost V. The *C. elegans* heterochronic gene lin-4 encodes small RNAs with antisense complementarity to lin-14. Cell. 3 Dec 1993;**75**(5):843-54. DOI: 10.1016/0092-8674(93)90529-y

[6] Wang Y, Shi C, Yang T, Zhao L, Chen J, Zhang N, et al. High-throughput sequencing revealed that microRNAs were involved in the development of superior and inferior grains in bread wheat. Scientific Reports. 2018;**8**. DOI: 10.1038/s41598-018-31870-z

[7] Chen C, Zeng Z, Liu Z, Xia R. Horticulture research small RNAs, emerging regulators critical for the development of horticultural traits. Horticultural Research. 2018;5:63. DOI: 10.1038/s41438-018-0072-8

[8] Rupaimoole R, Slack FJ. MicroRNA therapeutics: Towards a new era for the management of cancer and other diseases. Nature Reviews. Drug Discovery. 2017;**16**:203-221. DOI: 10.1038/nrd.2016.246

[9] Paul P, Chakraborty A, Sarkar D, Langthasa M, Rahman M, Bari M, et al. Interplay between miRNAs and human diseases. Journal of Cellular Physiology. 2018;**233**:2007-2018. DOI: 10.1002/jcp.25854

[10] Liang H, Zhang S, Fu Z, Wang Y, Wang N, Liu Y, et al. Effective detection and quantification of dietetically absorbed plant microRNAs in human plasma. The Journal of Nutritional Biochemistry. 2015;**26**:505-512. DOI: 10.1016/j.jnutbio.2014.12.002

[11] Samad AFA, Kamaroddin MF, Sajad M. Cross-kingdom regulation by plant microRNAs provides novel insight into gene regulation. Advances in Nutrition. 2020:1-15. DOI: 10.1093/advances/nmaa095

[12] Li Y, Bian Z, Liang X, Cai X, Yin Y, Wang C, et al. Exogenous plant MIR168a specifically targets mammalian LDLRAP1: evidence of cross-kingdom regulation by microRNA. Cell Res. Jan 2012;**22**(1):107-126. DOI: 10.1038/cr.2011.158

[13] Link J, Thon C, Schanze D, Steponaitiene R, Kupcinskas J, Zenker M, et al. Food-derived Xeno-microRNAs: Influence of diet and detectability in gastrointestinal tract—Proof-of-principle study. Molecular Nutrition & Food Research. 2019;**63**:1-11. DOI: 10.1002/mnfr.201800076

[14] Lukasik A, Zielenkiewicz P. Plant MicroRNAs-novel players in natural medicine? International Journal of Molecular Sciences. 2017;**18**. DOI: 10.3390/ijms18010009

[15] Cullen BR. Transcription and processing of human microRNA precursors. Molecular Cell. 2004;**16**:861-865. DOI: 10.1016/j.molcel.2004.12.002

[16] Zeng Y, Cullen BR. Structural requirements for pre-microRNA binding and nuclear export by exportin 5. Nucleic Acids Research. 2004;**32**:4776-4785. DOI: 10.1093/nar/gkh824

[17] Kim Y-K, Kim B, Kim VN. Re-evaluation of the roles of DROSHA, Exportin 5 , and DICER in microRNA biogenesis. Proceedings of the National Academy of Sciences. 2016;**113**:E1881-E1889. DOI: 10.1073/pnas.1602532113

[18] Gomes AQ, Nolasco S, Soares H. Non-coding RNAs: Multi-tasking molecules in the cell. International Journal of Molecular Sciences. 2013;**14**:16010-16039. DOI: 10.3390/ijms140816010

[19] Yu B, Yang Z, Li J, Minakhina S, Yang M, Padgett RW, et al. Methylation as a crucial step in plant microRNA biogenesis. Science. 2005;**307**:932-935

[20] Yu Y, Jia T, Chen X. The 'how' and 'where' of plant microRNAs. The New Phytologist. 2017;**216**:1002-1017. DOI: 10.1111/nph.14834

[21] Gulyaeva LF, Kushlinskiy NE. Regulatory mechanisms of microRNA expression. Journal of Translational Medicine. 2016;**14**:143. DOI: 10.1186/s12967-016-0893-x

[22] Chandradoss SD, Schirle NT, Szczepaniak M, Macrae IJ, Joo C. A dynamic search process underlies MicroRNA targeting. Cell. 2015;**162**:96-107. DOI: 10.1016/j.cell.2015.06.032

[23] Friedman RC, Farh KKH, Burge CB, Bartel DP. Most mammalian mRNAs are conserved targets of microRNAs. Genome Research. 2009;**19**:92-105. DOI: 10.1101/gr.082701.108

[24] Kang J-W, Baek H-A, Cho S-D, Lee J-S. Is use of micro-RNA–containing food feasible? Journal of Food Chemical and Nanotechnology. 2016;**2**:42-49

[25] Wang W, Liu D, Zhang X, Chen D, Cheng Y, Shen F. Plant MicroRNAs in Cross-Kingdom Regulation of Gene Expression. International Journal of Molecular Sciences. 10 Jul 2018;**19**(7):2007. DOI: 10.3390/ijms19072007

[26] Vidigal JA, Ventura A. The biological functions of miRNAs: Lessons from in vivo studies. Trends in Cell Biology. 2015;**25**:137-147. DOI: 10.1016/j.tcb.2014.11.004

[27] Iwasa J, Marshall WF, Karp G. Karp's cell and molecular biology: concepts and experiments (15 ed). New York city, United states: Wiley. 2016

[28] Achakzai HK, Barozai MYK, Din M, Baloch IA, Achakzai AKK. Identification and annotation of newly conserved microRNAs and their targets in wheat (Triticum aestivum L.). PLoS One. 10 Jul 2018;**13**(7):e0200033. DOI: 10.1371/journal.pone.0200033

[29] Mlotshwa S, Pruss GJ, MacArthur JL, Endres MW, Davis C, Hofseth LJ, et al. A novel chemopreventive strategy based on therapeutic microRNAs produced in plants. Cell Res. Apr 2015;**25**(4):521-524. DOI: 10.1038/cr.2015.25

[30] Rukov JL, Wilentzik R, Jaffe I, Vinther J, Shomron N. Pharmaco-miR: Linking microRNAs and drug effects. Briefings in Bioinformatics. 2014;**15**:648-659. DOI: 10.1093/bib/bbs082

[31] Luo Y, Wang P, Wang X, Wang Y, Mu Z, Li Q, et al. Detection of dietetically absorbed maize-derived

microRNAs in pigs. Scientific Reports. 2017;**7**:1-10. DOI: 10.1038/s41598-017-00488-y

[32] Li Z, Xu R, Li N. MicroRNAs from plants to animals, do they define a new messenger for communication?. Nutrition Metabolism (Lond). 2008;**15**:68. Available online: https://doi.org/10.1186/s12986-018-0305-8

[33] Skog J, Würdinger T, van Rijn S, Meijer DH, Gainche L, Curry WT, et al. Glioblastoma microvesicles transport RNA and proteins that promote tumour growth and provide diagnostic biomarkers. Nature Cell Biology. 2008;**10**:1470-1476. DOI: 10.1038/ncb1800

[34] Weber JA, Baxter DH, Zhang S, Huang DY, Huang KH, Lee MJ, et al. The microRNA spectrum in 12 body fluids. Clinical Chemistry. 2010;**56**:1733-1741. DOI: 10.1373/clinchem.2010.147405

[35] Cui J, Zhou B, Ross SA, Zempleni J. Nutrition, microRNAs, and human health. Advanced Nutrition. 2017;**8**:105-112. DOI: 10.3945/an.116.013839

[36] Liang G, Zhu Y, Sun B, Shao Y, Jing A, Wang J, et al. Assessing the survival of exogenous plant microRNA in mice. Food Science & Nutrition. 2014;**2**:380-388. DOI: 10.1002/fsn3.113

[37] Zhou Z, Li X, Liu J, Dong L, Chen Q, Liu J, et al. Honeysuckle-encoded atypical microRNA2911 directly targets influenza a viruses. Cell Research. 2015;**25**:39-49. DOI: 10.1038/cr.2014.130

[38] Zhou LK, Zhou Z, Jiang XM, Zheng Y, Chen X, Fu Z, et al. Absorbed plant MIR2911 in honeysuckle decoction inhibits SARS-CoV-2 replication and accelerates the negative conversion of infected patients. Cell Discovery. 2020;**61**:1-4

[39] Chin AR, Fong MY, Somlo G, Wu J, Swiderski P, Wu X, et al. Cross-kingdom inhibition of breast cancer growth by plant miR159. Cell Research. 2016;**26**:217-228. DOI: 10.1038/cr.2016.13

[40] Li M, Chen T, He JJ, Wu JH, Luo JY, Ye RS, et al. Plant MIR167e-5p inhibits enterocyte proliferation by targeting β-catenin. Cell. 2019;**8**:1-14. DOI: 10.3390/cells8111385

[41] Kumar D, Kumar S, Ayachit G, Bhairappanavar SB, Ansari A, Sharma P, et al. Cross-kingdom regulation of putative miRNAs derived from happy tree in cancer pathway: A systems biology approach. International Journal of Molecular Sciences. 2017;**18**:1-21. DOI: 10.3390/ijms18061191

[42] Patel M, Mangukia N, Jha N, Gadhavi H, Shah K, Patel S, et al. Computational identification of miRNA and their cross kingdom targets from expressed sequence tags of Ocimum basilicum. Molecular Biology Reports. 2019;**46**:2979-2995. DOI: 10.1007/s11033-019-04759-x

[43] Rakhmetullina A, Pyrkova A, Aisina D, Ivashchenko A. In silico prediction of human genes as potential targets for rice miRNAs. Computational Biology and Chemistry. 2020;**87**:107305. DOI: 10.1016/j.compbiolchem.2020.107305

[44] Sánchez-Romo D, Hernández-Vásquez CI, Pereyra-Alférez B, García-García JH. Identification of potential target genes in Homo sapiens, by miRNA of Triticum aestivum: A cross kingdom computational approach, Non-Coding RNA Res. 2002;**7**:89-97. Available online: https://doi.org/10.1016/J.NCRNA.2022.03.002

Chapter 14

Comparative Study between Herbal and Synthetic Antidepressant Drugs

Rizwana Bee, Mohammad Ahmad and Kamal Kishore Maheshwari

Abstract

According to the WHO report approximately 450 million people suffer from mental and behavioural disorder. Depression is one of the most common neurodegenerative disorders which arise due to the imbalance of neurotransmitters release at the synaptic cleft. A large number of synthetic drugs are being used as standard treatment for depression, they have many adverse effects that a limit the therapeutic treatment. Traditionally herbs are used for the treatment of depression which may offer advantage in terms of safety and tolerability, possibly by improvement in patient compliance. Herbal drugs are more commonly used because these have small amount of chemicals, these produced less side effects than standard drugs. Overall, this chapter presented an overview of the research that has been done on the many herbs, Mechanism of action involving monoamine reuptake, neuroreceptor binding and channel transporter function, and neural communication or HPA modulation. Several pharmaceutical companies are working on "triple" reuptake inhibitors that stop all three monoamines from being reabsorbed. Studies into the interplay of monoamine systems with other neurotransmitters (e.g., CRF, neurokinins, glutamate, and GABA etc.) will aid in the development of realistic, integrated neurochemical models of depression.

Keywords: depression, neurotransmitter, monoamine reuptake inhibitors, selective 5-hydroxytryptamine reuptake inhibitors *and Achyranthes aspera*

1. Introduction

Depression is a weakening disease and it is mostly affecting modern society. The world health organization forecasts that in 2022 depression will become the major common cause of loss of interest in the working in the entire world. Thus the research of depression is one of the most important way through which we can obtain new treatment of depression and improve the developed drugs which can work better for depressive individuals. It will also assist to develop and create new approaches that will be used for better treatment of depression. Chemical transmission is the major tool through which nerves communicate with each other. Now it is well known that the presynaptic and postsynaptic events are responsible for the plasticity and learning within the Central nervous system. Chemical transmission requires different types of steps including synthesis of the neurotransmitters, their storage in secretary vesicles, and their release into the synaptic cleft between presynaptic and postsynaptic cleft. The initial step of the synthesis of neurotransmitters is the facilitated transport of amino acids from blood to the brain, in the brain precursors are converted into neurotransmitters enzymatically. These are stored in the synaptic vesicles, and finally released into the synaptic cleft via calcium dependent process. The release rate of neurotransmitters determined the rate of firing of neurons which means that the drug alter the firing rate of neurons. This modification of neurons carried out the alteration of release of neurotransmitters. After this released neurotransmitters bind with somatodendritic auto receptors. Thus binding of neurotransmitter to auto-receptors is responsible for reducing the synthesis of neurotransmitters or additional release from the presynapse. The synaptic results of neurotransmitter are ceased via binding with specific receptors and reuptake into the pre-synapse. Neurotransmitters metabolized by monoamine oxidase enzymes in the presynapse [1].

2. Plant profile

Achyranthes aspera (family-Amarantheceae) is commonly known as Latjira in Hindi. The plant is used for the treatment of dysentery, fever and diabetes [2]. *A. aspera* is available as weed in whole India, Asia and many other parts of the world such as Mexico, Central America and Africa [3]. It is described as bitter, pungent, purgative, heating, laxative, stomachic, carminative and digestive and is also used for the treatment of bronchitis, heart disease, piles, itching abdominal problems, ascites, rheumatism, abdominal enlargement, rabies and also for enlarged cervical gland. It is use as folk medicine. It is also known as medicinal herb in different types of system of medicine in India. It is known by different names such as *Chirchita* (Hindi), *Apamarg* (Sanskirt), *Aghedi* (Gujrati), *Apang* (Bengali), *Nayurivi* (Tamil), *Kalalat* (Malayalam) [4]. This plant grows on road sides. It is also found as field boundaries and waste places as a weed throughout India up to an altitude of 2100 m and in South Andaman Islands [5]. The leaves extract of *A. aspera* having antifertility effect [6]. Methanolic extract of *A. aspera* shows wide varieties of pharmacological activities however, little is known about its anti-depressant activity. Most of the researches are not found its antidepressant activity by using open field test and forced swimming test, so the aim of present study to assess the anti-depressant activity of *A. aspera* extract against physically induced depression in rats, using open field test and forced swimming test apparatus [5]. *A. aspera* (Chirchita) belong to the family Amaranthaceae. Two different varieties of *A. aspera* are mentioned in Ayurvedic and Chinese medicines, 1st is red and 2nd is white [2].

Common name of *A. aspera:* [7].
Arabian: Atkumah, Na'eem, No'eem, Mahout, Wazer (Yemen).
Ayurvedic: Apamarg, Chirchita, Shikhari, Shaihkharika.
Bengali: Apang.
English: Prickly chaff flower, Hawai chaff flower, Devil's horse whip.
French: Achyranth a feuillers rudes, collant, Gendarme.
Gujrati: Safad Aghedo, Anghadi, Andhedi, Agado.
Hindi: Latjira, Chirchita, Lamchichra, Sonpur, Onga.
Indonesia: Jarong.

The methanolic extract of *A. aspera* showed the anxiolytic activity due the presence of its phytoconstitents viz. alkaloid, steroid and triterpenes. It could be used for the management of anxiety disorders because it is economically therapeutic agent [8]. Seed extract of *A. aspera* give the hypolipidemic activity which might be attributed to its phyto-constituents like saponin and flavonoids. Thus it showed the protective effect against HFF [9]. Leaves and stem parts of the *A. aspera* were converted into powder form and extracted with distilled water, which extract exhibited antimicrobial activities because of its many photochemical constituents including flavonoids and alkaloids [10]. The root extract of *A. aspera* has anticancer activity against different human cancer cell lines due the presence of its chemical constituents like alkaloid, flavonoids, phenolics and terpenoids [11]. The methanolic extract of it possess antiviral (antiherpes) activity because of its pure compound oleanolic acid. The OA of *A. aspera* showed the protective effect against both HSV-1 and HSV-2. Result showed that OA or methanolic extract of *Acyrantes aspera* act on the early stage of HSV replication [12]. It was also reported that its phytoconstituent (non- alkaloid fraction) significantly inhibits Epstein–Barr-virus which is a member of Herpesviride family [13]. The ethanolic extract of *A. aspera* seeds showed significant anti arthritic activity at various concentrations ranging from 10 to 1000 μg/ml [14]. The brewer's yeast induced pyrexia in rats used for the investigation of antipyretic activity of *A. aspera* extract. Regulation of body temperature requires a balance between production and loss of heat. The hypothalamus acts as a regulator for the set point at which body temperature is maintained [15]. The antiulcer activity of *A. aspera* demonstrated that the methanolic extract of *A. aspera* protects rats against ulcer by using pyloric ligation method. From the result it has been clear that the methanolic extract of *A. aspera* at a dose of 300 mg/kg shows maximum ulcer protection as compared to control group [16]. *A. aspera* contain different chemical constituents such as alkaloids, flavonoids, saponins, steroids and terpenoids. Its water soluble alkaloid achyranthine isolated via extraction possess anti-inflammatory activity [17]. The result showed that the ethanolic extract of *A. aspera* having antifertility activity. It also possesses the anti-zygotic, blastocytotoxic and antiovulatory activities [18]. Antiarthritic activity of *A. aspera* has been carried out by using most popular method, known as inhibition of protein denaturation. The ethanolic extract of *A. aspera* seeds showed significant anti-arthritic activity of various concentrations ranging from 10 to 1000 μg/ml [14]. Alkaloids of leaves of *A. aspera* plant determined with the help of thin layer chromatography. In this method silica gel aluminum used as stationary phase while chloroform used as mobile phase for the determination of alkaloids in the leaves of *A. aspera*. Measurement of alkaloid in the alkaloid fraction extract of leaves of *A. aspera* carried out using high-performance liquid chromatography. Alkaloids of *A. aspera* extract used for the treatment of different disorders such as in-vivo study of it demonstrated that the alkaloid of *A. aspera* cause apoptosis and healing in breast cancer cells in mice induced by benzopyrene. *A. aspera* consist of 13 different types of chemical constituents while alkaloids are major constituents of it. 53.36% alkaloids are present in the *A. aspera* [19].

3. Description and Distribution

A. aspera is a medicinal plant. It is found throughout India as an annual herb. It is also found in Asia and many parts of world such as Mexico, Central America and Africa. *A. aspera* consist of many antioxidants like alkaloids, terpenoids and saponins, which have various pharmacological properties. Different types of chemical constituents have been isolated from this plant by various techniques. All pharmacological properties and chemical constituents are used for the treatment of various human diseases. *A. aspera* globally available as a medicinal weed in Baluchistan, Ceylon, Tropical Asia, Africa, Australia and America. It is also present Shiv Bari and Himachal Pradesh. In India it is found in field boundaries and also present at the road sides. The plant grows to a height of 0.2 to 2.0 m. root is cylindrical, 0.1–1.0 cm in thickness. Root is yellowish- brown in color, which is of two types secondary and tertiary. Stem is square in shape and yellowish-brown in color. Leaves are simple, slightly acuminate, petiolate and ovate. Leaves contain anomocytic type of stomata on the lower epidermis. Flower is 8–30 cm long and 3–7 mm wide. It is bisexual greenish-white. It consists of 5 perianth segment, 5 stamens, short filament, 7 gynoecium bicarpellary, syncarpous, ovary superior, single ovule, style and single stigma. It is found in two different color red and white flower. Seeds are round at the base, which are brown in color [7]. The whole plant and seeds of *A. aspera* consist of an alkaline substance known as potash [20]. It is common herbal drug in Ayurvedic, Unani-Tibbi, Siddha, Allopathic, Homeopathic, Naturopathic and Home remedies [21]. It is useful for the treatment of cough, renal dropsy, fistula, scrofula, skin rash, nasal, infection, chronic malaria, impotence, fever, asthma, piles and snake bites [22].

4. Chemical constituents

*A. aspera*consist of different types of phytochemicals such as alkaloids, tannins, cardiac glycosides, steroids, flavonoids, terpenoids, reducing sugar and saponins. Saponins include ecdysterone, 20-hydroxy-ecdysone [23]. It consists of alkaloids such as three bisdesmosidic saponins (I-III), 20-hydroxy-ecdysone, quercetin 3-*O*-β-D-galactoside [24]. It possesses triterpenoids, which are β-D-glukopyranosyl-13-β-[*O*-α-L-rhamnopyranosyl-(1 → 3)-*O*-β-D-glucopyrauronosyloxy] machaerinate [25]. It is also a good source of ketones, including 36, 37-dihydroxyhenpentacontan-4-one, triacontanol, 36,47-dihydroxyhenpentacontan-4-one [26, 27]. Pentatriacontane, 6-penta-tri-acontanone, Hexa-triacontane, tritriacontane, these are found in the stem of *A. aspera* [27]. Leaves and stem leaves consist of different types of chemical constituents such as 20-hydroxy ecdysone, quercetin-3-*O*-β-D-galactoside, P-benzoquinone, hydroquinone, spathulenol, nerol, asarone and eugenol [28, 29]. Seeds of *A. aspera*contains a number of D-glucoronic acid, β-D-galactopyranosyl ester of D-glucoronic acid, oleanolic acid, amino acid, hentriacontane, 10-tricosanone, 10-octacosanone and 4-tritriacontanone [30]. It is also consist of various type of cyclicchain aliphatic fatty acids, fatty acid composition (lauric, myristi, palmitia, stearic, arachidic, behenic, oleic and linoleic acid) and oleonolic acid glycosides [α-L-rhamnopyranosyl-(1 → 4)-(β-D-glucopyranosyluronic acid)-(1 → 3)-oleonolic acid, α-L-rhamnopyranosyl-(1 → 4)-(β-D-glucopyranosyluronic acid)-(1 → 3)-oleonic acid-28-*O*-β-D-glucopyranoside [31, 32].

Acyranthine a water soluble alkaloid present in the *A. aspera* is responsible for various type of pharmacological activities like dilation of blood vessels, lowering of the blood pressure, depression of heart and increase the rate and amplitude of respiration. It is also consisting of another water soluble alkaloid known betain. Betain is isolated from the whole plant [33].

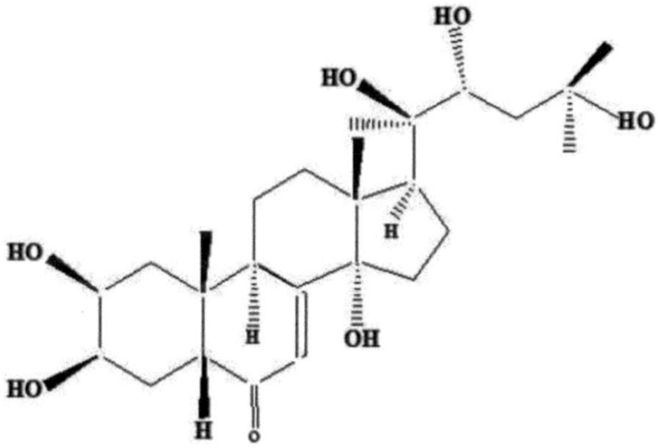

Ecdysterone

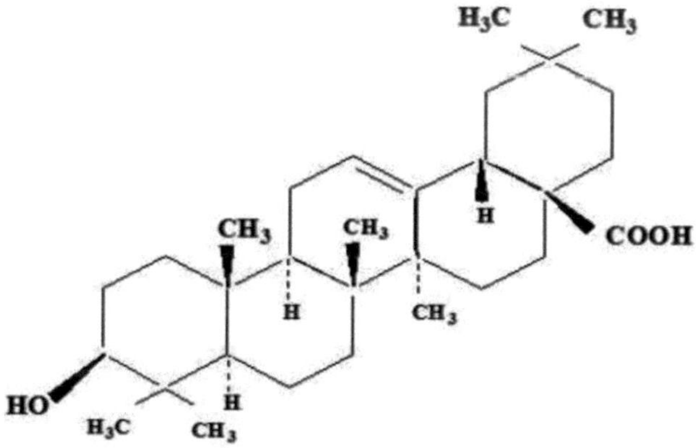

Oleanolic acid

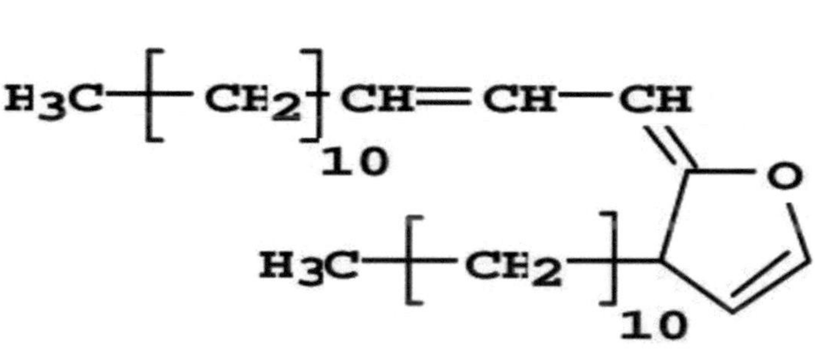

Cyclic chain aliphatic fatty acid

5. Medicinal uses

A. aspera shows a wide spectrum of pharmacological activities such as bitter, pungent, heating, laxative, stomachic, carminatives and improve appetite as well as useful in vomiting and heart disease. It is also used in various types of disease like pile, itching, abdominal pains, dyspepsia, dysentery and blood disease [34]. It is widely used for the treatment of many disorders, which are asthmatic cough, snakebite, hydrophobia, urinary calculi, rabies, influenza and gonorrhea. Its dried leaf powder mixed with honey is useful for the treatment of early stage of asthma [35]. Naayuruvi kuzhi thailum has been identified that *Acyrantes aspera* as the primary constituent comes under the Siddha system, which is used in the management of asthma [36]. Traditionally, this plant is used in the treatment of asthma and cough [37]. The root of *A. aspera* is used in whooping cough, tonsillitis [38, 39].

6. Pharmacological activities

The literature survey has shown that following pharmacological action of *A. aspera*.

6.1 Anti-parkinsonism activity

Parkinson disease is arising due to the degradation of dopamine- carrying neurons in the substantia nigra. The neuronal death occurs in PD is due to the damage of free radicals and lewy's bodies formation [40]. Levodopa is used as the first line drug for the treatment of Parkinson disease [41]. Powder of the whole plant of *A. aspera* is extracted by using hydro-alcoholic solvent and its get evaporated to a concentrate by rotary evaporator at 40°C [42]. 24 rats were divided into four groups (n = 6). Hydro-alcoholic extract at a dose of 200 and 400 mg/kg was administered to the rats before 30 minutes of haloperidol treatment for 20 days. In a study of anti-parkinsonism activity, the ant-parkinsonism effect of hydro alcoholic extract of *A. aspera* on haloperidol which is administered at a dose of 2 mg/kg via intraperitoneal route induced catatonia in rats. In haloperidol treated rats the motor coordination was studied by using rotarod test and hang test. The increase degree of catalepsy in haloperidol treated group was measured after 60 and 90 minutes of administration. The result has shown score of catalepsy was significantly decreased after 60 minutes with the test drug HA at a dose of 200 and 400 mg/kg. It is also demonstrated that group exhibited maximum reduction in the catalepsy, which is treated with 400 mg/kg. The results of rotarod test show that the retention time was reduced in the haloperidol treated group. The retention time significantly improved in HA treated group. Among these groups, maximum retention time was noted in the 400 mg/kg treated group [43].

6.2 Anxiolytic activity

Anxiolytic activity of *A. aspera*is due to the presence of its phytochemical constituents such as alkaloids, steroids and triterpenes. Benzodiazepines are the first line drug for the treatment of anxiety but these have lots of side effects like sedation, muscle relaxation, anterograde amnesia and physical dependence [44]. Methanolic extract of *A. aspera* was administered to the different groups (100, 300 and 600 mg/kg) by using different apparatus, hole board, open field, elevated plus maze and light dark test. Animals were treated with methanolic extract at a dose of 100, 300 and 600 mg/kg, p.o. shows significant and dose dependent increase in the number and duration of head poking as compared to control group. In open field test, animals treated with methanolic extract of *A. aspera*at a dose of 100, 300 and 600 mg/kg, p.o. in this test there was significant ($p < 0.01$) increase in rearing. The number of squares traveled by the animals also significantly ($p < 0.01$) increased when animals treated orally with methanolic extract of *A. aspera* at 300 and 600 mg/kg. Thus result was indicating a dose dependent anxiolytic activity of the plant extract. There was also significant ($p < 0.01$) increase the number of entries and time spent in the open arm of elevated plus maze of methanolic extract treated group at 100 to 600 mg/kg. Diazepam used as a standard drug. In the close arm of elevated plus maze, number of entries and time spent significantly ($p < 0.01$) decrease as compared to control group. The group of animal administered 600 mg/kg of methanolic extract of *A. aspera* was demonstrated higher number of entries and time spent in open arm than the standard drug. In the light and dark test, animals treated with methanolic extract of *A. aspera* at 300 and 600 mg/kg dose indicated significantly ($p < 0.01$) increase the time spent in lighted box, number of crossings and transfer latency. In the dark box significantly ($p < 0.01$) decrease the time spent [8].

6.3 Hypolipidemic activity

Alcoholic extract of the entire plant of *A. aspera* demonstrated hypoglycemic activity. Rats were divided into four groups each containing six animals. Consumption of fructose is responsible to increase body weight as a result of decreased insulin level in the blood. It is also responsible to decreased leptin production followed by an increase in the circulating nonesterified fatty acids, which decrease insulin sensitivity due to increasing the intramyocellular lipid content [45]. In the present study it was found that the HFF significantly increased TGL [46]. Saponins constituents of *A. aspera* extract are reported to increase the lipoprotein lipase which is responsible for the removal of circulating free fatty acids that results decrease the total cholesterol [47]. It is also reported saponins are effective as HMG-CoA reductase inhibitors [48]. It has reported that 100 mg/kg of *A. aspera* administered to the rats significant ($p < 0.001$) decrease in the level of VLDL and LDL with an increase in the levels of HDL were observed [9].

6.4 Antiulcer activity

Gastric ulcer is a pathological condition caused due to the imbalance between aggressive factors, such as gastric acid, pepsin, stimulation of vagus nerves, secretion of gastrin and increase in the number of parietal cells and protective factors like bicarbonate ion, mucus productivity, mucus secretion and prostaglandins. Literature survey has shown that its chemical constituents like flavonoids and triterpenoids are responsible for antiulcer activity [49]. The root part of *A. aspera* was extracted with methanol. Ulcer was induced by pylorus ligation method. Ranitidine is used as the standard drug for the comparison of methanolic extract of *A. aspera.* 300 mg/kg dose of MEAA showed 91.89% antiulcer activity. From the result it has clear that 300 mg/kg dose of MEAA shows maximum antiulcer activity than the control group. The lower dose of MEAA does not show antiulcer activity but at higher dose it shows ulcer protection activity [16].

6.5 Diuretic activity

Diuretics are the drugs which are used to increase the rate of urine flow. These are used to adjust the balance of body fluid [50]. It is reported that it consists of alkaloids, flavonoids, saponins, steroids and terpenoids [17]. The aqueous and alcoholic extract of leaves of *A. aspera* showed good diuretic activity. In this study it has clear that urine volume, cation and anion excretion was found to be increased, Na^+/K^+ ratio of 2.04 and 2.18 were obtained for aqueous and alcoholic extract respectively while the normal value for Na^+/K^+ ratio is reported to be 2.05–2.83 [51].

6.6 Antidiabetic activity

Diabetes is one of the most common disorders. About 30 million people suffer from diabetes in the world. It is occurring due the imbalance secretion of glucose and insulin. Insulin is used for maintaining blood glucose level. It is characterized by high blood glucose level, weight loss, extreme thirst and weakness. Alloxan administered to the animals for inducing diabetes. Alloxan administered to the animals for 30 days continuously. Animals were treated with ethanolic extract of *A. aspera* the blood glucose level was found to be increased by 123% and 128% on the 15th and 16th day of exposure respectively. After completion of exposure period the blood cholesterol level decrease was found to be 5.5% [52].

6.7 Antifertility activity

Protective effect of ethanolic extract of *A. aspera* against fertility is now being investigated including antizygotic activity, blastocytotoxic activity and abortifacient activity. The results showed the extract of *A. aspera* having antifertility and antiestrogenic effect in female rats. Administration of ethanolic extract of *A. aspera* to the animals at a dose of 200 mg/kg and 400 mg/kg significantly decrease in the duration of estrous & metesterous phase. Treated the animals with ethanolic extract of it at a dose of 200 and 400 mg/kg reduced the weight of ovaries than the control group [18].

6.8 Anti-inflammatory activity

The leaves of *A. aspera*are used for the treatment of dermatoligical disorder [53]. It was investigated that alcoholic extract of *A. aspera*has potential anti-inflammatory effect in Wistar rats at different doses such as 50, 100 and 200 mg/kg. Anti-inflammatory effect of *A. aspera* extract carried out by using carrageenan-induced paw edema (acute inflammatory model) and cotton pellet granuloma test (chronic inflammatory model). All the doses of alcoholic extract of *A. aspera* tested in carrageenan-induced paw edema caused a significant ($p < 0.05$) and decreased paw edema 32–40.5 compared to control group. In cotton pellet granuloma model, the concentration of *A. aspera* (50, 100 and 200 mg/kg) caused a significant ($p < 0.05$) and marked inhibition 34.6% of granuloma weight as compared to control group [54].

6.9 Antipyretic activity

In a study of anti-pyretic activity of crude extract of *A. aspera* was carried out by brewer's yeast-induced pyrexia in rats. Initially rectal temperatures were recorded. Administration of the yeast at a dose 10 mg/kg to the rats produced significant increase in rectal temperature 24 hours after yeast injection [55]. The methanolic extract of leaves of *A. aspera* consist of alkaloids, steroids, proteins, flavonoids, saponins, mucilage, carbohydrates and tannins. The methanolic extract was administered orally to different groups at a dose of 100 and 200 mg/kg by intra-peritoneal route. 0.3 ml of normal saline was administered to the control group. Paracetamol (150 mg/kg) used as a standard drug. The methanolic extract of *A. aspera* demonstrated significant ($p < 0.01$) antipyretic activity. The dose at a 200 mg/kg extract has shown a good antipyretic activity ($p < 0.01$) with all the doses used when compared to the control group [15].

6.10 Anthelmintic activity

Helminthiasis is one of the most popular disease and one of the most serious diseases [56]. Stem powder of *A. aspera* extracted with methanol and water. It was extracted by using maceration process. Its chemical constituents such as saponins A, saponins B, terpenoids and volatile oils showed anthelmintic activity. Albendazole used as a standard drug for the comparison of anthelmintic activity of *A. aspera.* Extract of it's used at different concentration (2.5, 5, 10 and 20 mg/ml) for testing anthelmintic activity which based on the determination of time of paralysis and time of death of the worms. All the methanolic extracts of *A. aspera* showed the better protection against the helminthiasis [57].

6.11 Antibacterial activity

Phytochemical components of *A. aspera* like flavonoids and alkaloids showed the antibacterial activity [58]. It is used for the treatment of urinary tract infections [59]. Five bacterial species used as a testing organism including *Pseudomonas aeruginosa*, Proteus *mirabillus* and *Enterococcus faecalis.* The leaf and stem of the *A. aspera* was extracted with organic solvent. 5 mg/ml concentration of the extract used as a testing agent and their activity measured by the determination of zone of inhibition as produced by antibiotic sensitivity method on Mueller-Hinton agar [10].

6.12 Antifungal activity

The antifungal activity of *A. aspera* was obtained by using aqueous & ethanolic extract of root of its. Clotrimazole (1% w/w) used as standard drug for the comparison of *A. aspera* extract. The study is carried out to determine the antifungal activity of the *A. aspera* root extract by agar well diffusion method [60]. Antifungal activity was obtained through the sabouraud dextrose agar medium against culture of *Trichophyton rubrum*. The microorganism containing culture was inoculated and these inoculated plates were maintained for 2 hours at room temperature to allow diffusion of the solution into the medium. These petridishes incubated 25° ± 1 for 7 days [61]. Antifungal activity determined through the inhibition of diameters of zone surrounding each of the walls. The result has shown that the zone of inhibition of ethanolic extract is 23 mm and zone of inhibition of aqueous extract is 19 mm taking 10 mg/ml of extract. Ethanolic extract of *Achyranthesaspera* shows good antifungal activity against *Trychophyton rubrum* than the aqueous extract [62].

6.13 Antiviral activity

Different types of compounds obtained from plant origin have been shown to exhibit antiviral activity against some virus including herpes simplex virus those chemical constituents which are having antiviral activity includes alkaloids, flavonoids, tannins, terpenes, saponins, quinines, polysaccharides, steroidal glycoside proanthocyanidin and proteins [63]. Herpes simplex virus is of two types HSV-1 and HSV-2. Acyclovir has been used for the treatment of viral disease since 1970 [64]. Other types of antiviral drugs used such as ganciclovir, foscarnet and cidofovir that target herpes-virus DNA polymerases [65]. In the study it was evaluate that the methanolic extract of *A. asperahaving* antiviral activity. Its constituent oleanolic acid also possessed antiherpes activity. The methanolioc extract of *A. asperawas* found to be weak anti-herpes activity (EC_{50} 64.4 μg/ml for HSV-1 and EC_{50} 72.8 μg/ml for HSV-2). On the other hand, oleanolic acid possessed potent anti-herpes virus activity against both HSV-1 (EC_{50} 6.8 μg/ml) and HSV-2 (EC_{50} 7.8 μg/ml) [12].

6.14 Other activities

Study shows the hydro-ethanolic, n-hexane and chloroform extracts of root of *A. aspera* were found to be effective for sperm immobilization, sperm validity and nuclear chromatin decondensation [66]. It has been demonstrated that the ethanolic extract of root of *A. asperaplant* exhibits post coital antifertility effect in female albino rats. According to their experimental study, the ethanolic extract of *A. aspera* at a dose 200 mg/kg showed 83.3% anti-implantation effect [67]. The methanolic extract of leaves of *A. aspera* is responsible for cancer chemo protective action. It is consisting of different chemical constituents, including alkaloid, non-alkaloid and saponins. It is demonstrated that the methanolic extract of *A. aspera* allow nephroprotective activity against lead acetate induced nephrotoxicity in male albino rats [68]. The research showed that ethanolic extract of *A. aspera* produce broncho-protective effect against toluene diisocyanate induced occupational asthma in wistar rats. In this the total and differential leucocytes count was carried out in blood and bronchoalveolar fluid. It is revealed that *A. aspera* treated rats did not show any airway abnormality [69]. Acyranthine, it is water soluble constituent of *Acyrantes aspera* which decreased blood pressure and heart rate. It is also responsible dilation of blood vessels and increased the rate and amplitude of respiration in dogs and frogs. The contractile effect of acyranthine alkaloid was found to be at 0.5 mg/ml on frog rectus abdominal muscle was less than that of acetylcholine (0.1 mg/ml) [33]. It is exhibited that the petroleum ether extract of *A. asperaat* a dose 200 mg/kg shows protective effect against allergic reaction in both milk induced leukocytosis and milk induced eosinophilia in mice. The antiallergic activity of *A. aspera* was found to be due to the presence of steroids such as β-sitosterol, ecdysone and ecdysterone [70]. It is demonstrated that the ethanolic and aqueous extracts of *A. aspera* used for wound healing activity. The wound healing activity was carried out by using two experimental wound models, first is excision wound model and second is incision wound model [71]. It has been demonstrated that stem extract of *A. aspera* shows anti-plasmodial effect [72].

7. Synthetic drugs

7.1 History of antidepressants

In the late 1940s two scientist Hafliger & Schindler were synthesized a series of more than 40 iminodibenzyl derivatives which are possibly used as antihistamine, sedatives, analgesics and anti-parkinsonism drugs. Out of this imipramine was found to be a dibenzazepine compound, which is different from the phenothiazines because of replacement of the sulfur with an ethylene bridge to produce a seven membered central ring analogous to the benzepine antipsychotic agents [73]. During clinical investigation of these phenothiazenes analogs, Kuhn was found to be imipramine relatively ineffective for the treatment of psychosis but it had a remarkable effect for the treatment of depression [74]. Tricyclic antidepressants showed quinidine like effect on cardiac conduction that can be harmful at overdose and these are used limited for the heart patients. This is the main reason that TCAs only limited used to the patient at any given time. The research of chemically related compound to imipramine was found to be multiple analogs that are common in clinical use in the United States. There were also yielded diabenzazepines, imipramine and its secondary metabolite desipramine, as well as its 3-chloro derivative cloimipramine, amitriptyline and its N-demethylated metabolite nortriptyline, doxepin (dibenzoxepine) and protriptyline. Dibenzazepines are similar to the phenothiazines chemically. The ethylene group of middle of imipramine is responsible for the dissimilar stereochemical properties and prevents conjugation among the rings. Secondary metabolite (desipramine) of imipramine is similar to imipramine as an antidepressant while it is also showing some dissimilarity from imipramine. It might be possible that desipramine responsible for therapeutic responses to imipramine but it is no more effective or rapidly acting than imipramine [75].

7.2 Monoamine oxidase inhibitors

Among the all clinically introduced drugs, monoamine oxidase inhibitors were found to be first drugs for the treatment of depression while these are replaced by tricyclic and other types of antidepressant drugs because these having more efficacies and less side effects than the monoamine oxidase inhibitors. Phenelzine, tranylcypromine and iproniazide are the example of monoamine oxidase inhibitors. That drug irreversibly inhibits the MAO-A and MAO-B enzymes [76].

7.3 Selective 5-hydroxytryptamine reuptake inhibitors

These drugs also called as selective serotonin reuptake inhibitors or SSRIs, including flouxetine, fluvoxamine, paroxetine, citalopram and sertraline. SSRIs are most commonly prescribed for the treatment of depression. These are showing selectivity for the 5-HT not for noradrenaline uptake. SSRIs produced less anticholinergic side effects than the tricyclic antidepressant drugs. They are equally effective as MAOIs and TCAs for treating the depression but in case of severe depression, less effective than TCAs [76].

7.4 Sites of action of antidepressant drugs

Diagram is showing noradrenergic (top) and serotonergic (bottom) nerve terminals. Sevsral types of drugs such as SSRIs, SNRIs and TCAs increase the availability

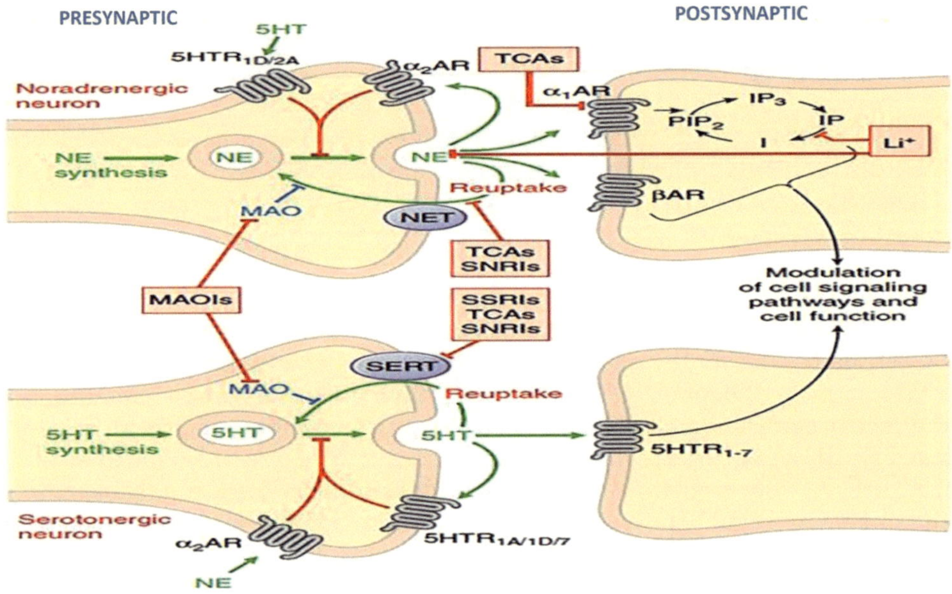

Figure 1.
Modulation of GPCR signaling and activation of protein kinase & ion channel.

of noradrenergic or serotonergic neurotransmitters at synaptic cleft by blocking the transporter of norepinephrine and serotonin neurotransmitter at presynaptic terminals. MAOIs used for the inhibition of catabolism of norepinephrine and serotonin. Some antidepressant drugs like trazodone has direct effects on serotonergic receptors. Antidepressant drugs are used for the treatment of chronic depression, desensitizes presynaptic autoreceptors and heteroreceptors. These are responsible for producing long lasting changes in monoaminergic neurotransmission. Effect of antidepressant drug on postsynaptic receptors, including modulation of GPCR signaling and activation of protein kinase & ion channel (See **Figure 1**) [75].

8. Conclusion

Different types of psychiatric problems, particularly sadness, depression and anxiety are afflicting an increasing number of people. These mental diseases not only have a negative impact on people's daily lives, but they also place a significant financial burden on society. The psychopharmacology of herbs has gotten a lot of attention in recent decades. Finally, it may be concluded that, *Achyrantes aspera* extract exert a protective effect against physically induced depression. It has been also proved that herbal drugs show lesser adverse effects as compared to synthetic drugs that's why *Achyranthes* aspera may be used for the treatment of depression as an herbal remedy.

Author details

Rizwana Bee[1], Mohammad Ahmad[2] and Kamal Kishore Maheshwari[3]*

1 Department of Pharmacy, Integral University Lucknow, India

2 Department of Pharmacology, Faculty off Pharmacy, Integral University Lucknow, India

3 Mahatma Jyotiba Phule Rohilkhand University, Bareilly, UP, India

*Address all correspondence to: kamalbareilly@yahoo.co.in

References

[1] Kuhar MJ, Couceyro PR, Lambert PD. Catecholamines. In: Siegel GJ, Agranoff BW, Albers L, Fisher SK, Uhler MD, editors. Basic Neurochemistry. Philadelphia, PA: Lippincott Williams & Williams; 2001. pp. 243-262

[2] Sutar NG, Sutar UN, Sharma YP, Shaikh IK, Kashirsagar SS. Phytochemical investigation and pharmacological screening of leaves of *Achyranthes aspera* L. as analgesic and antipyretic. Biosciences, Biotechnology Research Asia. 2008;5(2):841-844

[3] Dey A. *Achyranthes aspera* phytochemical and pharmacological aspects. International Journal of Pharmaceutical Sciences Review and Research. 2011;**9**(2):013

[4] Dwivedi S, Dubey R, Mehta K. *Achyranthes aspera* Linn. (Chirchita) a magic herb in folk medicine. Ethnobotanical Leaflets. 2008;**12**:670-676

[5] Gupta RK. Medicinal and Aromatic Plants. New Delhi: CBS Publishers and Distributors; 2010. pp. 1-15

[6] Parmar HK, Sharma D. Pharmacological and medicinal importance of *Achyranthes aspera*. International Journal of Pharmacy and Life Sciences. 2015;**6**(7):4627-4630

[7] Sharma V, Chaudhary U. An overview on indigenous knowledge of *Achyranthes aspera*. Journal of Critical Reviews. 2015;**2**(1):7-19

[8] Barua CC, Talukdar A, Begam SA, Borah P, Lakhar M. Anxiolytic activity of methanol leaf extract of *Achyranthes aspera* Linn in mice using experimental models of anxiety. Indian Journal of Pharmacology. 2012;**44**(1):63-67

[9] Malarvili T, Veerappan RM, Begum VH. Effect of *Achyranthes aspera* seeds on lipid profiles in selected tissues of rats fed with high dose of fructose. Journal of Pharmacy Research. 2011;**2**(6):1769-1771

[10] Pandey R, Samasivarao Y, Gurumurthy. Antibacterial activity of medicinal plants against pathogens from extracts of *Achyranthes aspera*. Med. Aromat. Plants 2013;**5**(2):1000135-1000136

[11] Singh S, Verma SK, Singh SK. In-vitro anticancer activity of *Achyranthes aspera* root extract against different human cancer cell lines. Biolife. 2017;**5**(1):119-122

[12] Mukharjee H, Ojha D, Bag P, Chandel HS, Bhattacharyya S, Chatterjee TK, et al. Anti-herpes virus activity of *Achyranthes aspera*, an Indian ethnomedicine and its triterpene acid. Microbiological Research. 2012;**168**(4):238-244

[13] Chakraborty A, Brantner A, Mukuinaka T, Nobukuni Y, Kuchido M, Konoshima T. Cancer chemo-preventive activity of *Achyranthes aspera* leaves on Epstien-Barr virus activation and two stage mouse skin carcinogenesis. Cancer Letters. 2002;**177**:1-5

[14] Sujhata K, Kavitha K, Manoharan S. Assessment of in-vitro anti-arthritic activity of *Achyranthes aspera*. World Journal of Pharmaceutical Sciences. 2014;**3**(6):894-901

[15] Goli V, Macharla SV, Gowrishankar NL, Dhanalakshmi C, Bhaskar J, Bhaskar KM. Anti-pyretic activity of *Achyranthes aspera* Linn. Pharmanest. 2011;**2**:204-206

[16] Deshmukh VN, Nehete JY, Shewale VV, Raghav NA, Gawande VT. Gastric antiulcer activity of *Achyranthes aspera* L. roots in pylorus ligated rats. Global Journal of Pharmacology. 2011;**5**(3):143-146

[17] Gokhale AB, Damre A, Kulkarni KR, Saraf MN. Preliminary evaluation of anti-inflammatory and anti-arthritic activity of *S. lappa, A. speciosa and A. aspera*. Phytomed. 2002;**9**(5):433-437

[18] Gurumani M, Blalmurugan K. Evaluation of antifertility potential of ethanolic extract of whole plant of *Achyranthes aspera* in female albino rats. International Journal of Current Pharmaceutical Research. 2014;**5**(1):31-36

[19] Meles DK, Wurlina and Adnyana, D.P.A. Measurement of alkaloids *Achyranthes aspera* Linn level using thin layer chromatography method and high-performance liquid chromatography. KnE Life Sciences. 2017;**3**:378-385

[20] Dhale DA, Bhoi S. Pharmacognostic characterization and phytochemical screening of *Achyranthes aspera* Linn. Current Agriculture Research. 2013;**1**(1):51-57

[21] Hasan S. Pharmacological and medicinal uses of *Achyranthes aspera*. International Journal of Environmental Science and Technology. 2014;**3**(1):123-129

[22] Banerji A, Chintalwar GJ, Joshi NK. Isolation of ecdysterone from Indian plants. Phytochemistry. 1971;**10**:2225-2226

[23] Kapoor VK, Singh H. Isolation of betain from *Achyranthes aspera* Linn. Indian Journal of Chemistry. 1966;**4**(10):461-463

[24] Michl G, Abebe D, Baukar F, Debella A, Kunert O, Schmid MG. New triterpenoids saponins from *Achyranthes aspera* Linn. Helvetica Chimica Acta. 2000;**83**(2):359-363

[25] Batta AK, Rangaswami S. Crystalline chemical components of some vegetable drugs. Phytochemistry. 1973;**12**:214-216

[26] Rastogi RP, Mehrotra BN. Compendium of Indian Medicinal Plants. Vol. 5(11). New Delhi: Central Drug Research Institute, Lucknow and National Institute of Science Communication and Information Resources; 2004. pp. 7-8

[27] Kunert O, Haslinger E, Schmid MG, Reiner J, Bucar F, Mulatu E, et al. Monatshefte Fur. Chem. 2000;**131**(2):195-204

[28] Rameshwar RD. Indian Perfumer. 2007;**51**(1):33-34

[29] Hariharan V, Rangaswami S. Structure of saponines A and B from the seeds of *Achyranthes aspera*. Phytochemistry. 1970;**9**:409-414

[30] Chauhan AS, Rawta GS, Singh CP. Phytochemical study of *Actranthes aspera* Linn. Asian Journal of Chemistry. 2002;**14**(2):1059-1061

[31] Vijyaraj R, Vidhya R. Biological activity of *Achyranthes aspera*. Asian Journal of Biochemical and Pharmaceutical Research. 2016;**1**(6): 2231-2560

[32] Neogi NC, Garg RD, Rathor RS. Pharmacological and medicinal uses of *Achyranthes aspera*. The Indian Journal of Pharmacy. 1970;**32**(2):43-46

[33] Agharkar SP. Medicinal Plants of Bombay Presidency. Jodhpur (India): Scientific Publication; 1991

[34] Singh V. Traditional remedies to treat asthma in northwest and trans

Himalayan regions in J. and K. state. Fioterapia. 1995;**56**(6):507-509

[35] Suresh A, Anandan T, Sivanandum G, Veluchamy G. A pilot study of Naayuruvi Kuzhi Thailam in Eraippunoi (bronchial asthma). Journal of Research in Ayurveda & Siddha. 1985;**6**:171-176

[36] Nadkarni KM. Indian Materia Medica. Vol. 1. Mumbai: Bombay Popular Prakashan; 2009. pp. 21-22

[37] Singh VK, Ali ZK. Folk medicines of Aligarh (Uttar Pradesh), India. Fitoterapia. 1989;**60**:483-490

[38] Anis M, Iqbal M. Medicinal plant lore of Aligarh, India. International Journal of Pharmacognosy. 1994;**30**:113-115

[39] Shibeshi W, Maconnen E, Zerihun L, Debella A. Effect of *Achyranthes aspera* on fetal abortion. Uterine and pituitary weights, serum lipids and hormones. African Health Sciences. 2006;**6**(2):108-112

[40] Akhtar MS, Iqbal J. Evaluation of hypoglycemic effect of *Achyranthes aspera*in normal and allaxon-diabetic rabbits. Journal of Ethnopharmacology. 1991;**31**(1):49-57

[41] Page C, Curtis M, Sulter M, Walker M, Hoffman B. Integrated Pharmacology. 2nd ed. New York: Elsevier; 2006. pp. 263-268

[42] Chitra V, Manasa K, Mythilia A, Tamilanban T, Gayathri K. Effect of hydro alcoholic extract of *Achyranthes aspera* on haloperidol induced Parkinson's disease in Wistar rats. Asian Journal of Pharmaceutical and Clinical Research. 2017;**10**(9):318-321

[43] Kaplan HI, Sadock BJ. Comprehensive Textbook of Psychiatry. New York: Lippincott Williams and Wilkins; 2005

[44] Virkamaki A, Korsheninnikova E, Seppala-Lindross A. Intramyo cellular lipid is associated with resistance to in-vivo insulin action on glucose uptake. Antilipolysis and early insulin signaling pathways in human skeletal muscles. Diabetes. 2001;**50**:2337-2343

[45] Reiser S, Powell AS, Scholfield DJ, Panda P, Fields M, Canary JJ. Day long glucose, insulin and fructose responses of hyperinsulinemic and non-hyperinsulinemic men adapted to diets containing either fructose of high-amylose corn starch. American Journal of Nutrition. 1989;**50**:1008-1014

[46] Guimaras PR, Galavo AMP, Batista CM, Azovedo GS, Oliveira RD, Lamounier RP, et al. Egg paint (*Solanum melongena*) infusion has modest and transitory effect on hypercholesteremic subjects. Brazilian Journal of Medical and Biological Research. 2000;**33**:1027

[47] Lee M, Bangerter FW, Deninno MP, Inskeep PB, Mc Carthy PA, Pettini JL, et al. Comparison of synthetic saponin cholesterol absorption inhibitors in rabbits. Evidence for a non stoichimetric, intestinal mechanism of action. Journal of Lipid Research. 1999;**40**:694-699

[48] Samara K, Mota L, Nunes GE, Pinto MEF, Ferreira AL, Monteiro AR, et al. Flavonoids with gastro-protective activity. Molecules. 2009;**14**:979-1012

[49] Agunu A, Abdulrehman EM, Andrew GO, Muhammed Z. Diuretic activity of the stem-bark extracts of steganotaenia araliaceahoehst. Journal of Ethnopharmacology. 2005;**96**:471-475

[50] Niranjan S, Alok KD, Mishra Soumya K, Priyanka G, Susri MS. Diuretic activity of *Achyranthes aspera* leaves extract. RJP. 2012;**3**(4):216-218

[51] Geetha K. Antidiabetic activity of *Achyranthes aspera* L. with alloxanised mice for the estimation of level of glucose and cholesterol. Asian Journal of Plant Science & Research. 2016;**6**(2):18-23

[52] Jayaweera DMA. Medicinal Used Plants in Ceylon, Part IV. National Science Council of Sri Lanka: Colombo, Sri Lanka; 1982. pp. 234-236

[53] Kumar VS, Sankar P, Varatharajan R. Anti-inflammatory activity of roots of *Achyranthes aspera*. Pharmaceutical Biology. 2009;**47**(10):973-975

[54] Vogel HG. Drug Discovery and Evaluation Pharmacological Assays. 2nd ed. New York: Springer; 2002. p. 716

[55] Choudhary GB. Phytochemical investigation and screening of anthelmintic activity of leafy extracts of various *Ocimum* (Tulsi) species. Journal of Pharmaceutical Sciences and Research. 2010;**3**(9):2140-2141

[56] Bharathi NM, Sravanthi V, Sujeeth S, Kalpana K, Santhoshi P, Pavani M. In-vitro anthelmintic activity of methanolic and aqueous extracts of *Achyranthes aspera* (Amaranthaceae). International Journal of Pharmaceutics. 2013;**3**(2):181-184

[57] Lai PK, Roy J. Antimicrobial and chemopreventive properties of herbs and spices. Current Medicinal Chemistry. 2004;**11**:1451-1460

[58] Eisenberg DM, Kessler RC, Foster C, Norlock FE, Calkins DR. Unconventional medicine in the United States. The New England Journal of Medicine. 1993;**328**:246-252

[59] Acumedia. Neogen corporation P.I. 7150, Rev. 04, October. www.google.com. 2008

[60] Aneja KR. Experiments in Microbiology Plant Pathology and Biotech. 4th ed. New Delhi: New Age International Publisher; 2007

[61] Mishra Kumar K, Dhongade Hemant J, Banarase Bhimrao N, Rajput Singh D. Evaluation of antifungal activity of roots of *Achyranthes aspera* for ringworm infection. European Journal of Pharmaceutical and Medical Research. 2016;**3**(2):318-320

[62] Chattopadhyay D, Chawla Sarkar M, Chatterjee T, Bag P, Chakrabarty S. Recent advancements for the evaluation of antiviral activities of natural products. New Biotechnology. 2009;**25**(5):347-368

[63] Whitley RJ, Roizman B. Herpes simplex virus infections. Lancet. 2001;**357**(9267):1513-1518

[64] Clercq ED. Antiviral drugs in current clinical use. Journal of Clinical Virology. 2004;**30**(2):115-133

[65] Paul D, De D, Ali KM, Chatterjee K, Nandi DK, Ghosh D. Comparative study on the spermicidal activity of organic solvent fractions from hydroethanolic extracts of *Achyranthes aspera* and *Stephania hernandifolia* in human and rat sperm. Contraception. 2010;**81**(4):355-361

[66] Vasudeva N, Sharma SK. Post-coital antifertility activity of *Achyranthes aspera* Linn. Root. Journal of Ethnopharmacology. 2006;**107**(2):179-181

[67] Jayakumar T, Sridhar MP, Bharathprasad TR, Ilayaraja M, Govindasamy S, alasubramanian, M.P. Experimental studies of *Achyranthes aspera* (L) preventing nephrotoxicity induced by lead in albino rats. Journal of Health Science. 2009;**55**(5):701-708

[68] Goyal BR, Mahajan SG, Mali RG, Goyal RK, Mehta AA. Beneficial effect of *Achyranthes apsera* Linn. in

toluene-di-isocyanate induced occupational asthma in rats. Global Journal of Pharmacology. 2007;**1**(1):6-12

[69] Datir FSB, Ganjare AB, Nirmal SA, Bhawar SB, Bharati DK, Patil MJ. Evaluation of antiallergic activity of the various extracts of the aerial parts of *Achyranthes aspera* Var. Porphyristachya (Wall.Ex Moq.) hook. Pharmacology. 2009;**3**:921-925

[70] Edwin S, Jarald E, Edwin DL, Jain A, Kinger H, Dutt KR, et al. Wound healing and antioxidant activity of *Achyranthes aspera* Linn. Pharmaceutical Biology. 2009;**46**(12):824-828

[71] Inbaneson SJ, Ravikumar S, Suganthi P. In-vitro anti-plasmodial effect of ethanolic extracts of coastal medicinal plants along Palk strait against *plasmodium falciparum*. Asian Pacific Journal of Tropical Biomedicine. 2012;**2**(5):364-367

[72] Goodman and Gilman. Goodman & Gilman's the Pharmacological Basis of Therapeutics. New York: McGraw-Hill; 9th ed1996. p. 432

[73] Kuhn R. The treatment of depressive states with G22355 (imipramine hydrochloride). The American Journal of Psychiatry. 1958;**115**:459-464

[74] Goodman and Gilman. Goodman & Gilman's the Pharmacological Basis of Therapeutics. New York: McGraw-Hill; 12th ed2011. p. 399

[75] Shih JC, Chen K, Ridd MJ. Monoamine oxidase from genes to behavior. Annual Review of Neuroscience. 1999;**22**:197-217

[76] Rang H, Dale M, Ritter J, Flower R. Rang & Dale's Pharmacology. 6th ed. Elsevier/Churchill Livingstone; 2007. pp. 560-580

Chapter 15

Phenolic Compounds and Antioxidant Activities of Eight Species of Fabaceae That Are Commonly Used in Traditional Medical Practices in the Republic of Suriname

Dennis R.A. Mans, Priscilla Friperson, Jennifer Pawirodihardjo and Meryll Djotaroeno

Abstract

The consumption of diets rich in antioxidants may minimize the chances of developing debilitating diseases such as cardiovascular, diabetic, inflammatory, neoplastic, and cognitive disorders. The Fabaceae or pea family is the third most species-rich plant family on Earth and includes more than 19,000 species in over 700 genera. Many species of Fabaceae are ingredients of staple diets and medicinal substances. This may be attributable to the presumably high content of antioxidants in these plants, particularly phenolic compounds. The Republic of Suriname (South America) harbors over 400 species of Fabaceae in more than 100 genera and has a rich ethnopharmacological tradition that also involves a number of Fabaceae species. In this chapter, we evaluated the literature to determine whether the traditional use of eight of the medicinally most commonly employed Surinamese species of Fabaceae may be associated with their phenolic content and antioxidant activity. Our results suggest that this may hold true for *Caesalpinia pulcherrima, Cajanus cajan, Clitoria ternatea, Desmodium adscendens, Lablab purpureus, and Tamarindus indica* but not for *Copaifera guyanensis* and *Dipteryx odorata*, the bioactivities of which mainly seem to be determined by terpenoids and coumarins, respectively, without an apparent involvement of antioxidant effects.

Keywords: Suriname, Fabaceae, traditional medicine, pharmacological activity, phytochemical composition, phenolic content, antioxidant activity

1. Introduction

Reactive oxygen species (ROS) are chemically unstable oxygen-containing molecules such as superoxide anions and hydroxyl radicals that are able to readily react with and inflict damage to cellular constituents such as nucleic acids, proteins, and lipids [1–3]. ROS are continuously formed in the body during metabolic reactions involving oxygen such as the mitochondrial electron transport chain, in activated white blood cells in order to eliminate bacteria and other invaders, and as products of various intracellular enzymatic reactions such as those catalyzed by nitric oxide synthase and xanthine oxidase, which yield nitric oxide radicals and superoxide radicals, respectively [1–3]. ROS are also produced following exposure of the body to various noxious agents ranging from car exhaust and cigarette smoke to γ-radiation and certain medical drugs [1–3].

ROS play important roles in the cells of the body, for instance, as elements of intracellular signaling pathways for several normal physiological functions including those associated with the regulation of immunity, cell differentiation, and longevity [4–6]. However, a buildup of these species may cause oxidative stress, cell and tissue injury, and cell death [4–6] and is probably at the basis of several ailments such as heart conditions, Alzheimer's disease, and cancer, as well as premature aging and cerebrovascular accidents [7–11]. For this reason, the body has a variety of innate antioxidant defense mechanisms to its disposal to mitigate potential damage by ROS, including enzymatic antioxidant systems (for instance, superoxide dismutase, catalase, and glutathione peroxidase) and non-enzymatic systems (for instance, bilirubin, glutathione, and certain vitamins) [12]. In addition to these innate defense systems, exogenous antioxidants provided through the diet and/or nutritional supplements may help protect the body from oxidative stress [13]. Thus, the consumption of compounds rich in antioxidants may decrease the risk of developing the abovementioned diseases [14–16].

An important class of plant-derived antioxidants is represented by phenolic compounds, secondary plant metabolites made up of one or more aromatic ring(s) coupled to one or more hydroxyl group(s) [17]. Phenolic compounds help protect plants from pathogens, animal and insect attack, as well as ultraviolet radiation; provide plants their characteristic colors; and contribute to the organoleptic properties of plants [18]. There are tens of thousands of plant phenolic compounds including the main dietary constituents flavonoids, phenolic acids, and tannins, in addition to coumarins, naphthoquinones, stilbenes, anthraquinones, and lignans [13, 17]. Their mitigating effect on oxidative stress has been attributed to their ability to eliminate potentially harmful oxidizing free radical species by acting as reducing agents, hydrogen donors, quenchers of singlet oxygen, or chelators of metal ions that catalyze oxidation reactions [13, 17].

The pea family Fabaceae is a large family of flowering plants that include various economically important plants such as the soybean *Glycine max* (L.) Merr., the cowpea *Vigna unguiculata* (L.) Walp.), and the peanut *Arachis hypogaea* L. [19, 20]. The Fabaceae family also includes many species that represent important sources of a wide variety of ethnobotanical medicines against a myriad of diseases (see, for instance, references [20, 21]). This may be attributable to their relatively high contents of various pharmacologically active constituents including phenolic compounds with antioxidant properties [22, 23]. In addition, the Fabaceae is considered a plant family that hyperaccumulates selenium, a key constituent of selenoproteins such as the antioxidant enzyme glutathione peroxidase [24].

The Republic of Suriname (South America) has a land area of roughly 165,000 km^2, about 80% of which consists of sparsely inhabited, dense, pristine, and highly biodiverse tropical rain forest [25]. Conversely, about 80% of the country's population of just over 600,000 lives in the relatively narrow northern coastal zone of the country [26]. Mostly because of the variety of habitats and the humid tropical temperature, the biodiversity in Suriname is high, encompassing roughly 5100 different plant species [27]. As in other parts of the world, the Fabaceae plant family represents a substantial part of Suriname's plant diversity, with estimations of over 400 different species in more than 100 genera from the northern coast all the way up to the expansive forested mountain ranges [28]. The Fabaceae are also ingredients of a large variety of traditional medicines in Suriname. So far, it is not clear whether this is because of their remarkably high phenolic content and antioxidant activity. In this chapter, we have addressed this topic by assessing whether the traditional uses and pharmacological activities of eight medicinally commonly employed Fabaceae in Surinamese traditional medicine may be associated with their phenolic content and antioxidant activity.

2. ROS and oxidative stress

ROS can be defined as oxygen-containing reactive species and include oxygen-free radicals with unpaired electrons such as superoxide, hydroxyl, peroxyl, and alkoxyl radicals, as well as non-radical species such as hydrogen peroxide, peroxynitrite, hypochlorous acid, and ozone [1–3]. Reactive nitrogen species (RNS) such as nitric oxide, peroxynitrite, and nitrogen dioxide radical, as well as reactive chlorine species (RCS) such as hypochlorous acid, are also classified as ROS [1–3]. As mentioned in the preceding section, ROS are able to readily react with and cause damage to biomolecules including proteins, lipids, and nucleic acids, leading to cell and tissue injury [4–6]. The high reactivity of ROS derives from the presence of a single unpaired electron in their outer orbit formed as a result of incomplete reduction of the oxygen metabolites [4–6].

ROS can be generated from either endogenous or exogenous sources. Endogenous sources of ROS are cellular organelles where oxygen metabolism is high, such as mitochondria, phagocytic cells, endoplasmic reticulum, and peroxisomes [12]. For instance, during oxidative phosphorylation in the mitochondria, the electron transport chain produces electrons for the reduction of molecular oxygen into superoxides. The superoxides are transformed into the much less reactive hydrogen peroxide by superoxide dismutase. However, when hydrogen peroxide interacts with ions of transition metals such as Fe^{2+} and Cu^{2+}, the most reactive ROS, hydroxyl radicals are formed through Fenton's reaction [29]. And phagocytized bacteria, bits of necrotic tissue, other harmful cells, and foreign particles are destroyed by macrophages and neutrophils by the so-called respiratory burst (or oxidative burst), involving the rapid release of superoxides and hydrogen peroxide following the supply of electrons by NADPH [30].

Other important endogenous (enzymatic) sources of ROS are the cytochrome P450 superfamily of enzymes that produce ROS during the detoxification and excretion of xenobiotics [31], cyclooxygenase and lipoxygenase that generate ROS from arachidonic acid [32], and xanthine oxidoreductase that produces superoxide anions during the breakdown of purines to uric acid [33]. And as mentioned before, in the Fenton and Haber-Weiss reactions, molecular oxygen is reduced to form superoxide anions, which dismutates to form hydrogen peroxide that can react with traces of iron or copper to form more highly reactive hydroxyl ions and subsequently hydroxyl radicals [34].

Exogenous sources of ROS are γ-radiation and UV radiation; air pollutants such as car exhaust, cigarette smoke, and industrial contaminants; peroxides, aldehydes, oxidized fatty acids, and transition metals in foods; a large variety of xenobiotics including toxins, pesticides, and herbicides; as well as various medical drugs such as narcotics, anesthetizing gases, and antineoplastic agents [1–3]. Gamma radiation, for instance, interacts with water molecules to form water radical cations and free electrons, which react with other water molecules to form highly active hydroxyl radicals, superoxides, and organic radicals. These ROS are then converted into organic hydroperoxides and hydrogen peroxide, which subsequently react with Fe^{2+} and Cu^{2+} ions, generating even more ROS, eventually resulting in massive damage to cellular biomolecules such as DNA, proteins, and lipids [35].

Iron and copper, along with cadmium, nickel, arsenic, and lead, not only generate ROS by Fenton or Haber-Weiss type reactions, but also by direct reactions with cellular constituents, producing, for example, thiol-type radicals [36]. For instance, arsenic induces the production of peroxides, superoxides, and nitric oxide and inhibits antioxidant enzymes such as glutathione-transferase, glutathione-peroxidase, and glutathione-reductase by binding to the sulfhydryl group [37]. And lead triggers lipid peroxidation and increases glutathione peroxidase concentration in brain tissue [38]. The free radicals generated from these reactions can affect DNA, with substitutions of some DNA bases such as guanine with cytosine, guanine with thymine, and cytosine with thymine [39].

An example of a medical drug that generates ROS is the antitumor antibiotic doxorubicin, both the antineoplastic activity and the cardiomyopathy of which are probably based on its reduction to a semiquinone-derivative that can autoxidize in the presence of oxygen and then produces superoxide anions following electron donation by oxidases such as mitochondrial NADPH and nitric oxide synthases [40].

3. Defenses against oxidative stress

At non-cytotoxic levels, ROS and their secondary electrophilic species perform important functions in the human body, among others, by acting as redox signaling messengers required for the normal physiological functioning of cells [41]. In general, ROS are messengers in the transduction of certain metabolic and environmental cues, which affect diverse signaling pathways, culminating in the activation of transcription factors and other proteins, determining cell fate [5]. A well-described example is redox signaling involving the oxidation of cysteine residues of proteins by hydrogen peroxide, and converting a thiolate anion in cysteine (Cys-S-) into the sulfenic form (Cys-SOH), causing the protein to undergo allosteric changes that alter its function [42]. The sulfenic form can be reduced to thiolate anions by the disulfide reductases thioredoxin and glutaredoxin, to return the protein function to its original state [43]. Comparable reversible ROS-operated mechanisms are involved in the regulation of several key signal transduction pathways such as the PI3K-AKT and RAS-MEK-ERK pathways involved in the promotion of cell proliferation, nutrient uptake, and cell survival [44, 45].

Whether ROS cause oxidative stress and cellular damage is determined by the net result of their production and elimination by antioxidant defenses. Thus, oxidative stress is a consequence of "a disturbance in the prooxidant to antioxidant balance in favor of the former, leading to potential damage" [3]. The antioxidant defenses prevent the formation of ROS or interrupt their propagation, eliminate ROS by scavenging them, slow down redox reactions by removing free-radical intermediates, inhibit oxidation reactions by being oxidized themselves, and repair the oxidized molecules [46]. These mechanisms can be distinguished into innate defense systems and exogenous antioxidants provided through the diet and/or nutritional supplements.

3.1 Innate antioxidant defenses

The innate antioxidant defenses of the body comprise enzymatic and non-enzymatic systems. The main enzymatic antioxidant systems are superoxide dismutase, catalase, and glutathione peroxidase. The metalloprotein superoxide dismutase catalyzes the dismutation of superoxides, that is, the formation of one molecule of oxygen and one molecule of hydrogen peroxide from two superoxides [47, 48]. Hydrogen peroxide can subsequently be converted into highly reactive hydroxyl radicals in the presence of transition metal ions such as Fe^{2+} or Cu^{2+} in the Fenton reaction, propagating the damage inflicted to cellular DNA, proteins, and lipids [47, 48]. Superoxide dismutase prevents this process through its three isoforms, cytosolic copper/zinc-superoxide dismutase (Cu/Zn-SOD, SOD_1), mitochondrial manganese superoxide dismutase (Mn-SOD, SOD_2), and extracellular copper/zinc-superoxide dismutase (Cu/Zn-EC-SOD, SOD_3) [47, 48]. The isoforms are located in distinct cellular compartments and/or have different metal components, but all three convert and neutralize superoxides as mentioned above [47, 48].

Catalase acts as a catalyst for the conversion of hydrogen peroxide into oxygen and water. It mitigates the effect of intracellular hydrogen peroxide [49]. Glutathione peroxidases are a family of at least eight oxidoreductases that contain seleno-cysteine in the active site [50, 51]. These enzymes catalyze the reduction of organic hydroperoxides into alcohol and water groups using reduced glutathione as a co-substrate [50, 51]. They can also catalyze the reduction of hydrogen peroxide to water and oxygen by oxidation of reduced glutathione to its disulfide [50, 51]. Oxidized glutathione can be reduced to glutathione by the enzyme glutathione reductase by using NADPH as a reducing substrate [50, 51]. In this way, glutathione peroxidase protects cells from oxidative damage and helps detoxify hydrogen peroxide [50, 51].

Non-enzymatic endogenous antioxidant mechanisms are, among others, bilirubin and albumin. Bilirubin is produced from the enzymatic degradation of hemoglobin and other heme proteins to first yield biliverdin, and then bilirubin following reduction of biliverdin by the enzyme biliverdin reductase [52]. Bilirubin prevents lipid oxidation by removing peroxyl radicals whereby it is oxidized itself to biliverdin, after which it is rapidly reduced by biliverdin reductase to bilirubin [52]. And serum albumin represents an abundant circulating antioxidant defense system [53]. It is able to bind transition metals such as copper and iron, preventing the formation of hydroxyl radicals *via* the Fenton reaction after their interaction with hydrogen peroxide, directly scavenge hydroxyl radicals, and bind and transport bilirubin, which then acts as an inhibitor of lipid peroxidation [53].

3.2 Exogenous defenses: dietary nutrients

Exogenous antioxidants are mainly derived from dietary sources and include, among others, a variety of phenolic compounds, essential minerals, vitamins, small peptides, and certain fatty acids [13]. Their health-promoting and preventive effects against diseases associated with oxidative stress are now well established [7–11]. The most common phenolic compounds in the diet are phenolic acids and various subclasses of flavonoids, which together account for on average 60 and 30%, respectively, of the total dietary intake of phenolic compounds [54].

Phenolic compounds are able to act as antioxidants in multiple ways, among others, because of their redox properties, which enable them to adsorb and neutralize free radicals, quench singlet and triplet oxygen, or decompose peroxides [55, 56]. These processes are accomplished by hydrogen atom transfer, transfer of a single electron, sequential proton loss electron transfer, or chelation of transition metals [55, 56]. In addition, phenolic compounds are able to act synergistically with other antioxidants such as ascorbic acid, β-carotene, and α-tocopherol [57] and are presumably also involved in the regulation of intracellular glutathione levels [58].

Other dietary constituents with antioxidant properties are certain essential minerals, vitamins, small peptides, and fatty acids. Copper, iron, manganese, zinc, and selenium are indirectly involved in the body's antioxidant defenses by enhancing the activities of antioxidant enzyme. For instance, selenium is a cofactor of glutathione transferase and other selenoproteins [59]. It has notable antioxidant activity [60] and may be beneficial in chronic conditions such as cancer [61], heart disease [62], and cognitive disorders [63]. And copper, zinc, and manganese are cofactors of superoxide dismutase [64].

Antioxidant vitamins such as ascorbic acid are able to quench ROS by donating electrons to them; α-tocopherol inhibits ROS generation, preventing lipid peroxidation of cellular membranes; thiamin is a cofactor of NADPH that is required for the production of glutathione reductase and the activity of catalase; and the retinol precursor β-carotene reacts with peroxyl, hydroxyl, and superoxide radicals [65, 66]. The common dietary small peptide glutathione is able to directly scavenge ROS [67]. And polyunsaturated fatty acids in, for instance, fish oil, are able to eliminate ROS and inhibit cellular processes that generate ROS, decreasing the risk of cardiovascular diseases by reducing triacylglycerol production in the plasma [68].

4. Fabaceae

4.1 Taxonomy

The pea family Fabaceae, also known as Leguminosae, is the third largest family of flowering plants after the Orchidaceae (orchid family) and the Asteraceae (aster family), representing about 7% of the global number of flowering plant species [69]. The Fabaceae consists of more than 700 genera and about 20,000 species of annual, biennial, or perennial trees, shrubs, herbaceous plants, vines, and lianas, which are encountered in all ecosystems throughout the world except Antarctica and the high Arctic [69, 70]. Most woody trees are found in tropical regions, while the herbaceous plants and shrubs are predominant outside the tropics [70]. Fabaceae members are readily recognizable by their fruits known as legumes or pods, which split open as they dry, releasing the seeds, and by their compound, stipulated leaves [71].

The leaves of many species (such as those of the common vetch *Vicia sativa* L.) have glands that produce nectar (extrafloral nectaries) through which they attract ants, which protect them from attacks by herbivores [72]. In other species (such as some in the genus *Acacia*), the stipules (outgrowths on both sides of the base of the leafstalk) are modified to tiny chambers called domatia, which accommodate "body guard" ants [73]. Many Fabaceae (such as species of groundnut in the genus *Apios*) also host symbiotic bacteria in their roots—called rhizobia—which convert atmospheric nitrogen into a form that they can use for their metabolism (such as nitrate or ammonia) in a process referred to as nitrogen fixation [74]. The flowers of most species are conspicuous and colorful to attract pollinator insects [71]. The ovary itself matures into a legume or pod that encloses the seeds [71].

The Fabaceae includes six subfamilies [75], namely the Faboideae (or Papilionoideae), Caesalpinioideae, Detarioideae, Cercidoideae, Dialioideae, and Duparquetioideae [75]. The largest subfamily is that of the cosmopolitan Faboideae that harbors 503 genera and about 14,000 species including species of milkvetch in the genus *Astragalus*, species of lupin in the genus *Lupinus*, and species of pea in the genus *Pisum* [75]. The pantropical subfamily Caesalpinioideae includes about 4400 species in 148 genera such as the peacock flower *Caesalpinia pulcherrima* (L.) Sw., the candle bush *Senna alata* (L.) Roxb., the shy plant *Mimosa pudica* L., and the soap pod *Senegalia tenuifolia* (L.) Britton & Rose [75].

The subfamilies Detarioideae and Cercidoideae are mainly tropical and include 84 genera and about 760 species, and 12 genera and about 335 species, respectively [75]. Well-known examples in the Detarioideae are the ornamental pride of Burma *Amherstia nobilis* Wall and the tamarind *Tamarindus indica* L. that bears edible fruit. Renowned species in the Cercidoideae are well-appreciated ornamentals such as the pom pom orchid tree *Bauhinia divaricata* L. and the Judas tree *Cercis siliquastrum* L. [75]. The 85 species in 17 genera of the subfamily Dialioideae are widespread throughout the tropics [75]. A well-known example is the western African velvet tamarind *Dialium cochinchinense* Pierre, the velvety black pods of which contain a vitamin-rich acidic pulp that is chewed to relieve thirst or macerated in water to produce a beverage [75]. The subfamily Duparquetioideae is the smallest, consisting of one genus and one species, the liana *Duparquetia orchidacea* Baill that is native to western and central Africa [75].

The five largest genera of the Fabaceae family are *Astragalus* (milkvetches, subfamily Faboideae; over 3000 species), *Acacia* (acacias, subfamily Caesalpinioideae; over 1000 species), *Indigofera* (true indigos, subfamily Faboideae; around 700 species), *Crotalaria* (rattlepods, subfamily Faboideae; around 700 species), and *Mimosa* (sensitive plants or touch-me-nots, subfamily Caesalpinioideae; around 400 species), which constitute about a quarter of all legume species [75].

4.2 Economic value

Together with cereals, some vegetables and fruits, roots and tubers, oil-bearing crops, and sugar crops, various Fabaceae have been a staple food for humans for millennia, and their use and subsequent domestication and cultivation have been critical to the development of human civilization settlements [76, 77]. There are records dating the use of several species and varieties of beans in Asia, the Americas, and Europe to about 6000 BC, when they were becoming an essential staple as a source of protein (see, for instance, references [78, 79]). Contributing to the importance of the Fabaceae to human civilization were their extraordinary diversity and abundance and the broad variety of other uses they can be put to, ranging from ornamentals to medicines [69, 70]. In fact, species of Fabaceae are still among the economically and culturally most important plants in the world, providing foods, natural fertilizers, and forage; medicines; ornamentals; as well as materials for the pharmaceutical, cosmetic, and textile industries (see, for instance, reference [80]).

Examples of Fabaceae that are food crops of global importance are *G. max* (soybean), *Phaseolus* (beans), *Pisum sativum* (pea), *Cicer arietinum* (chickpeas), *Medicago sativa* (alfalfa), *A. hypogaea* (peanut), *Ceratonia siliqua* (carob), and *Glycyrrhiza glabra* (liquorice) [81]. Notably, the Fabaceae plant family is the second most important economic producer of crop plants after the Poaceae, the rice family [80]. Furthermore, the ability of Fabaceae to fix atmospheric nitrogen makes them very suitable as natural fertilizers to replenish soil that has been depleted of nitrogen [82]. A few species used for this purpose are leadtrees (*Leucaena* spp.) and riverhemps (*Sesbania* spp.) [82]. The additional nitrogen they receive increases their protein content, making some of them (such as the alfalfa *M. sativa* L. as well as clovers (*Trifolium* spp.), vetches (*Vicia* spp.), and peanut-like species (*Arachis* spp.) suitable as fodder for livestock [83].

Examples of Fabaceae with therapeutic properties are gum Arabic from the gum acacia *Senegalia senegal* (L.) Britton that has antitussive and anti-inflammatory properties [84] and tragacanth from *Astragalus gummifer* Labill that can be used as a demulcent in burn wounds [85]. Other species of Fabaceae are used for the production of vegetable oils for cooking. Well-known examples are the oils extracted from the soya bean *G. max* [86] and the peanut *A. hypogaea* [87].

Still other Fabaceae members are industrially farmed to produce dyes. Examples are the logwood *Haematoxylon campechianum* L., the heartwood of which produces red and purple dyes such as the histological stain hematoxylin [88], and the true indigo *Indigofera tinctoria* L., the leaves of which give the blue dye indigotin [89]. Furthermore, the roots of species in the genus *Derris* such as *D. elliptica* found in Southeast Asia and the southwest Pacific islands are a source of the strong insecticide rotenone [90]. And well-known ornamentals are the cockspur coral tree *Erythrina crista-galli* L., the national tree of Argentina, and the national flower of Argentina and Uruguay [91], and the Chinese wisteria *Wisteria sinensis* (Sims) DC that is a much appreciated ornamental vine [92].

4.3 Phenolic compounds and antioxidant activity

In addition to the applications mentioned above, many species of Fabaceae are traditionally used for medicinal or invigorating purposes (as mentioned in Section 6 of this chapter). The pharmacological activities have been associated with the abundant presence in the plants of certain bioactive ingredients—particularly phenolic compounds such as phenolic acids, (iso)flavonoids, and anthocyanins—with relatively high antioxidant activity [93–96]. In fact, the phenolic compounds in many species of Fabaceae—mostly isoflavones such as genistein and daidzein—are involved in a variety of physiological and metabolic processes that are relevant to human health [97]. The seeds are often not only highly nutritious, but also contain the majority of the phenolics [97–102]. Several of the phenolics elicited high antioxidant potential, displaying the ability to scavenge free radicals, and the ability to interact with proteins [97, 98], as well as a diversity of pharmacological activities including, among others, anti-inflammatory, vasodilatory, analgesic, antimicrobial, anti-allergenic, cardioprotective, anti-atherogenic, anticarcinogenic, and immunomodulating activities [97, 98].

However, as mentioned before, the Fabaceae comprise almost 20,000 species, and much of the information on the antioxidant activity and phenolic content extrapolated to the entire plant family is based on investigations with a relative handful of species (see, for instance, references [22, 23, 103–106]). Nevertheless, despite variable antioxidant activities among species, these studies have suggested a good correlation between total phenolic content and antioxidant activity [22, 23, 103–106].

DOI: http://dx.doi.org/10.5772/intechopen.106076

The Fabaceae also constitute the greatest number of selenium-hyperaccumulating species, *that is*, plants that accumulate selenium in their cells at concentrations in excess of 1000 mg per kg dry weight [107]. Many selenium hyperaccumulators in this family belong to the genus *Astragalus* (milkvetches, subfamily Faboideae), the largest Fabaceae genus with over 3000 species of herbs and small shrubs [108]. The members of the much smaller genus *Neptunia* (subfamily Caesalpinioideae) also hyperaccumulate selenium [109].

5. The Republic of Suriname

5.1 Generalities

The Republic of Suriname is located on the northeast coast of South America, bordering the Atlantic Ocean and surrounded by French Guiana, Brazil, and Guyana (**Figure 1**). Roughly 80% of the approximately 600,000 inhabitants live in the capital city of Paramaribo and other urbanized areas in the northern coastal zone of the country (**Figure 1**). The remaining 20% resides in the rural-coastal areas and the southern-rural interior, which comprises approximately 90% of the country's land surface and largely consists of sparsely inhabited savanna and undisturbed, dense tropical rainforest with a very high animal and plant biodiversity [25, 26] (**Figure 1**).

Suriname's most important economic means of support are crude oil drilling, gold mining, agriculture, fisheries, forestry, and ecotourism [110]. These activities

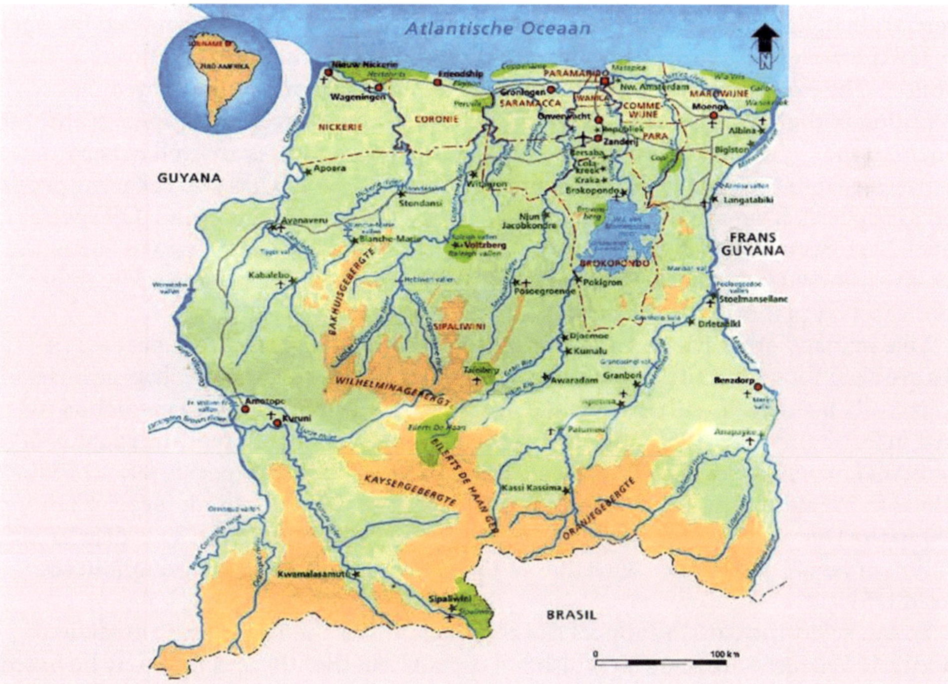

Figure 1.
Map of the Republic of Suriname. Circle in top left: suriname's location in South America.

substantially contributed to the gross domestic product in 2020 of about USD 3 billion [111], positioning Suriname on the World Bank's list of upper-middle-income economies [112]. Suriname's population is among the most varied in the world, comprising Amerindians (the original inhabitants of the country) as well as descendants from enslaved Africans, indentured laborers from Asia, and European settlers, as well as immigrants from various Latin American and Caribbean countries [113]. All ethnic groups have preserved much of their original culture and identity, still practicing the religion they were raised with, speaking the language from their country of origin, maintaining their specific perceptions of health and disease, and adhering to their ethnopharmacological traditions [114, 115].

As a result, the use of various forms of traditional medicine is deeply rooted in the country, despite the broad availability of affordable modern health care [114, 115]. This inclination, together with the easy access to raw plant material from Suriname's rich biodiversity, probably accounts for the frequent use of traditional herbal medications in the country, either alone or in conjunction with prescription medicines [114, 115]. As in many other regions throughout the world, parts from Fabaceae members are often used for preparing the traditional medicines. The botanical knowledge to identify useful and edible plants has probably been obtained from ancient knowledge from the country of origin, by exchanging information with other cultures, by observing other peoples and animals, and by trial and error [114, 115].

5.2 Fabaceae in Suriname

The Fabaceae plant family is the most common family in tropical rainforests and dry forests of the Americas and Africa [116]. This plant family is also abundantly present in Suriname, and all growth forms—from dwarf shrubs and broadleaf evergreen trees to lianas and plants with bulbs or rhizomes—can be encountered between the northern coastal plain and the heavily forested and mountainous interior of the country. The exact number of genera and species in Suriname is not known, but according to the Checklist of the Venezuelan Guiana, there were 1032 species and 146 genera in the Guiana Shield in the year 2007 [28]. These figures are well in accordance with those from the National Herbarium of Suriname, which has 146 Fabaceae genera and 531 species from the Guiana Shield in its repository, 132 genera and 429 species of which have been collected in Suriname [28]. Thus, the Fabaceae species in Suriname can be estimated to constitute roughly 10% of the total number of approximately 5100 vascular plants in the country.

Like in many other parts of the world, several of the Surinamese Fabaceae species are used for a diversity of medicinal purposes. These species of Fabaceae have extensively been dealt with in several comprehensive publications on medicinal plants used in Suriname [117–125], and their total amounted to about 60 of the roughly 800 medicinal plant species. Thirty-nine of the medicinal Fabaceae species (about 65%) belong to the subfamily Faboideae, 16 (about 25%) to the Caesalpinioideae, 4 (about 7%) to the Detarioideae, and only 1 (about 2%) to the Cercidoideae. This distribution is more or less in accordance with that of the Fabaceae subfamilies throughout the world [75].

So far, scientific data to support the health claims of the Surinamese medicinal species of Fabaceae are scant. It is also not certain whether these claims may be based on the relatively high content of phytochemicals with antioxidant activity of these plants that, as mentioned above, seems to be one of the hallmarks of this plant family.

For this reason, we consulted the literature for evidence implicating the phenolic antioxidants in the plants in their traditional claims of beneficial health effects as well as their pharmacological activities. Fabaceae members that are mainly used for religious and ritual and spiritual purposes (such as the rosary pea or kokriki *Abrus precatorius* L., the bushillo shimbillo or yaraní *Zygia inaequalis* (Humb. & Bonpl. ex Willd.) Pittier, and the shining rattlepod or ogri-aypesi *Crotalaria micans* Link. [van Andel and Ruysschaert, 2011]) have been left out of our selection. From the remaining plants, eight that have been most frequently mentioned as sources of traditional medicines in the abovementioned publications [117–125] are in detail addressed hereunder (see also **Table 1**).

Plant species	Traditional uses	Pharmacological activities	Antioxidant phenolic compounds
Caesalpinia pulcherrima (L.) Sw. (peacock flower; krerekrere)	Oral complaints; gynecological, obstetric, and genitourinary conditions; colds and fevers; gastrointestinal disorders	Antimicrobial, analgesic, anti-inflammatory, cytotoxic, antioxidant activities	Yes; flavonoids
Cajanus cajan (L.) Millsp. (pigeon pea; loangopesi)	Oral complaints; skin problems; inflamed eyes; antiparasitic; analgesic; diabetes mellitus; labor induction; anti-emetic; gastrointestinal disorders	Anti-inflammatory, antioxidant activities	Yes; flavonoids
Clitoria ternatea L. (butterfly pea; kembang telang)	Aphrodisiac; inflamed eyes; memory-enhancing and improving of cognitive functions; sedative, anxiolytic, and antidepressant	Antimicrobial, antipyretic, analgesic, anti-inflammatory, analgesic, antidiabetic, antioxidant activities	Yes; flavonoids
Copaifera guyanensis Desf. (copaiba; hoepelhout)	Oral complaints; skin problems; respiratory ailments; wound healing-stimulatory; inflammations; microbial infections; parasitic infections; genitourinary conditions; gastrointestinal disorders; diabetes mellitus, hypertension	Antimicrobial, antiparasitic, anti-inflammatory, wound healing-stimulatory, antioxidant activities	No; terpenoids
Desmodium adscendens (Sw.) DC. (glue sticks; konkruman)	Respiratory ailments; fever; rheumatism; inflammation; epilepsy; genitourinary conditions; gastrointestinal disorders; diabetes mellitus; hypertension	Anti-asthmatic, anti-anaphylactic, antihypertensive, antioxidant activities	Yes; flavonoids, anthocyanins, tannins

Plant species	Traditional uses	Pharmacological activities	Antioxidant phenolic compounds
Dipteryx odorata (Aubl.) Willd. (tonka bean; tonkaboon)	Hair care; colds, fever, respiratory ailments; analgesic; gastrointestinal disorders; genitourinary conditions; parasitic infections; aphrodisiac	Antimicrobial, antiviral, anticoagulant, anticancer, anti-inflammatory activities	Yes; coumarin analogues, but no apparent antioxidant activities
Lablab purpureus (L.) Sweet (hyacinth bean; kulibontyi)	Alcohol intoxication; aphrodisiac; fungal skin infections; hypertension; high cholesterol; diabetes mellitus	Anti-inflammatory, analgesic, antidiabetic, antimicrobial, antihypertensive, anticancer, antioxidant activities	Yes; flavonoids
Tamarindus indica L. (tamarind; tamarinde)	Gastrointestinal disorders; skin problems; wound healing-stimulatory; microbial infections; parasitic infections, inflammations; hypertension; genitourinary conditions	Anti-inflammatory, analgesic, antimicrobial, antiviral, antihypertensive, antidiabetic, anticancer, antioxidant activities	Yes; phenolic compounds like tannins as well as selenium, ascorbic acid, and ß-carotene

Table 1.
Antioxidant compounds of eight Fabaceae members from Suriname and association with pharmacological activity.

6. Health effects of some Surinamese Fabaceae and relationship with phenolic antioxidants

6.1 *Caesalpinia pulcherrima* (L.) Sw

The peacock flower or krerekrere *C. pulcherrima* (L.) Sw. (**Figure 2**) is an evergreen shrub that grows to 3 m tall and likely originates from Mexico and the Caribbean, but can now be encountered in all tropical and subtropical parts of the Americas. Its beautiful inflorescence in yellow, red, and orange has made it a generally valued ornamental plant and the national flower of the Caribbean island of Barbados. The mature seeds contain cyanide and are poisonous, but the immature seeds are edible after roasting [126]. As the taste seems reminiscent of that of peanuts, another Surinamese vernacular for *C. pulcherrima* is "jodenpinda," meaning "the peanut of the Jews," in reference to the colonial masters from Jewish ancestry on whose plantations the enslaved Africans had come to know the plant [127].

Preparations from various parts of *C. pulcherrima* are used as a mouthwash for teeth and gums; as an emmenagogue, to accelerate childbirth, and as a strong abortifacient; for treating colds and fevers; against gastrointestinal complaints such as diarrhea, constipation, and gall bladder problems; and to remedy urinary tract problems such as kidney stones [128, 129]. In Suriname, *C. pulcherrima* is used for the same purposes [118, 120, 125] but also for good fortune and to honor Mama Aisa, an important deity in Afro-Surinamese Winti religion [130].

Phytochemical investigations have revealed the presence of various bioactive constituents in *C. pulcherrima* including a variety of flavonoid compounds along with glycosides,

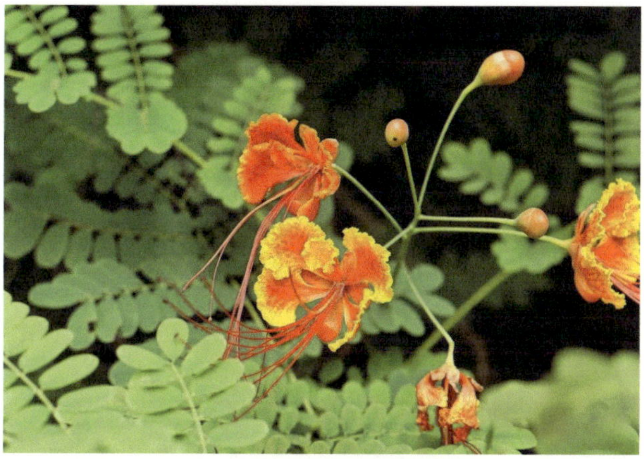

Figure 2.
Flower of the peacock flower or krerekrere Caesalpinia pulcherrima *(L.) Sw. (from: https://images.app.goo.gl/bqSv1gehtAQT11uk8).*

alkaloids, terpenoids, and sterols [131–133]. Some of these compounds have been associated with pharmacological activities such as antimicrobial, analgesic, anti-inflammatory, and cytotoxic activities, supporting some of the traditional uses of the plant [132–134].

Preparations from several parts of *C. pulcherrima* also exhibited substantial antioxidant activity [134–136]. Studies with this plant and other species of *Caesalpinia* have suggested that this activity may be associated with, among others, anti-inflammatory activity [135, 136], the inhibition of prostaglandin biosynthesis [135], the inhibition of nitric oxide production [136, 137], and/or the stimulation of superoxide dismutase and catalase activity [137]. These activities might be attributed to the phenolic compounds in the plant [136, 138, 139], supporting a role of these substances and their antioxidant activities in its apparent health-promoting effects.

6.2 *Cajanus cajan* (L.) Millsp.

The pigeon pea or loangopesi *C. cajan* (L.) Millsp. (**Figure 3**) is an erect, woody shrub that grows to a height of about 4 meters and that is native to the Old World [140]. It is not known in the wild but has been cultivated for centuries in tropical and subtropical regions of the world for its edible, protein-rich seeds, its medicinal properties, as well as its usefulness as fuel, a green manure, and for soil stabilization [140]. This plant is believed to have reached the New World including Suriname by means of the Trans-Atlantic slave trade at the end of the seventeenth century [141]. It grows relatively fast, is rather resilient, easily adapts to different soil and climatic conditions, and is drought-resistant [142], which makes it of utmost importance for food security in areas where rainfall is not reliable and droughts are likely to occur [143]. Not surprisingly, *C. cajan* has become part of the daily staple meals of millions of people throughout the world [140].

Humans have also used *C. cajan* since long medicinally, among others, for oral hygiene and treating oral complaints such as gingivitis and stomatitis, and ulcers and inflammations in the oral cavity, skin problems, as well as various chronic diseases such as diabetes mellitus [144–146]. In Suriname, the fresh leaf is squeezed into inflamed eyes [117] and incorporated into an infusion to facilitate childbirth [117] and to stop severe vomiting [118]. The potential therapeutic efficacy of these

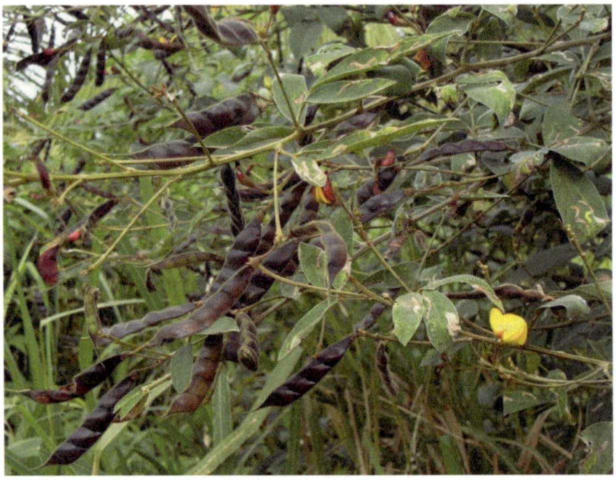

Figure 3.
Seedpods of the pigeon pea or loangopesi Cajanus cajan *(L.) Millsp. (from: https://images.app.goo.gl/k6pETr1KXfuioSte8).*

traditional remedies is partially supported by the results from pharmacological studies showing remarkable anti-inflammatory activity of preparations from several parts *C cajan* in both cell culture and animal models [147–150].

These observations have been attributed to the prevention of lipid peroxidation, the stimulation of endogenous antioxidant enzyme activities, and/or a decrease in the production of inflammatory cytokines [148–150]. The phytochemicals that have been held responsible for these activities were flavonoids [148–150], which was in accordance with the high phenolic content of *C. cajun* that included a diversity of flavonoids, tannins, coumarins, and stilbenes [147, 151]. Notably, flavonoid and phenolic contents of the plant samples correlated well with their individual antioxidant activity [149, 152]. Based on these data, *C. cajan* has been proposed as a candidate for skin care research and development [151].

6.3 *Clitoria ternatea* L.

The butterfly pea *Clitoria ternatea* L. is a perennial herbaceous climber that is native to tropical equatorial Asia, but can now also be found in Africa, Australia, and the Americas including Suriname. The genus name "*Clitoria*" has been derived from the presumed resemblance of the strikingly blue flowers with light yellow markings to the shape of human female genitals (**Figure 4**). This is also captured in the Indonesian/Malay vernacular of the plant "kembang telang," "kembang" meaning "blossoming," "swollen," or "extended," and "telang" meaning "blue-colored flower." The blue color of the flower is caused by its high content of ternatins, polyacylated derivatives of the anthocyanin delphinidin 3,3′, 5′-triglucoside [153]. It is used in south-eastern Asia as a natural coloring for rice dishes, desserts, hot and cold beverages, and textiles for making clothing. The attractive flower also makes the plant a well-appreciated ornamental in many parts of the world. Other notable chemical components in *C. ternatea* are cyclotides, exceptionally stable macrocyclic peptides present in all tissues of this plant [154]. These compounds are the bioactive molecules in a commercial eco-friendly insecticide developed from this plant [155].

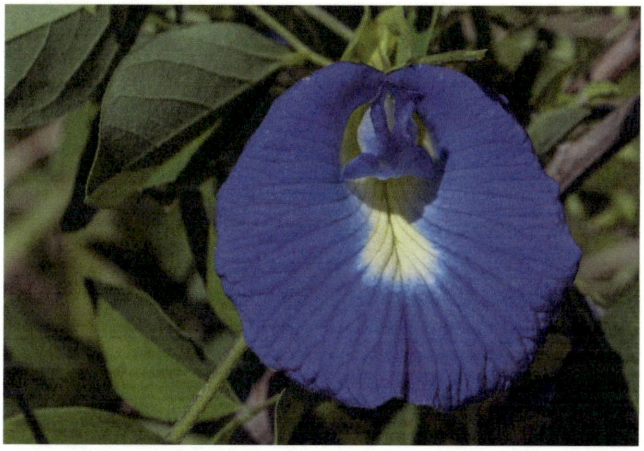

Figure 4.
Flower of the butterfly pea or kembang telang Clitoria ternatea *L. (from: https://images.app.goo.gl/dtytS8JnGZBEzhPg9).*

In traditional Chinese medicine, *C. ternatea* is used to increase female libido [156]. And in Indian Ayurveda, preparations from the plant are believed to enhance memory, improve cognitive function, control or prevent seizures, relieve stress, prevent or treat anxiety and depression, and exert calming and sedative effects [157]. These effects might be associated with the modulation of serotonin and acetylcholine metabolism in the brain [158]. In Suriname, *C. ternatea* is mainly used by the Javanese, who pour the diluted sap from the macerated leaf into inflamed eyes [118].

A variety of preclinical studies have shown that extracts from *C. ternatea* display a wide range of pharmacological activities including antimicrobial, antipyretic, anti-inflammatory, analgesic, diuretic, local anesthetic, antidiabetic, insecticidal, blood platelet aggregation-inhibiting, and vascular smooth muscle-relaxing properties [157, 159]. Many of these activities have been attributed to the presence of flavonols (in the form of flavonol glycosides) and anthocyanins in the plant [159]. These compounds could elicit some of the abovementioned pharmacological activities through their well-documented antioxidant effects [160, 161] or by contributing to the pharmacological activities of other bioactive compounds in the plant [159].

For instance, the anthocyanin delphinidin 3-sambubioside (from the dried calices of the roselle *Hibiscus sabdariffa* L.; Malvaceae) elicited anti-inflammatory activity in both cell and animal models [162], the synthetic cyclotide [T20K]kalata B1 delayed disease progression and diminished symptoms in a mouse model of multiple sclerosis [163], and the pentacyclic triterpenoid taraxerol isolated and purified from extracts of the transformed root somaclones of *C. ternatea* displayed encouraging anticancer properties [164]. Interestingly, the antioxidant properties of *C. ternatea* have commercially been utilized by including extracts from the flower in antiaging cosmetic products [165].

6.4 *Copaifera guyanensis* Desf.

The copaiba or hoepelhoutboom *Copaifera guyanensis* Desf. is an evergreen tree with a thick trunk that grows to about 25 m tall and that is indigenous to the swamps and rainforests of northern South America including Suriname (**Figure 5**). *C. guyanensis* is much in demand for the oleoresin in the grayish-brown bark of the trunk.

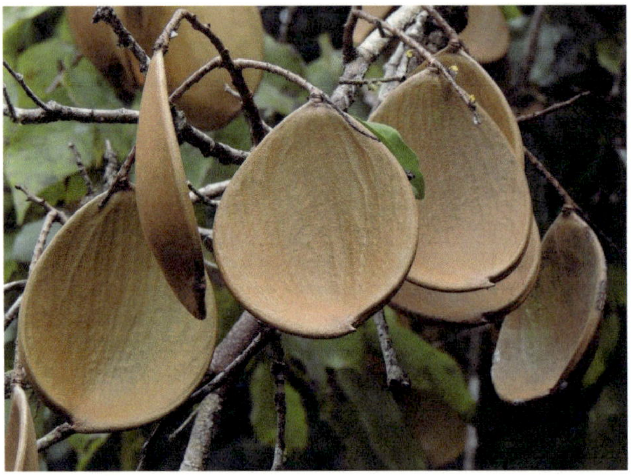

Figure 5.
Seedpods of the copaiba or hoepelhout Copaifera guyanensis *Desf. (from: https://images.app.goo.gl/G6iLQWMFEEfyPR8D8).*

The oleoresin is a transparent, yellow to light brown liquid consisting of a nonvolatile fraction and a volatile essential oil with a scent that has been described as woody, sweet, and balsamic [166, 167]. The oleoresin is harvested by drilling a hole in the trunk of the tree and collecting it with the help of a polyvinyl chloride pipe, after which the borehole is plugged in order for the tree to sufficiently recover to retap it a year later. The oleoresin is used in small amounts as a food additive and as a flavoring agent in foods and beverages and has officially been approved in the USA for these purposes (see, for instance, [168]). It is also an ingredient of perfumes, varnishes, and lacquers and used as a substitute for diesel oil [169–171]. Given the latter application, *C. guyanenesis* is also called "diesel tree." The flexible but tough heartwood has been used for preparing hoops to tightly press the staves of barrels against each other, achieving watertight containers to store sugar. Hence, the Surinamese vernacular "hoepelhout," literally meaning "wood for constructing hoops" [125].

C. guyanansis oleoresin (as well as that of other *Copaifera* species) has a very long history of medicinal use. In fact, the Amazonian Indigenous peoples have known the healing properties of the oleoresins for centuries from their observation that injured animals rubbed themselves on the tree's trunk to heal their wounds [169, 172]. This led to the use of the oleoresin against, among others, microbial infections and inflammations and as a disinfectant, styptic, and wound-healing stimulatory substance [166, 173]. Other indications of *C. guyanensis* oleoresin are a sore throat, tonsillitis, bronchitis, and tuberculosis; cystitis, kidney and bladder infections, vaginal discharge, and gonorrhea; stomach ulcers; as well as a variety of skin problems including insect bites, eczema, blisters, sores, and psoriasis [167, 169, 174]. *C. guyanansis* oleoresin has essentially the same traditional uses in Suriname, where, in addition, a tea from the bark is drunk against diabetes mellitus, hypertension, malaria, and jaundice [125].

The principle pharmacologically active ingredients in the volatile essential oil of *C. guyanensis* oleoresin are sesquiterpenes, most notably β-caryophyllene, while the nonvolatile fraction mainly consists of acid diterpenes such as copalic acid and kaurenoic acid [166, 173]. Particularly β-caryophyllene displayed substantial antiseptic, anti-inflammatory, and antimicrobial effects including activity against *Staphylococcus aureus* [166, 167, 175], a common cause of skin infections. For these reasons, the cosmetic industry extensively uses *Copaifera* oleoresins in anti-acne creams, formulations for treating stretch marks and scars, as well as shampoos, capillary lotions, soaps, and bathing foams [176]. β-Caryophyllene also selectively binds to the cannabinoid receptor 2 [177], which makes it an interesting candidate to relieve pain and inflammation [176, 178]. The diterpenes from *Copaifera* oleoresins reportedly elicited *in vitro* antibacterial, anti-inflammatory, antileishmanial, antitrypanosomal, and wound-healing stimulatory activities [179]. These findings substantiate some of the traditional uses of *C. guyanenesis*, but so far there are no convincing data on the usefulness of *Copaifera* oleoresins in the clinic (see, for instance, reference [178]).

There are also reports on antioxidant activity of *Copaifera* species. For instance, the oleoresin from *C. langsdorffii* Desf. elicited notable antilipoperoxidation, antioxidant, and anti-inflammatory activity in an experimental model of random skin flaps on rat dorsums [180]. In addition, the essential oil from *C. officinalis* L. seed reduced lipid oxidation, showing promise as a natural antioxidant to increase the shelf life of meat products [168]. This effect has tentatively been attributed to the phenolic compounds identified in the essential oil [168]. Phenolic compounds—particularly flavonoids—have also been detected in the fruit and leaf of several *Copaifera* species [181, 182]. However, at this moment, there is no hard evidence to associate phenolic compounds and their potential antioxidant activities with the traditional uses and pharmacological activities of *Copaifera* species.

6.5 *Desmodium adscendens* (Sw.) DC

The glue sticks *D. adscendens* (Sw.) DC is a creeping or ascending herbaceous perennial herb or low shrub that can grow up to 1 meter in height. It probably originates from Africa, but is now widespread in tropical areas of Asia, South and Central America, and the Caribbean. The presence of many small hooked hairs on the seedpods (**Figure 6**) makes them cling to clothing, body parts, as well as the feathers and coats of pollinating animals, ensuring a wide dispersal of the plant. Hence, the vernacular "glue stick" in English and "konkruman" ("informer") in Suriname: the sticky pods attaching to

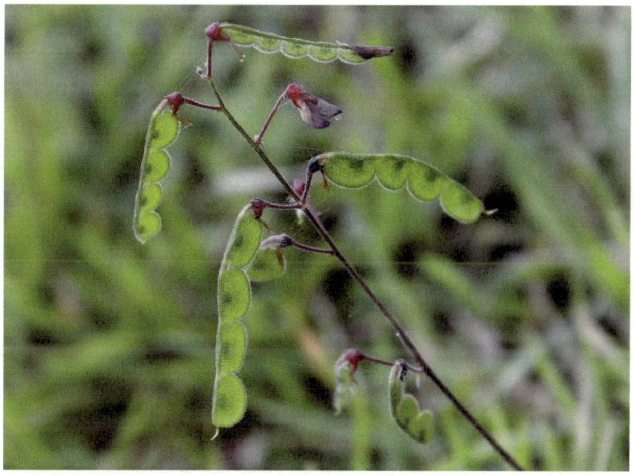

Figure 6.
Seedpods of the glue sticks or konkruman Desmodium adscendens *(Sw.) DC. (from: https://images.app.goo.gl/CoBQwXQrRHUgXq4e9).*

clothing betray the unapproved presence of the bearer "in the field," that is, away from home [183]. The plant is also believed to attract and hold fortune and prosperity while at the same time capturing and removing bad luck and disease [125].

Leaf, stem, and root of *D. adscendens* (as well as parts of the closely related species *Desmodium barbatum* (L.) Benth. and *Desmodium incanum* (Sw.) DC) have probably been used for thousands of years by native peoples of the Americas for a variety of health issues, including asthma and allergies; muscle cramp and back pain, rheumatism; venereal diseases, vaginal infections, and ovarian inflammation; epilepsy; hypertension; and diabetes mellitus [184, 185]. In Suriname, preparations from *D. adscendens* leaf, stem, and root are taken to relieve abdominal pain, fever, and painful urination associated with venereal diseases and as a remedy against diabetes mellitus and hypertension [124].

D. adscendens is rich in phenolic compounds including flavonoids, anthocyanins, and tannins, as well as reducing sugars, alkaloids, (soya)saponins, triterpenes, and amines [185, 186]. The meaningful pharmacological activities displayed by some of these compounds—such as anti-asthmatic and anti-anaphylactic activity [187, 188] and antihypertensive activity [183]—may support some of the traditional uses of the plant.

There are also reports associating the appreciable content of phenolic compounds with its antioxidant activity and some of its pharmacological effects. For instance, astragalin, the 3-O-glucoside of the flavonoid kaempferol, displayed antioxidant, anti-inflammatory, and anti-atopic dermatitis activity and attenuated lipopolysaccharide-induced inflammatory responses by suppressing the NF-κB signaling pathway [189]. Astragalin also elicited antibacterial activity [190], which may explain the abovementioned traditional uses of the plant for treating infections, venereal diseases, and wounds [124, 184, 185]. Moreover, leaf and whole-plant extracts from *D. adscendens* displayed ROS scavenging activity and antioxidant properties *in vitro* [186]. These preparations also protected an LLC-PK1 pig kidney epithelial cell line from glucose-induced oxidative stress [191] and hepatocytes from carbon-tetrachloride-induced injury and hepatitis C virus infection [192]. These observations support the possibility that the antioxidant properties and the phenolic compounds of *D. adscendens* may be associated with its potential therapeutic value.

6.6 *Dipteryx odorata* (Aubl.) Willd

The tonka bean or tonkaboon *D. odorata* (Aubl.) Willd. (**Figure** 7) is a large semi-deciduous tree with a small, rounded crown that generally grows up to 30 m tall and that is native to Central America and northern South America. The tree is sometimes cultivated but is mostly harvested from the wild for its seed that is rich in coumarin [193]. The tonka beans are black and wrinkled, and have a smooth, brown interior, and their high content of coumarin and several of its derivatives such as umbelliferone (7-hydroxycoumarin) give them a strong sweet and spicy fragrance that is reminiscent of vanilla and almond [193]. For this reason, coumarin is abundantly used in the perfume industry as a fragrance and in desserts and stews as a substitute for vanilla [194]. However, at large infused doses, coumarin may cause liver damage, hemorrhages, and paralysis of the heart [195]. It is therefore controlled as a food additive by many governments [194] and has even been banned in the USA [196]. Anticoagulant prescription drugs such as warfarin are based on 4-hydroxycoumarin that was initially isolated from *D. odorata* seed, but coumarin itself does not have anticoagulant properties [197]. Other non-medical applications of coumarins are their use as agrochemicals,

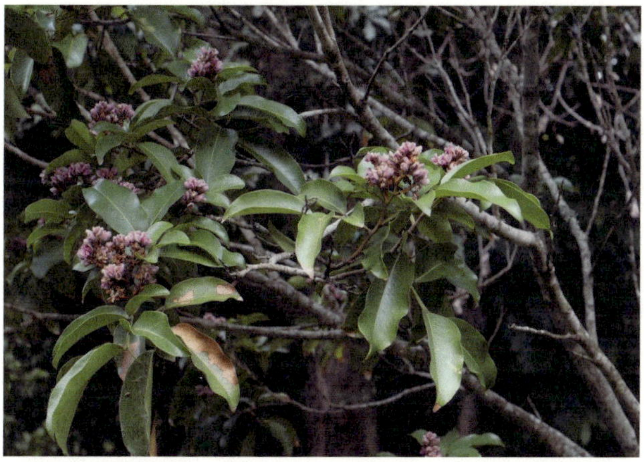

Figure 7.
Flowering tonka bean or tonkaboon Dipteryx odorata *(Aubl.) Willd. (from: https://images.app.goo.gl/Yy9nodcJhZr5mwvG9).*

materials for food processing, optical brighteners, and dispersed fluorescent and laser dyes (see, for instance, references [198, 199]).

Despite the safety concerns, the seed and various other parts of *D. odorata* are traditionally used, among others, to fortify the scalp and improve hair growth; as a remedy for colds, fever, coughing, asthma, and tuberculosis; for treating stomach pain and diarrhea; against dysentery and schistosomiasis; as an emmenagogue, and as an aphrodisiac [200, 201]. In Suriname, *D. odorata* seed is mainly used as an ingredient of products to treat hair loss, dandruff, and an itching scalp; against colds; and to command luck [125, 202].

Some of the traditional uses of *D. odorata* are supported by the results from studies with various coumarin analogues—from the seed as well as other parts of the plant—showing a wide range of pharmacological activities such as antimicrobial, antituberculosis, antiviral, anticoagulant, anticancer, anti-inflammatory, and antioxidant activities [194, 203]. In addition to coumarin, *D. odorata* seed contains various other bioactive flavonoids, particularly isoflavones [204], particularly in the endocarp [205] as well as some of its other parts [206, 207]. These compounds are known to elicit potent antioxidant activity [208] and are, similarly to coumarins, phenylpropanoid-derived natural products. However, so far, their presence in *D. odorata* has neither been associated with antioxidant activity nor with the traditional and pharmacological activities of preparations from the plant.

6.7 *Lablab purpureus* (L.) Sweet

The hyacinth bean *L. purpureus* (L.) Sweet (**Figure 8**) is an annual or short-lived perennial vine of approximately 6 m high that is presumably native to Africa and has been introduced in south-eastern Asia where it has been cultivated as early as 2500 BC [209]. Since then, it has been carried to many tropical and subtropical parts of the world including Suriname, where it has been brought by Hindustani indentured laborers around the end of the nineteenth century [124]. Hence, its Surinamese vernacular "kulibontyi," literarily meaning "the bean of the coolies," the epithet used for Hindustanis in that period. *L. purpureus* is commercially cultivated as an edible

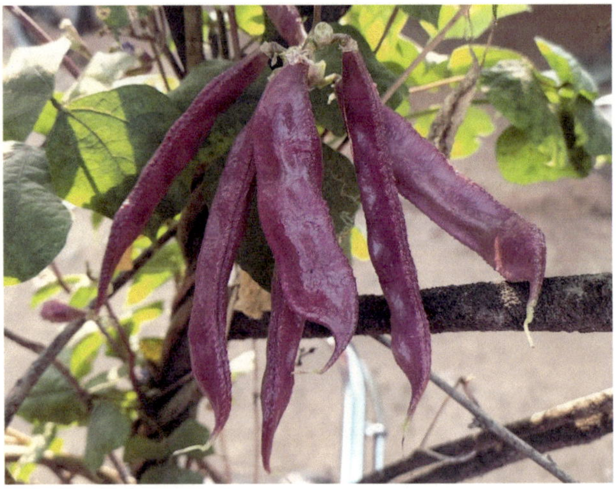

Figure 8.
Seedpods of the hyacinth bean or kulibontji Lablab purpureus *(L.) sweet (from: https://images.app.goo.gl/EpBr6jHWi2s63vEHA).*

plant, as forage for livestock, and as an ornamental. The seed is poisonous due to its high content of toxic cyanogenic glucosides and trypsine and must thoroughly be cooked to destroy the toxin before consumption [210].

Preparations from various parts of the plant are used for a wide range of medicinal applications, ranging from remedies for alcohol intoxication and insufficient libido to medications for hypertension, high cholesterol, and diabetes mellitus [211, 212]. In Suriname, this plant is mainly used by Hindustanis, who apply the macerated leaves as a poultice against the fungal skin infections pityriasis versicolor and ringworm [124]. Pharmacological studies have shown, among others, anti-inflammatory, analgesic, antidiabetic, antimicrobial, antihypertensive, and anticancer activities [213, 214]. These activities may be associated, at least in part, with the presence in the plant of a variety of pharmacologically active constituents including phenolic compounds such as the flavonoids isoflavone, kievitone, and genistein [212, 215, 216]. In studies with other plants, some of these compounds reportedly decreased the production and the release of arachidonic acid, the expression of cyclooxygenase-1, cyclooxygenase-2, and 15-lipooxygenase, as well as the production of downstream-situated inflammatory mediators such as nitric oxide and prostaglandin E2, eliciting anti-inflammatory activities [217–220]. Whether the phenolic compounds in *L. purpureus* also elicit these activities is not certain. But should that be the case, they can account for the traditional uses of the plant as well as the interest of the pharmaceutical industry to develop them to medicinal foods, nutraceuticals, and pharmaceuticals [211, 221].

6.8 *Tamarindus indica* L.

The tamarind or tamarinde *T. indica* is a long-living fruiting tree with a dense, spreading crown that can reach a height of 30 m. It is probably indigenous to tropical Africa where it grows in the wild. The tree has been cultivated for centuries in the tropics and subtropics as an ornamental plant, for its edible seedpods (**Figure 9**), and for its many medicinal uses. It has presumably been introduced in Suriname by enslaved Africans in the seventeenth century in order to fight diseases such as fever,

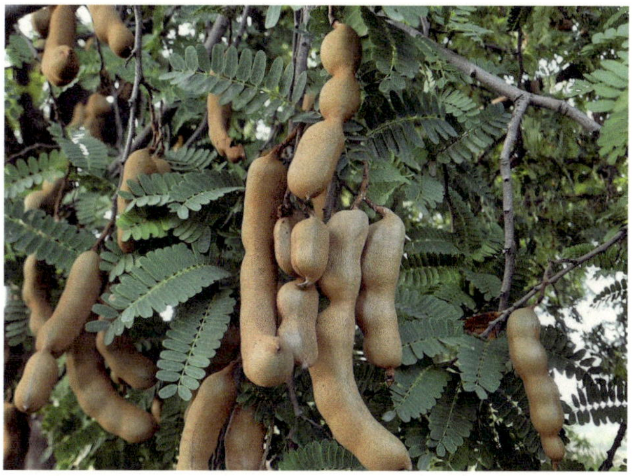

Figure 9.
Seedpods of the tamarind or tamarinde Tamarindus indica *L. (from: https://images.app.goo.gl/FJZ5FyY8UrNma1QUA).*

diarrhea, and worm infections on the slave ships [141]. *T. indica* produces pods with a hard, brown shell that contain about 10 seeds surrounded by a sour pulp that is rich in tartaric acid, acetic acid, and citric acid and is used in cooking, to flavor foods, in refreshing drinks, and as a key ingredient of Worcestershire sauce.

Preparations from *T. indica* leaf, seed, fruit, stem bark, and root are extensively used in folk medicine, among others, for treating abdominal complaints, to stimulate wound healing, to treat microbial and parasitic infections, against various skin diseases, to fight various inflammatory ailments, and as a remedy for hypertension and diabetes mellitus [222, 223]. In Suriname, *T. indica* preparations are used for the same conditions but also against menstrual pain and excessive vaginal discharge [117, 121]. Some of the traditional uses are supported by the results from pharmacological studies showing anti-inflammatory, analgesic, antimicrobial, antiviral, antihypertensive, antidiabetic, and anticancer activities in several laboratory models (see, for instance, references [224–226]).

Some of these activities may be attributable to the presence in the plant of pharmacologically active ingredients with notable antioxidant properties such as phenolic compounds [224–227] including tannins [227, 228], as well as selenium [229], and ascorbic acid and ß-carotene [228]. The antioxidant activity of *T. indica* preparations has been associated with, among others, their antidiabetic, hypolipemic, and antihypertensive effects in laboratory animals [230–232]. Thus, several of the traditional uses and pharmacological activities of *T. indica* may be partially associated with the presence in the plant of phenolic compounds with antioxidant activity.

7. Concluding remarks

Parts from species in the Fabacaeae plant family are among the most commonly used ingredients in Surinamese traditional medical practices and are employed for a wide diversity of medical indications. In this chapter, we have determined whether the abundant medicinal use of these plants may be associated with their phenolic content and antioxidant activity. This was based on the association of the Fabaceae family with these properties [93–102], even though phenolic antioxidants have been found in a relative handful of the roughly 20,000 plant species in this family that have scientifically been evaluated [93–102]. The plants assessed in the current chapter were *C. pulcherrima*, *C. cajan*, *C. ternatea*, *C. guyanensis*, *D. adscendens*, *D. odorata*, *L. purpureus*, and *T. indica* (**Table 1**). For six of these plants—*C pulcherrima*, *C cajan*, *C. ternatea*, *D. adscendens*, *L. purpureus*, and *T. indica*—the traditional uses and pharmacological activities could be attributed, at least in part, to their phenolic compounds (more specifically, their flavonoids) and the notable antioxidant activities of these substances (**Table 1**). However, the traditional uses and pharmacological activities of *C. guyanensis* mainly seemed to be determined by terpenoids which did not elicit antioxidant activity (**Table 1**). And those of *D. odorata* mainly seemed to involve coumarins, which, although classified as phenolic compounds, did not seem to act *via* antioxidant activity (**Table 1**). This argues against the characterization of the Fabaceae as "a plant family of antioxidant phenolic compounds" [93–102] and underscores the necessity to further explore this group of plants for other classes of phytochemicals and other so far unknown but potentially useful pharmacological activities.

Author details

Dennis R.A. Mans*, Priscilla Friperson, Jennifer Pawirodihardjo and Meryll Djotaroeno
Faculty of Medical Sciences, Department of Pharmacology, Anton de Kom University of Suriname, Paramaribo, Suriname

*Address all correspondence to: dennismans16@gmail.com

References

[1] Li R, Jia Z, Trush MA. Defining ROS in biology and medicine. Reactive Oxygen Species (Apex, NC). 2016;**1**:9-21. DOI: 10.20455/ros.2016.803

[2] Kumar V, Abdussalam A. A review on reactive oxygen and nitrogen species. Era's Journal of Medical Research. 2017;**4**:1-5

[3] Sies H, Jones DP. Reactive oxygen species (ROS) as pleiotropic physiological signalling agents. Nature Reviews: Molecular Cell Biology. 2020;**21**:363-383. DOI: 10.1038/s41580-020-0230-3

[4] Pham-Huy LA, He H, Pham-Huy C. Free radicals, antioxidants in disease and health. International Journal of Biomedical Sciences. 2008;**4**:89-96

[5] Schieber M, Chandel NS. ROS function in redox signaling and oxidative stress. Current Biology. 2014;**24**:R453-R462. DOI: 10.1016/j.cub.2014.03.034

[6] Bardaweel SK, Gul M, Alzweiri M, Ishaqat A, Salamat HA, Bashatwah RM. Reactive oxygen species: The dual role in physiological and pathological conditions of the human body. Eurasian Journal of Medicine. 2018;**50**:193-201

[7] Klaunig JE, Kamendulis LM. The role of oxidative stress in carcinogenesis. Annual Review of Pharmacology and Toxicology. 2004;**44**:239-267. DOI: 10.1146/annurev.pharmtox.44.101802.121851

[8] Markesbery WR, Lovell MA. DNA oxidation in Alzheimer's disease. Antioxidants & Redox Signaling. 2006;**8**:2039-2045. DOI: 10.1089/ars.2006.8.2039

[9] Elahi MM, Kong YX, Matata BM. Oxidative stress as a mediator of cardiovascular disease. Oxidative Medicine and Cellular Longevity. 2009;**2**:259-269. DOI: 10.4161/oxim.2.5.9441

[10] Cui H, Kong Y, Zhang H. Oxidative stress, mitochondrial dysfunction, and aging. Journal of Signal Transduction. 2012;**2012**:646354. DOI: 10.1155/2012/646354

[11] Shirley R, Ord EN, Work LM. Oxidative stress and the use of antioxidants in stroke. Antioxidants (Basel). 2014;**3**:472-501. DOI: 10.3390/antiox3030472

[12] Noori S. An overview of oxidative stress and antioxidant defensive system. Open Access Scientific Reports. 2012;**1**:413. DOI: 10.4172/scientificreports.413

[13] Balsano C, Alisi A. Antioxidant effects of natural bioactive compounds. Current Pharmaceutical Design. 2009;**15**:3063-3073. DOI: 10.2174/138161209789058084

[14] Caleja C, Ribeiro A, Barreiro MF, Ferreira ICFR. Phenolic compounds as nutraceuticals or functional food ingredients. Current Pharmaceutical Design. 2017;**23**:2787-2806. DOI: 10.2174/1381612822666161227153906

[15] Aune D, Keum N, Giovannucci E, Fadnes LT, Boffetta P, Greenwood DC, et al. Dietary intake and blood concentrations of antioxidants and the risk of cardiovascular disease, total cancer, and all-cause mortality: A systematic review and dose-response meta-analysis of prospective studies. The American Journal of Clinical Nutrition. 2018;**108**:1069-1091. DOI: 10.1093/ajcn/nqy097

[16] Jayedi A, Rashidy-Pour A, Parohan M, Zargar MS, Shab-Bidar S. Dietary antioxidants, circulating antioxidant concentrations, total antioxidant capacity, and risk of all-cause mortality: A systematic review and dose-response meta-analysis of prospective observational studies. Advances in Nutrition. 2018;**9**:701-716. DOI: 10.1093/advances/nmy040

[17] Minatel IO, Borges CV, Ferreira MI, Gomez HAG, Chen CYO, Lima GPP. Phenolic compounds: Functional properties, impact of processing and bioavailability. In: Soto-Hernandez M, Palma-Tenango M, del Rosario Garcia-Mateos M, editors. Phenolic Compounds—Biological Activity. London: IntechOpen; 2017. DOI: 10.5772/66368

[18] Babenko LM, Smirnov OE, Romanenko KO, Trunova OK, Kosakivska IV. Phenolic compounds in plants: Biogenesis and functions. Ukrainian Biochemical Journal. 2019;**91**:5-18. DOI: 10.15407/ubj91.03.005

[19] Isely D. Leguminosae and Homo sapiens. Economic Botany. 1982;**36**: 46-70. DOI: 10.1007/BF02858699

[20] Molares S, Ladio A. The usefulness of edible and medicinal Fabaceae in Argentine and Chilean Patagonia: Environmental availability and other sources of supply. Evidence-based Complementary and Alternative Medicine. 2012;**2012**:901918. DOI: 10.1155/2012/901918

[21] Macêdo MJF, Ribeiro DA, de Oliveira SM, de Macêdo DG, Macedo JGF, de Almeida BV, et al. Fabaceae medicinal flora with therapeutic potential in Savanna areas in the Chapada do Araripe. Northeastern Brazil. Revista Brasileira de Farmacognosia. 2018;**28**:738-750. DOI: 10.1016/j.bjp.2018.06.010

[22] Tungmunnithum D, Drouet S, Lorenzo JM, Hano C. Characterization of bioactive phenolics and antioxidant capacity of edible bean extracts of 50 Fabaceae populations grown in Thailand. Food. 2021;**10**:3118. DOI: 10.3390/foods10123118

[23] Jacob MCM, da Silva-Maia JK, Albuquerque UP, Pereira FO. Culture matters: A systematic review of antioxidant potential of tree legumes in the semiarid region of Brazil and local processing techniques as a driver of bioaccessibility. PLoS One. 2022;**17**:e0264950. DOI: 10.1371/journal.pone.0264950

[24] Tinggi U. Selenium: Its role as antioxidant in human health. Environmental Health and Preventive Medicine. 2008;**13**:102-108. DOI: 10.1007/s12199-007-0019-4

[25] Hammond DS. Forest conservation and management in the Guiana Shield. In: Hammond DS, editor. Tropical Rainforests of the Guiana Shield. Wallingford: CABI Publishing; 2005

[26] General Bureau of Statistics/Census Office. Results of the Eight General Census of Suriname. Demographic and Social Characteristics and Migration. Paramaribo: General Bureau of Statistics; 2013

[27] Ministry of Labor, Technological Development and Environment. Suriname. The Fourth National Report to the Convention on Biological Diversity. Paramaribo, Suriname: Ministry of Labor, Technological Development and Environment; 2012

[28] Berry PE, Weitzman AL. Checklist of the Plants of the Guiana Shield (Venezuela: Amazonas, Bolivar, Delta Amacuro; Guyana, Surinam, French Guiana). In: Funk VA, Hollowell TH,

Berry PE, Kelloff CL, Alexander SN, editors. Checklist of the Plants of the Guiana Shield (Venezuela: Amazonas, Bolivar, Delta Amacuro; Guyana, Surinam, French Guiana). Washington, DC: Smithsonian Institution; 2007

[29] Kowaltowski AJ, Castilho RF, Vercesi AE. Mitochondrial permeability transition and oxidative stress. FEBS Letters. 2001;**495**:12-15. DOI: 10.1016/s0014-5793(01)02316-x

[30] Thomas DC. The phagocyte respiratory burst: Historical perspectives and recent advances. Immunology Letters. 2017;**192**:88-96. DOI: 10.1016/j.imlet.2017.08.016

[31] McDonnell AM, Dang CH. Basic review of the cytochrome P450 system. Journal of the Advanced Practitioner in Oncology. 2013;**4**:263-268

[32] Ivanov I, Saam J, Kuhn H, Holzhütter HG. Dual role of oxygen during lipoxygenase reactions. The FEBS Journal. 2005;**272**:2523-2535. DOI: 10.1111/j.1742-4658.2005.04673.x

[33] Battelli MG, Polito L, Bortolotti M, Bolognesi A. Xanthine oxidoreductase in drug metabolism: Beyond a role as a detoxifying enzyme. Current Medicinal Chemistry. 2016;**23**: 4027-4036. DOI: 10.2174/0929867323666160725091915

[34] Thomas C, Mackey MM, Diaz AA, Cox DP. Hydroxyl radical is produced via the Fenton reaction in submitochondrial particles under oxidative stress: Implications for diseases associated with iron accumulation. Redox Report. 2009;**14**:102-108. DOI: 10.1179/135100009X392566

[35] Spitz DR, Azzam EI, Li JJ, Gius D. Metabolic oxidation/reduction reactions and cellular responses to ionizing radiation: A unifying concept in stress response biology. Cancer Metastasis Reviews. 2004;**23**:311-322. DOI: 10.1023/B:CANC.0000031769.14728.bc

[36] Sciskalska M, Zalewska M, Grzelak A, Milnerowicz H. The influence of the occupational exposure to heavy metals and tobacco smoke on the selected oxidative stress markers in smelters. Biological Trace Element Research. 2014;**159**:59-68. DOI: 10.1007/s12011-014-9984-9

[37] Hu Y, Li J, Lou B, Wu R, Wang G, Lu C, et al. The role of reactive oxygen species in arsenic toxicity. Biomolecules. 2020;**10**:240. DOI: 10.3390/biom10020240

[38] Lopes ACBA, Peixe TS, Mesas AE, Paoliello MMB. Lead exposure and oxidative stress: A systematic review. In: de Voogt P, editor. Reviews of Environmental Contamination and Toxicology. Cham: Springer; 2016. DOI: 10.1007/978-3-319-20013-2_3

[39] Jan AT, Azam M, Siddiqui K, Ali A, Choi I, Haq QM. Heavy metals and human health: Mechanistic insight into toxicity and counter defense system of antioxidants. International Journal of Molecular Sciences. 2015;**16**:29592-29630. DOI: 10.3390/ijms161226183

[40] Kong CY, Guo Z, Song P, Zhang X, Yuan YP, Teng T, et al. Underlying the mechanisms of doxorubicin-induced acute cardiotoxicity: Oxidative stress and cell death. International Journal of Biological Sciences. 2022;**18**:760-770. DOI: 10.7150/ijbs.65258

[41] Finkel T. Signal transduction by reactive oxygen species. The Journal of Cell Biology. 2011;**194**:7-15. DOI: 10.1083/jcb.201102095

[42] Rhee SG. Cell signaling. H_2O_2, a necessary evil for cell signaling. Science. 2006;**312**:1882-1883. DOI: 10.1126/science.1130481

[43] Winterbourn CC, Hampton MB. Thiol chemistry and specificity in redox signaling. Free Radical B iology & Medicine. 2008;**45**: 549-561. DOI: 10.1016/j.freeradbiomed.2008.05.004

[44] Meng TC, Fukada T, Tonks NK. Reversible oxidation and inactivation of protein tyrosine phosphatases *in vivo*. Molecular Cell. 2002;**9**:387-399. DOI: 10.1016/s1097-2765(02)00445-8

[45] Lee SR, Yang KS, Kwon J, Lee C, Jeong W, Rhee SG. Reversible inactivation of the tumor suppressor PTEN by H_2O_2. The Journal of Biological Chemistry. 2002;**277**:20336-20342. DOI: 10.1074/jbc.M111899200

[46] Gutteridge JMC, Halliwell B. Antioxidants in Nutrition, Health and Disease. Oxford: Oxford University Press; 1994

[47] Ighodaro OM, Akinloye OA. First line defence antioxidants-superoxide dismutase (SOD), catalase (CAT) and glutathione peroxidase (GPX): Their fundamental role in the entire antioxidant defence grid. Alexandria Journal of Medicine. 2018;**54**:287-293. DOI: 10.1016/j.ajme.2017.09.001

[48] Wang Y, Branicky R, Noë A, Hekimi S. Superoxide dismutases: Dual roles in controlling ROS damage and regulating ROS signaling. The Journal of Cell Biology. 2018;**217**:1915-1928. DOI: 10.1083/jcb.201708007

[49] Nandi A, Yan L-J, Jana CK, Das N. Role of catalase in oxidative stress- and age-associated degenerative diseases. Oxidative Medicine and Cellular Longevity. 2019;**2019**:9613090. DOI: 10.1155/2019/9613090

[50] Lubos E, Loscalzo J, Handy DE. Glutathione peroxidase-1 in health and disease: From molecular mechanisms to therapeutic opportunities. Antioxidants & Redox Signaling. 2011;**15**:1957-1997. DOI: 10.1089/ars.2010.3586

[51] Sarıkaya E, Doğan S. Glutathione peroxidase in health and diseases. In: Bagatini M, editor. Glutathione System and Oxidative Stress in Health and Disease. London: IntechOpen; 2020. DOI: 10.5772/intechopen.91009

[52] Moussa Z, Judeh Z, Ahmed S. Nonenzymatic exogenous and endogenous antioxidants. In: Das K, Das S, Biradar MS, Bobbarala V, Tata SS, editors. Free Radical Medicine and Biology. London: IntechOpen; 2019. DOI: 10.5772/intechopen.87778

[53] Roche M, Rondeau P, Singh NR, Tarnus E, Bourdon E. The antioxidant properties of serum albumin. FEBS Letters. 2008;**582**:783-1787. DOI: 10.1016/j.febslet.2008.04.057

[54] Spencer JP, Abd El Mohsen MM, Minihane AM, Mathers JC. Biomarkers of the intake of dietary polyphenols: Strengths, limitations and application in nutrition research. The British Journal of Nutrition. 2008;**99**:12-22. DOI: 10.1017/S0007114507798938

[55] Pereira DM, Valentão P, Pereira JA, Andrade PB. Phenolics: From chemistry to biology. Molecules. 2009;**14**:2202-2211. DOI: 10.3390/molecules14062202

[56] Zeb A. Concept, mechanism, and applications of phenolic antioxidants in foods. Journal of Food Biochemistry. 2020;**44**:e13394. DOI: 10.1111/jfbc.13394

[57] Croft KD. The chemistry and biological effects of flavonoids and phenolic acids. Annals of the New York Academy of Sciences. 1998;**854**:435-442. DOI: 10.1111/j.1749-6632.1998.tb09922.x

[58] Myhrstad MC, Carlsen H, Nordström O, Blomhoff R, Moskaug JØ. Flavonoids increase the intracellular glutathione level by transactivation of the gamma-glutamylcysteine synthetase catalytical subunit promoter. Free Radical Biology & Medicine. 2002;**32**:386-393. DOI: 10.1016/s0891-5849(01)00812-7

[59] Hariharan S, Dharmaraj S. Selenium and selenoproteins: Its role in regulation of inflammation. Inflammopharmacology. 2020;**28**:667-695. DOI: 10.1007/s10787-020-00690-x

[60] Schnabel R, Lubos E, Messow CM, Sinning CR, Zeller T, Wild PS, et al. Selenium supplementation improves antioxidant capacity *in vitro* and *in vivo* in patients with coronary artery disease. The SElenium Therapy in Coronary Artery disease Patients (SETCAP) Study. American Heart Journal. 2008;**156**(1201):e1-e11. DOI: 10.1016/j.ahj.2008.09.004

[61] Cai X, Wang C, Yu W, Fan W, Wang S, Shen N, et al. Selenium exposure and cancer risk: An updated meta-analysis and meta-regression. Scientific Reports. 2016;**6**:19213. DOI: 10.1038/srep19213

[62] Ju W, Li X, Li Z, Wu GR, Fu XF, Yang XM, et al. The effect of selenium supplementation on coronary heart disease: A systematic review and meta-analysis of randomized controlled trials. Journal of Trace Elements in Medicine and Biology. 2017;**44**:8-16. DOI: 10.1016/j.jtemb.2017.04.009

[63] Santos JR, Gois AM, Mendonça DM, Freire MA. Nutritional status, oxidative stress and dementia: The role of selenium in Alzheimer's disease. Frontiers in Aging Neuroscience. 2014;**6**:206. DOI: 10.3389/fnagi.2014.00206

[64] Reddi AR, Jensen LT, Naranuntarat A, Rosenfeld L, Leung E, Shah R, et al. The overlapping roles of manganese and Cu/Zn SOD in oxidative stress protection. Free Radical Biology & Medicine. 2009;**46**:154-162. DOI: 10.1016/j.freeradbiomed.2008.09.032

[65] Sinbad OO, Folorunsho AA, Olabisi OL, Ayoola OA, Temitope RJ. Vitamins as antioxidants. Journal of Food Science and Nutrition Research. 2019;**2**:214-235. DOI: 10.26502/jfsnr.2642-11000021

[66] Khadim RM, Al-Fartusie FS. Antioxidant vitamins and their effect on immune system. Journal of Physics Conference Series. 2021;**1853**:012065. DOI: 10.1088/1742-6596/1853/1/012065

[67] Minich DM, Brown BI. A review of dietary (phyto)nutrients for glutathione support. Nutrients. 2019;**11**:2073. DOI: 10.3390/nu11092073

[68] Saini RK, Prasad P, Sreedhar RV, Akhilender Naidu K, Shang X, Keum YS. Omega-3 polyunsaturated fatty acids (PUFAs): Emerging plant and microbial sources, oxidative stability, bioavailability, and health benefits—A review. Antioxidants (Basel). 2021;**10**:1627. DOI: 10.3390/antiox10101627

[69] Christenhusz MJM, Byng JW. The number of known plants species in the world and its annual increase. Phytotaxa. 2016;**261**:201-217. DOI: 10.11646/phytotaxa.261.3.1

[70] Schrire B, Lavin M, Lewis GP. Global distribution patterns of the Leguminosae: Insights from recent phylogenies. Biologiske Skrifter. 2005;**55**:375-422

[71] Glimn-Lacy J, Kaufman PB. Pea family (Fabaceae). In: Botany Illustrated. Introduction to Plants, Major Groups, Flowering Families. Boston: Springer; 2006

[72] Katayama N, Suzuki N. Role of extrafloral nectaries of *Vicia faba* in attraction of ants and herbivore exclusion by ants. Entomological Science. 2004;**7**:119-124. DOI: 10.1111/j.1479-8298.2004.00057.x

[73] Young TP,·Stubblefield CH, Isbell LA. Ants on swollen-thorn acacias: Species coexistence in a simple system. Oecologia 1997;109:98-107. DOI: 10.1007/s004420050063

[74] Parker MA. Relationships of bradyrhizobia from the legumes *Apios americana* and *Desmodium glutinosum*. Applied and Environmental Microbiology. 1999;**65**:4914-4920. DOI: 10.1128/AEM.65.11.4914-4920.1999

[75] The Legume Phylogeny Working Group (LPWG). A new subfamily classification of the Leguminosae based on a taxonomically comprehensive phylogeny. Taxon. 2017;**66**:44-77. DOI: 10.12705/661.3

[76] Purugganan MD. Evolutionary insights into the nature of plant domestication. Current Biology. 2019;**29**:R705-R714. DOI: 10.1016/j.cub.2019.05.053

[77] Schaal B. Plants and people: Our shared history and future. Plants, People, Planet. 2019;**1**:14-19. DOI: 10.1002/ppp3.12

[78] Zárate S. The archaeological remains of *Leucaena* (Fabaceae) revised. Economic Botany. 2000;**54**:477-499. DOI: 10.1007/BF02866547

[79] Rodríguez MF, Rúgolo de Agrasar ZE, Aschero CA. El uso de las plantas en unidades domésticas del sitio arqueológico Punta de la Peña, Puna Meridional argentina (Use of plants in domestic units at the archaeological site of Punta de la Peña 4, Puna in southern Argentina). Chungará. 2006;**38**:257-271. DOI: 10.4067/S0717-73562006000200009

[80] Gepts P, Beavis WD, Brummer EC, Shoemaker RC, Stalker HT, Weeden NF, et al. Legumes as a model plant family. Genomics for food and feed report of the cross-legume advances through genomics conference. Plant Physiology. 2005;**137**:1228-1235. DOI: 10.1104/pp.105.060871

[81] Shavanov MV. The role of food crops within the Poaceae and Fabaceae families as nutritional plants. IOP Conferfence Series: Earth and Environmental Science. 2021;**624**:012111. DOI: 10.1088/1755-1315/624/1/012111

[82] Al-Fredan MAA. Nitrogen fixing legumes in the plant communities. American Journal of Environmental Sciences. 2011;**7**:166-172

[83] Chimphango SBM, Gallant LH, Poulsen ZC, Samuels MI, Hattas D, Curtis OE, et al. Native legume species as potential fodder crops in the mediterranean renosterveld shrubland, South Africa. Journal of Arid Environments. 2020;**173**:104015. DOI: 10.1016/j.jaridenv.2019.104015

[84] Vasishth A, Guleria V. Potential of *Senegalia senegal* for gum arabic extraction. Indian Journal of Ecology. 2017;**44**:817-819

[85] Emam-Djomeh Z, Fathi M, Askari G. Gum tragacanth (*Astragalus gummifer* Labillardiere). In: Razavi SMA, editor. Emerging Natural Hydrocolloids: Rheology and Functions. Hoboken: Wiley; 2019. DOI: 10.1002/9781119418511.ch12

[86] De Almeida Chuffa LG, Vieira FR, da Silva DAF, Franco DM. Soybean seed oil: Nutritional composition, healthy

benefits and commercial applications. In: Varnham A, editor. Seed Oil. Hauppauge: Nova Science; 2015

[87] Sharma KK, Bhatnagar-Mathur P. Peanut (*Arachis hypogaea* L.). In: Wang K, editor. Agrobacterium Protocols. Methods in Molecular Biology. Vol. 343. Totowa: Humana Press; 2006. DOI: 10.1385/1-59745-130-4:347

[88] Ortiz-Hidalgo C, Pina-Oviedo S. Hematoxylin: Mesoamerica's gift to histopathology. Palo de Campeche (logwood tree), pirates' most desired treasure, and irreplaceable tissue stain. International Journal of Surgical Pathology. 2018;**27**:1066

[89] Wahyuningsih S, Ramelan AH, Wardani DK, Aini FN, Sari PL, Tamtama BPN, et al. Indigo dye derived from *Indigofera tinctoria* as natural food colorant. IOP Conference Series Materials Science and Engineering. 2017;**193**:012048. DOI: 10.1088/1757-899X/193/1/012048

[90] Zubairi SI, Sarmidi MR, Aziz RA. A study of rotenone from *Derris* roots of varies location, plant parts and types of solvent used. Advances in Environmental Biology. 2014;**8**:445-449

[91] De Mello LM, Lemos R, Marques A, Stefenon VM. Ancient and current distributions of *Erythrina crista-galli* L. (Fabaceae) in South America. Floresta e Ambiente. 2019;**26**:e11442017. DOI: 10.1590/2179-8087.114417

[92] Compton JA, Lack HW. The discovery, naming and typification of *Wisteria floribunda* and *W. brachybotrys* (Fabaceae) with notes on associated names. Willdenowia. 2012;**42**:219-240. DOI: 10.3372/wi.42.42207

[93] Meenu M, Kamboj U, Sharma A, Guha P, Mishra S. Green method for determination of phenolic compounds in mung bean (*Vigna radiata* L.) based on near-infrared spectroscopy and chemometrics. International Journal of Food Science and Technology. 2016;**51**:2520-2527. DOI: 10.1111/ijfs.13232

[94] Capistrán-Carabarin A, Aquino-Bolaños EN, García-Díaz YD, Chávez-Servia JL, Vera-Guzmán AM, Carrillo-Rodríguez JC. Complementarity in phenolic compounds and the antioxidant activities of *Phaseolus coccineus* L. and *P. vulgaris* L. Landraces. Foods. 2019;**8**:295. DOI: 10.3390/foods8080295

[95] Moloto MR, Phan ADT, Shai JL, Sultanbawa Y, Sivakumar D. Comparison of phenolic compounds, carotenoids, amino acid composition, *in vitro* antioxidant and anti-diabetic activities in the leaves of seven cowpea (*Vigna unguiculata*) cultivars. Food. 2020;**9**:1285. DOI: 10.3390/foods9091285

[96] Zhang Y, Meenu M, Yu H, Xu B. An investigation on phenolic and antioxidant capacity of under-utilized food legumes consumed in China. Food. 2020;**9**:438. DOI: 10.3390/foods9040438

[97] Singh B, Singh JP, Kaur A, Singh N. Phenolic composition and antioxidant potential of grain legume seeds: A review. Foodservice Research International. 2017;**101**:1-16. DOI: 10.1016/j.foodres.2017.09.026

[98] Mazur WM, Duke JA, Wähälä K, Rasku S, Adlercreutz H. Isoflavonoids and lignans in legumes: Nutritional and health aspects in humans. The Journal of Nutritional Biochemistry. 1998;**9**:193-200. DOI: 10.1016/S0955-2863(97)00184-8

[99] Kim IS. Current perspectives on the beneficial effects of soybean isoflavones and their metabolites for humans.

Antioxidants (Basel). 2021;**10**:1064. DOI: 10.3390/antiox10071064

[100] Alshehri MM, Sharifi-Rad J, Herrera-Bravo J, Jara EL, Salazar LA, Kregiel D, et al. Therapeutic potential of isoflavones with an emphasis on daidzein. Oxidative Medicine and Cellular Longevity. 2021;**2021**:6331630. DOI: 10.1155/2021/6331630

[101] Islam A, Islam MS, Uddin MN, Hasan MMI, Akanda MR. The potential health benefits of the isoflavone glycoside genistin. Archives of Pharmaceutical Research. 2020;**43**:395-408. DOI: 10.1007/s12272-020-01233-2

[102] Nakamoto M, Otsuka R, Tange C, Nishita Y, Tomida M, Imai T, et al. Intake of isoflavones reduces the risk of all-cause mortality in middle-aged Japanese. European Journal of Clinical Nutrition. 2021;**75**:1781-1791. DOI: 10.1038/s41430-021-00890-w

[103] Bakasso S, Lamien-Meda A, Lamien CE, Kiendrebeogo M, Millogo J, Ouedraogo AG, et al. Polyphenol contents and antioxidant activities of five *Indigofera* species (Fabaceae) from Burkina Faso. Pakistan Journal of Biological Sciences. 2008;**11**:1429-1435. DOI: 10.3923/pjbs.2008.1429.1435

[104] Godevac D, Zdunić G, Savikin K, Vajs V, Menković N. Antioxidant activity of nine Fabaceae species growing in Serbia and Montenegro. Fitoterapia. 2008;**79**:185-187. DOI: 10.1016/j.fitote.2007.10.001

[105] Khatun S, Kim T. Phenolic compound, antioxidant activity and nutritional components of five legume seed. American Journal of Biomedical Science and Research. 2021;**12**:328-334. DOI: 10.34297/AJBSR.2021.12.001767

[106] Rodríguez Madrera R, Campa Negrillo A, Suárez Valles B, Ferreira Fernández JJ. Phenolic content and antioxidant activity in seeds of common bean (*Phaseolus vulgaris* L.). Food. 2021;**10**:864. DOI: 10.3390/foods10040864

[107] Gupta M, Gupta S. An overview of selenium uptake, metabolism, and toxicity in plants. Frontiers in Plant Science. 2017;7:2074. DOI: 10.3389/fpls.2016.02074

[108] Alford ÉR, Lindblom SD, Pittarello M, Freeman JL, Fakra SC, Marcus MA, et al. Roles of rhizobial symbionts in selenium hyperaccumulation in *Astragalus* (Fabaceae). American Journal of Botany. 2014;**101**:1895-1905. DOI: 10.3732/ajb.1400223

[109] Harvey MA, Erskine PD, Harris HH, Brown GK, Pilon-Smits EAH, Casey LW, et al. Distribution and chemical form of selenium in *Neptunia amplexicaulis* from Central Queensland, Australia. Metallomics. 2020;**12**:514-527. DOI: 10.1039/c9mt00244h

[110] General Bureau of Statistics. 9th Environment Statistics Publication 2015-2019. Paramaribo: General Bureau of Statistics; 2020

[111] International Monetary Fund (2020). Suriname: At a Glance. Washington, DC: International Monetary Fund; 2022

[112] The World Bank Group. Data—Suriname. Washington, DC: World Bank Group; 2021

[113] International Organization for Migration. Suriname Migration Profile A Study on Emigration from, and Immigration into Suriname. Switzerland: International Organization for Migration; 2015

[114] Mans DRA, Ganga D, Kartopawiro J. Meeting of the minds:

Traditional herbal medicine in multiethnic Suriname. In: El-Shemy H, editor. Aromatic and Medicinal Plants—Back to Nature. Rijeka: InTech; 2017. DOI: 10.5772/66509

[115] Mans DRA. The use of medicinal plants in Suriname: The ethnopharmacological legacy of slavery and indentured labour. In: Menke H, Buckingham J, Gounder F, Kumar A, Hassankhan MS, editors. Social Aspects of Health, Medicine and Disease in the Colonial and Post-Colonial Era. New Delhi: Manohar; 2020

[116] Burnham RJ, Johnson KR. South American palaeobotany and the origins of neotropical rainforests. Philosophical Transactions of the Royal Society, B: Biological Sciences. 2004;**359**:1595-1610. DOI: 10.1098/rstb.2004.1531

[117] Stephen HJM. Geneeskruiden Van Suriname: Hun Toepassing in de volksgeneeskunde en in de magie (Herbal Medicines from Suriname: Their Applications in Folk Medicine and Wizardry). Amsterdam: De Driehoek; 1979

[118] May AF, Sranan oso dresi. Surinaams kruidenboek (Surinamese Folk Medicine. A Collection of Surinamese Medicinal Herbs). Paramaribo: De Walburg Pers; 1982

[119] Titjari. Famiri-encyclopedia foe da natoera dresi-fasi. Gezinskruidenboek van de natuurgeneeswijzen. Natuurgeneeswijzen uit het zonnige Suriname (Encyclopedia of Plant-based Forms of Treatment. Folk Medicines from Sunny Suriname). Amsterdam: Sangrafoe; 1985

[120] Heyde H. Surinaamse Medicijnplanten (Surinamese Medicinal Plants). 2nd ed. Paramaribo: Westfort; 1987

[121] Tjong AG. Het gebruik van medicinale planten door de Javanen in Suriname (The Use of Medicinal Plants by the Javanese in Suriname). Paramaribo: Instituut voor de Opleiding van Leraren; 1989

[122] Slagveer JL. Surinaams Groot Kruidenboek: Sranan Oso Dresie (A Surinamese Herbal: Surinamese Traditional Medicines). Paramaribo: De West; 1990

[123] Sedoc NO. Afrosurinaamse natuurgeneeswijzen: Bevattende meer dan tweehonderd meest gebruikelijke geneeskrachtige kruiden (Afro-Surinamese Natural Remedies: Over two hundred Commonly Used Medicinal Herbs). Paramaribo: Vaco Press; 1992

[124] Raghoenandan UPD. Een Ethnobotanisch Onderzoek onder de Hindustanen in Suriname (An Ethnobotanical Survey among Hindustanis in Suriname). Paramaribo: Anton de Kom Universiteit van Suriname; 1994

[125] Van Andel TR, Ruysschaert S. Medicinal and Ritual Plants of Suriname. Amsterdam: KIT Publishers; 2011

[126] Bhat R, Karim AA. Exploring the nutritional potential of wild and underutilized legumes. Comprehensive Reviews in Food Science and Food Safety. 2009;**8**:305-331. DOI: 10.1111/j.1541-4337.2009.00084.x

[127] Ostendorf FW. Nuttige planten en sierplanten in Suriname (Useful plants and Ornamentals in Suriname). Paramaribo: Landbouwproefstation in Suriname; 1962

[128] Pawar CR, Amol DL, Surana SJ. Phytochemical and pharmacological aspects of *Caesalpinia pulcherrima*. Journal of Pharmacy Research. 2008;**1**:131-138

[129] Elfahmi NV, Woerdenbag HJ, Kayser O. Jamu: Indonesian traditional herbal medicine towards rational phytopharmacological use. Journal of Herbal Medicine. 2014;**4**:51-73. DOI: 10.1016/j.hermed.2014.01.002

[130] Wooding CJ. Winti: een Afro-Amerikaanse godsdienst in Suriname. Een cultuurhistorische analyse van de religieuze verschijnselen in de Para (Winti: An African-American Religion in Suriname. A Cultural-Historical Analysis of Religious Phenomena in Para). Meppel: Krips Repro BV; 1972

[131] Srinivas KV, Rao YK, Mahender I, Das B, Krishna KVR, Kishore KH, et al. Flavanoids from *Caesalpinia pulcherrima*. Phytochemistry. 2003;**63**:789-793. DOI: 10.1016/s0031-9422(03)00325-x

[132] Zanin JL, de Carvalho BA, Martineli PS, dos Santos MH, Lago JH, Sartorelli P, et al. The genus *Caesalpinia* L. (Caesalpiniaceae): Phytochemical and pharmacological characteristics. Molecules. 2012;**17**:7887-7902. DOI: 10.3390/molecules17077887

[133] Anju V, Zachariah S. Phytochemical and pharmacological activities of *Caesalpinia pulcherrima*—An overview. International Journal of Pharmaceutical Research. 2013;**5**:6-13

[134] Pankaj N, Deepak N, Ranveer B. A review on phytochemical and pharmacological aspects of *Caesalpinia pulcherrima*. International Journal of Research in Ayurveda and Pharmacy. 2011;**2**:416-421

[135] Badami S, Geetha B, Sharma SV, Rajan S, Suresh B. Antioxidant activity of *Caesalpinia pulcherrima* heartwood. Biological & Pharmaceutical Bulletin. 2003;**26**:1534-1537

[136] Kumbhare MR, Sivakumar T, Udavant PB, Dhake AS, Surana AR. *In vitro* antioxidant activity, phytochemical screening, cytotoxicity and total phenolic content in extracts of *Caesalpinia pulcherrima* (Caesalpiniaceae) pods. Pakistan Journal of Biological Sciences. 2012;**15**:325-332. DOI: 10.3923/pjbs.2012.325.332

[137] Yodsaoue O, Karalai C, Ponglimanont C, Tewtrakul S, Chantrapromma S. Potential anti-inflammatory diterpenoids from the roots of *Caesalpinia mimosoides* Lamk. Phytochemistry. 2010;**71**:1756-1764. DOI: 10.1016/j.phytochem.2010.06.016

[138] Shukla S, Mehta A, John J, Singh S, Mehta P, Vyas SP. Antioxidant activity and total phenolic content of ethanolic extract of *Caesalpinia bonducella* seeds. Food and Chemical Toxicology. 2009;**47**:1848-1851. DOI: 10.1016/j.fct.2009.04.040

[139] Ighodaro A, Ogbeide OK. Antioxidant activity and assessment of total phenolic and flavonoid contents of *Caesalpinia pulcherrima* leaf extract and fractions. Journal of the Chemical Society of Nigeria. 2020;**45**:945-950

[140] Fuller DQ, Murphy C, Kingwell-Banham E, Castillo CC, Naik S. *Cajanus cajan* (L.) Millsp. origins and domestication: The South and Southeast Asian archaeobotanical evidence. Genetic Resources and Crop Evolution. 2019;**66**:1175-1188. DOI: 10.1007/s10722-019-00774-w

[141] Carney JA, Rosomoff RN. In the Shadow of Slavery. Africa's Botanical Legacy in the Atlantic World. Berkeley: University of California Press; 2009

[142] Bekele-Tesemma A. Profitable Agroforestry Innovations for Eastern Africa: Experience from 10 Agroclimatic Zones of Ethiopia, India, Kenya,

Tanzania and Uganda [Internet]. Nairabi: World Agroforestry Centre (ICRAF), Eastern Africa Region; 2007. Available from: http://apps.worldagroforestry.org/downloads/Publications/PDFS/B15073.pdf. [Accessed: June 10, 2022]

[143] Emefiene ME, Salaudeen AB, Yaroson AY. The use of pigeon pea (*Cajanus cajan*) for drought mitigation in Nigeria. Academic Journal of Interdisciplinary Studies. 2013;**2**:29-37. DOI: 10.5901/ajis.2013.v2n12p29

[144] Ganesan S. Traditional oral care medicinal plants survey of Tamil Nadu. Indian Journal of Natural Products and Resources. 2008;**7**:166-172

[145] Upadhyay B, Parveen DAK, Kumar A. Ethnomedicinal and ethnopharmaco-statistical studies of eastern Rajasthan, India. Journal of Ethnopharmacology. 2010;**129**:64-86. DOI: 10.1016/j.jep.2010.02.026

[146] Al-Saeedi AH, Hossain MA. Total phenols, total flavonoids contents and free radical scavenging activity of seeds crude extracts of pigeon pea traditionally used in Oman for the treatment of several chronic diseases. Asian Pacific Journal of Tropical Disease. 2015;**5**:316-321. DOI: 10.1016/S2222-1808(14)60790-8

[147] Pal D, Mishra P, Sachan N, Ghosh AK. Biological activities and medicinal properties of *Cajanus cajan* (L) Millsp. Journal of Advanced Pharmaceutical Technology & Research. 2011;**2**:207-214. DOI: 10.4103/2231-4040.90874

[148] Lai YS, Hsu WH, Huang JJ, Wu SC. Antioxidant and anti-inflammatory effects of pigeon pea (*Cajanus cajan* L.) extracts on hydrogen peroxide- and lipopolysaccharide-treated RAW264.7 macrophages. Food & Function. 2012;**3**:1294-1301. DOI: 10.1039/c2fo30120b

[149] Hassan EM, Matloub A, Aboutabl ME, Ibrahim NA, Mohamed S. Assessment of anti-inflammatory, antinociceptive, immunomodulatory, and antioxidant activities of *Cajanus cajan* L. seeds cultivated in Egypt and its phytochemical composition. Pharmaceutical Biology. 2015;**54**:1380-1391. DOI: 10.3109/13880209.2015.1078383

[150] Vo T-LT, Yang N-C, Yang S-E, Chen C-L, Wu C-H, Song T-Y. Effects of *Cajanus cajan* (L.) Millsp. roots extracts on the antioxidant and anti-inflammatory activities. The Chinese Journal of Physiology. 2020;**63**:137-148. DOI: 10.4103/CJP.CJP_88_19

[151] Tungmunnithum D, Hano C. Cosmetic potential of *Cajanus cajan* (L.) Millsp: Botanical data, traditional uses, phytochemistry and biological activities. Cosmetics. 2020;**7**:84. DOI: 10.3390/cosmetics7040084

[152] Sarkar R, Mandal N. Hydroalcoholic extracts of Indian medicinal plants can help in amelioration from oxidative stress through antioxidant properties. Journal of Complementary and Integrative Medicine. 2012;**9**:1553-1583. DOI: 10.1515/1553-3840.1583

[153] Terahara N, Saito N, Honda T, Toki K, Osajima Y. Acylated anthocyanins of *Clitoria ternatea* flowers and their acyl moieties. Phytochemistry. 1990;**29**:949-953. DOI: 10.1016/0031-9422(90)80053-J

[154] Nguyen GK, Zhang S, Nguyen NT, Nguyen PQ, Chiu MS, Hardjojo A, et al. Discovery and characterization of novel cyclotides originated from chimeric precursors consisting of albumin-1 chain a and cyclotide domains in the Fabaceae family. The Journal of Biological

Chemistry. 2011;**286**:24275-24287. DOI: 10.1074/jbc.M111.229922

[155] Mensah R, Leach D, Young A, Watts N, Glennie P. Development of *Clitoria ternatea* as a biopesticide for cotton pest management: Assessment of product effect on *Helicoverpa* spp. and their natural enemies. Entomologia Experimentalis et Applicata. 2015;**154**:131-145. DOI: 10.1111/eea.12263

[156] Fantz PR. Ethnobotany of *Clitoria* (Leguminosae). Economic Botany. 1991;**45**:511-520. DOI: 10.1007/BF02930715

[157] Mukherjee PK, Kumar V, Kumar NS, Heinrich M. The ayurvedic medicine *Clitoria ternatea*—From traditional use to scientific assessment. Journal of Ethnopharmacology. 2008;**120**:291-301. DOI: 10.1016/j.jep.2008.09.009

[158] Jain NN, Ohal CC, Shroff SK, Bhutada RH, Somani RS, Kasture VS, et al. *Clitoria ternatea* and the CNS. Pharmacology, Biochemistry, and Behavior. 2003;**75**:529-536. DOI: 10.1016/s0091-3057(03)00130-8

[159] Oguis GK, Gilding EK, Jackson MA, Craik DJ. Butterfly pea (*Clitoria ternatea*), a cyclotide-bearing plant with applications in agriculture and medicine. Frontiers in Plant Science. 2019;**10**:645. DOI: 10.3389/fpls.2019.00645

[160] Phrueksanan W, Yibchok-anun S, Adisakwattana S. Protection of *Clitoria ternatea* flower petal extract against free radical-induced hemolysis and oxidative damage in canine erythrocytes. Research in Veterinary Science. 2014;**97**:357-363. DOI: 10.1016/j.rvsc.2014.08.010

[161] Sushma NJ, Prathyusha D, Swathi G, Madhavi T, Raju BDP, Mallikarjuna K, et al. Facile approach to synthesize magnesium oxide nanoparticles by using *Clitoria ternatea*—Characterization and *in vitro* antioxidant studies. Applied Nanoscience. 2015;**6**:437-444. DOI: 10.1007/s13204-015-0455-1

[162] Sogo T, Terahara N, Hisanaga A, Kumamoto T, Yamashiro T, Wu S, et al. Anti-inflammatory activity and molecular mechanism of delphinidin 3-sambubioside, a *Hibiscus* anthocyanin. BioFactors. 2015;**41**:58-65. DOI: 10.1002/biof.1201

[163] Thell K, Hellinger R, Sahin E, Michenthaler P, Gold-Binder M, Haider T, et al. Oral activity of a nature-derived cyclic peptide for the treatment of multiple sclerosis. Proceedings of the National Academy of Sciences of the United States of America. 2016;**113**:3960-3965. DOI: 10.1073/pnas.1519960113

[164] Swain SS, Rout KK, Chand PK. Production of triterpenoid anti-cancer compound taraxerol in Agrobacterium-transformed root cultures of butterfly pea (*Clitoria ternatea* L.). Applied Biochemistry and Biotechnology. 2012;**168**:487-503. DOI: 10.1007/s12010-012-9791-8

[165] Kamkaen N, Wilkinson JM. The antioxidant activity of *Clitoria ternatea* flower petal extracts and eye gel. Phytotherapy Research. 2009;**23**:1624-1625. DOI: 10.1002/ptr.2832

[166] Veiga Junior VF, Rosas EC, Carvalho MV, Henriques MG, Pinto AC. Chemical composition and anti-inflammatory activity of copaiba oils from *Copaifera cearensis* Huber ex Ducke, *Copaifera reticulata* Ducke and *Copaifera multijuga* Hayne—A comparative study. Journal of Ethnopharmacology. 2007;**112**:248-254. DOI: 10.1016/j.jep.2007.03.005

[167] Leandro LM, de Sousa VF, Barbosa PCS, Neves JKO, da Silva JA,

da Veiga-Junior VF. Chemistry and biological activities of terpenoids from copaiba (*Copaifera* spp.) oleoresins. Molecules. 2012;**17**:3866-3889. DOI: 10.3390/molecules17043866

[168] Monteschio JO, de Vargas Junior FM, Alves da Silva AL, das Chagas RA, Fernandes T, Leonardo AP, et al. Effect of copaíba essential oil (*Copaifera officinalis* L.) as a natural preservative on the oxidation and shelf life of sheep burgers. PLoS One. 2021;**16**:e0248499. DOI: 10.1371/journal.pone.0248499

[169] Veiga VF Jr, Pinto AC. The *Copaifera* L. genus. Quimica Nova. 2002;**25**:273-286. DOI: 10.1590/S0100-40422002000200016

[170] Plowden C. The ethnobotany of copaiba (*Copaifera*) oleoresin in the Amazon. Economic Botany. 2004;**58**:729-733

[171] Santnna BMP, Fontes SP, Pinto AC, Rezende CM. Characterization of woody odorant contributors in copaiba oil (*Copaifera multijuga* Hayne). Journal of the Brazilian Chemical Society. 2007;**18**:984-989

[172] Veiga VF, Zunino L, Calixto JB, Patitucci ML, Pinto AC. Phytochemical and antioedematogenic studies of commercial copaiba oils available in Brazil. Phytotherapy Research. 2001;**15**:476-480. DOI: 10.1002/ptr.976

[173] Lucas FA, Kandrotas AL, Neto EN, de Siqueira CE, André GS, Bromerschenkel I, et al. Copaiba oil in experimental wound healing in horses. Ciencia Rural. 2017;**47**:e20151292. DOI: 10.1590/0103-8478cr20151292

[174] Pieri FA, Mussi MC, Moreira MAS. Óleo de copaíba (*Copaifera* sp.): Histórico, extração, aplicações industriais e propriedades medicinais (Copaíba oil (*Copaifera* sp.): History, extraction, industrial aplications and medicinal properties). Revista Brasileira das Plantas Medicinais. 2009;**11**:465-472. DOI: 10.1590/S1516-05722009000400016

[175] Santos AO, Ueda-Nakamura T, Dias Filho BP, Veiga Junior VF, Pinto AC, Nakamura CV. Antimicrobial activity of Brazilian copaiba oils obtained from different species of the *Copaifera* genus. Memórias do Instituto Oswaldo Cruz. 2008;**103**:277-281. DOI: 10.1590/s0074-02762008005000015

[176] Da Silva AG, Puziol Pde F, Leitao RN, Gomes TR, Scherer R, Martins ML, et al. Application of the essential oil from copaiba (*Copaifera langsdorfi* Desf.) for acne vulgaris: A double-blind, placebo-controlled clinical trial. Alternative Medicine Review. 2012;**17**:69-75

[177] Ceccarelli I, Fiorenzani P, Pessina F, Pinassi J, Aglianò M, Miragliotta V, et al. The CB2 agonist β-caryophyllene in male and female rats exposed to a model of persistent inflammatory pain. Frontiers in Neuroscience. 2020;**14**:850. DOI: 10.3389/fnins.2020.00850

[178] Hebert P, Barice EJ, Park J, Dyess SM, McCaffrey R, Hennekens CH. Treatments for inflammatory arthritis: Potential but unproven role of topical copaiba. Integrative Medicine (Encinitas, Calif.). 2017;**16**:40-42

[179] Da Trindade R, da Silva JK, Setzer WN. *Copaifera* of the neotropics: A review of the phytochemistry and pharmacology. International Journal of Molecular Sciences. 2018;**19**:1511. DOI: 10.3390/ijms19051511

[180] De Lima Silva JJ, Guimarães SB, da Silveira ER, de Vasconcelos PR, Lima GG, Torres SM, et al. Effects of *Copaifera langsdorffii* Desf. On

ischemia-reperfusion of randomized skin flaps in rats. Aesthetic Plastic Surgery. 2009;**33**:104-109. DOI: 10.1007/s00266-008-9263-2

[181] Adzu B, Balogun SO, Pavan E, Ascêncio SD, Soares IM, Aguiar RWS, et al. Evaluation of the safety, gastroprotective activity and mechanism of action of standardised leaves infusion extract of *Copaifera malmei* Harms. Journal of Ethnopharmacology. 2015;**175**:378-389. DOI: 10.1016/j.jep.2015.09.027

[182] Batista ÂG, Ferrari AS, da Cunha DC, da Silva JK, Cazarin CB, Correa LC, et al. Polyphenols, antioxidants, and antimutagenic effects of *Copaifera langsdorffii* fruit. Food Chemistry. 2016;**197**:1153-1159. DOI: 10.1016/j.foodchem.2015.11.093

[183] Mans DRA, Grant A, Pinas N. Plant-based ethnopharmacological remedies for hypertension in Suriname. In: Builders P, editor. Herbal Medicine. London: IntechOpen; 2017. DOI: 10.5772/intechopen.72106

[184] Rastogi S, Pandey MM, Rawat AKS. An ethnomedicinal, phytochemical and pharmacological profile of *Desmodium gangeticum* (L.) DC. and *Desmodium adscendens* (Sw.) DC. Journal of Ethnopharmacology. 2011;**136**:283-296. DOI: 10.1016/j.jep.2011.04.031

[185] Seriki SA, Odetola AO, Adebayo OF. Analysis of phytoconstituents of *Desmodium adscendens* in relation to its therapeutic properties. American Journal of Biomedical Science and Research. 2019;**2**:158-162. DOI: 10.34297/AJBSR.2019.02.000598

[186] Muanda FN, Bouayed J, Djilani A, Yao C, Soulimani R, Dicko A. Chemical composition and, cellular evaluation of the antioxidant activity of *Desmodium adscendens* leaves. Evidence-based Complementary and Alternative Medicine. 2011;**2011**:620862. DOI: 10.1155/2011/620862

[187] Addy ME, Burka JF. Effects of *Desmodium adscendens* fractions on antigen-and arachidonic acid-induced contractions of guinea pig airways. Canadian Journal of Physiology and Pharmacology. 1988;**66**:820-825

[188] Addy ME, Awumey EM. Effects of the extracts of *Desmodium adscendens* on anaphylaxis. Journal of Ethnopharmacology. 1984;**11**:283-292. DOI: 10.1016/0378-8741(84)90074-6

[189] Riaz A, Rasul A, Hussain G, Zahoor MK, Jabeen F, Subhani Z, et al. A bioactive phytochemical with potential therapeutic activities. Advances in Pharmacological Sciences. 2018;**2018**:9794625. DOI: 10.1155/2018/9794625

[190] Adeniyi BA, Izuka KC, Odumosu B, Aiyelaagbe OO. Antibacterial and antifungal activities of methanol extracts of *Desmodium adscendens* root and Bombax buonopozense leaves. International Journal of Biological and Chemical Sciences. 2013;**7**:185-194. DOI: 10.4314/ijbcs.v7i1i.15

[191] François C, Fares M, Baiocchi C, Maixent JM. Safety of *Desmodium adscendens* extract on hepatocytes and renal cells. Protective effect against oxidative stress. Journal of Intercultural Ethnopharmacology. 2015;**4**:1-5. DOI: 10.5455/jice.20141013041312

[192] Chuisseu PDD, Galani BRT, Younang NCK, Kouam AF, Simo BFN, Tchana AN, et al. Aqueous extracts of *Desmodium adscendens* (Fabaceae) possess *in vitro* antioxidant properties and protect hepatocytes from carbone tetrachloride-induced injury

and hepatitis C virus infection. Investigational Medicinal Chemistry and Pharmacology. 2020;**3**:36. DOI: 10.31183/imcp.2020.00036

[193] Sarker SD, Nahar L. Progress in the chemistry of naturally occurring coumarins. In: Kinghorn A, Falk H, Gibbons S, Kobayashi J, editors. Progress in the Chemistry of Organic Natural Products. Cham: Springer; 2017. DOI: 10.1007/978-3-319-59542-9_3

[194] Lončar M, Jakovljević M, Šubarić D, Pavlić M, Buzjak Služek V, Cindrić I, et al. Coumarins in food and methods of their determination. Food. 2020;**9**:645. DOI: 10.3390/foods9050645

[195] Loprinzi CL, Sloan J, Kugler J. Coumarin-induced hepatotoxicity. Journal of Clinical Oncology. 1997;**15**:3167-3168. DOI: 10.1200/JCO.1997.15.9.3167

[196] Abraham K, Wöhrlin F, Lindtner O, Heinemeyer G, Lampen A. Toxicology and risk assessment of coumarin: Focus on human data. Molecular Nutrition & Food Research. 2010;**54**:228-239. DOI: 10.1002/mnfr.200900281

[197] Matos MJ, Santana L, Uriarte E, Abreu AO, Molina E, Yordi EG. Coumarins—An important class of phytochemicals. In: Rao AV, Rao LG, editors. Phytochemicals—Isolation, Characterisation and Role in Human Health. London: IntechOpen; 2015. DOI: 10.5772/59982

[198] Hussain MI, Qamar Abbas S, Reigosa MJ. Activities and novel applications of secondary metabolite coumarins. Planta Daninha. 2018;**36**:e018174040. DOI: 10.1590/S0100-8358201836010001

[199] Pereira A, Martins S, Caldeira AT. Coumarins as fluorescent labels of biomolecules. In: Rao V, Mans D, Rao L, editors. Phytochemicals in Human Health. London: IntechOpen; 2019. DOI: 10.5772/intechopen.85973

[200] Bourdy G, DeWalt SJ, de Michel LRC, Roca A, Deharo E, Muñoz V, et al. Medicinal plants uses of the Tacana, an Amazonian Bolivian ethnic group. Journal of Ethnopharmacology. 2000;**70**:87-109. DOI: 10.1016/s0378-8741(99)00158-0

[201] De Oliveira PC, de Sou Q, BCdO. Traditional knowledge of forest medicinal plants of Munduruku Indigenous people—Ipaupixuna. European. Journal of Medicinal Plants. 2020;**31**:20-35. DOI: 10.9734/ejmp/2020/v31i1330309

[202] Van Andel T, Behari-Ramdas J, Havinga R, Groenendijk S. The medicinal plant trade in Suriname. Ethnobotany Research and Applications. 2007;**5**:351-372

[203] Venugopala KN, Rashmi V, Odhav B. Review on natural coumarin lead compounds for their pharmacological activity. BioMed Research International. 2013;**2013**:963248. DOI: 10.1155/2013/963248

[204] Sullivan G. Occurrence of umbelliferone in the seeds of *Dipteryx odorata* (Aubl.) Willd. Journal of Agricultural and Food Chemistry. 1982;**30**:609-610. DOI: 10.1021/jf00111a051

[205] Da Cunha CP, Godoy RLO, Braz FR. Isolation of flavonoids from *Dipteryx odorata* by high-performance liquid chromatography. Revista Virtual de Química. 2016;**8**:43-56. DOI: 10.5935/1984-6835.20160004

[206] Socorro MP, Pinto AC, Kaiser CR. New isoflavonoid from *Dipteryx odorata*. Zeitschrift für Naturforschung. 2003;**58B**:1206-1209

[207] Januário AH, Lourenço MV, Domézio LA, Pietro RCLR, Castilho MS, Tomazela DM, et al. Isolation and structure determination of bioactive isoflavones from callus culture of *Dipteryx odorata*. Chemical & Pharmaceutical Bulletin. 2005;**53**: 740-742. DOI: 10.1248/cpb.53.740

[208] Rüfer CE, Kulling SE. Antioxidant activity of isoflavones and their major metabolites using different *in vitro* assays. Journal of Agricultural and Food Chemistry. 2006;**54**:2926-2931. DOI: 10.1021/jf053112o

[209] Maass BL. Origin, domestication and global dispersal of *Lablab purpureus* (L.) Sweet (Fabaceae): Current understanding. Legume Perspectives. 2016;**13**:5-8

[210] Rasha MS, Abdel Atti KA. Effect of dietary hyacinth bean (*Lablab purpureus*) on broiler chicks performance. Research Journal of Agriculture and Biological Sciences. 2007;**3**:494-497

[211] Al-Snafi AE. The pharmacology and medical importance of *Dolichos lablab* (*Lablab purpureus*)—A review. IOSR Journal of Pharmacy. 2017;**7**:22-30

[212] Naeem M, Shabbir A, Ansari AA, Aftab T, Khan MMA, Uddin M. Hyacinth bean (*Lablab purpureus* L.)—An underutilised crop with future potential. Scientia Horticulturae. 2020;**272**:109551. DOI: 10.1016/j.scienta.2020.109551

[213] Habib MAM, Hasan R, Nayeem J, Uddin N, Rana S. Anti-inflammatory, antioxidant and cytotoxic potential of methanolic extract of two Bangladeshi bean *Lablab purpureus* L. sweet white and purple. International Journal of Pharmaceutical Sciences and Research. 2012;**3**:776-781. DOI: 10.13040/IJPSR.0975-8232.3(3).776-81

[214] Rai K, Rai N, Pandey-Rai S. Unlocking pharmacological and therapeutic potential of hyacinth bean (*Lablab purpureus* L.): Role of OMICS based biology, biotic and abiotic elicitors. In: Jimenez-Lopez J, Clemente A, editors. Legumes Research. Vol. 2. London: IntechOpen; 2021. DOI: 10.5772/intechopen.99345

[215] Qiaoyu L, Lingsheng D. Chemical study on the flower of *Dolichos lablab* L. Journal of China Pharmaceutical University. 1996;**27**:205-207

[216] Kala KB, Tresina Soris P, Mohan VR, Vadivel V. Nutrient and chemical evaluation of raw seeds of five varieties of *Lablab purpureus* (L.) Sweet. Advances in Bioresearch. 2010;**1**:44-53

[217] Turco I, Ferretti G, Bacchetti T. Review of the health benefits of faba bean (*Vicia faba* L.) polyphenols. Journal of Food and Nutrition Research. 2016;**55**:283-293

[218] Zhang Y, Pechan T, Chang SK. Antioxidant and angiotensin-I converting enzyme inhibitory activities of phenolic extracts and fractions derived from three phenolic-rich legume varieties. Journal of Functional Foods. 2018;**42**:289-297. DOI: 10.1016/j.jff.2017.12.060

[219] Zhu F, Du B, Xu B. Anti-inflammatory effects of phytochemicals from fruits, vegetables, and food legumes: A review. Critical Reviews in Food Science and Nutrition. 2018;**58**:1260-1270. DOI: 10.1080/10408398.2016.1251390

[220] Shi Y, Mandal R, Singh A, Pratap SA. Legume lipoxygenase: Strategies for application in food industry. Legume Science. 2020;**2**:e44. DOI: 10.1002/leg3.44

[221] Morris JB. Morphological and reproductive characterization in hyacinth bean, *Lablab purpureus* (L.) sweet germplasm with clinically proven nutraceutical and pharmaceutical traits for use as a medicinal food. Journal of Dietary Supplements. 2009;**6**:263-279. DOI: 10.1080/19390210903070830

[222] Havinga RM, Hartl A, Putscher J, Prehsler S, Buchmann C, Vogl CR. *Tamarindus indica* L. (Fabaceae): Patterns of use in traditional African medicine. Journal of Ethnopharmacology. 2010;**127**:573-588. DOI: 10.1016/j.jep.2009.11.028

[223] Menezes APP, Trevisan SCC, Barbalho SM, Guiguer EL. *Tamarindus indica* L. A plant with multiple medicinal purposes. Journal of Pharmacognosy and Phytochemistry. 2016;**5**:50-54

[224] De Caluwé E, Halamov K, van Damme P. *Tamarindus indica* L.: A review of traditional uses, phytochemistry and pharmacology. Afrika Focus. 2010;**23**:53-83

[225] Meher B, Dash DK, Roy A. A review on: Phytochemistry, pharmacology and traditional uses of *Tamarindus indica* L. World Journal of Pharmacy and Pharmaceutical Sciences. 2014;**3**:229-240

[226] Shaikh Z, Mujahid M, Bagga P, Khalid M, Noorul H, Nesar A, et al. Medicinal uses and pharmacological activity of *Tamarindus indica*. World Journal of Pharmaceutical Sciences. 2017;**5**:121-133

[227] Siddhuraju P, Vijayakumari K, Janardhanan K. Nutritional and antinutritional properties of the underexploited legumes *Cassia laevigata* Willd. and *Tamarindus indica* L. Journal of Food Composition and Analysis. 1995;**8**:351-162

[228] El-Siddig K, Gunasena HPM, Prasa BA, Pushpakumara DKNG, Ramana KVR, Vijayanand P, et al. Tamarind—*Tamarindus indica* L. Fruits for the Future 1. Southampton: Southampton Centre for Underutilized Crops; 2006

[229] Almeida MMB, de Sousa PHM, Fonseca ML, Magalhães CEC, Lopes MFG, de Lemos TLG. Evaluation of macro and micro-mineral content in tropical fruits cultivated in the northeast of Brazil. Ciência e Technologia de Alimentos. 2009;**29**:581-586

[230] Martinello F, Soares SM, Franco JJ, Santos AC, Sugohara A, Garcia SB, et al. Hypolipemic and antioxidant activities from *Tamarindus indica* L. pulp fruit extract in hypercholesterolemic hamsters. Food and Chemical Toxicology. 2006;**44**:810-818. DOI: 10.1016/j.fct.2005.10.011

[231] Bhutkar MA, Bhise SB. Anti-oxidative effect of *Tamarindus indica* in alloxan induced diabetic rats. International Journal of Research in Pharmaceutical and Biomedical Sciences. 2011;**2**:1006-1009

[232] Lim CY, Junit SM, Abdulla MA, Aziz AA. *In vivo* biochemical and gene expression analyses of the antioxidant activities and hypocholesterolaemic properties of *Tamarindus indica* fruit pulp extract. PLoS One. 2013;**8**:e70058. DOI: 10.1371/journal.pone.0070058

Chapter 16

Green Extraction Techniques for Phytoconstituents from Natural Products

Bincy Raj, Soosamma John, Venkatesh Chandrakala and Gajula Harini Kumari

Abstract

The use of green extraction techniques for extracting phytoconstituents from natural sources minimizes the amount of solvents needed and the amount of waste generated during the extraction process. Traditional extraction processes generate a lot of solvent waste, which causes a lot of environmental and health issues. Furthermore, by employing automated modern processes, exposure to solvents and vapor is reduced. Green extraction is based on the analytical procedures that employ less energy, allow the use of different solvents and sustainable natural products, and provide a safe and superior extract/product. According to a life cycle analysis of waste created in Active Pharmaceutical Ingredient (API) manufacturing plants, solvent-related waste accounts for 80% of the waste. In case other pharmaceutical companies generate equal amounts of solvent waste, addressing solvent selection, use, recovery, and disposal will go a long way toward tackling the issue. Solvent considerations will feature regularly in the case histories of the drug development process. Natural extracts comprise phytoconstituents such as proteins, lipids and oils, dietary fibres, carbohydrates, antioxidants, essential oils and fragrances, and colours, and can be found in wide variety of plant materials. In this chapter, we will discuss principles, techniques, and solvents used for green extraction techniques of phytoconstituents.

Keywords: green extraction, phytoconstituents, pharmaceuticals, solvents

1. Introduction

Medicinal plants are getting more demand because of their distinctive features as an abundant source of curative phytochemicals that may be used to develop new medications. Approximately 20% of all known plants have been employed in pharmacological investigations, positively improving the healthcare system by treating cancer and other ailments [1]. Many of these medicinal plants are good sources of phytochemicals like polyphenols, carotenoids, flavonoids, anthocyanins, and vitamins that possess antioxidant activities. Today, medicinal plants are finding diverse use in society from medicine to cosmetics, nutraceuticals, herbal drinks, herbal foods, and other articles in their daily uses. Plant phytoconstituents are created as secondary metabolites, which are produced through a variety of biological routes in secondary metabolism. The choice of solvents for extracting phytoconstituents from plants is critical. A suitable solvent has an appropriate extraction capacity as well as the ability to maintain the chemical structure of the desired molecules stable [2].

Green technologies are increasingly being employed in practically every scientific sector to promote ecologically acceptable activities that do little or no harm to humans. Ionic liquids, aqueous biphasic systems, and pressurized hot water have all become attractive research topics in recent years [3]. Traditional techniques of extracting phytoconstituents require the use of more powerful and toxic solvents (nonenvironmentally friendly), as well as more energy. Each method's extraction time varies, ranging from minutes to 7 days in the case of maceration [4]. Another problem is that none of the current plant processing methods meets all the economical, safety, and scalability requirements. Other concerns include security hazards, solvent toxicity, and the existence of solvent remnants in the extracts. The high cost of feedstock, the high cost of extracting desirable bioactive compounds, their comparatively low yield, and the resulting substantial concentration of residual waste biomass are the major roadblocks to commercially viable phytochemical production [5]. In many process sectors, microwave-assisted extractions like ultrasound-assisted extraction, pulsed electric field extraction, and molecular distillation have been reported. Green chemistry, as ecological and economic chemistry, could be one of the solutions to humanity's future [6]. The entire process of green extraction of phytoconstituents from natural sources is concluded in the **Figure 1**.

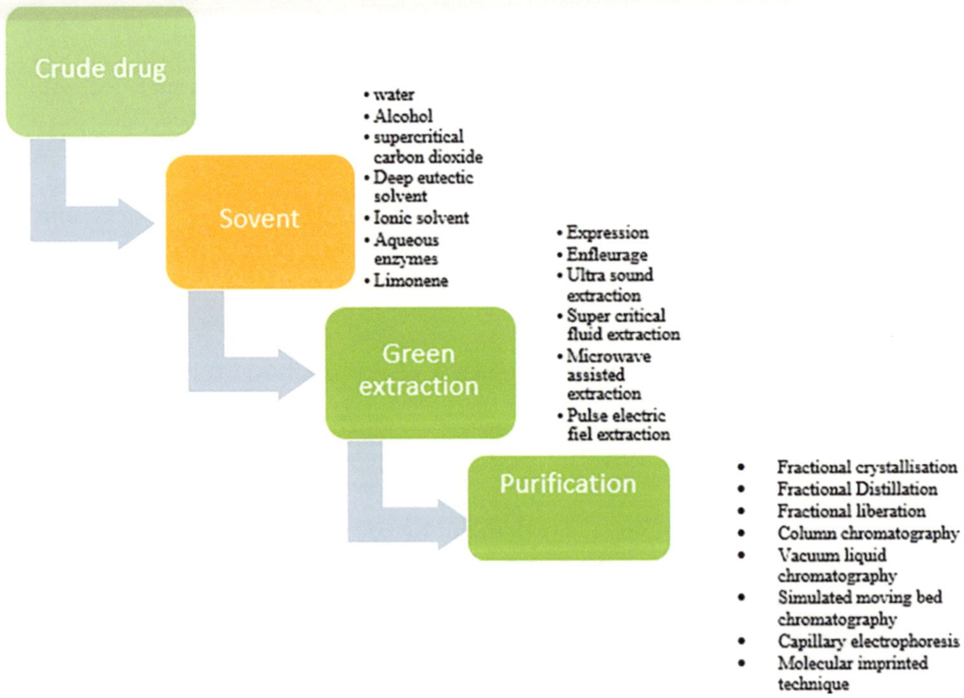

Figure 1.
Extraction of crude drugs using green solvent, green extraction process, and purification techniques.

2. Green extraction

A vast diversity of plants, animals, and microorganisms can produce a wide spectrum of chemical compounds with amazing health-care properties in nature. Science is steadily changing our world by finding the possibilities of natural products [7]. Natural product extraction has been practised since civilization. Extraction methods are used in the perfume, cosmetics, pharmaceutical, food, and chemicals sectors. Recent extraction technique advancements have mostly focused on creating solutions that employ lower solvents [8].

Soxhlet extraction, maceration, and hydro distillation (HD) are examples of traditional/conventional extraction processes. The choice of specific solvents has a considerable impact on any extraction rate. The polarity of the target biochemical is the most significant factor to consider, and when choosing a solvent, the solvent's molecular affinity for the solute, as well as its environmental friendliness, toxicity, and economic efficiency, must all be considered. Simple, safe, repeatable, low-cost, and adaptable to a variety of applications are all desirable characteristics in an extraction procedure. High-temperature extraction (e.g., Soxhlet technique, HD) has been shown to cause changes in the composition due to phytoconstituent degradation [9].

To circumvent the constraints of classic extraction procedures, green extraction techniques can be employed to extract phytoconstituents from plants. The majority of these include less harmful chemical synthesis, nontoxic chemicals, safe solvent aides, energy efficiency patterns, use of sustainable feedstock, fewer derivatives, catalysis, design to avoid deterioration, and time scheduling for pollution avoidance, hazardous air pollutants, and naturally safer chemistry for safety programs. The development of effective and selective technologies for extracting and isolating bioactive phytoconstituent is crucial. This article aims to provide a detailed overview of green solvents employed, as well as the methods for extracting and isolating natural compounds form natural sources. Green solvents can help to improve old procedures significantly, especially when incorporated with new and novel methodologies. Hydrolysis of cellulose from biomass with supercritical water and the extraction of hydrophobic compounds using supercritical CO_2 are few examples of green extraction process.

3. Solvent selection for green extraction

Solvents, their vapors, and mists have a variety of health impacts. Many contain narcotic properties, causing lethargy, dizziness, carcinogens, etc. Solvents irritate the eyes and respiratory system, as well as causing skin problems. High doses can cause unconsciousness and death in certain people. Petroleum-based solvents, which are mostly sourced from fossil fuels, are commonly utilized in various stages of the analytical process [10]. Solution preparation, extraction, and enrichment of phytoconstituents, washing of extracts, solvent exchange, sample preservation, dilution, cleaning of glassware, liquid desorption, derivatization, analytical separation, and detection are all activities that involve solvents in phytochemistry. A suitable solvent has an appropriate extraction capacity as well as the ability to maintain the chemical structure of the desired molecules stable.

3.1 Water

Water is one such "green" solvent that can have its properties changed by changing the temperature. Water's polarity allows it to be employed as an extraction solvent for both natural and inorganic substances that are aqueous soluble, like proteins, carbohydrates, and organic acids. Water is an important green solvent for the extraction of phytoconstituents. It has no harmful health or environmental consequences [11]. Furthermore, it is the safest and cheapest solvent. The technology used has an impact on the extractability of biologically active chemicals. Water is used as the only extractant in several ways, including decoction, infusion, and hydro distillation. Water as a solvent can be used in a variety of traditional and modern procedures. Extraction with pressurized hot water is one of the most promising new green extraction techniques and procedures, especially in a dynamic mode [11]. Water, on the other hand, has several drawbacks in terms of the less solubility of nonpolar molecules and energy required to enrich products. This difficulty can be overcome in part by employing supercritical water or a mixture of alcohol and water.

When using hydro distillation, high temperatures and long distillation times might cause volatiles to change and be lost. Supercritical water extraction (SWE) was shown to have a quicker extraction time, cheaper costs, and higher purity than hydro distillation. In terms of oxygenated components, SWE's products yielded higher valuable essential oil. To boost extraction yields, microwave-assisted extraction with water as a solvent has been proposed.

3.2 Alcohol

Alcohols like methanol, ethanol, and isopropyl alcohol have similar solvent properties such as solvent strengths, dielectrics, critical points, and hydrogen donating abilities. However, due to its nontoxic nature, ethanol has ascended to the top [12]. Alkanes (heptane, hexane) and simple alcohols (methanol, ethanol) are healthier for the environment than dioxane, acetonitrile, acids, formaldehyde, and tetrahydrofuran [13]. The main disadvantage of alcohol is that they are flammable and some of them are toxic (i.e., methanol). In addition, extended exposure to their vapors can also lead to health problems.

3.3 Supercritical carbon dioxide (CO_2)

CO_2 as a liquid or supercritical solvent possesses multiple features of an admirable green solvent. They are incombustible, nonpoisonous, nonenvironmentally harmful, plentiful, inexpensive, easy to produce, simple to eliminate from a product, do not add to smog, and do not contribute to global warming [14]. Purified CO_2 is produced, pressurized, and cooled to a liquid state at 20 psi and −20°C before being stored or transported in insulated bulk containers for use in a variety of liquid and supercritical CO_2 processes. The viscosity of CO_2 is extremely low, and supercritical CO_2 has negligible surface tension [15]. The strong diffusivity, along with the low viscosity, causes significant improvements in the condensed phases. Supercritical fluid extraction of a crude drug is achieved by passing supercritical CO_2 over a column packed drug material. Until the substrate is depleted, supercritical CO_2 travels over the column of packed material and dissolves soluble components. The loaded solvent is then transported through a separator, where the soluble components precipitate as pressure and temperature are reduced. The CO_2 is recirculated once it has been condensed. It is employed in the removal of caffeine from coffee and tea, the removing fatty material from cacao, the production of hops extracts, sesame seed oil, and pesticide extraction from rice. Under high pressure, SC CO_2 is used to extract triglycerides and volatile compounds. Volatile, triglyceride and phenolic chemicals etc. are extricated at high pressure (300–400 bars) with EtOH. Add water or alcohols like ethanol or iso-propyl-alcohol to the SC-CO_2 extraction has already been used to modify the polarity [16].

3.4 Deep eutectic solvents (DES)

DES is formed when the melting point of a mixture of substances is much lower than the melting points of the two constituents. A hydrogen bond donor (HBD) and a hydrogen bond acceptor (HBA) are required to build a DES system, and when mixed in the right proportions, they generate a novel "mesh" of hydrogen-bond-interconnected molecules with remarkable physicochemical features [17]. Their extraordinary physicochemical features (like ionic liquids) combined with remarkable green properties, low cost, and ease of handling are piquing researchers' attention in a variety of sectors. The eutectic composition of DESs is formed by heating and stirring two or more solid starting components to generate a transparent, viscous homogenous liquid. Other techniques involve grinding (combining and powdering solid components till clear liquid forms), evaporation (dissolving all starting elements in water and then removing the water via evaporation at reduced pressure), and freeze-drying (dissolving all starting components in water and then draining the water via evaporation at reduced pressure).

Among them, heating and stirring below the melting points of the individual constituents is possibly the most acceptable method [18]. Because DESs are nonflammable and nonvolatile, they are easier to store. They are also biodegradable, unlike standard organic solvents. Furthermore, DES manufacture is cost-effective, simple to run, and requires no modification, making their use on a broad scale possible. DESs can be made by mixing molecules derived from natural sources (e.g., glycerol and glucose), which makes them environmentally friendly. Within the HBD section, polymerized deep eutectic solvents (PDEs) are a novel category of DESs that can be polymerized [17].

The high viscosity of DES is a key disadvantage that can limit their usage as extraction solvents since it prevents the solvent from penetrating the extraction matrix. Although increasing the temperature of the extraction process helps reduce viscosity, this is not always the best solution because it consumes energy, and some heat-sensitive phytochemicals may not withstand the higher temperature. The addition of a co-solvent to the extraction medium is a straightforward technique to remedy this problem. Most of the time, this co-solvent is water, which keeps the process green; nevertheless, organic solvents like methanol have also been utilized. Alkaloids, phenolic acids, flavonoids, and saponins are all extracted using DES [19].

The DES is called natural deep eutectic solvents (NADES) when amino acids, organic acids, sugars etc. are used to make DES [20]. Due to the natural nature of its ingredients, NADESs are deemed environmentally beneficial and "readily biodegradable," and the resulting extracts can use in food, pharmaceutical, and cosmetics preparations. Because of their great stability and solubilization properties, NADES is ideal candidates to replace traditional solvents. NADESs combinations have efficiently extracted bioactive compounds including flavonoids, phenolic acids, alkaloids, natural pigments, sugars, peptides, and volatile components from natural matrices [21].

3.5 Ionic liquids (IL)

ILs were a type of organic salt that consisted of an organic cation (e.g., imidazolium, pyrrolidinium, pyrrolidinium tetra alkyl ammonium, pyrrolidinium tetra alkyl phosphonium) and an inorganic or organic anion (e.g., tetrafluoroborate, hexafluorophosphate, and bromide) that form of liquid below 100°C [22]. Because of their distinctive and construction dependent features, like low nucleophilicity, mixability with water or organic solvents, and good extractability, ILs have been frequently used [23]. A variety of organic and inorganic substances are perhaps enriched and separated using IL-based methods. As a result, they have been frequently used in food safety, drug testing, environmental monitoring, biological analysis, and other areas. The ability of ILs could be tailor-made for the extraction of alkaloids, flavonoids, terpenoids, phenylpropanoids, quinones, and other phytoconstituents from plants. A vast number of research organizations have also created IL-based silica and polymers that can improve the extraction/separation of target chemicals.

3.6 Aqueous enzymatic extraction (AEE)

Extraction is an important step in the isolation of bioactive chemicals from plant matter. However, because of the existence of complex cell wall polysaccharides including cellulose, hemicellulose, lignin, pectin alginate, and carrageenan, the extraction yield of bioactive chemicals is poor. Researchers are now considering modern methods of extracting these compounds because of the low specific gravity of bioactive compounds, the low productivity of the solvents used to extract these compounds, high energy, high durability, solvent residue in the extracts, and the decline in the quality of the final product, as well as environmental concerns [23]. The use of enzymes to extract bioactive chemicals from plants could be a viable substitute for traditional solvent extraction methods. Enzymes are excellent catalyzers for extracting, modifying, or synthesizing complex bioactive substances from nature. The natural ability of enzymes to accelerate reactions with perfect particularity, regiospecificity, and the ability to employ under gentle processing conditions in an aqueous medium facilitate enzyme-based extraction [24]. The use of enzymes for sugar extraction is a new topic that needs further research. To improve extraction processes, custom enzymes must be developed, either by biodiversity screening, genetic engineering perspective, or a mix of the two. From plant sources, enzyme-aided extraction can be utilized to obtain lipophilic, polyphenolic, and hydrophilic chemicals [25]. Factors including high enzyme production and downstream processing costs, extended incubation times, and an extra stage (de-emulsification) in the process are still preventing aqueous enzyme extraction from becoming commercially viable. Commercial enzyme production has been accelerated, and enzyme synthesis has now become more affordable. The downstream processing expenses could be reduced by using appropriate technology rather than the traditional technique [26].

3.7 Limonene

The predominant element of essential oils derived from citrus fruit peels is d-limonene, which belongs to the terpene family. Since its cleaner and degreaser properties were discovered and considered, d-limonene has sparked a surge of interest. In this sense, this chemical has been classified as a viable alternative to halogenated carbon hydrates or traditional degreasing chemicals commonly used in industry and households. Several authors have attempted to create a commercial application for d-limonene. Sustainable chemistry has generated a lot of study into the processing of renewable fuels due to the demand for environment-friendly techniques and products [27].

Because d-limonene has a higher boiling point (175°C) than n-hexane (69°C), it uses more energy to recover the solvent by evaporation. To minimize the difficulty of solvent recovery caused by high d-limonene's boiling point, a technique based on steam or hydro-distillation employing Clevenger can be used. Distilled water was added to the extracted oil and d-limonene mixture after Soxhlet extraction with d-limonene. D-limonene and extracted oil were separated using a Clevenger device and azeotropic water distillation at less than 100°C [28]. It is a valuable and practical method for determining the lipids and oils in olive seeds. Waste minimization, rapid operation, and energy saving are all possible with Soxhlet microwave-integrated with limonene and microwave Clevenger distillation [29]. Limonene has a dielectric constant that is very similar to that of hexane and has been used to extract rice bran oil, oil from olive leftovers, carotenoids from tomatoes or algae and, more recently, algal lipids from wet algae [30].

3.8 Solvent-free extraction

Solvent-free extraction of a variety of important natural products (essential oils, fragrances, edible oils, antioxidants, and other organic compounds) eliminates the price and threats correlated with large amounts of solvent. It minimizes the amount of wastewater after extraction and uses a fraction of the energy that a traditional solvent-solid extraction process does.

In 2008, Chemat et al. developed the MHG method, which uses *in situ* dielectric heating on plant cell water to stretch the structure and cause membrane and wall ruptures. As a result, plant matter is used to gather primary and secondary metabolites, as well as the water in the cells. The behavior described is known as hydro diffusion. Gravity then drops the diffused components into a container. A continuous condensation system is maintained using a perforated Pyrex disc. MHG has been used to extract pigments, aroma components, and antioxidants from a variety of natural sources on a lab and commercial scale [21].

4. Pre-treatment techniques

Crude drugs can be extracted in fresh or dried form. Grinding and drying of plant materials are examples of pre-preparation. This has an impact on the preservation of phytochemicals in final extracts. Air drying takes anywhere from 3 to 7 days. To optimize extraction operations and save energy, mechanical disruption pre-treatments can be employed alone or in combination. Bead milling, high-pressure homogenization, and hydrodynamic cavitation are all methods for mechanical disruption. The extraction of lipids has been demonstrated to be aided using a bead mill. Powdered samples, on the other hand, have a more homogenized and smaller particle size, developing in substantial surface contact with extraction solvents [31].

Nanotechnologies, including microwave, ultrasound, and pulse electric field, were found to improve operation efficacy as a pre-treatment before drying. After size reduction and before extraction, microwave pre-treatments upgraded the extraction of polyphenols, sugars, and other compounds. Pre-treatments with a pulsed electric field (PEF) improved extraction efficiencies in terms of yield and extract standard. PEF pre-treatment of rapeseed, apple, and sugar beet fruit extracts before mechanical expression resulted in higher yields [26]. Oven-drying is one more pre-extraction method that uses heat energy to eliminate moisture from substances. This procedure for preparing a sample is regarded as particular easiest and most rapid thermal processing method available for phytochemicals.

Costly drugs can be dried by freeze-drying. In freeze-drying before use, the sample is frozen at −80°C to −20°C to lyophilize any liquid (e.g., solvent, moisture) in the body samples. The mouth of the test tube or other container holding the sample is wrapped in needle-poked-parafilm to avoid sample loss during the operation. Freeze-drying resulted in a greater phenolic content compared to air-drying because most phytochemicals are preserved. This strategy is used to keep phytoconstituents safe. Freeze-drying, on the other hand, is a difficult process. Microwave drying is more expensive than traditional air drying. As a result, only fragile, heat-sensitive goods and high-quality materials are permitted [32].

5. Green technologies for extraction

The main goal of green extraction procedures is to obtain a rapid extraction, increased efficient energy usage, higher mass and heat transfer, smaller apparatus, and fewer processing stages [3]. Several novel alternatives to traditional techniques for obtaining target compounds from a variety of crude drugs have been proposed, such as ultrasound-assisted extraction (UAE), subcritical and supercritical fluid extraction (SFE), microwave-assisted extraction (MAE), and accelerated solvent extraction (ASE) [33]. These extraction methods, which are alternatives to traditional procedures, have piqued the curiosity of academics, who see future applications for recovering bioactive molecules from plants in less time using green solvents. Most of these new methods have already shown promise in extracting high-value chemicals, particularly natural antioxidants, from various sources such as plants or food processing by-products [34].

5.1 Expression

It is a physical technique in which pressure is employed to extract the oil or juice from a material. A tincture press was used to do this. When essential oils are temperature sensitive, this approach is used. It's used to extract essential oils from citrus peels like lemons and oranges. Squeezing any plant material at high pressures to extract oils or other liquids is known as expression. In remote rural locations, hand-operated presses or crushes are used, while in industrial hubs, massive mechanical presses are used. However, the products obtained are impure and frequently contain impurities such as water, mucoid particles, and cell tissues, making them murky, and pressing the volatile oil in plants completely is difficult. As a result, the crushed residue is frequently steam distilled to remove all volatile oils. Black soybean oil, for example, is frequently extracted using the low-temperature pressing process [31].

5.2 Effleurage (extraction with cold fat)

Enfleurage is the method of extracting aroma from flowers by absorbing it through contact with cold lipids. This method is used for fragrant flowers like jasmine and tuberose, which retain their unique aroma even after being plucked. To prevent fat odors from entering, fats should be saturated and odorless. It's best to use refined lard or beef suet. On both sides of a glass plate mounted on a rectangular hardwood frame or chassis, fat is thinly deposited. On a fat-coated chassis, fresh aromatic flowers are delicately stacked. Enfleurage produces far more floral oil than other processes.

5.3 Ultrasound extraction

Ultrasound extractions can now be finished in minutes with high reliability, reducing solvent consumption, clarifying control and work-up, improving final product purity, removing wastewater after treatment, and consuming only a fragment of the fossil energy required for a traditional extraction method [35]. USAE (ultrasound-assisted extraction) has been used to extract polyphenols from vegetable tissues, protein, sugar, and starch from cereals and legumes, oil, and flavor components. Extraction efficiency and rate are improved by sonication. It lowers the required temperature, saves solvents, and promotes the solubilization of the desired chemicals. Solubility is enhanced by a significant increase in the very temperature [36].

To extract phytochemicals from plants, both the cell wall and the cell membrane must be broken. Because of this, ultrasounds are used in ultrasound-assisted extraction for cell disintegration. Ultrasounds are sound waves that are above the human hearing range, with frequencies ranging from 20 kHz to a few gigahertz. Plant materials and liquids absorb the energy emitted by ultrasonic waves and convert it to heat. The frequency, intensity, and duration of ultrasonic therapy affect the amount of heat created in plant materials [37]. This heat energy debases proteins, destroys plant cells, and causes therapeutic substances to be released from plant cells. In most cases, the highest extraction rate is attained in the initial few minutes, which is also the most profitable time [38].

5.4 Super critical fluid extraction (SCFE)

The extraction of thermally labile chemicals is possible because of carbon dioxide's low critical temperature (304.1 K). It can replicate a variety of organic solvents by adjusting the density of SCF carbon dioxide. Because of its variable solvating strength, this feature allows for selective extraction, purification, and fractionation techniques. SCF carbon dioxide media provide the prime possibility for fractionation of reaction products and solvent separation, which can be performed by simply depressurizing the media. This is because SCF quickly penetrates and leaves solid matrices, compared to the use of organic solvents with a higher viscosity [39]. It has a broad variety of applications, including the extraction of common spices such as black pepper, celery seed, cumin, cinnamon, clove bud, and nutmeg. Extraction of Natural Colors: Paprika Pigments, etc. Dry Ginger, Saw Palmetto, Rosemary, and other botanicals are used to extract active ingredients. Forskolin, Turmerones—from Turmeric, *Oscimum sanctum,* Neem Leaf, and other plants; Cholesterol and other lipids are extracted from dried egg yolks. Hops are extracted to use in the beverage sector. Precipitation of Human Immunoglobulin G (IgG), viral deactivation, and other biochemical components. The main disadvantage of supercritical carbon dioxide extraction is the high cost of the device. Because supercritical carbon dioxide is nonpolar, polar co-solvents of 5% and 10% ethanol were added to change the polarity and improve solubility.

5.5 Microwave-assisted extraction

Nontraditional ways are more prominent when it comes to improving the quality and quantity of desired items. By directly linking microwave energy with the bulk reaction mixture, microwave irradiation creates efficient internal heating. The magnitude of energy transfer is determined by the molecules' dielectric characteristics. Radiation absorption and heating can be quite selective in this approach (Hoz et al.). The reduction in operating time and solvent use are two major benefits of microwave treatments. However, during microwave processing, acceleration in chemical reactions of target substances such as epimerization, oxidation, and polarization should be considered with dielectric heating.

Microwave-assisted extraction without solvents is a long-term technology for extracting and separating chemicals from natural plant resources. Microwave heating is directed at the moisture content of new material. Under microwave irradiation, plant cell water and charged molecules are stimulated; this internal alteration causes a significant amount of pressure to be imposed on plant cell walls, resulting in cell swelling. Due to the rupturing of plant cells, this swelling causes an increase in the mass transfer of solutes. As a result, phytochemical leaching from the plant cellular matrix into the extractant is facilitated during MAE [40]. The best extraction conditions were a microwave power of 150 W for 90 min. Concerning the efficiency and yield of essential oils, solvent-free microwave extraction was superior. As a result, increased rates of adsorption, diffusion, and separation of phytochemicals from the plant matrix into the extracting solvent are more likely [41].

An MAE can be performed using two different types of equipment. The apparatus runs at atmospheric pressure in the open mode, which is often coupled with a refluxing mechanism. Domestic microwaves are frequently modified to accommodate this model. The closed mode, on the other hand, allows for high-pressure operation. Pumping inert gas into the extraction chamber increases the pressure. During the heating of the extraction mixture, however, vapor pressure may generate a degree of pressure. Since these molecules were stable at microwave heating settings of up to 100°C for 20 min, this approach was confined to small-molecule phenolic compounds like phenolic acids (gallic acid and ellagic acid), quercetin, isoflavones, and trans-resveratrol. Due to compound oxidation, more MAE cycles (e.g., from 2 10 s to 3 10 s) resulted in a considerable reduction in phenolic and flavanone yields. Because tannins and anthocyanins are prone to temperature degradation, they may not be suitable for MAE [32].

Microwave-assisted hydro distillation (MAHD) is like standard hydro distillation, with the exception that the solvent is heated using microwaves. The solvent (typically water) and plant parts are placed inside a microwave oven (normally running at 2.45 GHz), and different output powers and reaction periods can be used to improve the extraction process. Again, using microwaves for the heating process speeds up the extraction of chemicals, requiring shorter timeframes to generate comparable amounts of extracts. Furthermore, the chemical makeup of extracts obtained by standard hydro distillation and MAHD is not comparable.

5.6 Pulsed electric field (PEF) extraction

In batch mode, the electric field strength (EFS) ranges from 100 to 300 V/cm, while in continuous mode, the EFS ranges from 20 to 80 kV/cm. An external electrical force is used in electro-permeabilization or electroporation to increase

DOI: http://dx.doi.org/10.5772/intechopen.105088

the permeability of cell membranes. The cell membrane is perforated by the formation of hydrophilic holes, which result in the opening of protein channels. When high-voltage electrical pulses are applied across the electrodes, the sample experiences a force per unit charge termed the electric field. The plant material is removed once the membrane loses its structural functioning [41]. Anthocyanin, carotenoids, lycopene, lutein, polyphenols, alkaloids, lactase, protein, polysaccharides, fat, oil, and other bioactive compounds are extracted using PEF. PEF-assisted extraction provides more bioactive component extracts, uses less energy, and takes less time to process, according to the study, resulting in the optimal process parameters [42].

6. Purification of phytoconstituents

The extracts, which contain numerous phytoconstituents, must be separated and purified further to obtain the fraction or pure phytoconstituents. The techniques utilized for isolation and purification from the extract are determined by the physical and chemical properties of the component to be separated. The physical approaches employed for this goal are as follows.

6.1 Fractional crystallization

The point of supersaturation in the solvent in which phytopharmaceuticals are soluble causes them to crystallize. The processes involved in the crystallization of phytoconstituents are slow concentration, slow evaporation, and chilling. Crystallization is an ideal purification procedure. It is operationally easy, very inexpensive, and may be done in quantities ranging from a few micrograms to hundreds of kilograms. The results are normally highly pure (unlike the mixes that can sometimes be obtained with distillation). Using chromatography to purify that much material is a nightmare. Another key point to remember about crystallization is that X-ray crystallography can be used to discover the structure of unknown molecules. With very few exceptions, X-ray crystallography is the gold standard for structure determination: if you can get a substance to crystallize, you can determine its structure. The only issue is that not all compounds crystallize, and finding circumstances that can preferentially recrystallize one chemical can take a long time [43].

6.2 Fractional distillation

This is a process of purifying phytoconstituents from a mixture. It's commonly used to separate hydrocarbons like crude oil, citral, and eucalyptol. Purification is accomplished by comparing the boiling points of the different substances. When heat is applied, the fractional distillation equipment is built in such a way that each chemical evaporates and separates at its boiling point. As a result, each fractionated chemical will condense and be collected separately via numerous syphons coupled to fractional distillation apparatus [44].

The fractional distillation method is based on differences in compound volatility and is affected by physicochemical properties of the components, as well as the pressure and temperature of the distillation process. The mass and energy transition between the fluid and vapor stages of the mixture has an impact on separation efficiency. Most terpenes are thermally unstable, dissolving, or oxidizing when exposed to high temperatures, light, or oxygen. As a result, the distillation technique is typically used at vacuum pressures to lower the vaporization temperature of the volatile mixture. Due to the boiling temperature reduction, the vacuum also slows processes such as thermal deterioration in temperature-sensitive chemicals. In the chemical industry, vacuum fractional distillation is used to separate compounds with extremely high boiling points that would need a lot of energy to separate under atmospheric pressure [45].

6.3 Fractional liberation

Fractional liberation separates some components from a mixture. The weakest base in the free salt is liberated first when an aqueous solution of alkaloid salts is treated with aliquots of alkali, followed by base liberation in ascending order of basicity. After each addition, shake the mixture with an organic solvent to get a fractionated sequence of bases. Organic acids that are soluble in water-immiscible solvents take a similar route. It is feasible to fractionally liberate acids in this case by adding mineral acids to a mixture of acid salts.

6.4 Chromatography

6.4.1 Column chromatography

Chromatography on a column separates and purifies phytochemicals on a laboratory and industrial scale without the use of complicated technology. The "eluent" is the liquid employed as the mobile phase, and the stationary phase is usually a solid or a liquid. The sample solution is supplied to a porous stationary phase, and the mobile phase is delivered at a greater pressure via the column, causing separation depending on the solute's affinity for the stationary phase. The development of HPLC (High-Performance Liquid Chromatography) was aided by the need for a higher degree of separation and faster analysis, which was met by refining the stationary phase packing material to a size of 3–10 m and eluent delivery via a high-pressure pump. Despite its extensive and time-consuming nature, commercial use of column chromatography is comparable to that of other techniques. The advantages of column chromatography include efficient sample handling regardless of the number or nature of the samples, the availability of a wide range of adsorbents, the selection and recyclization of a large solvent system, improved purity of the product, and minimal space requirements. Column chromatography has a few disadvantages, including the use of a large amount of mobile phase, compared to other techniques it is a complicated technique, time consumption, the requirement for an expert, and a greater cost of identifying the separated product.

6.4.2 Vacuum liquid chromatography (VLC)

The fundamental disadvantage of column chromatography is that it is a time-consuming technique; however, vacuum liquid chromatography can solve this problem. In vacuum chromatography, rather than using pressure, vacuum is employed to improve the flow rate and hence speed up the fractionation process. The stationary phase is usually 40–60 mesh particle size silica or reversed-phase silica, and the crude extracts are separated by gradient elution. TLC is a typical method for examining eluted fractions [43].

6.4.3 Simulated moving bed chromatography (SMB)

In the pharmaceutical sector, simulated moving bed (SMB) technology is an economical and eco-friendly process for purifying crude extracts and fractions [46]. It has a higher purity and yield than other techniques. A traditional Simulated Moving Bed system has 4–24 columns divided into four zones. In general, a four-column SMB should be sufficient for testing and optimizing purification conditions. Purification of sugars, proteins, monoclonal antibodies, separation of organic solvents, optical isomers, charged molecules, and desalting are all common applications. For the separation of crude medicines, the SMB technique utilizes extremely less solvent. The SMB technique is simple to adapt to a continuous process and can be integrated with other equipment such as evaporation. SMB, on the other hand, necessitates meticulous process control and is less adaptable than traditional elution chromatography.

6.5 Capillary electrophoresis (CE)

CE provides several advantages, including a smaller sample, high efficiency leads to shorter analysis time, cheap, environmental friendliness, reduced solvent usage, and a powerful tool appropriate for drug discovery [47]. CE is a new method for analyzing different phytochemical groups. Variations in mass to charge ratios are used to separate phytochemicals in capillary electrophoresis. Because borate can form compounds with the flavonoid nucleus' ortho dihydroxyl groups and the sugar's vicinal cis-dihydroxyl groups, borate buffers with a pH of 8–11 and a concentration of 25–200 mM are generally used [48].

Capillary zone electrophoresis (CZE) is the most basic characteristic, and it's been utilized to isolate a variety of target molecules, especially polyphenolic compounds like epicatechin, catechin, quercetin, gentistic acid, caffeic acid, gallic acid, trans-resveratrol, myricetin, and rutin from wine and grape samples. A CZE technique was also used to isolate antioxidants in Ginkgo leaf extracts. For the separation of anthocyanins in wine, a new CZE approach was developed recently [49]. Food analysis, environmental monitoring, clinical diagnostics, and pharmaceutical analysis have mostly used capillary electrophoresis. Since it allows the use of chirality selectors with limited aqueous solubility, nonaqueous capillary electrophoresis can be utilized to separate enantiomeric drugs. Furthermore, the low dielectric constant of organic solvents can let chiral counter-ions that have less selectivity in aqueous environments form ion pairs and therefore increase their selectivity. CE-MS is one of many multidimensional techniques used in the pharmaceutical and biotechnology industries, particularly for drug development. Because high resolution and structural and/or molecular weight information of an analyte may be collected along with using a mass spectrometer as a detector for CE splitting, could be useful. CE has various advantages (for example, high speed, efficiency, and low price); yet, combining CE with MS produces several problems. CE solvents, for example, are not accepted by MS.

6.6 Molecular imprinted technology

Molecular imprinting knowledge has been a prominent isolation method in the last years because of its distinctive qualities, such as high selectiveness, economical, and ease of preparation. Many correlative cavities with the memory of the template molecules' size, shape, and functional groups are produced when the template molecules are removed from the molecular imprinted polymer (MIP). As a result, the template molecule and its analogues will be able to recognize the MIP and adsorb it selectively. MIPs have been extensively used in the isolation of phytoconstituents and as sorbents for solid-phase extraction of herbal materials to enrich phytoconstituent components. MIP was made with methyl methacrylate as the monomer, solanesol as the template molecule, and ethylene glycol as the crosslinker by a suspension polymerization method. This technique is used for the purification of enriching in water extract of *Panax notoginseng*, solanesol from tobacco leaves, thermo-responsive magnetic MIP is used to isolate curcuminoids, curcumin, dimethoxy curcumin, and bisdemethoxycurcumin, from the TCM *Curcumae Longa* Rhizoma [50].

7. Conclusion

Plant materials go through several processes to acquire the necessary secondary metabolites and/or extract, including drying, extraction, separation, and purification. To produce better eco-friendly processes, the current investigation of the use of green solvents in the field of extraction needs more awareness for a greater perception of different factors such as innate solvent properties (polarity, viscosity, solubility, and pH), external factors (temperature, time, and solid-liquid ratio), and cytotoxicity. However, more study is needed on green or smart solvents that have high specificity for phytochemical compounds, as well as improved stability, recovery, and reduced operational costs. Until now, the framework has only been used to evaluate organic solvents. To expand the currently established techniques to new solvents, more study is required. This entails looking into novel waste-solvent treatment technologies as well as alternative solvent production techniques. Will the eventual transfer of DES/NADES-based extraction technologies to industrial sectors need further investments? Would their use result in a shorter lifespan for the extractors and the analytical tools required for their identification and quantification in the long run? All the questions are still open, and there are a lot of options for answers in the future.

Author details

Bincy Raj[1*], Soosamma John[2], Venkatesh Chandrakala[3] and Gajula Harini Kumari[3]

1 1Department of Pharmacognosy, College of Pharmaceutical Sciences, Dayananda Sagar University, Bangalore, India

2 Department of Pharmacognosy, East Point College of Pharmacy, Bidarahalli, Bangalore, India

3 Department of Pharmaceutics, East Point College of Pharmacy, Bidarahalli, Bangalore, India

*Address all correspondence to: bincympharm@gmail.com

References

[1] Abubakar AR, Haque M. Preparation of Medicinal Plants: Basic Extraction and Fractionation Procedures for Experimental Purposes. Journal of Pharmacy & Bioallied Sciences. 2020;**12**(1):1-10. https://doi.org/10.4103/JPBS. JPBS_175_19

[2] Chemat F, Abert-Vian M, Fabiano-Tixier AS, Strube J, Uhlenbrock L, Gunjevic V. Green extraction of natural products. Origins, current status, and future challenges. Trends in Analytical Chemistry. Elsevier. 2019;**118**:248-263

[3] Soquetta MB, Terra L d M, Bastos CP. Green technologies for the extraction of bioactive compounds in fruits and vegetables. CyTA—Journal of Food. 2018;**16**(1):400-412. DOI: 10.1080/19476337.2017.1411978

[4] Rodríguez De Luna SL, Ramírez-Garza RE, Serna Saldívar SO. Environmentally friendly methods for flavonoid extraction from plant material: Impact of their operating conditions on yield and antioxidant properties. Scientific World Journal. 2020;**2020**:1-38. DOI: 10.1155/2020/6792069

[5] Hamany Djande CY, Piater LA, Steenkamp PA, Madala NE, Dubery IA. Differential extraction of phytochemicals from the multipurpose tree, Moringa oleifera, using green extraction solvents. South African Journal of Botany. 2018;**115**:81-89. DOI: 10.1016/J. SAJB.2018.01.009

[6] Selvamuthukumaran M, Shi J. Recent advances in extraction of antioxidants from plant by-products processing industries. Food Quality and Safety. 2017;**1**(1):61-81. DOI: 10.1093/FQSAFE/FYX004

[7] Barbero GF, de Aguiar AC, Ferreiro-González M, Rostagno MA. Editorial: Exploring the potential of natural products through advanced techniques and green solvents. Frontiers in Chemistry. 2020;**0**:1166. DOI: 10.3389/FCHEM.2020.627111

[8] Chemat F, Vian MA, Cravotto G. Green extraction of natural products: Concept and principles. International Journal of Molecular Sciences. 2012;**13**(7):8615. DOI: 10.3390/IJMS13078615

[9] Blicharski T, Oniszczuk A. Extraction methods for the isolation of Isoflavonoids from plant material. Open Chemistry. 2017;**15**(1):34-45. DOI: 10.1515/CHEM-2017-0005

[10] SOLVENTS—International occupational safety & health information centre. n.d.. Available from: https://www.ilo.org/legacy/english/protection/safework/cis/products/safetytm/solvents.htm. [Accessed: September 9, 2021]

[11] Mihaylova D, Lante A. Water an eco-friendly crossroad in green extraction: An overview. The Open Biotechnology Journal. 2019;**13**(1):155-162. DOI: 10.2174/1874070701913010155

[12] Tekin K, Hao N, Karagoz S, Ragauskas AJ. Ethanol: A promising Green solvent for the deconstruction of lignocellulose. ChemSusChem. 2018;**11**(20):3559-3575. DOI: 10.1002/CSSC.201801291

[13] Capello C, Fischer U, Hungerbühler K. What is a green solvent? A comprehensive framework for the environmental assessment of solvents. Green Chemistry. 2007;**9**(9):927-934. DOI: 10.1039/B617536H

[14] Budisa N, Schulze-Makuch D. Supercritical carbon dioxide and its

potential as a life-sustaining solvent in a planetary environment. Life (Basel, Switzerland). 2014;**4**(3):331-340. DOI: 10.3390/life4030331

[15] Mayadevi S. Reactions in supercritical carbon dioxide. Indian Journal of Chemistry. 2012;**51**:1298-1305

[16] Vandeponseele A, Draye M, Piot C, Chatel G. Subcritical water and supercritical carbon dioxide: Efficient and selective eco-compatible solvents for coffee and coffee by-products valorization. Green Chemistry. 2020;**22**(24):8544-8571. DOI: 10.1039/D0GC03146A

[17] Skarpalezos D, Detsi A. Deep eutectic solvents as extraction media for valuable flavonoids from natural sources. Applied Sciences. 2019;**9**(19):4169. DOI: 10.3390/APP9194169

[18] Ishaq M, Gilani MA, Afzal ZM, Bilad MR, Nizami A-S, Rehan M, et al. Novel poly deep eutectic solvents based supported liquid membranes for CO_2 capture. Frontiers in Energy Research. 2020;**0**:272. DOI: 10.3389/FENRG.2020.595041

[19] Duan L, Dou L-L, Guo L, Li P, Liu E-H. Comprehensive evaluation of deep eutectic solvents in extraction of bioactive natural products. ACS Sustainable Chemistry and Engineering. 2016;**4**(4):2405-2411. DOI: 10.1021/ACSSUSCHEMENG.6B00091

[20] Paiva A, Craveiro R, Aroso I, Martins M, Reis RL, Duarte ARC. Natural deep eutectic solvents—Solvents for the 21st century. ACS Sustainable Chemistry and Engineering. 2014;**2**(5):1063-1071. DOI: 10.1021/SC500096J

[21] Chemat F, Vian MA, Ravi HK, Khadhraoui B, Hilali S, Perino S, et al. Review of alternative solvents for green extraction of food and natural products: Panorama, principles, applications and prospects. Molecules (Basel, Switzerland). 2019;**24**(16). DOI: 10.3390/MOLECULES24163007

[22] Xiao J, Chen G, Li N. Ionic liquid solutions as a green tool for the extraction and isolation of natural products. Molecules: A journal of synthetic chemistry and natural product chemistry. 2018;**23**(7). DOI: 10.3390/MOLECULES23071765

[23] Ghandahari Yazdi AP, Barzegar M, Sahari MA, Ahmadi Gavlighi H. Optimization of the enzyme-assisted aqueous extraction of phenolic compounds from pistachio green hull. Food Science and Nutrition. 2019;**7**(1):356-366. DOI: 10.1002/FSN3.900

[24] Puri M, Sharma D, Barrow CJ. Enzyme-assisted extraction of bioactives from plants. Trends in Biotechnology. 2012;**30**(1):37-44. DOI: 10.1016/J.TIBTECH.2011.06.014

[25] Saad N, Louvet F, Tarrade S, Meudec E, Grenier K, Landolt C, et al. Enzyme-assisted extraction of bioactive compounds from raspberry (*Rubus idaeus* L.) pomace. Journal of Food Science. 2019;**84**(6):1371-1381. DOI: 10.1111/1750-3841.14625

[26] Ummat V, Sivagnanam SP, Rajauria G, O'Donnell C, Tiwari BK. Advances in pre-treatment techniques and green extraction technologies for bioactives from seaweeds. Trends in Food Science & Technology. 2021;**110**:90-106. DOI: 10.1016/J.TIFS.2021.01.018

[27] Aissou M, Chemat-Djenni Z, Yara-Varón E, Fabiano-Tixier AS, Chemat F. Limonene as an agro-chemical building block for the synthesis and extraction of bioactive compounds. Comptes Rendus Chimie.

2017;**20**(4):346-358. DOI: 10.1016/J. CRCI.2016.05.018

[28] Virot M, Tomao V, Ginies C, Chemat F. Total lipid extraction of food using d-limonene as an alternative to n-hexane. Chromatographia. 2008;**68**(3-4):311-313. DOI: 10.1365/ S10337-008-0696-1

[29] Virot M, Tomao V, Ginies C, Visinoni F, Chemat F. Green procedure with a green solvent for fats and oils' determination. Microwave-integrated Soxhlet using limonene followed by microwave Clevenger distillation. Journal of Chromatography A. 2008;**1196-1197**(1-2):147, 152. DOI: 10.1016/J. CHROMA.2008.04.035

[30] Golmakani M-T, Mendiola JA, Rezaei K, Ibáñez E. Pressurized limonene as an alternative bio-solvent for the extraction of lipids from marine microorganisms. Journal of Supercritical Fluids. 2014;**92**:1-7. DOI: 10.1016/j. supflu.2014.05.001

[31] Feng W, Li M, Hao Z, Zhang J. Analytical Methods of Isolation and Identification. In: Rao V, Mans D, Rao L, editors. Phytochemicals in Human Health [Internet]. London: IntechOpen; 2019 [cited 2022 May 26]. Available from: https://www.intechopen. com/chapters/68108. DOI: 10.5772/ intechopen.88122

[32] Nn A. Citation: Azwanida NN (2015) A review on the extraction methods use in medicinal plants, principle, strength and limitation. Medicinal & Aromatic Plants. 2015;**4**(3):196. DOI: 10.4172/2167-0412.1000196

[33] Tiwari BK. Ultrasound: A clean, green extraction technology. TrAC Trends in Analytical Chemistry. 2015;**71**:100-109. DOI: 10.1016/J. TRAC.2015.04.013

[34] Fraterrigo Garofalo S, Tommasi T, Fino D. A short review of green extraction technologies for rice bran oil. Biomass Conversion and Biorefinery. 2021;**11**(2):569-587. DOI: 10.1007/S13399-020-00846-3

[35] Esclapez MD, García-Pérez JV, Mulet A, Cárcel JA. Ultrasound-assisted extraction of natural products. Food Engineering Reviews. 2011;**3**(2):108-120. DOI: 10.1007/S12393-011-9036-6

[36] Green SA. Green Chemistry: Progress and Barriers. Physical Sciences Reviews. 2016;**1**(10):1-7. DOI:10.1515/ psr-2016-0072

[37] Aihua S, Xiaoyan C, Xiaoguang Y, Jiang F, Yanmin L and Juhua Z. Applications and Prospects of Ultrasound-Assisted Extraction in Chinese Herbal Medicine. Open Access Journal of Biomedical Science. 2019;**1**(1):5-15. OAJBS.ID.000103. DOI: 10.38125/OAJBS.000103

[38] Esclapez MD, García-Pérez JV, Mulet A, Cárcel JA. Ultrasound-Assisted Extraction of Natural Products. n.d. Food Eng Rev 2011;**3**:108-120. DOI: 10.1007/ s12393-011-9036-6

[39] Ramsey E, Sun Q, Zhang Z, Zhang C, Gou W. Mini-review: Green sustainable processes using supercritical fluid carbon dioxide. Journal of Environmental Sciences. 2009;**21**(6):720-726. DOI: 10.1016/ S1001-0742(08)62330-X

[40] Ameer K, Shahbaz HM, Kwon J-H. Green extraction methods for polyphenols from plant matrices and their byproducts: A review. Comprehensive Reviews in Food Science and Food Safety. 2017;**16**(2):295-315. DOI: 10.1111/1541-4337.12253

[41] Masota NE, Vogg G, Heller E, Holzgrabe U. Comparison of extraction

efficiency and selectivity between low-temperature pressurized microwave-assisted extraction and prolonged maceration. Archiv der Pharmazie. 2020;**353**(10):2000147. DOI: 10.1002/ARDP.202000147

[42] Thulasidas JS, Varadarajan GS, Sundararajan R. Pulsed electric field for enhanced extraction of intracellular bioactive compounds from plant products: An overview. Novel Approaches in Drug Designing & Development. 2019;**5**(2):0026-0031. DOI: 10.19080/NAPDD.2019.05.555657

[43] Natural Product Isolation (2) - Purification Techniques, An Overview. (n.d.). Available from: https://www.masterorganicchemistry.com/2016/08/12/natural-product-isolation-2-purification-of-crude-mixtures-overview/. [Accessed: September 17, 2021]

[44] Abubakar AR, Haque M. Preparation of medicinal plants: Basic extraction and fractionation procedures for experimental purposes. Journal of Pharmacy & Bioallied Sciences. 2020;**12**(1):1. DOI: 10.4103/JPBS.JPBS_175_19

[45] Silvestre WP, Medeiros FR, Agostini F, Toss D, Pauletti GF. Fractionation of rosemary (*Rosmarinus officinalis* L.) essential oil using vacuum fractional distillation. Journal of Food Science and Technology. 2019;**56**(12):5422. DOI: 10.1007/S13197-019-04013-Z

[46] Cong J, Lin B. Separation of liquiritin by simulated moving bed chromatography. Journal of Chromatography A. 2007;**1145**(1-2):190-194. DOI: 10.1016/J.CHROMA.2007.01.088

[47] Gackowski M, Przybylska A, Kruszewski S, Koba M, Mądra-Gackowska K, Bogacz A. Recent applications of capillary electrophoresis in the determination of active compounds in medicinal plants and pharmaceutical formulations. Molecules. 2021;**26**(14):4141. DOI: 10.3390/MOLECULES26144141

[48] Vaher M, Koel M. Separation of polyphenolic compounds extracted from plant matrices using capillary electrophoresis. Journal of Chromatography A. 2003;**990**(1-2):225-230. DOI: 10.1016/S0021-9673(02)02013-7

[49] Tsao R, Deng Z. Separation procedures for naturally occurring antioxidant phytochemicals. Journal of Chromatography B. 2004;**812**:85-99. DOI: 10.1016/j.jchromb.2004.09.028

[50] Zhang Q-W, Lin L-G, Ye W-C. Techniques for extraction and isolation of natural products: A comprehensive review. Chinese Medicine. 2018;**13**(1):1-26. DOI: 10.1186/S13020-018-0177-X

Chapter 17

Pharmacological, Biopesticide, and Post-Harvest Loss Management Application of Jimsonweed (*Datura stramonium*)

Melaku Tafese Awulachew

Abstract

Datura stramonium is one of the most intriguing, in part because of its well-known therapeutic and psychoactive properties in the treatment of many diseases. Datura species have been found to exhibit a variety of biological activity. Insecticide, fungicide, antioxidant, antibacterial, hypoglycemic, and immune response boosting properties have been linked to the genus' species. These effects are linked to the existence of secondary metabolites such as terpenoids, flavonoids, with anolides, tannins, phenolic compounds, and tropane alkaloids, which are the most prevalent atropine and scopolamine in the genus Datura. Ingestion of Jimson weed produces the toxidrome of anticholinergic intoxication. Understanding and recognizing the classic signs and symptoms of anticholinergic intoxication can help clinicians evaluate persons presenting with Jimson weed poisoning. Moreover, this review is to identify the most important phytochemical substances extracted from the Jimsonweed and to characterize their biological activity for health effect and biopesticide application. Biopesticides are less harmful than chemical pesticides because they do not leave harmful residues, generally target one specific pest or a small number of related pests rather than broad spectrum chemical pesticides that affect other beneficial insects, birds, mammals, or non-target species, are effective in smaller quantities, decompose quickly and do not cause environmental problems, and are often cheaper. In conclusion, *Datura stramonium*, beside its medicinal value, can applicable for biopesticide application and for postharvest loss control of insects such as weevil.

Keywords: *Datura stramonium*, phytochemical components, pharmacological potential, biopesticide, weevil

1. Introduction

By 2050, the world's population is predicted to reach over 10 billion people; more than half of this increase will occur in Africa, resulting in an additional 1.3 billion people on the continent. As a result, more people will need to be nourished in the next decades, and more food and vaccines will be required around the world than previously. The

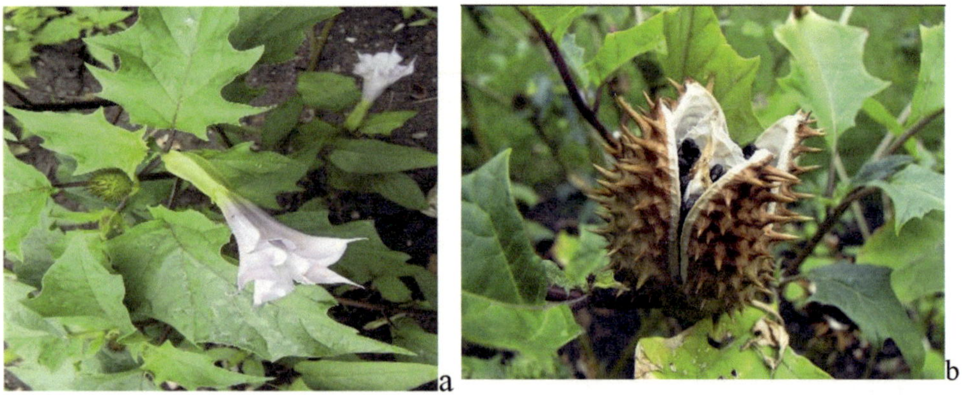

Figure 1.
Datura stramonium. a: Datura plant (leaves and flowers); b: D. stramonium Plant (leaves and fruit).

phytochemical and ethnopharmacological properties of the Jimson plant have always piqued people's curiosity [1]. The genus has 14 species of annual herbs and perennial shrubs ranging in height from 1 to 1.5 meters, with straight stems, thorny fruits, foul-smelling leaves, and highly scented trumpet-shaped flowers that bloom at the stem forks [2]. *Datura* plants thrive in nitrogen-rich soils and soils that have been disturbed by human activity, such as agricultural soils, roadsides, and animal pens [3]. Steroids, phenolic compounds, fatty acids, with anolides, and lactones are the most common components; however, the genus is best recognized for producing tropane-type alkaloids [4]. Therefore, this chapter aims to identify the main phytochemical components isolated from the Jimson weed (*Datura stramonium*) and describe their activity against biopesticides and medicinal effect, with an emphasis on the relevant literature.

2. Overview of Jimson weed

Jimson weed is a wild-growing herb that contains belladonna alkaloids. There have recently been reports of teens intentionally ingesting Jimson marijuana for hallucinogenic purposes. These individuals present to the emergency department with physical indications of atropine intoxication, mental problems, and hallucinations. A positive history, if available, and detection of anticholinergic symptoms are required for diagnosis. It is crucial to distinguish between lysergic acid diethylamide consumption and schizophrenia. Both central and peripheral signs of Jimson weed intoxication can be reversed by physostigmine, an anticholinergic drug. Ingestion of *Datura stramonium* is fairly common and can lead to intoxication and to anticholinergic manifestations that are potentially dangerous (**Figure 1**).

3. Phytochemical components and pharmacological potential of Jimson weed

The phenolic compounds (metabolites) present are linked to the biological functions assigned to the genus Datura. Plants create these chemicals in both their primary and secondary metabolism [5]. Plants' primary metabolites play a direct role in their growth, development, and reproduction, whereas secondary metabolites play an ecological role [6]. Different classes of phenolic compounds, such as terpenoids, flavonoids [7], steroids [8, 9], lectins [10, 11], glycosides, fatty acids, saponins [12], tannins [13], phenolic compounds [14], withanolides [15], and various volatile terpenes [16, 17], have been identified in *Datura* species.

3.1 Phenolic compounds

In methanolic and hydroalcoholic extracts, the existence of distinct classes of phenolic compounds in the genus Datura has been demonstrated. Flavonoids, tannins, and glycosidic phenolic substances are found in *D. metel* and *D. stramonium* [12].

In diverse solvent fractions such as ethyl acetate, butanol, hexane, chloroform, and methanol, Hossain et al. [14] investigated the existence of phenolic compounds in *D. metel*. Gallic acid, vanilic acid, quercetin, and ferulic acid were identified as the primary phenolic components in the methanolic extracts of *D. metel* roots and leaves [18].

On the other hand, LC-ESI-MS/MS analysis of the methanolic extract of *D. innoxia* aerial organs revealed the presence of 20 distinct phenolic compounds, with (−)-epicatechin, (+)-catechin, hyperoside, and p-coumaric acid being the most abundant metabolites detected [19].

3.1.1 Withanolides

Withanolides are steroidal lactones that have been identified from various Solanaceae genera [20]. Biological actions such as anti-inflammatory, antioxidant, anticancer, insecticide, antifood, and immunosuppressive characteristics have been found for these substances [20]. Within the genus *Datura (daturalactones)*, various withanolides have been identified and described, distinguishing themselves by having an epoxy in the lactone ring [21]. Five with anolides were discovered in the aerial portions (flowers, leaves, and stems) of *D. quercifolia Kunth* that have modest cytotoxic and prooxidant effects, as well as acetylcholinesterase inhibitory activity [22].

D. metel leaves have yielded a number of previously unknown withanolides, two of which exhibit anti-inflammatory properties [23]. In addition, 13 others with anolides were isolated from *D. metel* flowers and showed immunosuppressive properties against splenocyte proliferation in mice, as well as activity *in vitro* against human gastric adenocarcinoma cell proliferation (SGC-7901), human hepatoma (HepG2), and human breast cancer cell proliferation (HepG2) (MCF-7) [24].

3.1.2 Terpenes

Datura produces volatile substances that protect plants from herbivore harm by having varying quantities and types of glandular and non-glandular trichomes [25]. *D. wrightii* contains 17 volatile chemicals, the majority of which are sesquiterpenes (**Figure 2**), such as limonene, linalool, (E)-3,8-dimethyl-1,4,7-nonatriene (DMNT), and (E)—ocymene, with (E)—caryophyllene being the most common [25].

3.1.3 Lectins

D. stramonium and other Solanaceae have been found to contain lectins, a category of carbohydrate-specific binding proteins [26]. The biological role of lectins is controversial, albeit due to their toxicity in both mammals and insects, a defensive role for plants has been hypothesized [27].

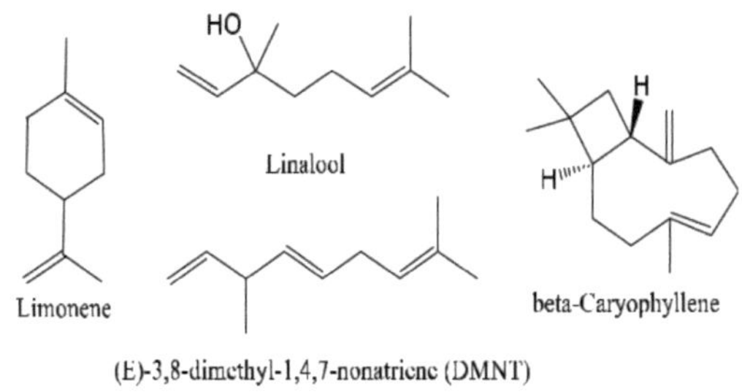

Figure 2.
Structure of some isolated volatile compounds (terpenes) in the genus Datura in response to insect damage.

The chitin-binding lectin *D. stramonium* agglutinin (DSA) has been isolated and purified from *D. stramonium* seeds [28]. In diabetic patients, the use of *D. stramonium* agglutinin in lectin microarrays has been used to identify kidney diseases. The amount of nacetyl-D-glucosamine (GlcNAc) coupled to (−1,4)-linked N-acetyl-D-glucosamine identified by lectin *D. stramonium* agglutinin (DSA) was significantly higher in individuals with diabetic nephropathy, according to the results of lectin microarrays [29].

3.1.4 Alkaloids

Datura has a diverse phytochemical makeup of tropane-type alkaloids, which are the plant's most potent chemicals [30, 31].

Tropane alkaloids, in particular, are a collection of roughly 200 alkaloids with a tropane ring (N-methyl-8-azabicyclo in their chemical structure, with L-ornithine as the major precursor) [32]. Atropine (hyoscyamine) and scopolamine (hyoscine) are the most prevalent alkaloids in the genus *Datura* [33].

The alkaloid fraction of *D. ceratocaula* revealed 36 compounds with a distinctive mass fragmentation spectrum, with atropine being the most abundant alkaloid in seed and scopolamine being the most abundant alkaloid in flowers [34]. Atropine and scopolamine were found in similar abundances in *D. ferox*, with 0.32 g of scopolamine per 100 g of dry plant material [35].

Scopolamine and atropine were the major alkaloids, with quantities changing based on the region of the plant [36]. The most abundant alkaloids in *D. quercifolia* are tropinone, tropine, pseudotropine, atropine, and scopolamine [37].

In the species *D. stramonium*, at least 67 tropane alkaloids (**Table 1**) have been found in various sections of the plant. Tropine, 3-tigloyloxy-6-propionyloxy-7-hydroxytropane, and 3,6-ditigloyloxy-7-hydroxytropane [38] have been identified as the most prevalent, alongside atropine and scopolamine. Okwu and Igara [39], on the other hand, discovered one steroidal alkaloid in *D. metel* that had antibacterial activity.

3.2 The biological functions of the Datura

3.2.1 Insecticide action

Different writers have looked at the insecticidal and repellant properties of *Datura* species. In contact and spray application experiments, leaf extracts of *D. metel* (acetone, water, and petroleum ether) have been shown to exhibit insecticidal and insect repellent activity against a variety of insect species. In organic extracts of

Alkaloid	Specie	Organ
Scopolamine	All	Roots, leaves, flowers, and seeds
Atropine	All	Roots, leaves, flowers, and seeds
3-Tigloyloxy-6,7-dihydroxytropane	*Datura stramonium*	Roots
Apoatropine	*Datura stramonium*	Roots, leaves, flowers, and seeds
3-Tigloyloxy-6-hydroxytropane	*Datura stramonium*	Roots
Hyoscyamine	*Datura quercifolia*	Roots, leaves, flowers, and seeds
3α-Tigloyloxy-6-isovaleroyloxy-7-hydroxytropane	*Datura stramonium*	Roots
3,6-Ditigloyloxy-7-hydroxytropane	*Datura stramonium*	Roots
Scopolamine	*Datura stramonium*	Roots, leaves, flowers, and seeds
Tropine	All	Roots, leaves, flowers, and seeds
3-acetoxynortropane	*Datura quercifolia*	Roots

Table 1.
Most abundant tropane alkaloids identified in the genus Datura [33, 37, 38].

D. metel, EC50 values of 12,000 ppm for grasshoppers and 11,600 ppm for red ants were found [31]. In the case of *D. stramonium*, pesticide activity has been assessed in non-polar extracts in adult individuals and larvae of various insects, both by contact and by food [27].

The larvicidal efficacy of *D. stramonium* aqueous root extract was tested on two mosquito species and found to be between 50 and 100 percent larval mortality at 100 percent concentration of the extracts 24 hours after treatment [40]. Different quantities of an aqueous extract of *D. stramonium* leaves and seeds were shown to be effective against flea beetles, a common maize pest [41].

The toxic effect of acetone extracts from *Datura inoxia* was evaluated against *Tribolium castaneum*, *Trogoderma granarium*, and *Sitophilus granarius*, where the plant extracts were observed in addition to the inhibition of enzymes acetylcholinesterase, carboxylesterase, acid phosphatases, and alkaline phosphatases (ALP) in toxicity test survivors [41].

3.2.2 Herbicidal

In aqueous and methanolic extracts, *D. metel* has shown possible herbicidal efficacy against "noxious weed parthenium," with the root showing superior effects to the stems, with both extracts reducing weed germination as well as stem development in individuals of a few weeks [1]. Similarly, germination inhibition was seen in methanolic and hexane root extracts of *D. metel* when it was tested for herbicide action against Phalaris minor.

Sakadzo et al. [42] found that an aqueous extract of *D. stramonium* inhibited root development, plumule length, and dry matter amount in *Amaranthus hybridus* and Tegetes minuta, with herbicidal effects both pre- and post-emergence.

3.2.3 Acaricide activity

The methanolic extracts of *D. stramonium* leaves and seeds showed acaricidal effects, with 98 percent mortality of adult Tetranychus urticae Koch (spider mites) in the leaf extract and 25 percent mortality in the seed extract, with a direct relationship between concentration and mortality rate for the leaf extracts but not for the seed extracts [7].

In adult mite immersion trials, an ethanolic extract from *Datura stramonium* leaves caused 20% mortality against *Rhipicephalus microplus* (Asian blue tick) [43]. *In vitro* experiments showed that the methanolic extract of *D. stramonium* inhibited the oviposition of Rhipicephalus (Boophilus) microplus by 77% [44].

3.2.4 Antifungal activity

Three members of the genus, *D. discolor, D. metel, and D. stramonium*, were tested for antifungal activity. Ethanolic and methanolic extracts from D. discolor stems and leaves were combined with culture medium to prevent the growth of Aspergillus flavus, Aspergillus niger, Penicillium chrysogenum, Penicillium expansum, Fusarium moniliforme, and Fusarium poae [12].

Rhizoctonia solani was inhibited by aqueous and methanolic extracts of *D. metel* leaves. D. metel's methanolic extract was up to 35 percent more toxic than the other 15 species investigated, preventing mycelial growth and being used in agriculture (herbicide, acaricide, insecticide) and medicine (antibacterial, cytotoxic, or antioxidant) production of sclerotium [15].

Furthermore, extracts of all parts of *D. metel* in various solvents (hexane, chloroform, acetone, and methanol) showed antifungal activity against three Aspergillus species: *A. fumigatus*, *A. niger*, and *A. flavus*, with the chloroform fraction having the lowest inhibitory concentration (MIC) of 625.0 g/mL [45].

The growth inhibition of five fungal species: *A. flavus*, *A. niger*, Alternaria solani, Fusarium solani, and Helianthus sporium used to assess the antifungal efficacy of methanol extracts from the leaves, seeds, stems, and roots of *D. inoxia* [46].

The antifungal activity of *D. stramonium* extracts on *Candida albicans* was stronger in aqueous extracts (74 percent), while methanol and chloroform extracts had good inhibitory activities (69 percent and 65 percent, respectively) [47].

3.2.5 Antibacterial activity

D. stramonium leaf and fruit extracts with different polarity solvents were tested against five pathogenic bacteria, with the extracted methanol and chloroform fractions from both leaves and fruits showing growth suppression of all tested microorganisms at various doses. All isolated fractions from the fruits efficiently inhibited the growth of *Pseudomonas aeruginosa* and Klebsiella pneumonia. The chloroform extract of leaves showed the greatest growth inhibition (77%) against *K. pneumonia* [47].

Using the paper disk diffusion method and ampicillin as a positive control, antibiotic activity of methanolic extracts (80%) of *Datura inoxia* against *Bacillus subtilis*, *Staphylococcus aureus*, and *Escherichia coli* was determined. Except for *E. coli* (2.5 g/mL), the results showed action against all bacteria at the greatest concentration of the extracts [48].

In the paper disk diffusion method, however, methanolic, ethanolic, and aqueous extracts of *D. stramonium* showed antibacterial activity against gram-positive and gram-negative bacteria. With a minimum inhibitory concentration of 25% w/v, ethanolic extract of leaves inhibited the growth of bacteria in *P. aeruginosa, K. pneumoniae*, and *E. coli* [49]. At 2.5, 1.25, and 0.75 mg/mL, the methanolic leaf extract showed antibacterial activity against gram-positive bacteria such as *Staphylococcus haemolyticus, S. aureus*, *Shigella dysenteriae*, and *Bacillus cereus*, as well as gram-negative bacteria such as *P. aeruginosa*, K. *pneumoniae, and E. coli* [13].

3.2.6 Antioxidant activity

Aqueous extracts of *D. metel* stems, roots, and leaves had antioxidant activity ranging from 23.8 to 49.3% [50]. *D. stramonium* methanolic extract had IC50 values of 35.3, 10.5, and 49.36 g/mL for radical DPPH, superoxide, and radical cation ABTS, respectively [51]. In comparison with *D. metel*, the antioxidant capacity and concentration of phenolic compounds and flavonoids, as well as the higher antioxidant capacity (221.25 1.06 mg EPA/g), were tested in *D. innoxia*, which had significantly higher values in all assays [52]. The presence of the maximum number of phenolic components, including flavonoids and tannins, in *D. metel* leaf methanol extract exhibited the highest antioxidant capacity in a DPPH purification test against other solvents and plant parts [53].

3.2.7 Hypoglycemic activity

The hypoglycemic action of *D. metel* seeds was investigated by adding pulverized seeds to the food of rats with induced diabetes, which resulted in a considerable decrease in blood glucose levels after 8 hours [54]. Although a hydromethanolic extract of *D. stramonium* root was tested in diabetic mice and found to have no substantial hypoglycemic effect, the extract considerably lowered blood glucose levels in diabetic by orally loaded mice at relatively large doses (100, 200, and 400 mg/kg) [55]. The antihyperglycemic effects of *D. inoxia* methanolic leaf extract were seen in -glucosidase, –amylase, lipase, and urease [56].

3.2.8 Cytotoxic activity

The ethyl acetate portion of the ethanolic extract of *D. metel* flowers was tested against cancer cell lines and found to be cytotoxic against the A549 (tongue), BGC-823 (gastric), and K562 (leukemia) cell lines [57]. Similarly, methanolic extracts of *Datura stramonium* seed were found to be cytotoxic to MCF7 (breast cancer) cells, with a cytotoxicity of 66.84 percent at 599 μg/mL [51]. These findings were similar to those reported by Gupta et al. [58], who investigated the cytotoxic effects of methanolic extracts of *D. stramonium* leaves on A549 and MCF7 cells, finding considerable immune stimulation [59]. The methanolic leaf extract of *D. innoxia* revealed a possible cytotoxic impact on MCF-7 human breast cancer cell lines, with an IC50 of 93.73 g/mL [59].

Rhinoxia B, a phytosterol isolated from *D. inoxia* leaf extracts, was found to have antiproliferative activity against human colon adenocarcinoma cells, HCT 15, with an IC50 of 4 M [58].

3.2.9 Other activities

Datura has anticholinergic (mydriatic, antispasmodic), anesthetic, analgesic, sedative-hypnotic, anti-parkinsonian, and aphrodisiac qualities due to the presence of tropane alkaloids. Tropane alkaloids' actions are linked to a competitive antagonist of muscarinic receptors. Some tropane alkaloids and derivatives, on the other hand, have exhibited differing affinities to the nicotinic acetylcholine receptor, albeit to a lesser amount, and are in some cases partial agonists [60]. Tropane alkaloids' nervous system effects are also linked to the action of monoaminergic neurotransmitters, as tropane alkaloids exhibit varying degrees of affinity for monoaminergic transporters [61].

4. Discussion

4.1 Jimson plant in Ethiopia

Ethiopia is primarily found in the tropical and subtropical regions of the world. As a result, the climatic conditions are favorable for the growth of the Jimson plant, and around 35–45 percent of Ethiopia's climate is suited for the Jimson plantation. In Ethiopia, Jimson plant has been seen in a number of locations. Oromia, Gambella, Somalia, Southern Nations, Nationalities and Peoples, Sidama, and Amhara [28] are just a few of the locations where it can be found.

4.1.1 Biopesticide based on atropine

In 1850, a Belgian chemist named Jean Servial Stas was the first to successfully isolate an alkaloid poison, extracting nicotine from the tissues of the murdered Gustave Fougnie with a mixture of acetic acid and ethyl alcohol. To keep pests away from plants and crops, Jimson seed is used as a pesticide. This method is effective against insecticide-resistant pests while causing no harm to beneficial insects. Jimson oil and seed extracts, which are used to make pesticides, are known to have germicidal and antibacterial capabilities, making them useful for protecting plants from various pests. One of the most significant differences between Jimson-based insecticides and their synthetic counterparts is that they do not leave any residue on the plants. Jimson insecticides are frequently employed in agriculture because they serve an important role in pest management. There has been a noticeable movement worldwide from synthetic pesticides to non-synthetic pesticides, owing to widespread understanding of the synthetic pesticides' adverse effects not just on plants and soil, as well as other living organisms.

Because atropine has multiple modes of action, insect species are unlikely to develop resistance to it based on just one. Most synthetic pesticides, on the other hand, target the insect's nervous system, and resistance to one chemical leads to resistance to all others that use the same response pathway. Atropine has long been thought to be an environmentally beneficial insect pest management strategy for plant protection.

4.1.2 The effect of atropine on pest growth regulation

The ability of Jimson products to control insect proliferation is a fascinating feature. The insect larva feeds and sheds its old skin as it grows. Ecdysis, or molting, is the process of shedding old skin and is controlled by an enzyme called ecdysones. The action of ecdysones is reduced when Jimson components, particularly atropine, enter the body of the larva, causing the larva to fail to molt, remain in the larval stage, and eventually perish. The larva will only perish after entering the pupal stage if the atropine concentration is not high enough. If the concentration is any lower, the adult that emerges from the pupa will be completely deformed and sterile [62].

4.1.3 Feeding prevention's atropine effect

An insect larva will seek to feed on a leaf if it is sitting on it. The maxillary glands are responsible for this particular eating trigger. As a result, peristalsis in the alimentary canal is accelerated, and the larva becomes hungry and begins feeding on the leaf's surface. Because atropine antagonizes the muscarine-like activities of acetylcholine and other choline esters, if the leaf is treated with a Jimson product, it will act as an antimuscarinic agent. The insect does not feed on the atropine-treated surface as a result of this perception. Its swallowing ability is also impaired [63].

4.1.4 Atropine has an anti-oviposition action

Another way atropine keeps pests at bay is by stopping females from laying eggs. When seeds in storage are covered with atropine or crude Jimson oil, this ability is known as oviposition prevention, and it comes in useful. The insects will no longer feed on them after this treatment. Further damage to the grains will be prevented, and the female will be unable to lay eggs throughout her life cycle's egg-laying period.

4.2 Anticholinergic poisoning from Jimson weed

4.2.1 Poisoning symptoms and signs

Symptoms begin to appear shortly after consumption [64]. The dryness of the mouth is the initial symptom, followed by a strong need to drink. The pupils then dilate, resulting in hazy vision. The skin appears flushed and heated. The face, neck, and chest may be affected by an atropine rash, which is more common in youngsters. Swallowing, talking, and peeing may be challenging for the patient. Tachycardia and palpations become more noticeable. Fever is common in children and can reach dangerously at high levels. Various behavioral and mental symptoms are reported depending on the amount of stramonium consumed. The patient is anxious, restless, and bewildered. His exuberance and hyperactivity may make him prone to muscle weakness and incoordination. Memory and orientation are disrupted, visual hallucinations are widespread, and mania and delirium are possible side effects. Coma and convulsions have been seen at larger doses, and cardiac and respiratory collapse can lead to death [64]. The psychosis usually passes in 12 hours, whereas the clinical abnormalities pass in 24 to 26 hours. The condition, on the other hand, can last up to 48 hours [64].

4.2.2 Diagnosis

A positive history of Jimson marijuana consumption is unquestionably beneficial in determining the diagnosis. In the absence of such information, the diagnosis is based on the recognition of paralysis of organs innervated by parasympathetic nerves, as well as strange mental symptoms. Intoxication with stramine must be distinguished from intoxication with lysergic acid diethylamide (LSD) and schizophrenia. Dilated pupils, tachycardia, and fever are all physical manifestations of Jimson marijuana and LSD [32]. However, the latter does not usually have a dry mouth or a flushed appearance. Goose pimples also emerge with LSD toxicity due to the sympathomimetic action. Another historically reported diagnostic method is to identify atropine in the patient's urine by placing a drop of urine in the eye of a cat and observing pupillary dilatation [32].

4.2.3 Treatment

Even if it has been several hours following intake, induced emesis is indicated. If the patient refuses to cooperate, an Ewald tube should be used to perform a stomach lavage to remove any leftover Jimson weed contents. The belladonna alkaloids cause decreased gastrointestinal motility and can stay in the stomach for long periods of time, despite their normally quick absorption. To bind unabsorbed material, roughly 5 mg of activated charcoal should be given *via* the tube once the gastric lavage has become clear. The patient is subsequently administered a cathartic, such as magnesium sulfate, to increase intestinal transit time and decrease absorption. To keep the agitated patient from hurting himself or others, physical restraints may be required. The stimulation will be kept to a minimum in a quiet, gloomy atmosphere.

Any fever should be treated with the appropriate antipyretics. When toxicity is present, hospitalization is recommended. Physostigmine inhibits the enzyme acetylcholinesterase as an anticholinesterase drug, allowing acetylcholine to accumulate at the neuroreceptor site. Physostigmine crosses into the CNS and reverses hallucinations and mental symptoms because of its tertiary amine structure [65]. If the diagnosis is correct, both central and peripheral effects should be reversed within minutes of injection if the diagnosis is correct. Neostigmine and pyridostigmine bromides are also anticholinesterase drugs, but they do not penetrate the CNS since they are quaternary amines.

4.3 Pharmacological activities (medicinal significance of *Datura stramonium*)

The World Health Organization estimates that four billion people, or about 80% of the world's population, already use herbal medicine for some component of primary health care. Plants produce a large number of secondary metabolites, which are a major source of many pharmacological medications [66]. *D. stramonium* is an effective cure for a variety of human illnesses, including ulcers, wounds, inflammation, rheumatism and gout, sciatica, bruising and swellings, fever, asthma, bronchitis, and toothache, according to Ayurvedic medicine. *D. stramonium* is used in a variety of folk medicine therapies [67]. Seeds with palm oil were used externally for insect bites and stings, and the juice of the leaves in heated milk was used to expel intestinal worms, especially cestodes When *Datura stramonium* leaves are combined with mustard oil, they can be used to treat skin problems. The juice of flower petals is used to treat earaches, and the seeds are used to treat coughs, fevers, and asthma. Seeds are smoked because of their narcotic properties [68]. Datura leaves, coupled with *Cannabis sativa* leaves and Neopicrorhizascrofulariflora stems, are mashed with water and applied to alleviate headaches in Western Nepal. Datura seeds are pulverized with rice grains and consumed orally for indigestion treatment. Fresh leaves are warmed and frequently placed on an injured body part before retiring to bed in portions of Central Nepal for the purported analgesic effect. Seeds are used as a tonic and febrifuge in India. Native Americans have utilized Datura seeds as a euphoric stimulant for many years when the leaves of *Datura stramonium* are mixed with mustard oil. It has been utilized as a medicinal agent in the United Kingdom since the 1800s [69].

4.3.1 Anticancer properties

At a therapeutic dose of 0.05 to 0.1 g, *D. stramonium* was found to have anticancer properties against human epidermal carcinoma of the nasopharynx. However, while utilizing Datura as an anticancer treatment, caution should be exercised because serious anticholinergic effects can develop [70].

4.3.2 Women's infertility

Datura flowers are an effective treatment for female infertility. The dried powder of Datura flowers is administered with honey 10 days after menstruation in a dosage of 120 mg. It is administered over a period of 5 to 7 days. This treatment is successful in cases of infertility caused by unknown factors [71].

4.3.3 Poisoning with organophosphates

Datura stramonium, which contains atropine and other anticholinergic chemicals, is an effective treatment for OP's central cholinergic symptoms. Following a severe organophosphate poisoning, Bania et al. [72] observed that DS seed extracts were beneficial. DS seeds were boiled in water to generate a 2 mg/mL atropine solution, which was then given to male rats as a single intraperitoneal injection 5 minutes before the subcutaneous administration of 25 mg/kg dichlorvos. In a rat model of severe organophosphate poisoning, pretreatment with Datura seed extract greatly enhanced survival.

4.3.4 Anti-asthmatic effects

D. stramonium includes a number of alkaloids with anticholinergic and bronchodilating properties, including atropine and scopolamine. Atropine and scopolamine expand bronchial smooth muscle and alleviate asthmatic episodes by inhibiting muscarinic receptors (especially the M2 receptors) on airway smooth muscle and submucosal gland cells. According to Charpin et al. [73], cigarette is an efficient bronchodilator in asthmatic patients with minor airway blockage when *D. stramonium* is used as an antiasthmatic.

When a mother uses *D. stramonium* for asthma, the fetus is exposed to it, which causes a continuous release of acetylcholine and desensitization of nicotinic receptors, which can lead to lasting damage to the fetus [74].

4.3.5 Analgesic effects

The hot plate and formalin tests were used to assess the analgesic impact of alcoholic Datura seed in acute and chronic pain. When the extracts were given intraperitoneally to the rats, they relieved pain in a dose-dependent manner, with ED50s of 25 and 50 mg/kg in hot plate and formalin tests, respectively [75].

4.3.6 Antiepileptic activity

Rats were continuously administered one of three herbal treatments, *S. lateriflora*, *G. sempervirens*, and *D. stramonium*, through water supply for 30 days, 1 week after status epilepticus was induced by a single injection of lithium (3 mEq/kg) and pilocarpine (30 g/kg), according to Peredery and Persinger [76]. During the treatment period and an additional 30 days when just tap water was administered, the number of spontaneous seizures per day was recorded for each rat during a 15-minute observation time. During therapy, rats given a dilute solution of the three herbal fluid extracts had no seizures. When the therapy was discontinued, the rats experienced a similar number of spontaneous seizures as the controls.

4.3.7 Antimicrobial effect

The bactericidal activity of methanol extracts of the aerial portion of DS against gram-positive bacteria was dosage dependent [48]. Sharma et al. [77] claimed that DS was highly efficient as a vibriocidal against Vibreo cholerae and Vibreo parahaemolyticus strains. The MIC value of acetone extracts of DS was in the range of 2.5–15 mg/mL, making them effective as broad spectrum vibriocidal agents.

4.3.8 Antifungal effect

The fungicidal properties of acetone extracts reveal the potential of *D. stramonium* seeds as a natural source of antifungal agent, according to Mdee et al. [78]. DS extracts have MICs ranging from 1.25 to 2.50 mg/mL.

4.3.9 Insecticidal effect

The odor of the Datura plant functions as a repellant for a variety of insects and pests. Under laboratory conditions, Kurnal et al. [79] found that ethanol extracts of *D. stramonium* leaf and seed have substantial acaricidal, repellant, and oviposition deterrent effect against adult two-spotted spider mites (Tetranychusurticae). After 48 hours, leaf and seed extracts at concentrations of 167.25 and 145.75 g/L (applied using a Petri leaf disc-spray tower method) killed 98 percent and 25 percent of spider mite adults, respectively. These findings imply that *D. stramonium* may be useful in the treatment of two-spotted spider mites.

4.3.10 Dosage

D. stramonium is generally administrated at a dose of 60–185 mg powder for leaf and 60–120 mg powder for seed [80].

5. Conclusion

Datura species are among the oldest plants used in traditional medicine, according to legend. Because of its psychoactive properties, it has been a source of major cultural traditions. The impacts of Jimson plants have been examined in numerous general biological activities, such as pesticide, fungicide, and antibacterial, among others, based on this cultural knowledge. Plants are utilized for a variety of purposes, including food, shelter, fiber, tan, gum, oil, and latex. They are high in minerals, antioxidants, vitamins, carbs, and proteins, and as a result, they have an immunomodulatory effect. *Datura stramonium* is a wild plant with a variety of medical and pharmacological qualities that have been used to treat cancer, rheumatism, ear discomfort, headaches, wounds, burns, stress, depression, insomnia, asthma, boils, and inflammation, according to this review. Pharmaceutical firms make *Datura stramonium* as herbal or botanical medications for a variety of ailments; however, it is not utilized in its native form due to its fatal effect. Furthermore, research into plant components has led to research into more critical biological activities such as cancer cell cytotoxicity. The relevance of studying secondary metabolites of the genus *Datura* has resulted in significant biological discoveries. However, new research continues to uncover new metabolites with potential biological activity in a variety of systems, establishing the genus as a valuable source of chemicals with novel pharmaceutical applications. This ability of Jimson products to control insect proliferation is a fascinating feature. The insect larva feeds and sheds its old skin as it grows. Overall, besides its medicinal value, Jimson weed can applicable for biopesticide application and for post-harvest loss control such as weevil.

Author details

Melaku Tafese Awulachew
School of Chemical and Bio-Engineering, Chemical Engineering Graduate Program, Addis Ababa Institute of Technology, Ethiopia

*Address all correspondence to: melakutafese12@gmail.com; melaku.tafese@aait.edu.et

References

[1] Ibrahim M, Siddique S, Rehman K, Husnain M, Hussain A, Akash MSH, et al. Comprehensive analysis of phytochemical constituents and ethnopharmacological investigation of genus Datura. Critical reviews™ in eukaryotic. Gene Expression. 2018;**28**(3):223-276

[2] Nayyar MS, Hanif MA, Mjaeed MI, Ayub MA, Rehman R. Chapter 16 – Datura. Medicinal Plants of South Asia; 2020. pp. 207-216

[3] Hernández J, Montes-Osuna N, Cariñanos P. The genus Datura L. (Solanaceae) in Mexico and Spain– ethnobotanical perspective at the interface of medical and illicit uses. Journal of Ethnopharmacology. 2018;**219**:133-151

[4] Khan W, Subhan S, Shams DF, Afridi SG, Ullah R, Shahat AA, et al. Antioxidant potential, phytochemicals composition, and metal contents of Datura alba. Hindawi Biomedical Research International. 2019;**2019**:1-9

[5] Nain J, Bhatt S, Dhyani S, Joshi N. Phytochemical screening of secondary metabolites of Datura stramonium. International Journal of Current Pharmaceutical Research. 2013;**5**(2):151-153

[6] Anulika NP, Ignatius EO, Raymond ES, Osasere O, Hilda A. The chemistry of natural product. Plant Secondary Metabolites. 2016; **4**(August):1-8

[7] Kumral NA, Çobanoğlu S, Yalcin C. Acaricidal, repellent and oviposition deterrent activities of Datura stramonium L. against adult Tetranychus urticae (Koch). Journal of Pest Science. 2010;**83**(2):173-180

[8] Mai NT, Cuc NT, Anh HLT, Nhiem NX, Tai BH, Yen PH, et al. Two new guaiane sesquiterpenes from Datura metel L. with anti-inflammatory activity. Phytochemistry Letters. 2017;**19**:231-236

[9] Haegi L. Taxonomic account of Datura L. (Solanaceae) in Australia with a note on Brugmansia Pers. Australian Journal of Botany. 1976;**24**(3):415-435

[10] Carlini CR, Grossi-de-Sá MF. Plant toxic proteins with insecticidal properties. A review on their potentialities as bioinsecticides. Toxicon. 2002;**40**(11):1515-1539

[11] Kilpatrick DC, Yeoman MM. Purification of the lectin from Datura stramonium. Biochemical Journal. 1978;**175**(3):1151-1153

[12] Al-Snafi AE. Medical importance of Datura fastuosa (syn: Datura metel) and Datura stramonium-a review. IOSR Journal of Pharmacy. 2017;**7**(2):43-58

[13] Gupta AK, Ahirwar NK, Shinde N, Choudhary M, Rajput YS, Singh A. Phytochemical screening and antimicrobial assessment of leaves of Adhatoda vasica, Azadirachta indica and Datura stramonium. UK Journal of Pharmaceutical and Biosciences. 2013;**1**(1):42-47

[14] Hossain MA, Al Kalbani MSA, Al Farsi SAJ, Weli AM, AlRiyami Q. Comparative study of total phenolics, flavonoids contents and evaluation of antioxidant and antimicrobial activities of different polarities fruits crude extracts of Datura metel L. Asian Pacific Journal of Tropical Disease. 2014;**4**(5):378-383

[15] Kagale S, Marimuthu T, Thayumanavan B, Nandakumar R,

Samiyappan R. Antimicrobial activity and induction of systemic resistance in rice by leaf extract of Datura metel against Rhizoctonia solani and Xanthomonas oryzae pv. Oryzae. Physiological and Molecular Plant Pathology. 2004;**65**(2):91-100

[16] Aboluwodi AS, Avoseh NO, Lawal AO, Ogunwande IA, Giwa AA. Chemical constituents and antiinflammatory activity of essential oils of Datura stramonium L. Journal of Medicinal Plant Studies. 2017;**5**(1):21-25

[17] Hare JD, Sun JJ. Production of induced volatiles by Datura wrightii in response to damage by insects: Effect of herbivore species and time. Journal of Chemical Ecology. 2011;**37**(7):751-764

[18] Javid M, Aziz A, Azhar MF, Qayyum A. Antioxidant, antibacterial, phytochemical composition of leaves and roots extracts of Datura alba. Zeitschrift Fur Arznei-& Gewurzpflanzen. 2017;**22**(4):165-168

[19] Benabderrahim MA, Sarikurkcu C, Elfalleh W, Ozer MS. Datura innoxia and Dipsacus laciniatus: Biological activity and phenolic composition. Biocatalysis and Agricultural Biotechnology. 2019;**19**(2):101163

[20] Veleiro AS, Cirigliano AM, Oberti JC, Burton G. 7- Hydroxywithanolides from Datura ferox. Journal of Natural Products. 1999;**62**(7):1010-1012

[21] Bandhoria P, Gupta VK, Sharma VK, Satti NK, Dutt P, Suri KA. Crystal structure of 6α, 7α: 24α, 25α-Diepoxy-5α, 12α-dihydroxy1-oxo-20S, 22R-witha-2-enolide isolated from Datura quercifolia leaves. Analytical Sciences: X-ray Structure Analysis Online. 2006;**22**:169-170

[22] Jasso C, Nieto-Camacho A, Ramírez-Apan M, Martínez M, Maldonado E. Antioxidant, cytotoxic, and acetylcholinesterase inhibitory activities of withanolides from Datura quercifolia. Planta Medica International Open. 2020;**7**(02):e68-e72

[23] Tan J, Liu Y, Cheng Y, Sun Y, Pan J, Guan W, et al. New withanolides with anti-inflammatory activity from the leaves of Datura metel L. Bioorganic Chemistry. 2020;**95**(103541):1-12

[24] Liu Y, Guan W, Lu ZK, Guo R, Xia YG, Lv SW, et al. New sesquiterpenoids from the stems of Datura metel L. Fitoterapia. 2019;**134**:417-421

[25] Hare JD. Variation in herbivore and methyl jasmonate-induced volatiles among genetic lines of Datura wrightii. Journal of Chemical Ecology. 2007;**33**(11):2028-2043

[26] Crowley JF, Goldstein IJ. Datura stramonium lectin: Isolation and characterization of the homogeneous lectin. Federation of European Biochemical Societies. 1981;**130**(1):149-152

[27] Maheshwari NO, Khan A, Chopade BA. Rediscovering the medicinal properties of Datura sp.: A review. Journal of Medicinal Plants Research. 2013;**7**(39):2885-2897

[28] CGIAR. Annual report, Indonesia. Research Program on Forests, Trees and Agroforestry. 2012

[29] Yang BY, Zhou YQ, Liu Y, Lu ZK, Kuang HX. Entkaurane diterpenoids from the pericarps of Datura metel L. acted on the vascular endothelial cells via TRPC6 and NF-κB protein. Medicinal Chemistry Research. 2018;**27**(1):115-121

[30] Kuganathan N, Ganeshalingam S. Chemical analysis of Datura metel leaves and investigation of the acute toxicity on grasshoppers and red ants. Journal of Chemistry. 2011;**8**(1):107-112

[31] Ali A, Ahmad F, Biondi A, Wang Y, Desneux N. Potential for using Datura alba leaf extracts against two major stored grain pests, the khapra beetle Trogoderma granarium and the rice weevil Sitophillus oryzae. Journal of Pest Science. 2012;**85**(3):359-366

[32] Cohen S. LSD side effects and compli' cations. Journal of Nerve and Mental Developments. 1960;**130**:30-40

[33] El Bazaoui A, Bellimam MA, Soulaymani A. Nine new tropane alkaloids from Datura stramonium L. identified by GC/MS. Fitoterapia. 2011;**82**(2):193-197

[34] Berkov S. Alkaloids of Datura ceratocaula. Zeitschrift für Naturforschung C. 2003;**58**(7-8):455-458

[35] Kovatsis A, Flaskos J, Nikolaidis E, Kotsaki-Kovatsi VP, Papaioannou N, Tsafaris F. Toxicity study of the main alkaloids of Datura ferox in broilers. Food and Chemical Toxicology. 1993;**31**(11):841-845

[36] Anju D, Ratan L. Phytochemical and pharmacological status of Datura fastuosa Linn. International Journal of Research Ayurveda Pharmacology. 2011;**2**(1):145-150

[37] Dupraz JM, Christen P, Kapetanidis I. Tropane alkaloids in transformed roots of Datura quercifolia. Planta Medica. 1994;**60**(2):158-162

[38] Berkov S, Zayed R, Doncheva T. Alkaloid patterns in some varieties of Datura stramonium. Fitoterapia. 2006;**77**(3):179-182

[39] Okwu DE, Igara EC. Isolation, characterization and antibacterial activity of alkaloid from Datura metel Linn leaves. African Journal of Pharmacy and Pharmacology. 2009;**3**(5):277-281

[40] Olofintoye LK, Simon-Oke IA, Omoregie OB. Larvicidal properties of Datura stramonium (jimson weed) and Nicotiana tabaccum (tobacco) extracts against the larvae of (Anopheles and Culex) mosquitoes. African Research Review. 2011;**5**(2):337-344

[41] Ali K, Shuaib M, Ilyas M, Hussain F, Arif M, Ali S, et al. Efficacy of various botanical and chemical insecticides against flea beetles on maize (Zea maize L.). PSM Veterinary Research. 2017;**2**(1):6-9

[42] Sakadzo N, Pahla I, Muzemu S, Mandumbu R, Makaza K. Herbicidal effects of Datura stramonium (L.) leaf extracts on Amaranthus hybridus (L.) and Tagetes minuta (L.). African Journal of Agricultural Research. 2018;**13**(34):1754-1760

[43] Ghosh S, Tiwari SS, Srivastava S, Sharma AK, Nagar G, Kumar KA, et al. In vitro acaricidal properties of Semecarpus anacardium fruit and Datura stramonium leaf extracts against acaricide susceptible (IVRI-I line) and resistant (IVRI-V line) Rhipicephalus (Boophilus) microplus. Veterinary Science Research Journal. 2015;**101**:69-74

[44] Shyma KP, Gupta JP, Ghosh S, Patel KK, Singh V. Acaricidal effect of herbal extracts against cattle tick Rhipicephalus (Boophilus) microplus using in vitro studies. Parasitology Research. 2014;**113**(5):1919-1926

[45] Sharma GL. Studies on antimycotic properties of Datura metel. Journal of Ethnopharmacology. 2002;**80**(2-3):193-197

[46] Kalim M, Hussain F, Ali H, Ahmad I, Iqbal MN. Antifungal activities of methanolic extracts of Datura inoxia. PSM Biological Research. 2016;**1**(2):70-73

[47] Bakht J, Qureshi M, Iqbal A, Shafi M. Effect of different solvent extracted samples from the leaves and fruits of Datura stramonium on the growth of bacteria and fungi. Pakistan Journal of Pharmaceutical Sciences. 2019;**32**(1):177-184

[48] Eftekhar F, Yousefzadi M, Tafakori V. Antimicrobial activity of Datura innoxia and Datura stramonium. Fitoterapia. 2005;**76**(1):118-120

[49] Banso A, Adeyemo S. Phytochemical screening and antimicrobial assessment of Abutilon mauritianum, Bacopa monnifera and Datura stramonium. Journal of Biochemistry. 2006;**18**(1):39-42

[50] Monira KM, Munan SM. Review on Datura metel: A potential medicinal plant. Global Journal of Research on Medicinal Plants & Indigenous Medicine. 2012;**1**(4):123-132

[51] Iqbal S, Sivaraj C, Gunasekaran K. Antioxidant and anticancer activities of methanol extract of seeds of Datura stramonium l. Free Radicals & Antioxidants. 2017;**7**(2):184-189

[52] Bhardwaj K, Kumar S, Ojha S. Antioxidant activity and FT-IR analysis of Datura innoxia and Datura metel leaf and seed methanolic extracts. African Journal of Traditional, Complementary and Alternative Medicines. 2016;**13**(5):7-16

[53] Alabri THA, Al Musalami AHS, Hossain MA, Weli AM, AlRiyami Q. Comparative study of phytochemical screening, antioxidant and antimicrobial capacities of fresh and dry leaves crude plant extracts of Datura metel L. Journal of King Saud University-Science. 2014;**26**(3):237-243

[54] Murthy BK, Nammi S, Kota MK, Rao RK, Rao NK, Annapurna A. Evaluation of hypoglycemic and antihyperglycemic effects of Datura metel (Linn.) seeds in normal and alloxan-induced diabetic rats. Journal of Ethnopharmacology. 2004;**91**(1):95-98

[55] Belayneh YM, Birhanu Z, Birru EM, Getenet G. Evaluation of in vivo antidiabetic, antidyslipidemic, and in vitro antioxidant activities of hydromethanolic root extract of Datura stramonium L. (Solanaceae). Journal of Experimental Pharmacology. 2019;**11**:29-38

[56] Bagewadi ZK, Muddapur UM, Madiwal SS, Mulla SI, Khan A. Biochemical and enzyme inhibitory attributes of methanolic leaf extract of Datura inoxia mill. Environmental Sustainability. 2019;**2**(1):75-87

[57] Pan Y, Wang X, Hu X. Cytotoxic withanolides from the flowers of Datura metel. Journal of Natural Products. 2007;**70**(7):1127-1132

[58] Gajendran B, Durai P, Varier KM, Chinnasamy A. A novel phytosterol isolated from Datura inoxia, RinoxiaB is a potential cure colon cancer agent by targeting BAX/Bcl2 pathway. Bioorganic and Medicinal Chemistry. 2019;**28**(2) 115242:2-18

[59] Gupta A, Kumar S, Mahindroo N, Saini RV. Bioactive fraction from Datura stramonium Linn. Promotes human immune cells mediated cytotoxicity towards lung and breast cancer cells. Pharmacognosy Journal. 2016;**8**(5):435-438

[60] Pin F, Vercouillie J, Ouach A, Mavel S, Gulhan Z, Chicheri G, et al. Design of α7 nicotinic acetylcholine receptor ligands in quinuclidine, tropane and quinazoline series. Chemistry, molecular modeling, radiochemistry, in vitro and in rats evaluations of a

[18 F] quinuclidine derivative. European Journal of Medicinal Chemistry. 2014;**82**:214-224

[61] Carroll FI, Gray JL, Abraham P, Kuzemko MA, Lewin AH, Boja JW, et al. 3-Aryl-2-(3′-substituted-1′, 2′, 4′-oxadiazol-5′- yl) tropane analogs of cocaine: Affinities at the cocaine binding site at the dopamine, serotonin, and norepinephrine transporters. Journal of Medicinal Chemistry. 1993;**36**(20):2886-2289

[62] Juss A, Porfirio Emerenciano D, Aparecida Medeiros Maciel M. Humberto Xavier JúniorF, de Fátima Vitória de Moura M. phytochemical and pharmacological aspects of meliaceae and Azadirachta indica. International Journal of Latest Research Science Technology. 2015;**4**(4):128-135 http://www.mnkjournals.com/ijlrst.htm

[63] Djibril D, Mamadou F, Gérard V, Codou Geuye M-D, Oumar S, Luc R. Physical characteristics, chemical composition and distribution of constituents of the neem seeds (Azadirachta indica a. Juss) collected in Senegal. Research Journal of Chemistry Science. 2015;**5**(7):52-58

[64] Goodman LS, Gilman A. The Pharmacological Basis of Therapeutics. New York: The MacMillan Company; 1975

[65] Duvoisin RC, Katz R. Reversal of central anticholinergic syndrome in man by physostigmine. Journal of the American Medical Association. 1968;**206**:1963-1965

[66] Davidson-Hunt I. Ecological ethnobotany: Stumbling toward new practices and paradigms. MASA J. 2000;**16**:1-13

[67] Kirtikar KR, Basu BD. Indian Medicinal Plants. 2nd ed. Vol. III. International Book Distributors: Dehradun; 1999. pp. 1783-1787

[68] Egharevba RKA, Ikhatua MI. Ethno-medical uses of plants in the treatment of various skin diseases in Ovia north east, Edo state, Nigeria. Research Journal of Agriculture and Biological Sciences. 2008;**4**(1):58-64

[69] Rajbhandari KR. Ethnobotany of Nepal. Kathmandu: Kishor Offset Press Private Limited; 2001. pp. 142-143

[70] Balachandran P, Rajgopal G. Cancer-an Ayurvedic perspective. Pharmacological Research. 2005;**51**(1): 19-30

[71] Kadam SD, Chavhan SA, Shinde SA, Sapkal PN. Pharmacognostic review on Datura. International Journal of Pharmacognosy & Chinese Medicine. 2018;**2**(4):000145

[72] Bania TC, Chu J, Bailes D, O'Neill M. Jimson weed extract as a protective agent in severe organophosphate toxicity. Academic Emergency Medicine. 2004;**11**(4):335-338

[73] Charpin D, Orehek J, Velardocchio JM. Bronchodilator effects of antiasthmatic cigarette smoke (Datura stramonium). Thorax. 1979;**34**(2):259-261

[74] Pretorius E, Marx J. Datura stramonium in asthma treatment and possible effects on prenatal development. Environmental Toxicology and Pharmacology. 2006;**21**(3):331-337

[75] Khalili Najafabadi M, Atyabi SM. Evaluation of analgesic effect of Datura stramonium seed extract in hot plate and formalin tested on male rats. International Journal of Medicinal and Aromatic Plants. 2004;**20**(3):309-322

[76] Peredery O, Persinger MA. Herbal treatment following postseizure induction in rat by lithium pilocarpine: Scutellarialateriflora (skullcap), Gelsemiumsempervirens (Gelsemium) and Datura stramonium (jimson weed) may prevent development of spontaneous seizures. Phytotherapy Research. 2004;**18**(9):700-705

[77] Sharma A, Patel VK, Chaturvedi AN. Vibriocidal activity of certain medicinal plants used in Indian folklore medicine by tribals of Mahakoshal region of Central India. Indian Journal of Pharmacology. 2009;**41**(3):129-133

[78] Mdee LK, Masoko P, Eloff JN. The activity of extracts of seven common invasive plant species on fungal phytopathogens. South African Journal of Botany. 2009;**75**(2):375-379

[79] Kurnal NA, Çobanoğlu S, Yalcin C. Acaricidal, repellent and oviposition deterrent activities of Datura stramonium L. against adult Tetranychusurticae (Koch). Journal of Pest Science. 2010;**83**(2):173-180

[80] Khare CP. Indian Medicinal Plants. Vol. 203. Delhi: Rajkamal Electric Press; 2007

Chapter 18

Rose Hip as a Nutraceutical

Ditte Christina Lustrup and Kaj Winther

Abstract

From ancient times, rose hip has been used as food source and as part of herbal remedies. Modern research has confirmed that rose hip, especially when containing seeds and shells, reduces pain and improves daily activity in animal models and in patients with osteoarthritis. The effect size on pain is comparable to that observed with nonsteroidal anti-inflammatory agents and superior to that obtained with paracetamol. For example, treatment with a subspecies of *Rosa canina* (Lito) resulted in 50% reduction in intake of pain killers. There are also strong indications that conditions such as rheumatoid arthritis, aging skin, and wrinkles benefit from treatment with rose hip. Cardiovascular diseases, especially where hyperlipidemia plays a major role, can be treated with rose hip, since a modest reduction of blood cholesterol levels as well as kidney and liver protection has been reported with the treatment. Variation in efficacy and amount of active ingredients in the different species, as well as with different ways of production, should be recognized. Rose hip can be collected from nature. It takes 5–7 *Rosa canina* berries to produce the daily dose of 5 gram of mixed shell-seed powder.

Keywords: Rosa canina, rose hip, seeds, shells, anti-inflammatory, antioxidant, vitamin C, collagen

1. Introduction

Rose hip is the pseudo-fruit of the wild rose (genus *Rosa* L.), the ancestor of the cultivated rose that is one of the most important flowers of the floricultural industry [1]. The genus *Rosa* includes over 100 different species that are found in many parts of the world, including North and South America, Europe, Asia, the Middle East [2], as well as in some parts of Africa [3, 4]. While most species originate from Asia, some are native to Europe, northwest Africa, and North America [5]. Wild roses are widespread in nature and are generally hardy plants capable of growing in many different environments. Some species flourish close to the sea, growing in sandy soil, while others are more common in the lowlands, inland, or in mountain regions [2, 6]. Their fruits can be harvested from late summer to early spring, depending on the specific type, climate, geographical location, and weather. The appearance, size, and taste of rose hips vary from species to species. While some are small such as medium-sized blueberries, others such as the fruits of *Rosa rugosa* can be as big as a large-sized strawberry, weighing up to 30 grams [author's own experience]. Often, the fruits are orange red in color. However, there are also yellow-green varieties, such as the fruits from *Rosa roxburghii*, or dark purple to almost black fruits from *Rosa pimpinellifolia*. Shape-wise, they vary from oval to flat or round to regular round fruits (**Figure 1**).

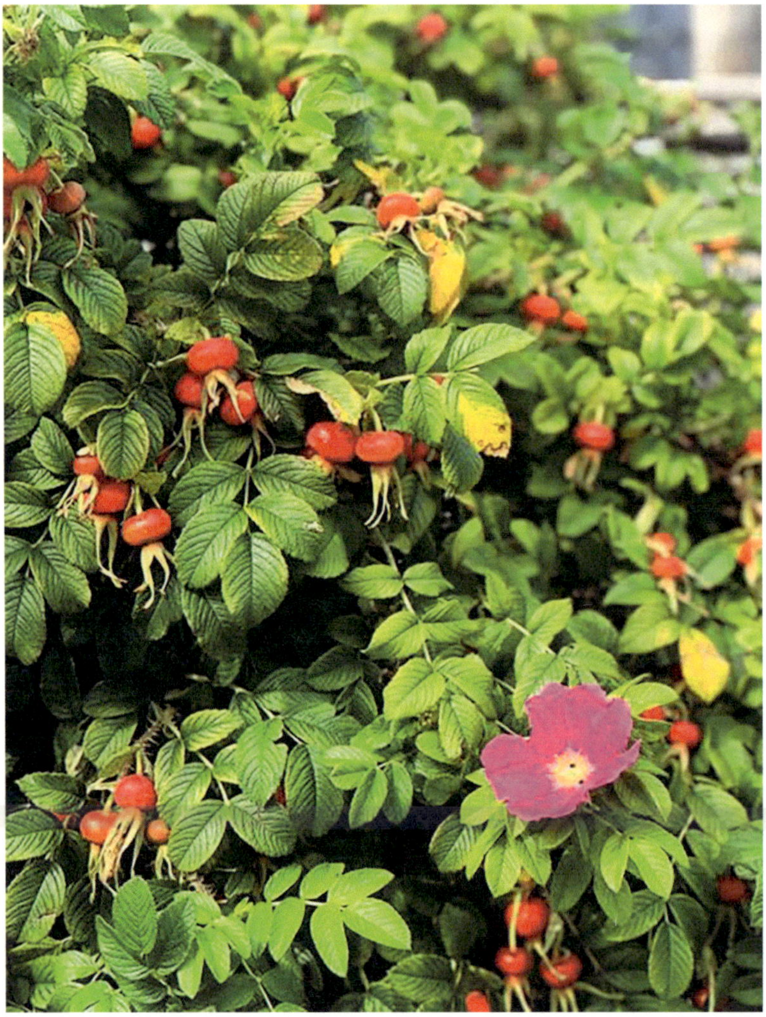

Figure 1.
Rosa rugosa berries. One flower is seen in the right lower corner.

2. Rose hip in food and folk medicine

Throughout history, the fruits of the wild roses have been gathered and consumed as food by many different cultures worldwide, especially in the colder regions [2, 3, 6–12]. For example, in North America, rose hips were an important food source during starvation in the winter, where many fruits and berries were no longer available. Specifically, the indigenous people of Canada consumed the raw fruits, as well as boiled them to make tea. Further up north in Alaska, the Inuits mixed rose hip fruits with water, seal oil, and a sweetener to make a pudding [7]. In Europe, many countries with a long history of using rose hips include Portugal, where rose hips were consumed raw as snacks [9]; Turkey, as tea [10]; Hungary, where people made rose hip wine or dried and ground the fruits and used them as substitute for wheat flour during famine [11]; Russia, where fresh rose hips were added directly to pies, dessert fillings, compote, and brandy, or used roasted fruits of *Rosa canina* as substitutes for coffee [3]. Indeed, according to findings from old Swiss pile buildings, the rose hip fruits were gathered along with other wild foods and used in the younger stone age by people in Switzerland (3710–3677 BC) [8]. In China, some types of rose hips were important ingredients of fermented beverages [12].

Though modern agricultural and health practices have reduced the need for harvesting wild food in large parts of the world, rose hips still play a role in many food cultures. In several European countries, rose hips collected from natural sources are commonly consumed in the form of tea, jam, drinks, wine, and jelly [13]. In Sweden, "Nypon Soppa," a traditional Swedish rose hip soup, has been popular for centuries, and in Poland, people use rose hips as filling in their traditional cake "paczki," a doughnut cake with fruit jam filling. In Turkey, the fruits can be found in juice [14] and food products such as rose hip marmalade and syrup [2]. In Portugal, they are used as children's snacks [9]. Rose hips are also some of the most gathered fruits in Russia, where they are consumed as tea and as ingredients in bread [3].

Besides their culinary use in food products, rose hips can be found as an ingredient in different health supplements [15]. Rose hips from different *Rosa* species have been widely used in traditional folk medicine. The native Americans in North America used rose hips from *Rosa pratincola* for eye- and stomach problems [16], and in China, fruits from *Rosa roxburghii* have been eaten for their detoxifying and heat-clearing effects [12]. In Europe, the fruits from *R. canina* and other species have been commonly consumed to strengthen the immune system and thereby prevent or treat the common cold, flu, and minor infectious disease [10, 17]. In Turkey, a rose hip decoction was used as remedy against diabetes [18] and bronchitis [19], while dried rose hips are used in the treatment of diseases in the liver, bladder, and kidneys in Poland [6]. In Romania and Italy, people have used the fruits from *R. canina* against diarrhea [20], and in Spain, the fruits have been consumed as an astringent and antianemic [21]. In the Middle East, rose hips have been utilized as diuretic [10, 17] and as a remedy against high blood pressure and kidney stones [17]. Apart from the abovementioned applications, rose hips have also been consumed to treat constipation [10]; chronic pain and ulcers [6]; fever and bloody cough [17]; menstrual pain and discomfort [10, 17]; dyspnea [22]; as well as for several anti-inflammatory diseases [23], including rheumatism [22].

Currently, standardized and cultivated rose hips form the basis of an herbal remedy, which consists mainly of powdered dried fruits from *Rosa canina* that is widely sold and consumed to reduce pain associated with arthritis [6]. Rose hips are also used in cosmetics [15] and skin care products. Although this chapter focuses on the fruits of the *Rosa* species, it is worth mentioning here that other parts of the plants such as the roots, petals, and flowers have also been used in traditional medicine [17].

3. The biology of the *Rosa* species

The best characterized species of the *Rosa* genus are *Rosa canina* L. and *Rosa rugosa* Thunb. Whereas the fruits from *R. canina* have been mostly used in traditional medicine, the *R. rugosa* variety is better known for its larger and well-tasting rose hips. Both species are currently used in the production of food products [15, 24], and in some countries, including Denmark, they are grown on an industrial scale [25].

3.1 *Rosa rugosa* Thunb

Rosa rugosa is a small shrub forming dense thickets. It has large white or pink flowers (8–10 cm across) and yields slightly flat round orange fruits, which are some of the largest among rose hips [25]. *R. Rugosa* is also known as Rugosa rose or Japanese rose [6], Beach rose, or Wrinkled rose, deriving the latter name from its distinctive wrinkled leaves. The species originated in Asia, where roots have been used in traditional medicine for many years [24]. It was first introduced to Europe in 1796 as an ornamental plant [26]. However, after 1845, it became a garden escape in many areas, such that it can now be found growing wild in 16 countries including Denmark, Norway, Sweden, Belgium, Austria, the European part of Russia, Germany, and Poland [26]. *R. rugosa* hips can be harvested from late July to early December.

R. rugosa is a strong and hardy plant, capable of living under harsh conditions, including along coastal areas. It easily out-matches other species and its dense shrubs can rapidly spread over larger areas, with the exclusion of many local species. For this reason, *R. rugosa* is considered an invasive species in many European countries. In Denmark, the plant is currently being removed in some areas by the local environmental agencies. However, as indicated by Skrypnik et al, it might be worth considering the rich nutritional content and potential health benefits of this species when discussing whether it should be removed from the environment or not [27].

3.2 *Rosa canina* L.

Rosa canina, also known as the dog rose or dog brier, is a large shrub capable of growing up to 2.7 meter (9 feet) in height [28]. *R. canina* has been used as a medicinal plant since ancient times, where it was first described by Pliny the Elder (23–79 BC), who observed it being used as an antidote against dog bites among French tribes. Hence its name, *Rosa canina* [23]. R. canina is native to Asia and to Europe where it is the most common of the *Rosa* species [28, 29]. It also grows in the wild in North

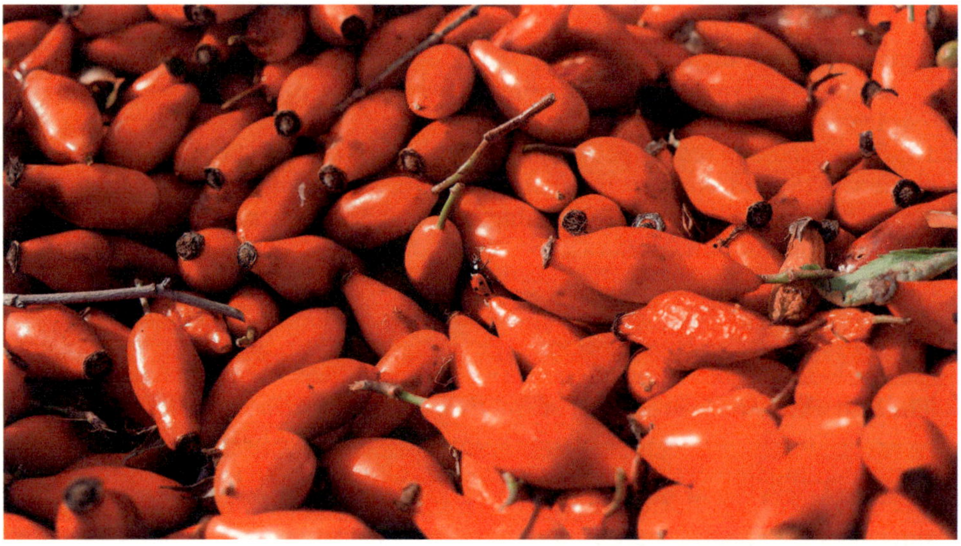

Figure 2.
Ripe berries from Rosa canina L just after harvesting.

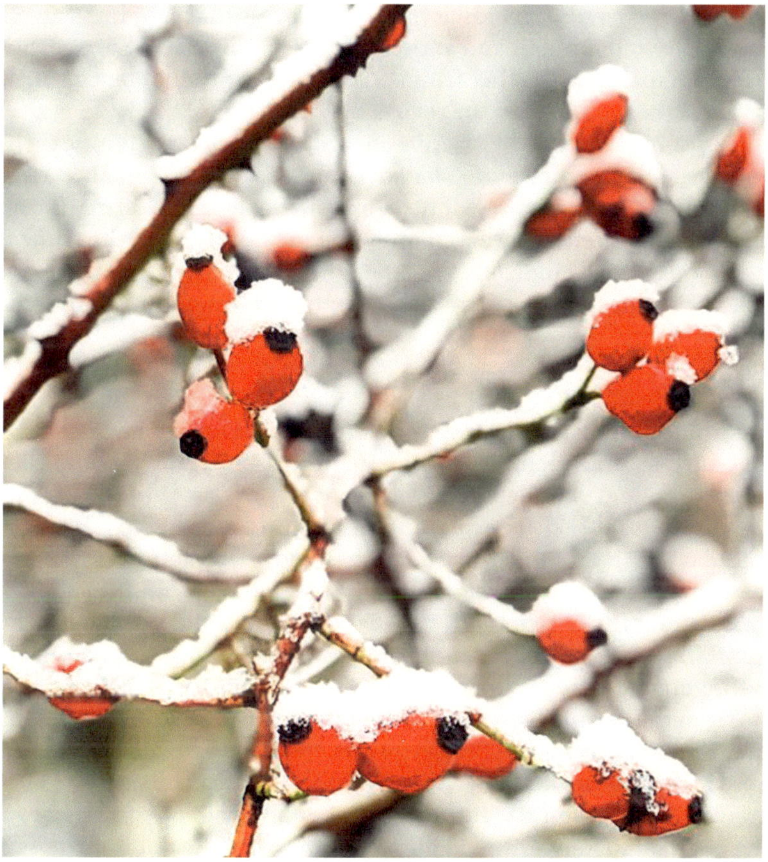

Figure 3.
Rosa canina L in snow. Most berries and fruits from other bushes and trees have fallen during this period and are rotting long before Christmas. In February you can still find intact rose hips. Something must preserve them.

America [29], Africa, Australia, and New Zealand, where it has been naturalized [28]. In addition to growing inland, the species can be found in mountain regions [22]. In contrast to *R. rugosa*, the fruits from *R. canina* are significantly smaller, deeper red in color, and oval-shaped. For more information about the biology of *R. canina*, see the review by Winther et al. (**Figure 2**) [23].

The flowers of *R. canina* start blooming from early summer until the end of the season. As such, rose hips from *R. canina* can be harvested from fall until early March, which is quite exceptional considering that most other fruits and berries are not available during the winter. Refer **Figure 3** for *R. canina* rose hips still on rose bushes in the winter. This could explain why the fruits are so appreciated in the colder northern regions of the earth.

4. Nutritional content of rose hips

Rose hips are known to contain high amounts of nutrients and bioactive substances that positively impact health. The fruits are particularly rich in vitamins, especially vitamin C, A, and E, as well as carotenoids (including beta-carotene and lycopene), essential fatty acids [30], polyphenols (including flavonoids, proanthocyanidins, catechins), triterpene acid, galactolipid [27], and antioxidants. They also have a noticeable content of dietary fiber compared with other fruits [31]. Regarding the content of bioactive compounds in rose hip seeds, refer the review by Winther et al. [23].

The content of nutrients and bioactive compounds can vary significantly depending on the species [2], ripening state, and environmental factors such as location and growth conditions [27]. Therefore, all rose hips are not equal in terms of their nutritional and bioactive contents. In this chapter, the focus will be on the fruits from *R. canina* and *R. rugosa*, with emphasis on some of the substances that these two species are particularly rich in, such as, vitamin C, specific carotenoids, and antioxidants.

4.1 Vitamin C

Rose hips are some of the richest sources of vitamin C among fruits and vegetables. The water-soluble vitamin is a vital micronutrient, and longer periods of deficiency results in scurvy, a deadly disease that earlier cost the lives of millions of people around the world [32]. The amount of vitamin C needed to prevent scurvy is small (10 mg/day) [33], and the disease is rare in today's societies. However, during times of food crisis or war, when most of the cultivated fruits and vegetables are scarce, access to vitamin-C-rich food, such as rose hips, could play an important role in the prevention of scurvy. For example, during World War II, this was the case in the United Kingdom, where blockages on the sea traffic made it difficult to import citrus fruits from the warmer colonies, rose hips became the country's main sources of vitamin C. For this reason, the British government encouraged people to gather and consume rose hips growing in the wild, to avoid an outbreak of scurvy [34].

In the human body, vitamin C influences many different physiological functions, acting as an important antioxidant and a cofactor in the biosynthesis of neurotransmitters, carnitine, and collagen [35]. The vitamin is also essential to the immune system, where it is found in high concentrations in the leukocytes, the body's immune cells. When these cells are activated by ongoing infections, the local quantity of vitamin C raises many folds. In neutrophils, vitamin C is thought to act as an antioxidant, protecting the immune cells from self-destruction by the reactive oxygen species (ROS) they produce in their fight against foreign pathogens, such as viruses or bacteria [33]. Furthermore, a clinical trial showed that supplementation with dietary vitamin C, given in the form of kiwi fruits, could enhance the function of the neutrophils, by stimulating their movement toward the site of infection [36]. In line with this finding, another study indicated that when patients with impaired immune systems, who were experiencing recurring infections, were given adequate amounts of vitamin C in their diet, their infections ceased [37]. Vitamin C also impacts other aspects of our health such as our cognitive functions [38], mood and energy, and common symptoms of low vitamin C intake includes irritability, fatigue, and decreased antioxidant capacity [35].

The daily recommendation for vitamin C varies greatly from country to country, with 40 mg/day in India and the United Kingdom, to 110 mg/day in Germany and France [39]. However, some authors argue that the body needs 200 mg/day to sustain good health [33, 40]. The vitamin C content in rose hips differs among *Rosa* species (**Table 1**) [48]. Furthermore, the vitamin content varies also with other factors such as growth location [27, 41] and the ripening state of the fruits [27, 30]. Generally, fruits from *R. rugosa* generally contain high amounts of vitamin C, from 600–1090 mg/100 g dried fruits [25, 31, 42, 43]. In *R. canina* the vitamin content varies significantly, from

Food	Vitamin C in mg/100 g
Kakadu-plum, raw	2300–3150
Rose hip, Canina, raw	274–2700
Acerola, raw	1677
Rose hip, Rugosa, raw	600–1090
Blackberries, raw	181
Red pepper, raw	179
Kale, raw	169
Sea buckthorn, raw	131
Lemon peel	129
Broccoli, raw/boiled	111/40
Strawberry, raw	67
Kiwi, raw	63
Orange, raw	54
Lemon, raw	49
Potato, raw/boiled	26/8

Sources: [31, 41–47].

Table 1.
Vitamin C content in selected berries, fruits and vegetables.

274 to 2700 mg/100 g [41, 44, 45]. By contrast, in the few studies, where the content of vitamin C was compared in both strains, *R. canina* was found to contain significantly lower levels of the vitamin, as compared with the levels in *R. rugosa* [6, 27, 30].

4.2 Carotenoids

Rose hips from *R. rugosa* and *R. canina* are rich in carotenoids, including beta-carotene and lycopene—plant color pigments that give fruits and vegetables their characteristic orange and red color [15]. Both carotenoids have well-known antioxidant effects [35], with lycopene being the most potent antioxidant among carotenoids [49]. Moreover, beta-carotene is a precursor for the biosynthesis of vitamin A, a fat-soluble antioxidant that is vital for our sight and skin. The vitamin is also essential for the immune system, such that one of the signs of vitamin A deficiency is an impaired resistance to infections [35]. While beta-carotene is the most abundant carotenoid in fruits and vegetables, lycopene-rich foods are fewer in number [50, 51]. Lycopene has recently gained a lot of attention in the field of health science, and a growing number of studies have linked the intake of this carotenoid with a decreased risk of cardiovascular disease [49, 52]. A meta-analysis from 2017 supports this indication of carotenoids by concluding that an increased intake of lycopene-rich food, including tomato products, could have a positive effect on blood pressure and endothelial function [53].

The content of beta-carotene and lycopene varies significantly in rose hips from both *R. canina* and *R. rugosa*. The fruits from *R. rugosa* have been shown to contain circa 11,4 mg/100 g of total beta-carotene [31], which is one of the highest contents among fruits and vegetables, ranking higher than carrots (9,7 mg/100 g). The beta-carotene content in *R. canina* fruits varied in one study from 1,2 to 2,9 mg/100 g (measured as (all-E)-beta-carotene) [54], which is significantly lower. However, in a comparative study with both species, the amount of beta-carotene (measured as (all E)-beta-carotene) was higher in *R. canina* fruits; 4.2 mg/100 g, compared with *R. rugosa* fruits; 3.2 mg/100 g [15].

It should also be noted that in the comparative study with both *R. rugosa* and *R. canina*, their content of (all-E)-lycopene ranged from 7.4 to 7.9 mg/100 g [15], which is higher than other well-known lycopene rich foods such as tomatoes (0.7–4.2 mg/100 g), pink guava (5.2–5.5 mg/100 g), and like that in watermelon (2.3–7.2 mg/100 g) [51]. In another study, fruits from *R. canina* had a significantly higher content of (all-E)-lycopene and total lycopene, ranging from 9 to 22.9 mg/100 g and 12.9–35 mg/100 g [54]. The amount of lycopene is known to vary significantly in fruits and vegetables. Factors that affect the content include ripeness of the fruits, quality of the soil, and weather temperature [51].

4.3 Antioxidants

Rose hips are an exceptional source of antioxidants. In a study where over 3100 foods from around the world were tested, rose hip from *R. canina* was one of the foods with the highest antioxidant content among berries, fruits, and vegetables (**Figure 4**) [55]. In another study where rose hips from different species were compared, the fruits from *R. rugosa* had a slightly lower antioxidant content than fruits from *R. canina* [29].

Dietary antioxidants protect the cells and tissue against free radicals and radical oxygen species (ROS). ROS are a group of highly reactive chemicals containing oxygen that are produced either exogenously or endogenously, during normal biological functions such as immune response, cell differentiation, growth, and proliferation. Overactivity of ROS has been associated with a wide variety of human disorders, such as chronic inflammation, age-related diseases, and cancers.

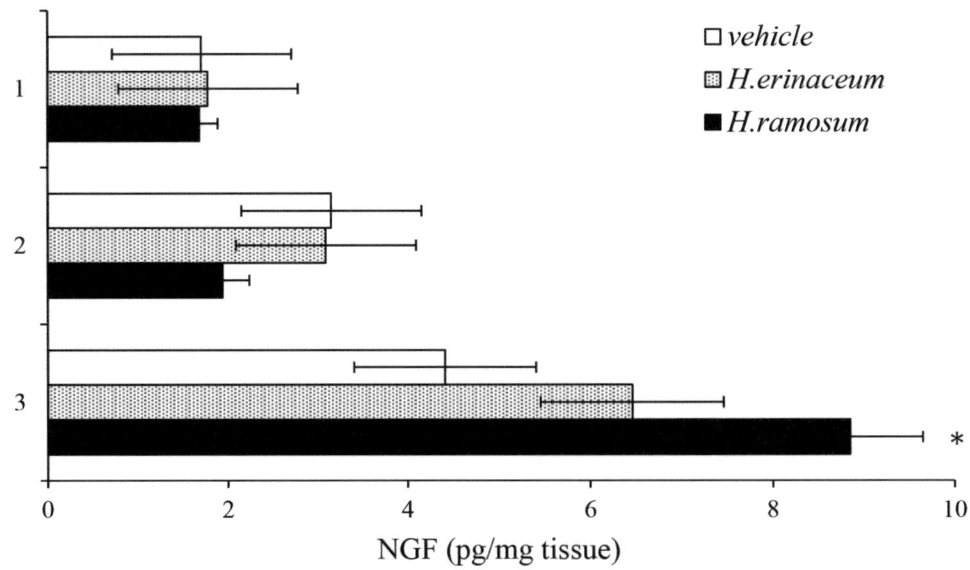

Figure 4.
Antioxidant content of different foods and drinks (mmol/100 g). The content of antioxidants is measured by the FRAP-method. Sources: [55, 56].

An example of this is seen in the bloodstream where vitamin C, along with other antioxidants, protects LDL-cholesterol, thus preventing the fatty acid molecule from getting stuck the arteries, in an event that can ultimately lead to arteriosclerosis [57]. ROS are constantly produced in the body, creating a demand for a steady supply of antioxidants from the diet to keep the reactive species in check. An imbalance of ROS and antioxidants, which results in an excess of the ROS, can lead to oxidative stress, a condition akin to overactivity of ROS [35] and therefore, any of the human disorders [49]. Some of the main antioxidants found in rose hips from the two species include vitamin C, E, and A, beta-carotene, lycopene, and flavonoids. **Figure 4** shows the antioxidant content in *R. canina* fruits and other selected foods measured by the FRAP-method (Ferric Reducing Ability of Plasma), one of several ways of measuring the antioxidant content in foods.

5. Rose hip as a medicinal plant

As mentioned previously, rose hips are used worldwide as folk medicine and sometimes also as food. In this section, the focus is on the medicinal properties of the fruits. Prescription medicine that is purchased from a drug store often has documented dose dependency, indicating that the more you take of the remedy, the more impact there will be on the body. An interesting question is—can such dose dependency be shown for an herbal remedy like rose hip? It should also be stated that whatever is indicated for rose hip as regards the effect on different diseases, is only relevant for the subspecies being considered or tested, as such effects may not be relevant for other rose hip subspecies. Furthermore, the active ingredients in the shells of the rose hips are very different from that within the seeds (**Figure 5**) [23]. A product consisting of shells alone can therefore have very different content regarding the amount of different active ingredients when compared with a product consisting of seeds alone or the combination seeds and shells—not to speak about preparations made from the leaves or roots of rose hip [23]. The content of active ingredients, besides what is related to differences within species and subspecies [15, 58], is also dependent of where the plant is grown—on the soil, number of hours with sun and altitude [41] as earlier stated.

The best method for demonstrating the medicinal properties of drugs is the randomized, double-blinded, placebo-controlled study. Unfortunately, established pharmaceutical companies are rarely interested in herbal remedies. Therefore, much of the research on the different species of rose hip has been performed only in animal models or in *in vitro* systems. Due to the huge variations in rose hip species and subspecies, as regards their content of active ingredients, the version of rose hip species/subspecies tested and sometimes also the manufacturing process will be stated. So far, the temperature at which the rose hips are dried during the manufacturing process of the herbs has been found to be very important [23]. This insight was first made by a Danish farmer, Erik Hansen, who recognized that he often lost his farm animals (e.g., cattle or horses), when their body temperature went above 42°C for a few hours. Upon coupling this observation with the knowledge that some of his friends also died when their body temperature went beyond 42°C even for short periods, Erik Hansen postulated that likewise, maintaining the rose hips to temperatures above 40°C for hours during the drying process would also be detrimental for the bioactive components in the fruits that have beneficial health effects. Hence, he invented and standardized a new method for storing rose hip for the winter season. In this process, the rose hips are never heated to more than 40°C. Moreover, the seeds and shells are separated and dried separately before milling, resulting in a rose hip powder, which

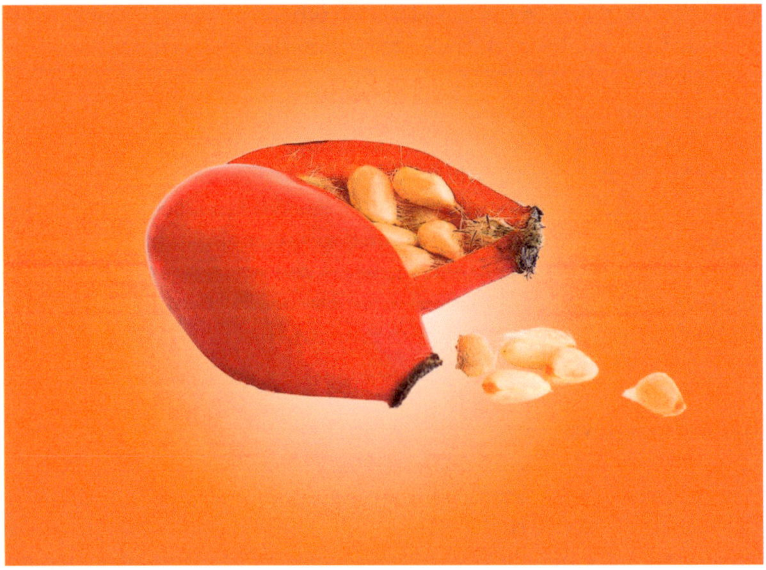

Figure 5.
One rose hip fruit with seeds exposed.

still contains all that was in the fruit on the day of harvest, except for the well-known itching hairs, which are removed. Eating the powder containing seeds and shells is therefore like eating a rose hip fruit picked from a bush. Refer **Figure 6** for the dried seeds and shells before and after the milling process. This methodology is in sharp contrast to rose hip products from Chile (a major exporter of rose hip worldwide), where the seeds are often removed from the fruits, before drying them at high temperatures resulting in powders, which are more brownish in color [23]. Only very few rose hip preparations have been tested in well-designed clinical trials. But there are many different preparations available in the health stores. However, the content of active ingredients is very dependent on how the powder (if powder) was produced and if an extraction, then how was the extraction methodology, for that particular product. In addition, one should consider whether the preparations include shells or seeds only or a combination of seeds and shells.

5.1 Can administration of rose hips improve the immune system?

As previously indicated, there are numerous claims in folk medicine worldwide, that rose hip improves the functions of the human immune system. Not surprisingly therefore, the anti-inflammatory effects of *Rosa canina,* subspecies Lito, (referred to in some studies as Hyben Vital), which contains both seeds and shells dried at low temperatures, have been shown to have anti-inflammatory properties when tested in humans. It was also documented that the preparation contained a compound capable of inhibiting the chemotaxis of neutrophil leucocytes *in vitro* and in lowering the levels of the anti-inflammatory marker, C-reactive protein (CRP), in human volunteers treated with rose hip at high doses for a month [59]. Likewise, in a study on volunteers with osteoarthritis and treated with the same rose hip powder at low dose (5 gram daily) for 3 months, CRP was significantly reduced when comparing the

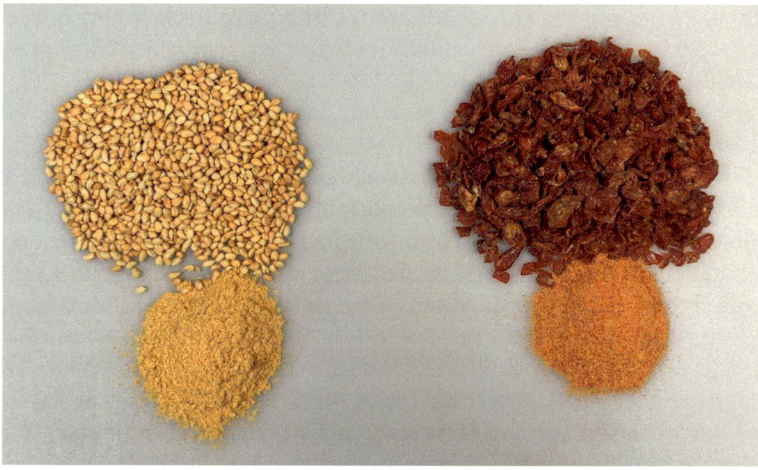

Figure 6.
Seeds and shells from rose hip dried at low temperature and then milled.

rose hip–treated group with placebo [60]. A significant reduction in the inflammatory marker—erythrocyte sedimentation rate (ESR) was also observed in the test group of a placebo-controlled study, where 5 gram of the same *R. canina* species was administered to rheumatoid patients for 6 months [61]. It is interesting to note that in these two studies, administration of a preparation composed of only the shells of rose hip did not cause significant changes in CRP levels [62, 63].

Another interesting query was: will rose hip treatment influence the likelihood of catching a flu or the common cold during the winter season? This was investigated in a clinical study, where rose hip shells (2 grams dispensed in liquid form) of the Lito subspecies or placebo were administered daily to 120 middleclass volunteers from the autumn season, for a total of 6 months. After 2 months of treatment, there was a statistically significant reduction in the number of volunteers catching a cold in the actively treated group when compared with placebo. In addition, the different symptoms related to colds were significantly reduced as the result of rose hip treatment. There was no statistically significant change in the likelihood of getting the flu. The levels of the inflammatory marker, CRP, were also not affected in this study [63].

It would be interesting if more studies were available on the effects of rose hip treatment on the immune system, especially as regards the studies involving rose hip preparations consisting of both seeds and shells. Preliminary results currently available suggest that the anti-inflammatory properties of rose hip formulations containing both seeds and shells may be stronger than preparations with shells alone. It is interesting to note that the number of colds was also influenced by elderberry, which has much in common with rose hip regarding bioactive ingredients [64].

5.2 Can rose hip treatment impact cardiovascular disease, hyperlipidemia, or glucose metabolism?

Hyperlipidemia and disturbances of glucose metabolism can predispose to cardiovascular disease, which is still a main killer worldwide [65]. A rose hip preparation based solely on powdered rose hip shells from Chile, administered for 6 weeks, at a daily dose of 40 gram in apple juice, citric acid, and sugar was tested in a randomized, placebo-controlled study.

In the actively treated group, there was a statistically significant 3.4% reduction in systolic blood pressure, while total cholesterol and LDL cholesterol fell by 4.9 and 6.0%, respectively [66]. There was no change in glucose tolerance or markers of inflammation between the treatment and placebo groups. Testing a pure shell liquid product from subspecies *Rosa canina* Lito [60] in a far lower dose (2 gram daily) for 6 months revealed a 4% drop in total cholesterol, when comparing groups. Blood pressure tended to decline because of active treatment. In accordance with these findings, a statistically significant reduction in total cholesterol of 8% and a statistically significant improvement in HDL cholesterol of 2% were observed in two other randomized placebo-controlled clinical trials, while testing a combined shell-seed rose hip powder, of the subspecies Lito, for 3 and 6 months, respectively [60, 67]. The dosage tested was 5 gram of dry rose hip powder daily. Rose hip powder (species and shell/seed content not defined) was shown to exert antiatherosclerotic effects by reducing atherosclerotic plaque formation in mice [68]. At present, there are no studies available focusing on plaque formation in humans. We were not able to find any indication of an impact on glucose metabolism from any subspecies of rose hip—not even when rose hip was tested in the high dose of 40 g of shells [66] or 40 grams of seeds daily (personal communication, Kaj Winther). For that reason, we assume that rose hip does not affect blood glucose levels.

In conclusion: It seems that rose hip can modify lipid metabolism. This can possibly be related to the shells as shell-only powders [62, 66] as well as combined shell/seed powders [60, 67] were able to improve the lipid profile. Such declines were not observed when testing a seed only product in high concentration (personal communication, Kaj Winther). Seeds from rose hip contain high amounts of polyunsaturated fatty acids, among them omega-3 and omega-6. Omega 3 and omega 6 acids [69] possibly supported by certain antioxidants may explain why rose hip powders containing also seeds [59–61] show more anti-inflammatory property than shells-only products [62, 63, 66]. It has not been possible to find any indications of an impact from any version of rose hip on glucose metabolism in humans although a few animal studies look promising.

5.3 Effect of rose hip on obesity

During the last decades, obesity rates have exploded among the young and the elderly, so that we have a worldwide epidemic. The mass movements of people from the rural areas into cities have caused great changes in lifestyles and diets. So many people now sit in front of their computers, as compared with carrying out physical work. These changes in lifestyle and the accompanying diseases confer great costs to the society. To control the obesity epidemic, there is a now a great focus on diets and food supplements. Seeds from rose hip contain high amounts of tiliroside, not present in the shells [23]. In a study performed on mice, Niomiya et al [70] found that extract of the seeds of *Rosa canina* that was rich in tiliroside, as well as pure tiliroside isolated from *Rosa canina*, significantly reduced body weight and visceral fat gain after a treatment period of 14 days or less. In the same period, a reduction in plasma triglyceride and fatty acids was also observed. Not surprisingly, these desirable alterations were ascribed to tiliroside. Later the same group of researchers designed a randomized, placebo-controlled and double-blinded study on humans in which they showed that rose hip seed extract containing tiliroside given daily for 3 months resulted in a significant reduction in abdominal visceral fat, body weight, and body mass index [71]. It was therefore concluded by the authors that rose hip seeds can be useful for the treatment of obesity in humans.

5.4 Effect of rose hip on osteoporosis

Loss of bone strength or osteoporosis has improved during the last century, possibly due to a combination of changes in our diet and our general reduction in physical activity. Osteoporosis is a serious threat to the public health system as loss of bone strength can lead to bone fractures and disabilities and in the elderly loss of height, due to loss of strength of thoracic and lumbar vertebrae. Such loss of height can limit important body functions and thereby quality of life. Bone formation is regulated by osteoblasts, which improves bone formation and osteoclasts, which facilitates destruction of calcified tissue (break down of bone structure). ROS (reactive oxygen species) are produced by osteoclasts, and ROS improves the destruction of collagen strands, which are important in bone remodeling [72, 73]. An increase in oxidants can also activate proteolytic enzymes such as elastases and metal proteinases resulting in a further damage of bone extracellular matrix [71]. Therefore, supplementation with antioxidants can support the restauration of bone mineral density (BMD). In a rat model, blueberries, rich in antioxidants, were shown to reduce the loss of BMD especially in the tibial and femoral area [71]. Extracts of different versions of rose hip have a phytochemical profile close to that of blueberry and have been suggested to play a role in preventing bone loss [74]. Indeed, rose hip was rated in the top three regarding antioxidant concentration when testing berries worldwide. And rose hip was rated at least three times more potent than blueberry (**Figure 4**) [74, 75]. In addition, rose hip also contains abundant amounts of vitamin C [23] (only one berry, Cockatoo Plum well known in Australia, is superior to rose hip regarding vitamin C content), as detailed in **Table 1**. Vitamin C (ascorbic acid) is an important player in regulating osteoblast differentiation and is important for secreting procollagen and stable collagen, which is needed for the growth of connective tissue and bone tissue [76].

Another argument for a positive role for rose hip treatment in osteoporosis is that the fruits contain a high number of polyphenols [77, 78], which are known to reduce bone loss resulting from oxidative stress [79]. A clinical study on humans showed that a subspecies of *Rosa canina* (Lito) was able to improve wrinkles of the skin [80], and it was further documented in human cartilage cells from the knee that the same rose hip subspecies supported the formation of collagen [81].

In summary: Rose hip is a very strong antioxidant, and there are indications that antioxidants can improve BMD in animal models. Rose hip can also improve bone quality from the impact of its rich sources of vitamin C, which improves the formation of collagen. Terpenes, abundant in rose hip, have also been proven to reduce bone loss, and rose hip (Lito) was also shown, in human knee cells, to inhibit the formation of MMP-1 (a metalloproteinase) known to impact bone loss. So even we still need a well-designed and large-scale clinical trial to document the impact of rose hip on bone density in humans—there are many indications that rose hip can support bone quality.

5.5 Effect of rose hip on arthrosis and rheumatoid arthritis

One of the larger limitations of quality of life in the elderly is osteoarthritis, which is present in more than 60% of people above 50 years of age. Osteoarthritis is often recognized in the hip, knee, spine, or hand and can reduce quality of life from simply the pain, which occurs from joints where the cartilage is disrupted and also from the inflammation, which can follow the destruction of cartilage.

Limitations in joint movements and pain can reduce the amount of physical activity and in the long run lead to a decline in muscular mass. It becomes more difficult to climb a staircase, ride a bicycle, or to enter a car. This can result in a reduction in social activities and finally a more limited lifestyle [79]. Treatment of osteoarthritis is initially often simply to try and cure symptoms such as pain. First choice of pain cure can be painkillers such as paracetamol and/or nonsteroidal anti-inflammatory agents (NSAIDs). Later on, synthetic opioids (Tramadol) may follow [82]. However, such medication does not repair the reason for pain (cartilage which is destructed). Painkillers only treat symptoms—and on the side—they have side effects such as gastrointestinal bleeding, heart problems, and liver damage [83–87]. Literally, what health professionals are often doing is that they place a bucket on the loft, to catch the water dripping from the destroyed roof instead of repairing the hole in the roof by placing a new roof tile. So, any herbal remedy, which reduces pain and even better also supports the restauration of cartilage, is of high interest in osteoarthritis.

Rheumatoid arthritis is a chronic, inflammatory, and autoimmune disease affecting the joints and also shortening life. Most common symptoms are pain, swollen joints, stiffness of joints, and loss of function. The initial treatment is usually disease-modifying antirheumatic drugs (DMARDs) often supported with pain killers such as paracetamol or nonsteroidal anti-inflammatory drugs (NSAIDs), which as earlier described have side effects. So, any herbal remedy, which can reduce pain and even better support repairment of the body, is of value also in rheumatoid arthritis.

Osteoarthritis is the disease in which rose hip (*Rosa canina*) has been tested the most, as we were able to find a total of six randomized, placebo-controlled, double-blinded clinical studies performed in humans. Five of these studies tested a powdered version of *Rosa canina* subspecies Lito, containing seeds as well as shells dried at very low temperature [23]. The background for this methodology was, as earlier discussed, that heating to more than about normal body temperature might destroy active ingredients in seeds and shells. These five studies focused on osteoarthritis of the hip, knee, and hand. The sixth study was focusing on osteoarthritis of the knee and was based on a product consisting of powdered shells only originating from Chile without any seeds added. The temperature during the preparation procedure was not given, but presumably it was high as most products from Chile are heavily heated [23]. Finally, there was a meta-analysis based on the shell and seed version of rose hip. There were two studies on rheumatoid arthritis, both placebo-controlled and based on the seed and shell version of rose hip.

If not stated, the treatment period was invariably 3 month and the dosage 5 gram daily of powdered rose hip containing seeds and shells served in capsules.

When focusing on osteoarthritis using the combined seed and shell powder, there was a significant reduction in reported pain and stiffness in all five studies [60, 67, 88–90]. In addition, there was also an improvement in general well-being and daily activity such as climbing a staircase, visiting the toilet, or entering a car. The improvement in daily activity was possibly the result of less pain and less stiffness in joints [60, 67, 88–90]. It is interesting to note that in four of the five studies, one study [60] was presented as a dose finding study, indicating dose dependency, there was a significant reduction in the consumption of rescue medication such as paracetamol, tramadol, or NSAIDs [67, 88–90]. This is of some interest as the volunteers in all studies were told not to change the consumption of rescue medication—even though they did so.

See details in **Figure 7**.

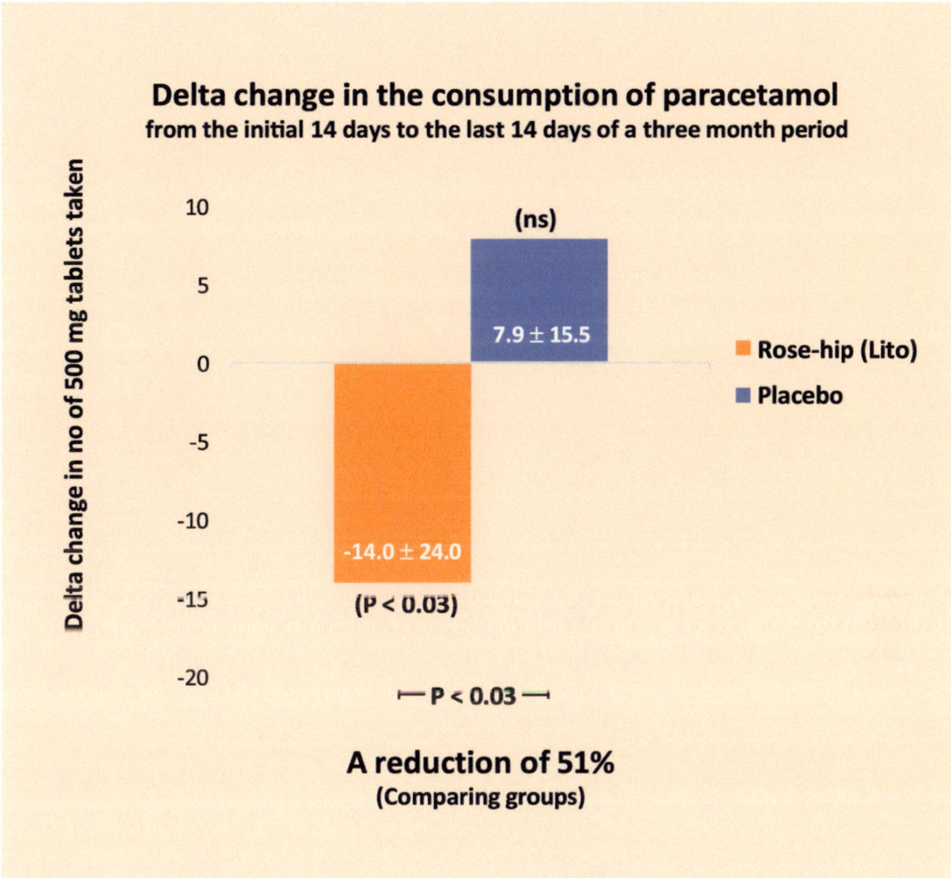

Figure 7.
Delta change in the consumption of 500 mg paracetamol tablets. The delta change is the delta value of the first fourteen days minus that of the last 14 days of a three-month treatment period.

When testing the shells only powder (2.225 gram daily), there were no impacts on what patients reported on symptoms such as pain, stiffness, daily activity, or quality of life and neither on the consumption of rescue medication. However, some improvements in knee function could be detected when using gait analyzing in a motor function laboratory [63].

A meta-analysis indicated that the Lito rose hip subspecies significantly reduced pain in osteoarthritis and that the effect size was better than what was observed for paracetamol [91] and comparable to what was seen for NSAIDs [92, 93]. Details are shown in **Figure 8**.

One of the two studies on rheumatoid arthritis only lasted for 1 month, and results were not conclusive [94]. The other study lasted for 6 month, and after 3 month there was a statistically significant improvement in daily activity scores, which was maintained also after 6 months of treatment. After 6 months, there was a further statistically significant improvement in patients as well as doctor's evaluation of disease severity and in quality of life using SF questionnaires [61].

In summary: There are strong indications that the combination of seeds and shells from subspecies of *Rosa canina* exerts a reduction in pain and an improvement in daily

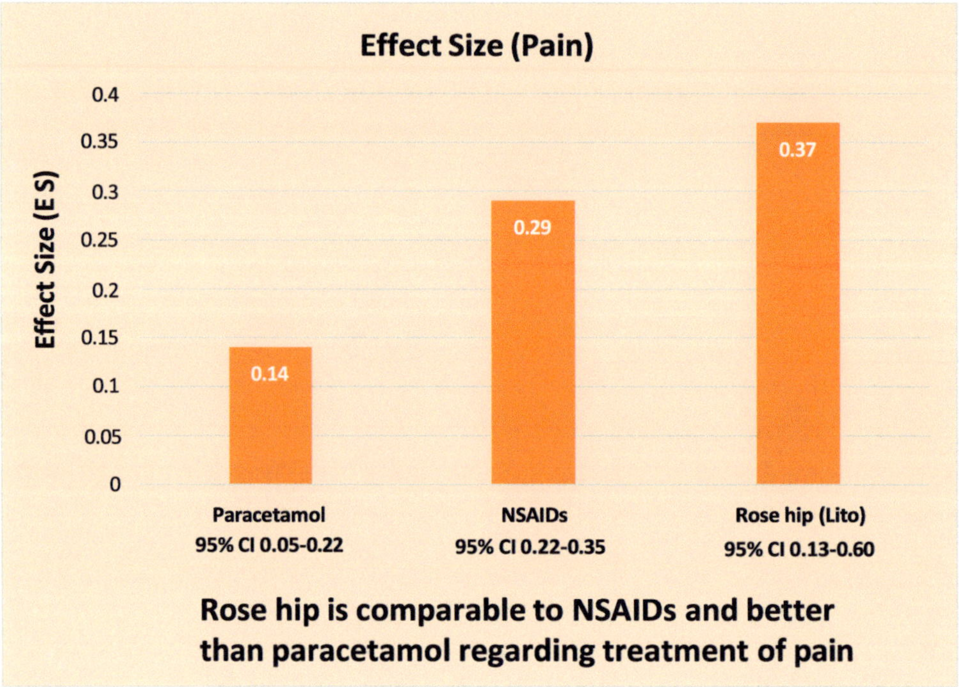

Figure 8.
Effect size of Rosa canina (Lito) right panel, to that of NSAIDs (mid panel) and that of paracetamol (left panel). It should be recognized that the Effect Size of rose hip is close to three times higher than that of paracetamol.

function in osteoarthritis and that the same remedy can be of some benefit to sufferers of rheumatoid arthritis [61, 91]. Other subspecies including subspecies from *Rosa rugosa* can have similar effects; this however remains to be established. From the present evidence it seems clear that both shells and seeds are needed as a study on shells-only did not show any impact on the pain and discomfort reported by patients [63].

However, the biochemical background for the beneficial effects of *Rosa canina* still remains to be fully elucidated. It was encouraging to note that C-reactive protein (CRP) fell in two studies on osteoarthritis [59, 60]. In a study on rheumatoid arthritis, there was a significant reduction in sedimentation rate, an inflammatory marker [61]. Again, no such changes in inflammatory markers were seen testing shells-only powders [62, 63]. From the insight we have today, it seems that a certain molecule, a galactolipid named GOPO, which acts as an anti-inflammatory agent, is important [95]. The high amount of natural vitamin C, present in *Rosa canina*, and easily absorbed [96] can play an important role for restoring collagen. Also, linoleic and alpha-linolenic acids, which contribute to the COX-1 and COX-2 inhibitory effects observed in rose hip together with triterpene acids, can add some clarification [97, 98]. And finally, the reduction in the synthesis of MMP-1 responsible for the breakdown of collagen can play an important role [81].

5.6 Rose hip for managing renal disturbances

The kidneys can be damaged in diseases such as diabetes and hypertension. In addition, the formation of stones in the kidneys gives rise to painful and dysfunctional condition. Acute kidney injury is defined as a disorder with disruption of kidney function leading to renal failure. Two major reasons for acute kidney injury are inflammation and oxidative stress. A correlation between a reduction in oxidative stress and a reduction in renal failure was observed in a study where rats with induced acute kidney injury were fed *Rosa canina* [99]. Similar results involving ameliorating renal failure were also observed in another group of rats treated with *Rosa laevigata* [100], as well as in rats suffering diabetes [101, 102].

Prevention strategies for avoiding calcium oxalate nephrolithiasis (kidney stones) are important and on demand. *Rosa canina* extracts have been tested and shown to reduce the number of calcium oxalate calculi and prevent nephrolithiasis in treated rats [103]. On the other hand, human studies for the effects of rose hip treatment on kidney dysfunction are lacking. However, it was encouraging to note that serum creatinine, a marker of kidney function, significantly improved in a human study with *Rosa canina* Lito [59].

5.7 Rose hip in liver protection

As we earlier stated from our search on folk medicines, rose hip has been claimed to act as a detoxifier. So, are there any indications that rose hip can support the liver? Hepatic injury (liver toxicity) is often characterized by lipid peroxidation, the production of free radicals, and a reduction in antioxidant enzyme activity. Among blood analyses, which can describe to what extend the liver is injured, there are serum alanine transaminase (ALT) and serum aspartate transaminase (AST). Due to our lifestyle, which for many include overeating, consumption of high amounts of alcohol and for some people also sometimes the consumption of different versions of medicine—foods and food supplies, which can protect the liver, has drawn increasing attention. In a study on rats where liver injury was induced, *Rosa canina* restored the abovementioned marker enzymes as well as histopathological alteration caused by the injury. The authors of the paper found a reduction in ALT and AST as the result of treatment and suggested that *Rosa canina* may exert its liver restoring capacity from its content of antioxidants and phenolic compounds [104]. In another study on diabetic rats testing the impact of *Rosa rugosa* on accumulation of fat in the liver, there was also a reduction in ALT and AST as the result of treatment together with a reduction in fat accumulation in the liver [105]. In a study on humans, consuming 45 gram daily of powdered *Rosa canina* from the subspecies Lito containing seeds and shells, given for 1 month, did not affect ALT [59]. However, treating 40 g daily of pure seed powder from the same subspecies for a full 3-month period resulted in a statistically significant drop in ALT (personal communication, K. Winther). This may indicate that also compounds related to rose hip seeds can be important when discussing the protection of the liver, and possibly 1 month of treatment is too short a timeframe when testing the impact of an herbal remedy on liver protection in humans.

In conclusion: From the literature available, it seems like different families of rose hip can be of interest when developing a treatment or a diet, which exerts some liver protection.

5.8 Rose hip for treating skin disorders and aging

Chronic inflammatory skin disorders (dermatitis) are common in humans of all ages, and we all get facial wrinkle as we get older than 50 years of age. Anti-inflammatory remedies can reduce the numbers and depth of wrinkles. The two main factors that determine aging of the skin are a) aging associated with time and b) aging resulting from exposure to UV, also known as "photo aging." The combination of these two factors results in loss of functionality of the skin as a barrier against "the outer world." Therefore, dryness, wrinkles, and spots (melanomas) occur. Consequently, protecting the aging skin with anti-inflammatory agents and antioxidants is very important [106].

An extraction of the root of *Rosa multiflora* was recently reported to improve dermatitis in an animal model via COX-2 inhibition. *Rosa multiflora* root extract that is rich in tannins was also shown to be antiallergic by lowering the number of eosinophil leucocytes in another animal model [107, 108]. Interestingly, quercetin isolated from *Rosa canina* was found to lower the melanin content in mouse melanoma cells, while oral administration of rose hip reduced skin pigmentation in guinea pigs [109, 110].

One human study demonstrates that a *Rosa canina* subspecies can influence skin wrinkles, the moisture of the skin, as well as skin elasticity [80]. The study was double-blinded and randomized, lasted 8 weeks, and included 34 volunteers. The effects of *Rosa canina* Lito were compared with a well-known antiwrinkle remedy, Astaxanthin. After 8 weeks of treatment, there was a significant reduction in the depth of crow feet wrinkles as the result of oral rose hip treatment. Similarly, skin moisture and skin elasticity were also significantly improved. The impact was comparable with that of Astaxanthin, which is a strong antioxidant containing the carotenoid pigment. Carotenoid pigment is also found in the rose hip preparation used [23], which is a strong antioxidant too, and rich in several xanthins and able to inhibit the synthesis of MMP-1, an enzyme responsible for the breakdown of collagen [81]. Such strong antioxidant may help to protect collagen and elastin from free radicals formed by UV-induced oxidation, which is responsible for skin aging [109, 110]. It is indeed interesting to note that the actual version of rose hip has been documented to improve collagen [81] and symptoms of osteoarthritis [67, 89–91]. In osteoarthritis as well for the skin, collagen plays a very central role. Another aspect of rose hip impact on the skin is GOPO and its anti-inflammatory property [59, 97]. GOPO was shown to inhibit the chemotaxis of neutrophils and the production of interleukins [59]. Inflammation is a key factor of particular interest as UV radiation is known to result in cell destruction and inflammation. Anti-inflammatory agents therefore have their place as a treatment. It should also be remembered that rose hip seeds and oil from these seeds are used to restore burn injury and restore scars in South America. As earlier stated, seeds from rose hip are also rich in poly unsaturated fatty acids (PUFA), among them linoleic acid and alpha linolenic acid [99], both major constituents of the barrier function of the epidermis [111, 112].

When human erythrocytes are stored in a blood bank, they can normally be stored for up to 5 weeks before the hemoglobin starts to leak out through the erythrocyte membranes as an indicator that the membranes are now disintegrating (getting older). Eighteen healthy volunteers were given 45 gram daily of rose hip powder (Lito) containing seeds and shells for 4 weeks and compared with a group of controls. It was shown that the leak of hemoglobin from red cells, in these volunteers, when stored in a blood bank, was significantly reduced because of treatment with rose hip [80]. Details are shown in **Figure 9**. This was evident after 14 days of treatment and remained for the entire treatment period. This indicates that cell membranes from human erythrocytes, when stored in a blood bank, survive longer before they disintegrate if

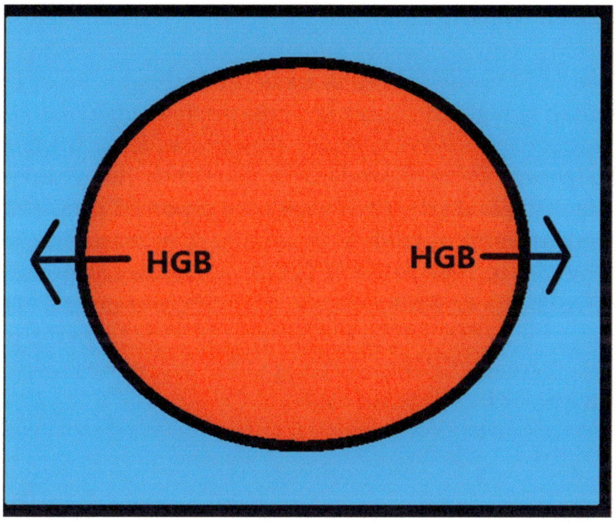

Figure 9.
Hemoglobin is leaking out through the erythrocyte membrane as the result of disintegration over time (aging) of the membrane. If human volunteers are treated Rosa canina this leak of hemoglobin is lowered indicating that membranes are now more resistant to disintegration.

volunteers have been treated rose hip the latest month before blood sampling. There is improved longevity of the red cell membranes as the result of rose hip treatment.

In summary: rose hip can influence wrinkles, moisture, and elasticity of the skin, as well as add to the longevity of red blood cells stored in a blood bank. The mechanism behind these properties is believed to be dependent on the antioxidant activity, as seen in the ability of rose hip to suppress the activity of matrix metalloproteinase 1 (MMP-1) that is involved in the breakdown of extracellular matrix and in particular, tissue remodeling. The result of MMP-1 suppression is also supportive to collagen. Anti-inflammatory capacity and certain fatty acids that are present in the seeds and shells are also thought to play an important role here.

5.9 Rose hip and diseases related to the gastrointestinal tract

Antiulcerogenic activity from "folk remedies" has often been reported, and in this connection, *Rose canina* L is also mentioned [113]. An antiulcerogenic effect from *Rosa canina* extracts was discovered in a rat model. It was later shown that *Rosa canina* can prevent gastric mucosa erosion and the associated hemorrhagic ulcer formation [114]. Extracts from the leaf of *Rosa canina* were also reported to have significant antidiarrheal activity, as well as significantly reduce the intestinal transit time in another animal study [115]. In a clinical trial on humans suffering either Morbus Crohn or Ulcerative colitis, it was documented that the combined seed and shell powder from *Rosa canina* (Lito) significantly lowered symptoms from Morbus Crohn but not symptoms from Ulcerative colitis [116]. One reason for that phenomenon can be that the rose hip version used in the experiment could inhibit neutrophil chemotaxis [59]. Excessive neutrophil activity is involved in the pathogenesis of Morbus Crohn.

In conclusion: Rose hip is interesting when focusing on the gastrointestinal tract, especially by impacting the gastro microbiome. However, more clinical studies in humans need to be available before making any conclusions.

5.10 Antiproliferative effects of rose hip

The involvement of ROS and free radicals in the pathogenesis of certain human diseases also including aging and cancer is increasingly recognized [117], and there are an increasing number of papers in which *Rosa canina* L has been tested on different cell lines in the laboratory. Such studies include colon, lung, and prostate cell lines in which cell proliferation and apoptosis have been reported [118, 119]. However, we were not able to find any clinical studies performed in humans that specifically focus on the impact of any rose hip species including *Rosa canina* on the survival rate among humans suffering from cancer. And as we do not want to create false hopes in people experiencing such a serious disease, our statement is: That from the present knowledge and insight it is too early to discuss the possible impact rose hip treatment might have on proliferative disorders in humans.

6. Conclusion

Rose hip is a very fascinating medicinal plant, which deserves much attention. It can grow on very poor soil, and it is a source of very potent antioxidant and anti-inflammatory agents. It is also a rich source of vitamins—especially vitamin C. Several clinical studies have established that rose hip is very effective for the treatment of osteoarthritis in humans and also in some animal models. Very important, dose dependency, one of the cornerstones when evaluating prescription medicine, has been documented for a subspecies of rose hip [60]. There are also indications that conditions such as rheumatoid arthritis, cardiovascular disease, and skin diseases including wrinkles can benefit from rose hip treatment. However, there are many different *Rosa* species that produce rose hips with varying contents of active compounds. Only careful comparative evaluation will establish which species are most promising. Currently, it seems like a certain subspecies of *Rosa canina* Lito is very promising. There is still a tremendous amount of research to be done before we have a clearer pattern. But for sure, rose hip is a medicinal plant with a long and fascinating history. When discussing anti-inflammatory diets and anti-inflammatory plants especially it is interesting to note that in osteoarthritis a subspecies of *Rosa canina* was able to reduce the consumption of rescue medication by up to 50%. This means that we can eat in a different way and possibly, spare governmental health expenditure for medicine. It has been very interesting to be part of this research.

Acknowledgements

We thank Claude Mona for excellent secretarial assistance.

Author details

Ditte Christina Lustrup and Kaj Winther*
Department of Nutrition, Exercise and Sports, University of Copenhagen, Denmark

*Address all correspondence to: kaha@nexs.ku.dk

References

[1] Senapati K, Rout GR. Study of culture conditions for improved micropropagation of hybrid rose. Horticultural Science. 2008;**35**(1):27-34

[2] Ercisli S. Chemical composition of fruits in some rose (Rosa spp.) species. Food Chemistry. 2007;**104**:1379-1384

[3] Shikov AN et al. Traditional and current food use of wild plants listed in the russian pharmacopoeia. Frontiers in Pharmacology. 2017;**8**:841

[4] Ghazghazi H et al. Phenols, essential oils and carotenoids of Rosa canina from Tunisia and their antioxidant activities. African Journal of Biotechnology. 2010;**9**(18):2709-2716

[5] Britannica T. Editors of Encyclopaedia. "rose". Encyclopedia Britannica. 2021. Available from: https://www.britannica.com/plant/rose-plant [Accessed: April 15, 2022]

[6] Czyzowska A et al. Polyphenols, vitamin C and antioxidant activity in wines from *Rosa canina* L. and *Rosa* rugosa Thunb. Journal of Food Composition and Analysis. 2015;**39**:62-68

[7] Kuhnlein HV, Turner NJ. Traditional Plant Foods of Canadian Indigenous Peoples: Nutrition, Botany and Use. Second ed. Australia, Canada, The Netherland, United Kingdom: Gordon and Breach Publishers; 1996

[8] Karg S, Märkle T. Continuity and changes in plant resources during the Neolithic period in western Switzerland. Vegetation History and Archaeobotany. 2002;**11**:169-176

[9] Barros L et al. Strawberry-tree, blackthorn and rose fruits: Detailed characterization in nutrients and phytochemicals with antioxidant properties. Food Chemistry. 2010;**120**: 247-254

[10] Ayati Z et al. Phytochemistry, traditional uses and pharmacological profile of Rose Hip: A review. Current Pharmaceutical Design. 2018;**24**:1-24

[11] Dénes A et al. Wild plants used for food by Hungarian ethnic groups living in the Carpathian Basin. Acta Societatis Botanicorum Poloniae. 2012;**81**(4):381-396

[12] Hong L et al. Ethnobotany of wild plants used for starting fermented beverages in Shui communities of southwest China. Journal of Ethnobiology and Ethnomedicine. 2015;**11**:42

[13] Polumackanycz M et al. Phenolic composition and biological properties of wild and commercial Dog Rose fruits and leaves. Molecules. 2020;**25**:5272

[14] Günes M. Pomological and phenological characteristics of promising rose hip (Rosa) genotypes. African Journal of Biotechnology. 2010;**9**(38):6301-6306

[15] Al-Yafeai A et al. Characterization of carotenoids and vitamin E in *R. rugosa* and *R. canina*: Comparative analysis. Food Chemistry. 2018;**242**:435-442

[16] Phillips KM et al. Nutrient composition of selected traditional United States Northern Plains Native American plant foods. Journal of Food Composition and Analysis. 2014;**34**:136-152

[17] Ayati Z et al. Genus Rosa/ a review of ethnobotany, phytochemistry and traditional aspects according to Islamic Traditional Medicine (ITM). Advances

in Experimental Medicine and Biology. 2021;**1308**:353-401

[18] Polat R, Satıl F. An ethnobotanical survey of medicinal plants in Edremit Gulf (Balıkesir–Turkey). J Ethnopharmacol. 2012;**139**(2):626-641

[19] Ugulu I, Baslar S, Yorek N, Dogan Y. The investigation and quantitative ethnobotanical evaluation of medicinal plants used around Izmir province, Turkey. Journal of Medicinal Plants Research. 2009;**3**(5):345-367

[20] Pieroni A, Quave CL, Giusti ME, Papp N. "We are Italians!": The hybrid ethnobotany of a Venetian diaspora in Eastern Romania. Human Ecology. 2012;**40**(3):435-451

[21] Rivera D, Obon C, Inocencio C, et al. The ethnobotanical study of local Mediterranean food plants as medicinal resources in Southern Spain. Journal of Physiology and Pharmacology. 2005;**56**(1):97-114

[22] Arnold N et al. A contribution to the flora and ethnobotanical knowledge of Mount Hermon, Lebanon. Flora Mediterranea. 2015;**25**:13-55

[23] Winther K et al. Bioactive ingredients of rose hips (Rosa canina L.) with special reference to antioxidative and antiinflammatory properties: In vitro studies. Botanics: Targets and Therapy. 2016;**6**:11-23

[24] Olech M et al. Biological activity and composition of teas and tinctures prepared for Rosa rugosa Thunb. Central European Journal of Biology. 2012;7(1):172-182

[25] Olech M et al. Multidirectional characterization of chemical composition and health-promoting potential of *Rosa rugosa* hips. Natural Product Research. 2017;**31**(6):667-671

[26] Weidema I. NOBANIS—Invasive Alien Species Fact Sheet –*Rosa rugosa*. From: Online Database of the European Network on Invasive Alien Species. 2006: NOBANIS www.nobanis.org. Available from: https://www.nobanis.org/globalassets/speciesinfo/r/rosa-rugosa/rosarugosa.pdf [Accessed: April 2022]

[27] Skrypnik L et al. Evaluation of the rose hips of *Rosa canina* L and *Rosa rugosa* thunb. as a valuable source of biological active compounds and antioxidants on the Baltic Sea Coast. Polish Journal of Natural Sciences. 2019;**34**(3):395-413

[28] Engels G, Brinckmann J. Herbalgram: Dog rose hip Rosa Canina Family: Rosceaea. The Journal of the American Botanical Council. 2016;**111**:8-9

[29] Koczka N et al. Total polyphenol content and antioxidant capacity of rose hips of some Rosa species. Medicines. 2018;**5**:84

[30] Medveckiene B et al. The effect of ripening stages on the accumulation of carotenoids, polyphenols and vitamin C in rosehips species/cultivars. Applied Science. 2021;**11**:6761

[31] DTU Foods public food database. Rose hip. Food Database, version 4. 2019. Available from: https://frida.fooddata.dk/food/27langen

[32] Worrall S. A nightmare disease haunted ships during age of discovery. National Geographics. 2017. Available from: https://www.nationalgeographic.com/science/article/scurvy-disease-discovery-jonathan-lamb [Accessed: April 2022]

[33] Elste V et al. Emerging evidence on Neutrophil motility supporting its usefulness to define vitamin C intake requirements. Nutrients. 2017;**9**:503

[34] Pavek PLS. Plant guide for dog rose (*Rosa canina* L.). Pullman, WA: USDA-Natural Resources Conservation Service; 2012

[35] Nordic Council of Ministers. Nordic Nutrition Recommendation 2012, Integrating Nutrition and Physical Activity. Narayana Press, 2014. 5th edition

[36] Bozonet M et al. Enhanced human neutrophil vitamin C status, chemotaxis and oxidant generation following dietary supplementation with vitamin C-Rich SunGold Kiwifruit. Nutrients. 2015;7:2574-2588

[37] Levy R et al. Vitamin C for the treatment of recurrent furunculosis in patients with impaired neutrophil functions. The Journal of infectious diseases. 1996;**173**:1502-1505

[38] Covarrubias-Pinto A et al. Old things new view: Ascorbic acid protects the brain in neurodegenerative disorders. International Journal of Molecular Science. 2015;**16**:28194-28217

[39] Carr CA, Lykkesfeldt J. Discrepancies in global vitamin C recommendations: A review of RDA criteria and underlying health perspectives. Critical Reviews in Food Science and Nutrition. 2021;**61**(5):742-755

[40] Lykkesfeldt J et al. Authors' perspective: What is the Optimum Intake of Vitamin C in Humans? Food Science and Nutrition. 2012;**2**:815-829

[41] Oprica L et al. Ascorbic acid content of rose hip fruits depending on altitude. Iranian Journal of Public Health. 2015;**44**(1):138-139

[42] National Institute for Health and Welfare. Rosehip, Rosa rugosa. Fineli Food Composition Database Release 19 (March 3, 2018), 2019. Available from: https://fineli.fi/fineli/en/elintarvik-keet/11007

[43] Al-Yafeai A et al. Bioactive compounds and antioxidant capacity of *Rosa rugosa* depending on degree of ripeness. Antioxidants. 2018;7:134

[44] Kazaz S et al. Variations in chemical compositions of Rosa damascena Mill. and *Rosa canina* L. fruits. Czech Journal of Food Science. 2009;**27**(3):178-184

[45] Demir F, Özcan M. Chemical and technological properties of rose (*Rosa canina* L.) fruits grown wild in Turkey. Journal of Food Engineering. 2001;**47**:333-336

[46] Mann J. Essentials of Human Nutrition. Oxford: Oxford University Press; 2017

[47] USDA, Food Data Central, SR legacy, released 2018. Acerola, (west Indian cherry), raw. Available from: https://fdc.nal.usda.gov/fdc-app.html#food-details/171686/nutrients

[48] Kaack K, Kuhn BF. Evaluation of rose hip species for processing of jam, jelly and soup. Tidsskr. Planteavl. 1991;**95**:353-358

[49] Przybylska S, Tokarczyk G. Lycopene in the prevention of Cardiovascular diseases. International Journal of Molecular Sciences. 2022;**23**:1957

[50] Mueller L, Boehm V. Antioxidant activity of beta-carotene compounds in different in vitro assays. Molecules. 2011;**16**:1055-1069

[51] Imran M et al. Lycopene as a natural antioxidant used to prevent human health disorders. Antioxidants. 2020;**9**:706

[52] Burton-Freeman BM, Sesso HD. Whole food versus supplement: Comparing the clinical evidence of tomato intake and lycopene supplementation on

cardiovascular risk factors. Advances in Nutrition. 2014;**5**:457-485

[53] Cheng HM et al. Tomato and lycopene supplementation and cardiovascular risk factors: A systematic review and meta-analysis. Atherosclerosis. 2017;**257**:100-108

[54] Böhm V et al. Rose hip—A new source of lycopene? Molecular Aspects of Medicine. 2003;**24**:385-389

[55] Carlsen MH et al. The total antioxidant content of more than 3100 foods, beverages, spices, herbs and supplements used worldwide. Nutrition Journal. 2010;**9**(3):1-11

[56] Carlsen HM, et al. The Antioxidant Food Table. 2010. Available from: http://www.Biomedcentral.com/content/supplementary/1475-2891-9-3-S1.pdf

[57] Institute of Physical Education and Nutrition. Radicals—what are free radicals (Danish). 2022. Copenhagen University. Available from: https://nexs.ku.dk/forskning/vidensbanken/radikaler/ [Accessed: April 15, 2022]

[58] Roman I, Stanila A, Stalina S. Bioactive compounds and antioxidant activity of *Rosa canina* L biotypes from spontaneous flora of Transylvania. Chemical Central Journal. 2013;**7**:73-85

[59] Kharazmi A, Winther K. Rose hip inhibits chemotaxis and chemiluminesence of human peripheral blood neutrophils in vitro and reduces certain inflammatory parameters in vivo. Inflammopharmacology. 1999;**7**(4):377-386

[60] Marstrand K, Warholm L, Pedersen F, Winther K. Dose dependent impact of rose-hip powder in patients suffering from osteoarthroitis of the hip and or knee—A Double Blind, Randomized, Placebo Controlled, Parallel Group, Phase III Study. International Journal of Complementary and Alternative Medicine. 2017;**7**(1):1-9

[61] Willich SN, Rossnagel K, Roll S, Wagner A, Mune O, Erlendson J, et al. Rose hip herbal remedy in patients with rheumatoid arthritis—A randomized controlled trial. Phytomedicine. 2010;**17**(2):87-93

[62] Winther K, Warholm L, Campbell-Tofte J, Marstrand K. Effect of *Rosa canina* L (Rose hip) on cold during winter season in a middleclass population: A randomized, double-blinded, placebo-controlled trial. Journal of Herbal Medicine. 2018;**43**:34-41

[63] Ginnerup-Nielsen E, Christensen R, Bliddal H, Zangger G, Hansen L, Henriksen M. Improved gait in persons with knee related mobility limitations by a rosehip food supplement: A randomized, double-blind, placebo-controlled trial. Gait and Posture. 2015; **42**(3):340-347

[64] Tiralongo E, Wee SS, Lea RA. Elderberry supplementation reduces cold duration and symptoms in air-travvellers: A Randomized, Double-blind, Placebo-Controlled Clinical Trial. Nutrients. 2016;**8**:182-197

[65] Lastra G, Sowers JR. Obesity and cardiovascular disease: Role of adipose tissue, inflammation, and the renin-angiotensin-aldosteron system. Hormone Molecular Biology and Clinical Investigation. 2013;**15**:49-57

[66] Anderson U, Berger K, Høgberg A, Landin-Olsson M, Holm C. Effects of rose hip intake on risk markers of type 2 diabetes and cardiovascular diseases: A randomized, double-blind, cross-over investigation in obese persons.

European Journal of Clinical Nutrition. 2012;**66**:585-590

[67] Rein E, Kharazmi A, Winther K. A herbal remedy, Hyben Vital (stand. Powder of a suibspecies of Rosa canina fruits), reduces pain and improves general wellbeing in patients with osteoarthrosis—A double-blind, placebo-controlled, randomized trial. Phytomedicine. 2004;**11**:383-391

[68] Cavalera M, Axling U, Rippe C, Swärd K, Holm C. Dietary rose hip exertrs antiatherosclerotic effects and increase nitric oxide-mediated dilatation in ApoE-null mice. The Journal of Nutritional Biochemistry. 2017;**44**:52-59

[69] Raiciu AD, Popescu M, Ivopol GC, Bordei N, Alexandru G, Crisan I, et al. Therapeutic applications of vegetable oils and GC-MS evaluation of omega 3, omega-6 and omega-9 amounts in six oleaginous plants. Review Chim. 2016;**67**:2449-2453

[70] Ninomiya K, Matsuda H, Kubo M, Morikawa T, Nishida N, Yoshikawa M. Potent anti-obese principle from *Rosa canina*: Structural requirements and mode of action of trans-tiliroside. Bioorganic and Medicinal Chemistry Letters. 2007;**17**:3059-3064

[71] Nagatomo A, Nishida N, Fukuhara I, Noro A, Kozai Y, Sato H, et al. Daily intake of rose hip extract decreases abdominal visceral fat in preobese subjects: A randomized, double-blind, placebo-controlled clinical trial. Diabetes Metabolism Syndrome Obesity. 2015;**8**:147

[72] Banfi G, Iorio EL, Corsi MM. Oxidative stress, free radicals and bone remodeling. Clinical Chemistry and Laboratory Medicine. 2008;**46**:1550-1555

[73] Scheweita S, Khoshhal K. Calcium metabolism and oxidative stress in bone fractures: Role of antioxidants. Current Drug Metabolism. 2007;**8**:519-525

[74] Devareddy L, Hooshmand S, Collins JK, Lucas EA, Chai SC, Arjmandi BH. Blueberry prevents bone loss in ovariectomized rat model of postmenopausal osteoporosis. Journal of Nutritional Biochemistry. 2008;**19**:694-699

[75] Halvorsen BL, Holte K, Myhrstad MCW, Barikmo I, Hvattum E, Remberg SF, et al. A systematic screening of total antioxidants in dietary plants. Journal of Nutrition. 2002;**132**:461-471

[76] Bernabei R, Mattone AM, Ortolani E, Lande F, Marzetti E. Screening, diagnosing and treatment of osteoporosis: A brief review. Clin Cases in Mineral and Bone Metabolism. 2014;**11**:201-207

[77] Fecka I. Qualitative and quantitative determination of hydrolysable tannins and other polophenols in herbal products from Meadowsweet and Dog Rose. Phytochemical Annal. 2009;**20**:177-190

[78] Hvattum E. Determination of Phenolic compounds in rose hip (*Rosa canina*) using liquid chromatography coupled to electrospray ionization tandem mass spectrometry and diode-array detection. Rapid Communication and Mass Spectrum. 2002;**16**:655-662

[79] Hubert PA, Lee SG, Chun OK. Dietary polyphenols, berries and are related bone loss: A review based on human, animal and cell studies. Antioxidants. 2014;**3**:144-158

[80] Phetcharat L, Wongsuphasawat K, Winther K. The effectiveness of a standardized rose hip powder, containing seeds and shells of Rosa canina, on cell longevity, skin wrinkles, moisture, and elasticity. Clinical Inrvervention in Aging. 2015;**10**:1-8

[81] Schwager J, Hoeller U, Wolframs S, Richard N. Rose hip and its constituents galactolipids confer cartilage protection by modulating cytokine and chemokine expression. BMC Complementary and Alternative Medicine. 2011;**11**:105

[82] Dieppe PA, Lohmander LS. Pathogenesis and management of pain in osteoarthritis. Lancet. 2005;**365**(9463): 965-973

[83] Vane JR, Botting RM. Anti-inflammatory drugs and their mechanisms of Action. Inflammation Research. 1998;**47**(2):78-87

[84] Griffin MR, Piper JM, Daugherty JR, Snowdon M, Roy WA. Non-steroidal anti-inflammatory drug use and increased risk for peptic ulcerdisease in elderly persons. Annals of Internal Medicine. 1991;**114**(4):257-263

[85] Silverstein JE, Faich G, Goldstein JL, Simon LS, Pincus T. Gastrintestinal toxicity with celecoxib vs nonsteroidal antiinflammatory drugs for osteoarthritis and rheumatoid arthritis. JAMA. 2000;**113**(25):1247-1255

[86] Gislason GH, Jacobsen S, Rasmussen JN, Rasmussen S, Buch P. Risk of death or reinfarction associated with the use of selective cyclooxygenase-2 inhibitors and nonselective nonsteroidal anti-inflammatory drugs after acute myocardial infarction. Circulation. 2006;**113**(25):2906-2913

[87] Roderigues G, Hernandes-Diaz S. Relative risk of upper gastrointestinal complications among users of acetaminophen and non-steroidal anti-inflammatory drugs. Epidemiology. 2001;**12**(5):570-576

[88] Warholm O, Skaar S, Hedman E, Mølmen HM, Eik L. Placebo-Controlled Clinical Trial. Current Therapeutyic Research. 2003;**64**(1):21-31

[89] Winther K, Apel K, Thamsborg G. A powder made from seeds and shells of a rose-hip subspecies (*Rosa canina*) reduces symptoms of knee and hip osteoarthritis: A randomized, double-blind, placebo-controlled clinical trial. Scandinavian Journal of Rheumatology. 2005;**34**:302-308

[90] Winther K, Campbell-Tofte J, Hansen P. Rose Hip Powder that contains the natural amount of shells and seeds alleviate pain in osteoarthritis of the dominant hand—Ramdomized, Double-Blind, Placebo-Controlled, Cross-over Clinical Trial. Open Journal of Rheumatology and Autoimmune Diseases. 2013;**3**:172-130

[91] Christensen R, Bartels EM, Altman RD, Astrup A, Bliddal H. Does the hip powder of Rosa canina (rosehip) reduce pain in osteoarthritis patients?—A meta-analysis of randomized controlled triasls. Osteoarthritis and Cartillage. 2008;**16**:965-972

[92] Verkleij SPJ, Luijsterburg PAJ, BohnenAM,KoesBW,Bierma-ZeinstraSMA. NSAIDs vs acetaminophen in knee and hip osteoarthritis: A systematic review regarding hetyerogeity influencing the outcomes. Osteoarthrosis and Cartilage. 2011;**19**:921-929

[93] Pelletier J-P, Martel-Pelletier J, Rannou F, Cooper C. Efficacy and safety of Oral NSAIDs and analgesics in the management of osteoarthritis: Evidence from real-life setting trials and surveys. Seminars in Arthritis and Rheumatism. 2016;**45**:22-27

[94] Kirkeskov B, Christensen R, Bügel S, Bliddal H, Danneskiold-Samsøe B, Christensen LP, et al. The effects of rose hip (Rosa canina) on plasma antioxidative activity and C-reactive protein in patients with rheumatoid arthritis and normal

controls: A prospective cohort study. Phytomedicine. 2011;**18**:953-958

[95] Larsen E, Kharazmi A, Christensen LP, Christensen SB. An anti-inflammatory galactolipid from Rose hip (*Rosa canina*) that inhibits chemotaxis of human peripheral blood neutrophils in vitro. Journal of Natural Production. 2003;**66**:994-995

[96] Winther K, Kharazmi A, Hansen ASV, Falk-Rønne J. The absorption of natural vitamin C in horses and anti-oxidative capacity: A randomized, controlled study on trotters during a three month intervention period. Comparative Exercise Physiology. 2012;**8**(3/4):195-201

[97] Jäger AK, Petersen KN, Thomasen G, Christensen SB. Isolation of linoleic and alpha-linolenic acids as COX-1 and COX-2 inhibitors in rose hip. Phytotherapy Research. 2008;**22**:982-984

[98] Saaby L, Jäger AK, Moseby L, Hansen EW, Christensen SB. Isolation of immunomodulatory Triterpene Acids from a Staqndardized Rose Hip Powder (*Rosa canina* L). Phytotherapy Research. 2011;**25**:195-201

[99] Ashtiyani SC, Najafi H, Jalalvandi S, Hosseinei F. Protective effect of the total flavonoids from *Rosa canina* L fruit extracts on renal disturbances induced by reperfusion injury in rats. Iraniam Journal of Kidney Diseases. 2013;**7**:290

[100] Zhao L, Xu L, Tao X, Han X, Yin L, Qi Y, et al. Protective effect of the total flavonoids form Rosa Laevigata michx fruit on renal ischaemia-reperfusion injury through suppression of Oxidative stress and inflammation. Molecules. 2016;**21**:952

[101] Kashihara M, Haruna Y, Kondeti K, Kanwar Y. Oxidative stress in diabetic nephropathy. Curr Med Chem. 2010;**17**: 4256-4269

[102] Zhou Y, Liao Q, Luo Y, Qing Z, Zhang Q, He G. Renal protective effect of Rosa Laevigata michx. By the inhibition of oxidative stress in streptozotocin-induced diabetic rats. Molecular Medicine Reports. 2012;**5**:1548-1554

[103] Tayefi-Nasrabadi H, Sadigh-Eteghad S, Aghdam Z. The effect of the hydroalcoholic extract of *Rosa canina* L Fruits on experimentally nephrolithisic whistar rats. Phytotherapy Research. 2012;**26**:78-85

[104] Sadeghi H, Hosseinzadeh S, Touri MA, Ghavamzadeh M, Barnak MJ. Hepatoprotective effect of Rosa canina fruit extract against carbon tetrachloride induced hepatoxicity in rat. Avicenna Journal of Phytomedicine. 2016;**6**:181

[105] Liu L, Yasen M, Tang D, Ye J, Aisa A, Xin X. Polyphenol-enriched extract of *Rosa rogusa* Thumb regulates lipid metabolism in diabetic rats by activation of AMPK parthway. Biomed and Pharmacother. 2018;**100**:29-35

[106] Rittie L, Fisher GJ. Natural and sun-induced aging of human skin. Cold Springer and Harbor Perspective Medicine. 2015;**5**:a015370

[107] Wang D, Beck LA. Immunologic targets in atopic dermatitis and emerging therapies: An update. American Journal of Clinical Dermatology. 2016;**17**:425-443

[108] Parl KH, Jeong MS, Park KJ, Choi YW, Seo SJ, Lee MW. Topical application of Rosa multiflora root extract improves atopic dermatitis-like skin lesions induced by mite antigen in NC/NGA mice. Biological Pharm Bulletin. 2014;**37**:178-183

[109] Pillaiyar T, Manickam M, Namasivayam V. Skin whitening agent: Medical chemistry perspectives of tyrosinhase inhibitors. Journal of

Enzyme Inhibition and Medicinal Chemistry. 2017;**32**:403-425

[110] Fujii T, Ikeda K, Saito M. Inhibitory effects of rose hip (*Rosa canina* L) on melanogenesis in mouse melanoma cells and on pigmentation in brown guinea pigs. Bioscience, Biotechnology, and Biochemistry. 2011;**75**:489-495

[111] Wertz PW. Epidermal lipids. Seminars in Dermatology. 1992;**11**: 106-113

[112] Öscan M. Nutrient composition of Rosa canina L. Seed and oils. Journal of Medicinal Food. 2002;**5**(3):137-140

[113] Gürbüz I, Üstün O, Yesilada E, Sezik E, Kutsal O. Antiulcerogenic activity of some plants used as folk remedy in Turkey. Journal of Ethnopharmacy. 2003;**88**:93-97

[114] Rao A, Gurfinkel D. The Bioactivity of saponins: Triterpenoid and steroidal glycosides. Drug Metabolism and Drug Interact. 2000;**17**:211-236

[115] Meli R, Di Carlo G, Capasso F. Inhibitory action of quercetin on essential transit in mice. Phytotherapy Research. 1990;**4**:201-202

[116] Bütner S, Jacobsen O, Andersen JR, Winther K. The Impact of a astandardized powder made from a subtype of Rose-hip on IBDQ symptom score in patients with Chrons`s Disease or Ulcerative Cholitis. Scandinavian Journal of Gastroenterology. 2004;**39**(240):39

[117] Tumbas VT, Canadanovic-Brunet JM, Cetojevic DD, Cetkovic GS. Effect of rosehip (*Rosa canina* L) phytochemicals on stable free radicals and human cancer cells. Journal of Science Food and Agriculture. 2012;**92**(6):1273-1281

[118] Jemenez S, Gascon S, Luquin A, Laguna M, Ancin-Azpilicueta C, Rodriquez-Yoldi MJ. Rosa canina extracts have antiproliferative and antioxidant effects on Caco-2 human colon cancer. Plos One. 2016;11(7):e0159136. DOI: 10.1371/journal.pone.0159136

[119] Kilinc K, Demir S, Turan I, Mentese A, Orem A, Sonmez M. Rosa canina extract has antiproliferative and proapoptotic effects on human lung and prostate cancer cells. Nutrition and Cancer. 2019;**72**(2):273-282

Chapter 19

Mulberry as a Valuable Resource for Food and Pharmaceutical Industries: A Review

Ritwik Acharya, Trisha Bagchi and Debnirmalya Gangopadhyay

Abstract

Mulberry is a fast growing hardy perennial woody plant belonging to the genus *Morus* of the family Moraceae. There are more than 60 species of the genus *Morus* found in the subtropical, tropical and temperate regions of Asia, Africa and North America. Cultivation of mulberry is highly economical since the leaf produced by mulberry is extensively used for feeding the silkworm, *Bombyx mori* for silk production. Mulberry possessing valuable nutritional and phytochemical constituents can serve as highly nutritious food for human with high therapeutic values. Mulberry fruit is rich in carbohydrate, protein and dietary fiber and an important foodstuff for the preparation of several value added items like jams, jellies, wines and syrups. Mulberry leaf has been identified as an excellent resource for the development of protein rich food products with natural antioxidant. Extracts of leaf, stem, twig, root and bark of mulberry are reported to have potential antimicrobial, anti-inflammatory, antioxidant, anti-hyperglycaemic, anticancer and anti-tyrosinase inhibition activity. Though mulberry is grown commercially in many countries for sericulture, its potential to be utilized as food for human consumption is not well recognized. The paper reviews the importance of mulberry as a valuable resource for various food, cosmetic, beverage and pharmaceutical industries.

Keywords: food, mulberry, nutritional constituents, Phytomedicine, value addition

1. Introduction

Mulberry (Genus: *Morus*; Family: Moraceae) is an economical and widespread woody plant. In the Asian countries mulberry is widely cultivated for its leaf to feed the monophagous silkworm (*Bombyx mori* L.). The silkworm (*B. mori* L.) only naturally feed on mulberry leaf which makes mulberry the most vital component of sericulture industry that provides employment to a large number of people of India, China, Bangladesh, Pakistan, and many other Asian countries [1]. Other than sericulture it has an enormous economic value leads to its several unique and special features. Each single parts of mulberry plant can be used for various purposes. In India it is popularly known as 'Kalpa Vriksha' for its multipurpose utilities [2].

Main elements that determine the nutritional quality of any edible plant products are the qualitative and quantitative presence of protein, carbohydrate, dietary fiber and types of vitamin present inside the product; mulberry plant can be highly rated in this context [2]. Mulberry fruits in fresh condition contain carbohydrate which is present either in the form of simple sugars or in the form of starch, soluble and insoluble fibers. They are low in calorie value and high in water content. Iron, vitamin C, decent amount of potassium, vitamin E and K are predominantly found present in the fruits. They are also rich in plant compounds, like anthocyanins, that contribute to their color and positive health effects. Fruits can also improve the blood sugar level, can lower the amount of blood cholesterol, and can help in preventing fatty liver disease. Fruits are also found effective in decreasing the oxidative stress which can reduce the risk of cancer. Leaves of mulberry are also excellent food stuffs as they show nearly the same properties as the fruit. Recent findings mentioned that mulberry leaves contain high amount of bioactive compounds which mainly includes alkaloids, flavonoids, γ-aminobutyric acid (GABA) and phenolic acids [3]. These compounds are effectively involved with antioxidation property [4, 5], as it lowers glycemia [6, 7] minimizes hypertension [8], prevents atherosclerosis, [9] and also shows anti-inflammation property [10]. Bioactive compounds like 1-deoxynojirimycin (DNJ), found in mulberry, seems to be a powerful inhibitor of α-glycosidase and has also shown potential therapeutic capacity for minimizing many diseases, particularly type II diabetes [11, 12]. Recent investigations also explored the very interesting tyrosinase inhibition activity of mulberry. In this regards, white mulberry (*Morus alba*), black mulberry (*Morus nigra)* and red mulberry (*Morus rubra*) are the most accepted worldwide species of the genus *Morus* [2].

Unani, Ayurveda, and Chinese systems of medicine traditionally recognize almost all mulberry varieties for their several pharmacological properties. *M. nigra* fruits are considered as one of the most important components having anti-cancerous properties and popularly known as 'Tuti Aswad or Toot Aswad' in Unani literature [13]. Traditional medicine practitioners consider mulberry as one of the most efficient

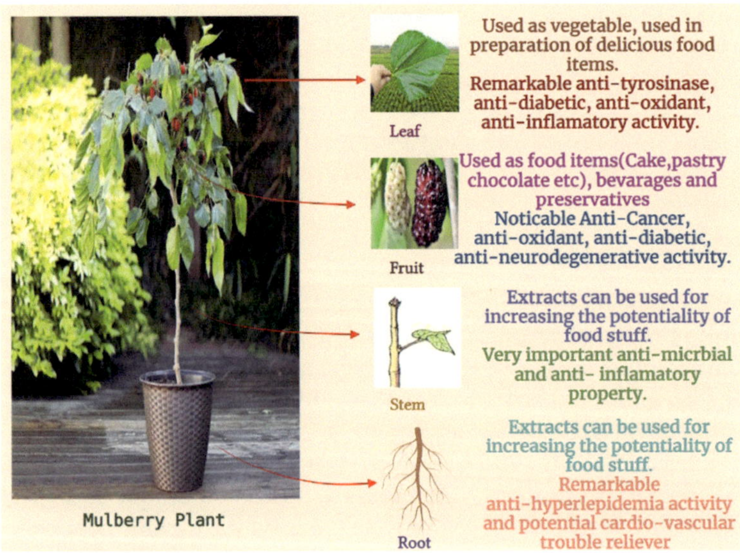

Figure 1.
Overview of importance of mulberry in food and pharmaceutical industry.

plant in the treatment of blood pressure, dental diseases, constipation, helminthic complications, diabetes, hypertension, anemia and arthritic pain [2].

Valuable constituents in mulberry plant; mainly the fruits and leaves categorizes it as a plant which can perfectly be placed in the category of a functional food that not only useful to human health but also having proper basic nutritional function [14]. The Ministry of Health of China in 1985, declared *M. alba* as the first medicinally significant edible fruit [15]. Both leaves and fruits of *M. alba* are also considered as food and drugs along with its primary considerations [16].

The population of Earth been never before as huge as it is today [17]. Rise of nutrient deficiencies is also tied with this population growth has become a serious global crisis, predominantly in the areas where the diet lacks variety. Cheap, easily available, nutritious and pharmaceutically influential plant resources are seems to be the solution of this global crisis. In this context the current review attempts to provide an insight into the potential of mulberry as a valuable resource for food and pharmaceutical industries. An overview of importance of mulberry in food and pharmaceutical industry is shown in **Figure 1**.

2. Geographical distribution of mulberry

Worldwide appreciable availability of any biological resource is extremely important from its exploitation point of view especially for the food and pharmaceutical industries. Presently, Mulberry is distributed in all regions between 50^{0}N Lat. and 10^{0}S Lat., and from sea level to 4000 m altitudes [18, 19], including Asia, Europe, North and South America, and Africa (**Figure 2**). American continent has four mulberry species (*M. insignis, M. celtidifolia, M. corylifolia*, and *M.mexicana*). In India, four mulberry species are reported; among them *M. alba* and *M. indica* are domesticated whereas *M. serrata* and *M. laevigata* grow wildly in the Himalayan territory [1]. China has 24 species but only four species has been spotted for its massive exploitation in sericulture (*M. alba, M. multicaulis, M.atropurpurea*, and *M. mizuho*).

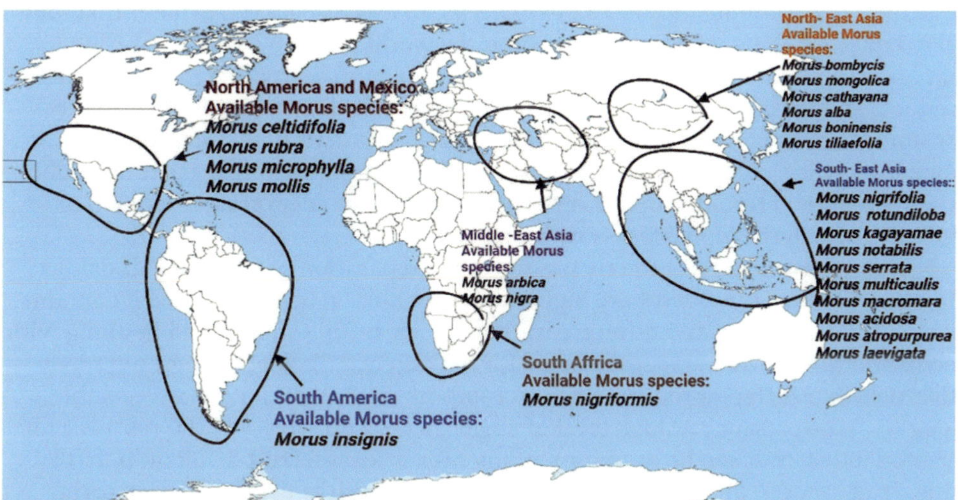

Figure 2.
Geographical distribution of mulberry along with zone wise available species.

Only *M. alba, M. bombycis*, and *M. latifoila* are in use in Japan though presence of 19 species has been recorded there. In Africa, presence of *M. mesozygia* has been reported from humid, sub-humid, and semi-arid areas [20].

3. Botanical description of mulberry plant

Before any sort of investigations of a plant it is extremely urgent to go through its overall botanical details. Mulberry is a perennial, fast growing, woody, deciduous, deep and wide rooted plant [21]. Generally the height of Mulberry plant is approximately 5-6 feet from the ground level [22]. Stem of mulberry is cylindrical in shape with milky sap and fissured bark [23]. Mulberry leaves are generally 5-7.5 cm long and 6-10 cm wide, but they vary widely in their size and shape. Leaves are mostly deeply lobed or having serrate margins; leaf apex is mostly acute with cordate or truncate base. Basal nerves are generally 3; near the margins lateral nerves are forked. Flowers are yellowish green in color with chromosome number 2n = 28. There are differentiations between female and male spikes shape and size in mulberry. Male spikes (catkins) are cylindrical and broad where as female spikes (catkins) are ovoid and stalked, and female spikes (catkins) shorter than male spikes (catkins). Mulberry fruits are arranged longitudinally around the central axis in cluster of small fruits similar with blackberry or loganberries. Mulberry fruits are white to pinkish white in color and during the time of ripening it becomes purple or black in color. Fruits contain many drupes which are enclosed in a fleshy perianth, upto 5 cm long, sub-globose or ovoid in shape. Ovary of mulberry is unicellular with presence of a bifid stigma [2].

4. Mulberry as a potential food resource

Increasing consumer demand has been one of the driving forces in exploration of new natural food resources, keeping in mind that the food product must satisfy both basic dietary requirements and health benefits. In this respect it is evident that mulberry fruits are already famous throughout the world for their mouth-watering taste that makes it suitable to consume either in fresh or as an ingredient in value-added products and for culinary uses (**Table 1**). It is gradually becoming popular to the consumers not only because of their taste but also due to its high nutritional importance along with low calorie value. Opportunity of exploiting other parts of mulberry as processed food resource is also very high. This has led to increased demand of mulberry also in the food processing industries.

Mulberry fruits can be directly used for the preparation of jam and soft drinks [33]. Fresh fruits of mulberry are highly rated for human health because it contains vitamins, amino acids, and different minerals such as Zn, Ca, Mn, and Fe along with pectin and fibrin. Mulberry leaf is used for making tea, dhokla, pakoda and many other delicious different foodstuffs [34]. Mulberry is already a popular vegetable, along with the presence of high level of sugar makes mulberry an ideal resource for the food industry. It can be used for making breads, cakes, fruit drink pulp, fruit wine, fruit sauce, fruit powder and also chocolate. Fresh or dried or frozen forms of mulberry fruits can be utilized to produce different kinds of tonic, wine, syrups, amaretto. Mulberry seeds also can be used to produce oil. Unripe and immature mulberry fruits can be used for chutney preparation [35]. Famous Turkish food 'Kome'

Food items	Uses	Reference
Squash	Fruits of *M. alba* used for the preparation of spiced squash and appetizer.	Hamid and Thakur, 2017 [24].
Pastry	Buckwheat flour, hulls, inulin and chokeberry along with *M. alba* extraction used for the production of pastry which is rich in fiber and low in calorie.	Komolka *et al.*, 2016 [25].
Chocolate	From dried *M. nigra* fruit obtained anthocyanins can be used in chocolate preparation.	Gultekin-Ozguven *et al.*, 2016 [26].
Pasta	Extraction of *M. nigra* having hypoglycaemic effect, it reduces the glycemic index is vastly used to produce pasta.	Yazdankhah *et al.*, 2019 [27].
Minced meat	Shelf life of minced meat increased by methanolic extraction of mulberry leaves.	Yazdankhah *et al.*, 2019 [27].
Yogurt	Anthocyanins of *M. rudra* acts as a coloring agent of strawberry flavored yogurt.	Byamukama *et al.*, 2014 [28].
Probiotics	For the isolation and culture of lactic acid forming bacteria *M. alba* silage is very important. These bacteria can stabilize the gastrointestinal tract microbial flora.	Jan *et al.*, 2021 [2].
Fruit jam	Mixed fruit jam prepared based on ratios of 70:30 rosella and mulberry fruit extract.	Wongchalat and Chatthongpisut., 2016 [29].
Cup cake	The concentrated amount of *M. alba* paste used to prepared cupcakes.	Jan *et al.*, 2021 [2]
Syrup	For the preparation of syrup *M. alba* fruit used and it can be stored for 6 months under refrigerated condition.	Thakur *et al.*, 2017 [30].
Vinegar	*M. alba* is exploited to prepare vinegar.	Karaagac *et al.*, 2016 [31].
Alcholic beverage	Fruit of *M. alba* used to produce alcoholic beverage and also used as a raw material to brew fruit wine.	Daris-Martin *et al.*, 2003 [32].

Table 1.
Uses of mulberry in preparation of food items, beverages and as preservative.

and 'Pestil' is prepared by mixing walnut, honey and flour with mulberry [36, 37]. Mulberry juice kept under a cold storage at a particular temperature for six months to one year has proven effective for healthy skin and in prevention of throat infection [38]. Mulberry paste popularly known as 'sangshengao' used to make tea in China and it also found effective in improving liver and kidney function, vision and hearing. Use of dehydrated mulberry fruit as a sweetening agent in black tea is extremely popular among the Iranian people. In some specified regions of China young leaves of mulberry is in use as vegetables [2]. Mulberry fruit powder can be consumed as an anti-aging substance as it protects the cell from the aging effect. It also stabilizes cholesterol level and increases the carbohydrate absorption capacity of the human digestive system. Over-ripened mulberry fruits are used to produced Mulberry wine, this also known as a 'lady's drink' in Europe. Anthocyanin obtained from of *M. rubra* used for yogurt coloration having no difference with strawberry brand yogurt [28]. *M. alba* extract can be used to produce pastry along with Buckwheat flour, buckwheat hulls, chokeberry and inulin [25]. Shelf life of minced meat can be increased with the help of methanolic extraction of mulberry plant [27]. *M. alba* fruits can also be used to prepare spiced squash and appetizers [24].

5. Pharmaceutical and therapeutic importance of mulberry

Mulberry having exclusive therapeutic properties that are primarily due to their indigenous chemicals along with their anti-oxidant, anti-diabetic, anti-hypertensive, anti-cancer, hepatoprotective properties, and many more. Most important and relevant pharmaceutical ability of mulberry to improve human health and well-being is discussed in this section (**Table 2**).

5.1 Anti-cancer activity

Across the globe different forms of cancer is the most fatal disease. Many types of medicines are available in the market for the treatment of cancer but the number of successful and safe drug is very few. Anthocyanins extracted from the *M. alba* fruit shows an invasion in human lung metastatic A549 carcinoma cells. Flavonoids isolated from the leaves of this plant acts as a cancer inhibiting profile agent [22]. From root bark of mulberry Albanol A (Mulberrofuran G) can be extracted which induce potent cytotoxicity in HL60 (Human Leucamia Cell line) by inhibiting topoisomerase II activity [14, 39]. *M. alba* leaf extract shows anti- proliferative lectin induced cell death by apoptosis in human breast cancer (MCF-7) and colon cancer (HCT-15) by inducing DNA fragmentation and morphological changes. Flavanone glycosides present in the root bark of *M. alba* having anti-proliferation activity against human ovarian cancer in H0-8910 cells [2].

5.2 Anti-hyperlepidemia

Obesity develops due to unusual fat deposition which is a risk for the human health. It is one of the serious problems across the globe because it can increase the chance of cardiac failure, cancer, diabetes and many other diseases. Daily consumption of *M. alba* fruit found effective in lowering the total cholesterol (TC) and lipoprotein levels in blood of both young and senior citizens. *M. alba* leaves extract which is DNJ rich if taken before meals can help to reduced the lipoproteins and triglycerides [2]. The root bark of *M. alba* plays an important role as inhibitor of the LDL (Low density lipo_protein) anthrogenic alternation and also act as a hypo-chlesterolemic element [22].

5.3 Anti-diabetic

Diabetes mellitus is characterized by high glucose levels (Blood sugar) which is a type of metabolic disorder. Insulin secretion, or insulin action or both can be defective in response to the high blood sugar (glucose) levels in this disease. Type 2 diabetes have two features- low gradic chronic inflammatory and the insulin resistance. Cardiovascular diseases and many other multi organ disorders can be developed by type 2 diabetes. Leaves of *M. alba* helps to decrease the blood glucose level and also prevents potential histo-pathological alterations in pancreas and kidneys which is observed in brown rats, in a recent experiment [14]. Soluble extract of *M. alba* fruit found effective in decreasing fasting blood glucose (FBG) and glycosylated serum protein (GSP) in STZ induced diabetic mice. In STZ induced diabetic rats *M. alba* stem bark also helps in the alternation of glutathione and insulin levels [2, 16, 40].

Pharmaceuticals importance of mulberry	Specis	Parts used	Major findings	Ref.
Anti-oxidant	*M. alba* *M. nigra*	Twigs, Bark Fruit Leaves Stem	• Twigs, bark consists morin, maclurin that is important for inflammatory responses, and nervous system functioning. • Scavenging activities against super oxide and anion radicals. • Shows strongest protective effect on H_2O_2-induced injury. • Moracin extracted from leaves it shows anti-oxidant activities. • Stem extract shows anti-oxidant activity that increase superoxide and NO scavenging activity.	Kadam *et al.*, 2019 [14], Wang *et al.*, 2014 [16], Jan *et al.*, 2021 [2].
Anti- Cancer	*M. alba*	Fruit Root bark Leaves	• Fruits containing anthocyanin shows an invasion against human lung metastatic. • Albanol A that isolated from root bark that induced potent cytotoxicity in Human Leucamia cell line • Anti-proliferation activity against human ovarian cancer. • Anti-proliferative lectin induced cell death in human breast cancer. • Flavonoids present in leaves that acts as a cancer inhibiting profile agent.	Khalid *et al.*, 2021 [22], Kadam *et al.*, 2019 [14], Naowaratwattana *et al.*, 2010 [39]
Anti-hyperlepidemia	*M. alba*	Fruit Leaves Root bark	• It can help to decrease cholesterol and lipoprotein. • DNJ extraction from leave help to reduce lipoproteins and triglycerides serum level. • Inhibit the LDL anthrogenic alternation.	Khalid *et al.*, 2021 [22].
Anti- Diabetic	*M. alba*	Leaves Fruits Stem bark	• Help to decrease blood glucose levels observed in brown rat. • Help to decrease fasting blood glucose (FBG) and glycosylated serum protein in diabetic mice. • Alternation of glutathione and insulin levels in STZ induced diabetic rats.	Kadam *et al.*, 2019 [14], Wang *et al.*, 2017 [16] Alanazi *et al.*, 2017 [40]
Anti-Inflammatory	*M. alba*	Leaves Stem Fruit Root	• Reduce the production of cytokine and pro-inflammatory mediators. • Inhibit NO production shows anti-inflammatory effect. • Presence of anthocyanins that can inhibit pro-inflammatory effect of cytokine in mice. • Inhibit histamine release and act as a natural source of anti-histamine and anti-allergic agent.	Park *et al.*, 2013 [10] Jan *et al.*, 2021 [2].

Pharmaceuticals importance of mulberry	Specis	Parts used	Major findings	Ref.
Anti-microbial	*M. mesozygia* *M. alba* *M. nigra*	Bark Stem bark Fruit	• Used for the micro-organisms associated infections. • Antimicrobial activity against *Enterococcus faecalis, E. coli, S. aureus*. • Prevent growth of *S. mutans*.	Kuete *et al.*, 2009 [41], Fukai *et al.*, 2005 [42], Thabti *et al.*, 2014 [43], Budiman *et al.*, 2017 [44].
Neurodegenerative action	*M. alba*	Fruit	• Protect against oxidative stress-induced apoptosis. • Fruit containing rutin, anthocyanin have impact on Parkinson's disease	Kim *et al.*, 2010 [45].
Hepatoprotective	*M. mesozygia* *M. indica*	Twigs	• Glycoprotein protects against CC14 induced liver damage. • In experimental rats it help to decrease the activity of gastric mucosal injury.	Kadam *et al.*, 2019 [14].
Activity against Skin disease	*M. alba*	Leaf	• Help in the inhibition of mammalian tyrosinase, melanin synthesis effects. • It also contain carotenoids that can help to decrease age spot, blemishes effect on skin.	Chang *et al.*, 2011 [46]. Kadam *et al.*, 2019 [14].
Cardiovascular activity	*M. alba*	Root bark	• Helps to reduce blood pressure, cholesterol level. • Morusinol present in the root bark helps to prevent collagen and arachidonic acid. • Reveratrol, a flavonoid acts as a vasodilator.	Doi *et al.*, 2000 [47]. Kadam *et al.*, 2019 [14].

Table 2.
Pharmaceutical importance of mulberry.

5.4 Anti- inflammatory

In some particular tissues presence of some microorganisms like bacteria, viruses, and fungi and their circulation in blood can cause complex vascular biological problems known as inflammation. If within a certain time period it is not diagnosed properly then it can cause severe health complications and also can cause some acute chronic diseases such as- cardiovascular disease, cancer and rheumatoid arthritis. Leaf extract of *M. alba* helps to reduce production of cytokine and pro-inflammatory mediators by nuclear factor- κB (NF-κB) activation suppression [10]. Twigs and root bark of mulberry consists maclurin, morin, resveratrol and isoquercitrin and the fruits of mulberry contains other essential fatty acids like palmitic, linoleic and oleic acids which are also important for inflammatory responses [14]. Stem extract of *M. alba* can inhibit NO production by suppressing both Inos mRNA and protein which shows an inflammatory effect. Anthocyanin present in the fruits of *M. nigra* shows an anti-inflammatory effect by inhibiting pro-inflammatory cytokine which is experimentally proven in mice. Root extract of *M. alba* is potential anti-histamine and anti-allergic natural drug resource as it successfully inhibits the histamine release and systemic allergic reaction [2].

5.5 Anti-oxidant

Different parts of mulberry consists variety of phytochemicals that have the potential of anti-oxidant properties. Moracin available in mulberry fruits help to prevent oxidative stress [14]. Fruit extract of *M. alba* showed radical-scavenging activities against anion radicals and superoxide that increases the level of antioxidants [16]. Moracin which can also be extracted from the leaves of *M. alba* shows better antioxidant activity better than other anti-oxidants like resveratrol. Stem of *M. alba* increase NO scavenging and superoxide activity. Fruits of *M. nigra* show the strongest protective effect against H_2O_2-induced oxidative injury in PC12 cells [2].

5.6 Anti-microbial

Anti-microbial property of mulberry is also well known. The bark of *M. mesozygia* used for the treatment of micro-organism associated infections [41]. Flavonoids isolated from *M. alba* shows positive response in the treatment of antiviral and antifungal diseases [14]. Hydro-methanolic stem bark extract of *M. alba* shows anti-microbial activity against *Enterococcus faecalis*, *Escherichia coli*, *Staphylococcus aureus* and *Salmonella typhimurium* [42–44]. Similarly, ethanolic extract of *M. nigra* prevent the growth of *Staphylococcus epidermidis*, and *Propionibacterium acnes.* Fruits of *M. alba* contain the anti-bacterial compound Morin which strongly inhibits *Streptococcus mutans*. The juice of *M. nigra* contain anti-microbial properties against *Bacillus spizizenii* and *Pseudomonas aeruginosa*. Vinegar produced from *M. alba* shows potential antimicrobial action against *Erwinia carotovora, Streptococcus pyogenes, Bacillus cereus* and anti-fungal activities against *Candida albicans* [2].

5.7 Neurodegenerative actions

For treating cognitive disorders and different types of neuronal dysfunction medicinal plants play an important role and mulberry is one of the most prominent among them. Polyphenolics, alkaloids found in *M. alba* can improve cognitive function and delay in neural-degeneration [45]. Mulberry fruits' lycophilised ethanolic extract can protect against oxidative stress-induced apoptosis in neural cells by the enhancement of the antioxidant enzymes production. In mulberry fruit rutin, quercetin anthocyanins are found present which have an impact on Parkinson's disease (PD) by interfering MPTP-induced dopaminergic neuronal damage and bradykinesia [2, 45].

5.8 Hepatoprotective

A few bioactive compounds obtained from the twigs of *M. mesozygia* esspecially shows the hepatoprotective activities. From *M. indica* a glycoprotein (MIL) is purified which protects against CC14 induced liver damage. In CC14 treated mice MIL found decreasing the activity of Lactate dehydrogenase (LDH), thiobarbituric acid-reactive substances (TBARS), and alanine aminotransferase (ALT). *M. alba* extract found effective in decreasing the activity gastric mucosal injury in rats [14].

5.9 Activity against skin problem due to anti-tyrosinase property

Use of tyrosinase inhibitors is getting huge importance in the cosmetic industry due to their skin-whitening effects. Tyrosinase can be used as a whitening agent as it is a copper-containing primary regulatory multifunctional enzyme that is responsible for the biosynthesis of melanin and determines the color of the skin. Deposition of excessive melanin causes numerous dermatological disorders, such as melasma and age spots [48]. Twigs and roots of mulberry can be utilized as natural agents to react against the tyrosinase activity in cosmetics [49]. In a recent experiment, *M. alba* fruit ethanolic extract has been utilized to formulate an emulsion-based cream to observe its clinical effect on skin melanin, moisture content and erythema for eight weeks. The formulated cream shown significant decrease in melanin content without causing any sort of skin irritation [50]. Betulinic acid ($C_{30}H_{48}O_3$) which has been successfully isolated from *M. alba* (hexane extract of stem and root bark) can be utilized as a whitening agent owing to its tyrosinase inhibitory activity [51]. Ethanolic extract of *M. nigra* shows excellent tyrosinase inhibition activity and also can be exploited for the formulation of peel-off mask and for acne treatment [44, 45]. Mulberries can help to reduce skin problems such as spots and blemishes appears with age and also provides healthier and shiny appearance to skin and hair. From the above discussion, it is clear that mulberry exhibits remarkable tyrosinase inhibition activity, hence can be included as a necessary component of cosmetic products and de-pigmentation agents for the treatment of disorders like hyper-pigmentation.

5.10 Cardiovascular activity

M. alba mostly used in eastern countries to treat cardiovascular diseases. Chinese people also use *M. alba* for decreasing blood pressure which can lead to cardiovascular disorder. It also helps to reduce serum cholesterol, hypertension and also prevents artherosclerosis [47]. From the root bark of *M. alba* morusinol is extracted which prevents collagen and arachidonic acid which induces TXB2 formation in cultured platelets known as the main causative agent of congestive cardiac failure. Mulberries contain Reveratrol, which is a very important flavonoid is found to increase the formation of Nitric oxide (NO) that acts as a vasodilator. Richness of flavanoids and vitamin C makes mulberry also ideal for treating other cold, flu-like problems [14].

6. Conclusion

Best way to find out the solution of hunger and pharmaceutical demand is the discovery and exploitation of new biological resources. Products from natural resources are now being re-emphasized to encounter these issues. Connection between the health and diet is very clear and consumers are now-a-days very much concern about their health. The solution of rural hunger and helping them to come out of the nutritional deficiency is not only a matter of deep concern. Investigating these connections has drawn the attention of the scientists in exploration of biological functional foods and pharmaceuticals, which can dominate the global nutrition market. The current review attempts to point out the potentiality of mulberry species in different areas and it is clear that mulberry is a versatile plant from both food and pharmaceutical aspects with huge possibilities. Mulberry is a jewel of food industry. Being low in calories, this plant can be exploited in the preparation of hypo-caloric foodstuffs and also can be added as a new ingredient to enhance the functional properties of different popular foods. Products like jam, jelly, wine, vinegar, tea, syrup, squash and many more are successfully formulated from mulberry that aids industrialists for further effective utilization of its fruits, leaves and other plant parts. Mulberry is also among the major ingredients in many traditional formulations sold worldwide. In addition to its exceptional usage in the food industry, recent studies have revealed that *Morus* species and their bioactive phytochemicals are having important biomedical activities, including anti-diabetic, antioxidants, anti-obesity, hypo-lipidemic, antihypertensive, and anti-atherosclerosis, etc. Tyrosinase inhibition activity of mulberry is comparable with kojic acid that makes it a wonderful ingredient in cosmetics. Different isolated chemical compounds like maclurin and morin, oxyresveratrol from different parts of *M. alba* shows potential tyrosinase inhibition activity. There are still some unidentified biological novel compounds present in mulberry that require proper exploration. Proper investigation, exploration and exploitation of mulberry in both food and pharmaceutical industry having the potentiality of creating a history.

7. Recommendations

Sericulture is mainly known as a women friendly enterprise, because of the high percentage of involvement of rural women which is about 53.45% of the total employment generated in silk industry. Though broad involvement of rural women are significantly high in the silk industry, but the involvement of tribal people is still scanty [52] which should be considered for extension for financial support and development of small scale industries, mainly in the developing countries. It is the most important fact that the main concentration of the sericulture industry moves around the silkworm feeding, cocoon generation and silk rearing. The proper exploitation of the mulberry in terms of food product and pharmacologically potent substance is still far from the goal. Lack of proper infrastructure for cocoon production and reeling often becomes a barrier for the cultivation of mulberry plant, because *B. mori* moth can only feed upon the fresh and juicy mulberry leaves [53]. Rural people will be able to overcome these constrains if they will be properly trained about the other economic importance of mulberry.

In this context, it is highly recommendable that proper training, campaigning, infrastructure and market development along with broad research and development projects on proper scientific exploitation of mulberry other than feeding the silkworm is absolutely essential and urgent.

Acknowledgements

Authors are grateful to the Hon'ble Vice Chancellor of Raiganj University, India for providing necessary facilities. This research did not receive any specific grant from funding agencies in the public, commercial, or not-for-profit sectors.

Conflict of interest

The authors declare no conflict of interest.

Author details

Ritwik Acharya, Trisha Bagchi and Debnirmalya Gangopadhyay*
Department of Sericulture, Raiganj University, Raiganj, West Bengal, India

*Address all correspondence to: deb_ganguly2003@yahoo.com

References

[1] Vijayan K, Tikader A, Weiguo Z, Nair CV, Ercisli S, Tsou CH. Morus. In: *Wild Crop Relatives: Genomic and Breeding Resources*. Berlin, Heidelberg: Springer; 2011. pp. 75-95

[2] Jan B, Parveen R, Zahiruddin S, Khan MU, Mohapatra S, Ahmad S. Nutritional constituents of mulberry and their potential applications in food and pharmaceuticals: A review. Saudi Journal of Biological Sciences. 2021;**28**(7):3909-3921

[3] Yu Y, Li H, Zhang B, Wang J, Shi X, Huang J, et al. Nutritional and functional components of mulberry leaves from different varieties: Evaluation of their potential as food materials. International Journal of Food Properties. 2018;**21**(1):1495-1507

[4] Arabshahi-Delouee S, Urooj A. Antioxidant properties of various solvent extracts of mulberry (Morus indica L). Leaves Food Chemical. 2007;**102**(4): 1233-1240

[5] Katsube T, Imawaka N, Kawano Y, Yamazaki Y, Shiwaku K, Yamane Y. Antioxidant flavonol glycosides in mulberry (Morus alba L.) leaves isolated based on LDL antioxidant activity. Food Chemistry. 2006;**97**(1):25-31

[6] Asano N, Oseki K, Tomioka E, Kizu H, Matsui K. N-containing sugars from Morus alba and their glycosidase inhibitory activities. Carbohydrate Research. 1994;**259**(2):243-255

[7] Jeszka-Skowron M, Flaczyk E, Jeszka J, Krejpcio Z, Król E, Buchowski MS. Mulberry leaf extract intake reduces hyperglycaemia in streptozotocin (STZ)-induced diabetic rats fed high-fat diet. Journal of Functional Foods. 2014;**8**:9-17

[8] Yang NC, Jhou KY, Tseng CY. Antihypertensive effect of mulberry leaf aqueous extract containing γ-aminobutyric acid in spontaneously hypertensive rats. Food Chemistry. 2012;**132**(4):1796-1180

[9] Harauma A, Murayama T, Ikeyama K, Sano H, Arai H, Takano R, et al. Mulberry leaf powder prevents atherosclerosis in apolipoprotein E-deficient mice. Biochemical and Biophysical Research Communications. 2007;**358**(3):751-756

[10] Park E, Lee S-M, Lee JE, Kim J-H. Anti-inflammatory activity of mulberry leaf extract through inhibition of NF-κB. Journal of Functional Foods. 2013;**5**:178-186

[11] Hu XQ, Jiang L, Zhang JG, Deng W, Wang HL, Wei ZJ. Quantitative determination of 1-deoxynojirimycin in mulberry leaves from 132 varieties. Industrial Crops and Products. 2013;**49**:782-784

[12] Hu XQ, Thakur K, Chen GH, Hu F, Zhang JG, Zhang HB, et al. Metabolic effect of 1-deoxynojirimycin from mulberry leaves on db/db diabetic mice using liquid chromatography–mass spectrometry based metabolomics. Journal of Agricultural and Food Chemistry. 2017;**65**(23):4658-4667

[13] Venkatesh KR, Chauhan S. Mulberry: Life enhancer. Journal of Medicinal Plants Research. 2008;**2**(10):271-278

[14] Kadam RA, Dhumal ND, Khyade VB. The mulberry, Morus alba (L.): The medicinal herbal source for human health. International Journal of Current Microbiology Applied Science. 2019;**8**(4):2941-2964

[15] Yuan Q, Zhao L. The mulberry (Morus alba L.) fruit - a review of characteristic components and health benefits. Journal of Agricultural and Food Chemistry. 2017;**65**(48):10383-10394

[16] Wang S, Liu XM, Zhang J, Zhang YQ. An efficient preparation of mulberroside a from the branch bark of mulberry and its effect on the inhibition of tyrosinase activity. PLoS One. 2014;**9**(10):e109396

[17] Leisinger KM, Schmitt K, Pandya-Lorch R. Six billion and counting: Population growth and food security in the 21st century. Washington, D.C.: International Food Policy Research Institute; 2002

[18] Tutin GT. Morus L. In: Tutin GT, Burges NA, Chater AO, Edmondson JR, Heywood VH, Moore DM, Valentine DH, Walters SM, Webb DA, editors. Flora Europa, Psilotaceae to Platanaceae. 2nd ed. Vol. 1. Australia: Cambridge University Press; 1996

[19] Machii H. A list of genetic mulberry resources maintained at National Institute of sericulture and entomological science. Misc Publications National Seric Entomology Science (Japan). 1999;**26**:1-77

[20] Le Houerou HN. The role of browse in the management of natural grazing lands. In: Le Houerou HN, editor. Browse in Africa, the current state of knowledge. Ethiopia: International Livestock Centre for Africa; 1980. pp. 329-338

[21] Wani MY, Mir MR, Baqual MF, Ganie NA, Bhat ZA, Ganie Q. Roles of mulberry tree. The Pharma Innovation. 2017;**6**(9):143-147

[22] Khalid N, Fawad SA, Ahmed I. Antimicrobial activity, phytochemical profile and trace minerals of black mulberry (Morus nigra L.) fresh juice. Pakistan Journal of Botany. 2011;**43**(6):91-96

[23] Rahman AHMM. Khanom a. *taxonomic and ethno-medicinal study of species from Moraceae (mulberry) family i n Bangladesh Flora*. Research in Plant Sciences. 2013;**1**:53-57

[24] Hamid H, Thakur NS. Development of appetizer (spiced squash) from mulberry (Morus alba L.) and its quality evaluation during storage. Journal of Applied and Natural Science. 2017;**9**(4):2235-2241

[25] Komolka P, Gorecka D, Buszka KS, Golinska AJ, Dziedzic K, Waszkowiak K. Sensory qualities of pastry products enriched with dietary fiber and polyphenolic substances. *Acta Scientiarum Polonorum, Technologia*. Alimentaria. 2016;**15**(2):161-170

[26] Gültekin-Özgüven M, Karadağ A, Duman Ş, Özkal B, Özçelik B. Fortification of dark chocolate with spray dried black mulberry (Morus nigra) waste extract encapsulated in chitosan-coated liposomes and bioaccessability studies. Food Chemistry. 2016;**201**:205-212

[27] Yazdankhah S, Mohammad H, Mohammad HA. The antidiabetic potential of black mulberry extract-enriched pasta through inhibition of enzymes and glycemic index. Plant Foods for Human Nutrition. 2019;**74**:149-155

[28] Byamukama R, Andima M, Mbabazi A, Kiremire BT. Anthocyanins from mulberry (*Morus alba*) fruits as potential natural colour additives in yoghurt. African Journal of Pure and Applied Chemistry. 2014;**8**(12):182-190

[29] Wongchalat R, Chatthongpisut R. Nutritional value and anthocyanins

of mulberry and Roselle mixed fruits jam. Applied Mechanics and Materials. 2016;**855**:65-69

[30] Thakur NS, Kumar P, Thakur A. Development of syrup from mulberry (Morus alba L.) and its quality evaluation under ambient and refrigerated storage conditions. International Journal of Bio-Resource & Stress Management. 2017;**8**(1):116-121

[31] Karaagac RA. An investigation of antimicrobial properties and antioxidant activities of mulberry vinegar which is naturally produce In Uzundere and Ispir (Erzurum). Journal of Pharmaceutical Biology. 2016;**6**(1):34-39

[32] Darias-Martín J, Lobo-Rodrigo G, Hernández-Cordero J, Díaz-Díaz E, Díaz-Romero C. Alcoholic beverages obtained from black mulberry. Food Technology and Biotechnology. 2003;**41**(2):173-176

[33] Ghosh A, Gangopadhyay D, Chowdhury T. Economical and environmental importance of mulberry: A review. International Journal of Plant and Environment. 2017;**3**(2):51-58

[34] Srivastava S, Kapoor R, Thathola A, Srivastava RP. Nutritional quality of leaves of some genotypes of mulberry (Morus alba). International Journal of Food Sciences and Nutrition. 2016;**57**(5-6):305-313

[35] Jalikop SH, Kumar R, Shivashankara KS. Variability in mulberry (Morus spp.) accessions for plant and fruit traits and antioxidant properties. Acta Horticulturae. 2011;**890**(890):267-272

[36] Yildiz O. Physicochemical and sensory properties of mulberry products: Gümüşhane pestil and köme. Turkish Journal of Agriculture and Forestry. 2013;**37**(6):762-771

[37] Eecisli S, Orhan E. Chemical composition of white (*Morus Alba*), red (*Morus Rubra*), and black (*Morus Nigra*) mulberry fruits. Food Chemistry. 2007;**103**(4):1380-1384

[38] Buhroo ZI, Bhat M, Kamili AS, Ganai N, Bali GK, Khan IL, et al. Trends in development and utilization of sericulture resources for diversification and value addition. Journal of Entomology and Zoology Studies. 2018;**6**(4):601-615

[39] Naowaratwattana W, De-Eknamkul W, De Mejia EG. Phenolic-containing organic extracts of mulberry (Morus alba L.) leaves inhibit HepG2 hepatoma cells through G2/M phase arrest, induction of apoptosis, and inhibition of topoisomerase IIα activity. Journal of Medicinal Food. 2010;**13**(5):1045-1056

[40] Alanazi AS, Anwar MJ, Alam MN. Hypoglycemic and antioxidant effect of morus alba l. stem bark extracts in streptozotocin-induced diabetes in rats. Journal of Applied Pharmacy. 2017;**9**(234):2

[41] Kuete V, Fozing DC, Kapche WFGD, Mbaveng AT, Kuiate JR, Ngadjui BT, et al. Antimicrobial activity of the methanolic extract and compounds from *Morus mesozygia* stem bark. Journal of Ethnopharmacology. 2009;**124**(3):551-555

[42] Fukai T, Kaitou K, Terada S. Antimicrobial activity of 2-arylbenzofurans from Morus species against methicillin-resistant Staphylococcus aureus. Fitoterapia. 2005;**76**(7-8):708-711

[43] Thabti I, Elfalleh W, Tlili N, Ziadi M, Campos MG, Ferchichi A. Phenols, flavonoids, and antioxidant and antibacterial activity of leaves and stem bark of *Morus* species.

International Journal of Food Properties. 2014;**17**:842-854

[44] Budiman A, Aulifa DL, Kusuma ASW, Kurniawan IS, Sulastri A. Peel-off gel formulation from black mulberries (Morus nigra) extract as anti-acne mask. National Journal of Physiology, Pharmacy and Pharmacology. 2017;**7**(9):987-994

[45] Kim J, Yun EY, Quan FS, Park SW, Goo TW. Central administration of 1-deoxynojirimycin attenuates hypothalamic endoplasmic reticulum stress and regulates food intake and body weight in mice with high-fat diet-induced obesity. Evidence-based Complementary and Alternative Medicine. 2017;**2017**:1-11

[46] Chang LW, Juang LJ, Wang BS, Wang MY, Tai HM, Hung WJ, et al. Antioxidant and antityrosinase activity of mulberry (Morus alba L.) twigs and root bark. Food and Chemical Toxicology. 2011;**49**(4):785-790

[47] Doi K, Kojima T, FUJIMOTO, Y. Mulberry leaf extract inhibits the oxidative modification of rabbit and human low density lipoprotein. Biological and Pharmaceutical Bulletin. 2000;**23**(9):1066-1071

[48] Mukherjee PK, Biswas R, Sharma A, Banerjee S, Biswas S, Katiyar CK. Validation of medicinal herbs for anti-tyrosinase potential. Journal of Herbal Medicine. 2018;**14**:1-16

[49] Li HX, Park JU, Su XD, Kim KT, Kang JS, Kim YR, et al. Identification of anti-melanogenesis constituents from Morus alba L. leaves. Molecules. 2018;**23**(10):2559

[50] Akhtar N, Hisham J, Khan HMS, Khan BA, Mahmood T, Saeed T. Whitening and antierythemic effect of a cream containing Morus alba extract. Hygeia Journal for Drugs and Medicines. 2012;**4**(1):97-103

[51] Nattapong S, Omboon L. A new source of whitening agent from a Thai mulberry plant and its betulinic acid quantitation. Natural Product Research. 2008;**22**(9):727-734

[52] Dewangan SK, Sahu KR. Participation of tribal women in sericulture in two tribal block of Raigarh District, Chhattisgarh, India. Asian Journal of Agriculture & Life Sciences. 2017;**2**(1):13-22

[53] Srinivasa G, Sarangi RN, Geetha GS, Rahmathulla VK, Geethadevi RG. Factors influencing the cocoon yield and sericultural income. Indian Journal of Sericulture. 2004;**43**(1):42-45

Chapter 20

Ginkgo biloba: A Potential Anti-Cancer Agent

Jian-Shu Lou, Die Hu, Hao-Jie Wang, Li-Ping Zhao, Jun-Hu Hu and Zhao-Huang Zhou

Abstract

Ginkgo biloba is generally considered as safe herbal extract in clinical application. Ginkgo Folium is a living fossil plant, which has been used in record by over few thousands of years. The extract of *G. biloba*, has been used extensively for the treatment of diseases related to the central nervous system and psychiatric disorders. Recently, different lines of evidence indicated that *G. biloba* exhibited anti-cancer effects. The potential therapeutic effect may due to antioxidant, anti-angiogenic and gene regulatory actions. In addition, Ginkgo Folium was studied in pharmacodynamic interactions induced by herb-drug interactions. These studies indicated that *G. biloba* usually exhibits synergistic effect. The extracts derived from *G. biloba* exhibits promising anticancer effect, including flavonoids, ginkgolide, and phenolic acids etc. This chapter will discuss the anticancer effect and mechanism of extracts derived from various parts of *G. biloba*, the possible usage as an adjuvant therapy in cancer treatment, and the development of *G. biloba* as potential novel anticancer drugs.

Keywords: *Ginkgo biloba*, cancer, natural products, herbal extract

1. Introduction

Almost everyone talks about cancer discoloration, and no matter what kind of cancer it is, it can be life-threatening. But fortunately, cancer can also be treated, in addition to mastering the rhythm of life, you can also choose Chinese herbal medicine to strengthen the immunity and enhance the ability to anti-cancer. The active gradients from several plants have anticancer effect, such as Elemene, vincristine and ginsenosides [1–6]. Elemene, isolated from the volatile oil of traditional Chinese medicine Curcuma wenyujin, has broad-spectrum anticancer activities and mild side effects. Vincristine is derived from periwinkle, which is used for the treatment of acute lymphoblastic leukemia, breast cancer. Ginsenosides is extracted from ginseng. Ginseng has been regarded as a famous traditional Chinese medicine since ancient times. After treatment with ginsenosides, ginsenosides inhibited cancer cell proliferation, invasion, and migration in several cancers, such as breast, brain, liver, gastric, and lung cancer [5].

In recent years, more and more studies have shown that *G. biloba* also has antitumor effects. *G. biloba* appeared on earth more than 200 million years ago and is the only living species in the order Ginkgoales [7–9]. Once *G. biloba* was growing everywhere on earth, but it became nearly extinct during the last ice age, and only survived in Asia. *G. biloba* has been used as a medicinal plant for a long time. It was firstly recorded in "Shennong Ben Cao Jing, but the medicinal value of ginkgo leaves recorded from the Song Dynasty. The medical use of *G. biloba* was first recorded in "Ben Cao Gang Mu" by Li Shizhen in Ming Dynasty [10]. *G. biloba* leaves are fan-shaped, flat, and have an indentation in the middle, giving birth to a species name "Biloba," a Latin word meaning bi-lobed [11]. Male flower pollens are carried by the wind to the female tree, which produces ovules that fertilize and grow into seeds. *G. biloba* takes 15 to 20 years to produce fruits, which have a rancid, nasty odor. However, the seeds contain certain mild toxic chemicals [12–14]. *G. biloba* has been a beloved plant in Asian countries as an ornamental tree in the gardens and as a medicinal plant, particularly in China, Korea, and Japan [15, 16].

Scientists from Japan and Germany made pioneering and important contributions to research and development. The development history of *G. biloba* fully embodies the determination of innovation and has become a model for the research and development of traditional Chinese medicine and botanic medicine. In 1929, the Japanese first isolated a flavonoid from *G. biloba* leaves [17]. In the 1960s, Dr. Schwab firstly extracted the active ingredients (ginkgo flavone and terpenoid lactone) from Chinese *G. biloba* leaves, which were processed into tablets. These active ingredients quickly became the first world's plant medicine, which were listed as the third generation of *G. biloba* leaves preparation. In 1972, Dr. Willmar Schwabe Company developed EGb761, a patent extract of *G. biloba* leaves. EGb761 contains 24% flavonoids and 6% terpenoids, which is widely used today [18]. From the 1920s to the 1930s, Chinese herbal medicine research upsurge, medical scholars began to analyze the chemical components of G. biloba, pharmacodynamics and toxicology research, with G. biloba tablet, known as the first generation of preparation. In the 1970s, Germany, France and other European countries carried out in-depth research on *G. biloba* leaves. Flavonoids and lactones extracted *G. biloba* have therapeutic effects on cardiovascular and cerebrovascular diseases [19]. In the 1990s, Professor Xie Delong, director of Shanghai Institute of Traditional Chinese Medicine, discovered a safer and more effective combination than the German ginkgo leaf invention patent, and innovated the process to raise the clear effective component of the extract to more than 50%, which was listed as the fifth generation of ginkgo leaf preparation.

At present, flavonoids (quercetin, kaempferol, isorhamnetin, lignin, etc.) and terpenoids (ginkgolide A, Ginkgolide B, ginkgolide C, ginkgolide J, etc.) have been found to be active pharmacological components in *G. biloba* [20]. It is recorded in Chinese Pharmacopoeia that *G. biloba* has the effects on promoting blood circulation and removing stasis, clearing collaterals and relieving pain, strengthening lungs and relieving asthma, removing turbidity and lowering lipids, and is used to treat blood stasis and blocking collaterals, chest paralysis and heartache, stroke hemiplegia, lung deficiency, cough and asthma, hyperlipidemia and other diseases [21–23]. In recent years, studies have also found that the pharmacological effect of *G. biloba* lies in the synergistic effect of various components, rather than a component to play a determined role. Studies have shown that *G. biloba* extract plays a significant role in the treatment of Alzheimer's disease, neurodegenerative diseases, brain dysfunction, eye diseases, cardiovascular diseases and other diseases. Moreover, recent studies have shown that extract from different part of *G. biloba* may also be useful in treating cancer [24].

2. Anticancer effect of extracts derived from various parts of *G. biloba*

Plants have provided a rich source of therapeutic agents and bases for synthetic drugs. *G. biloba* is dioecious. Male ginkgo biloba release pollen in spring to fertilize the female ginkgo biloba, which produces a large amount of ginkgo drup-like seeds in fall [25]. The seeds of *G. biloba* have been used for the treatment of cancer thousands of years ago in China [26], which is first mentioned in herbals in the Yuan dynasty. Mature ginkgo seeds covered with a fleshy thick outer layer, which named as exocarps, or seed coat, sarcotesta in some research papers. Seed mainly consists of mesosperm, membranous endopleura and kernel. The mesosperm is hard and white shell. The innermost layer of the seed is membranous endopleura, which is red and consists of 1–2 layers of parenchymal cells. The kernal of *G. biloba* is fleshy and pale yellowish-green, consisting of endosperm and embryo, which is an edible part of the seed. The leaves of *G. biloba* (*Ginkgo folium*) are fan-shaped, which are unique among seed plants.

Studies reported that extract or active ingredient from different parts of *G. biloba,* including seeds, exocarps, kernel and flowers exert anticancer effect. In recent years, the anticancer effect of *Ginkgo folium* was extensively reported. We summarized the current reports on the anticancer effect and potential mechanism of the extracts from the different parts of *G. biloba.*

2.1 The anticancer effect of *G. biloba* seeds

G. biloba seeds have been used in traditional Chinese medicine for centuries. The seeds have orange flesh shell, which are toxic as raw forms. The annual global yield of seeds is over 14 kt, more than 90% of which is produced in China [27]. As a traditional Chinese medicinal material, the ginkgo seeds have been used for clinical diseases such as asthma, coughs, cancers and etc. *G. biloba* seeds formed by the development of a fertilized ovule, contains an embryo and nutrient reserves that enable a new plant to grow. Only a few researches on the anticancer effects of *G. biloba* seeds extract. *G. biloba* seeds extracts positively induce cytochrome P450 (CYP) 1B1 expression, inhibiting the proliferation of breast cancer cells [28]. In this vitro study, polysaccharide derived from *G. biloba* seeds was isolated by ethanol fractionation, which decrease the percentages of G2-M cells, inhibiting the hepatoma cells proliferation. In addition, *G. biloba* seeds polysaccharides also make microvilli thinner and form apoptosis bodies on and around the spherical cells to promote apoptosis in hepatoma cells. While the hepatoma cells without *G. biloba* seeds polysaccharide treatment were of shuttle shape and small proportion of cells was of spherical shape [29].

2.2 The anticancer effect of *G. biloba* exocarps extract

G. biloba exocarp is the outermost layer of seeds, which was also called seed coat or sarcotesta in some studies. Exocarp was previously regarded as a waste material. It smells of rancid butter, causesing air pollution. Phenolic acid in exocarp can contaminate soil and poison fish and shrimp [30, 31]. Exocarp is rich in nutrients: the percent of polysaccharide is 10% and ginkgolic acids is more than 4%. Recently, constituents extracted from the exocarp shows antitumor effect [32].

The extracts prepare from the exocarps of *G. biloba* (GBEE) enhanced the ratio of Bax/Bcl-2. Meantime, the translocation of Bax/Bcl-2 to mitochondria was also increased accompanied by the release of cytochrome C. Consequently, the protein expression of cleaved-caspase-3, Fas, FasL, p-p38, and the mRNA levels of Fas were all increased, finally inducing apoptosis in lewis lung carcinoma cells (LLC). In vivo study further demonstrated the anticancer effect of GBEE on LLC [33]. GBEE increased the activation of acidic vacuole, the content of Atg5 protein and the ratio of LC3-II/LC3-I protein by AMPK induced inactivation on mTOR/p70S6k, which promoted the formation of autophagosomes in LCC, finally it induced autophagic cell death in LCC [34].

Despite of the directly effect on inducing cancer cell death, GBEE can also suppress the processes of angiogenesis and metastasis. It was reported that GBEE inhibited tumor metastasis in LLC mice model, characterized by the suppression on CD34 and microvessel density (MVD). This anti-metastasis effect might be due to the inhibition on angiogenesis, which mediated by downregulation on Wnt/β-catenin- vascular endothelial growth factor (VEGF) signaling pathway, including the inhibition on Wnt3a, β-catenin, VEGF, VEGF2 and p-AKT/AKT [35]. The suppression of GBEE on CD34 and MVD was also found in B16 melanoma. Meanwhile, GBEE attenuated the mRNA and protein levels of VEGF, hypoxia inducible factor-1α (HIF-1α), vascular endothelial growth factor receptor 2 (VEGFR2), p-PI3K and p-Akt. Finally, it exerted antiangiogenesis by inhibiting PI3K/Akt/HIF-1α/VEGF signaling pathways [36]. *G. biloba* exocarp extracts also have anti-metastasis effect in skin cancer via perturbing the expression of p-PI3K, p-Akt, NF-κB, and MMP-9 [37].

The polysaccharides isolated from *G. biloba* exocarp (GBEP) had therapeutic effect on cancer patients [33, 38, 39]. For instance, the area of tumors in patients with GBEP capsules were significantly reduced. Meanwhile, the ultrastructural of tumor cells in these patients observed by transmissional electron microscope revealed that abundant heterochromatins were observed in nuclei, swollen mitochondria and dilated rough endoplasmic reticulum were observed in cytosol, indicating apoptosis was triggered by GBEP [40]. The anticancer effect of GBEP was demonstrated in tumor bearing mice [39]. The mechanism involved in the anticancer effect of GBEP was illustrated in gastric cancer. GBEP downregulated the expression of c-myc and bcl-2, upregulated the level of c-fos genes, which inhibited proliferation and induced apoptosis on gastric cancer [40].

Botanical constituents extracted from the exocarp of *G. biloba* promoted ROS generation, which inducing G0/G1 phase arrest, apoptosis and autophagy in colon cancer cells. RT-qPCR analysis showed that Ginkgolic acid (GA) decreased Cyclin D1, CDK2, CDK4, and Cyclin E1 mRNA levels. The study also found that decreased p-mTOR, pp70s6k and p-pras40 protein levels induced by GA were reversed by NAC pretreatment [41]. GA extracted from the *G. biloba* exocarp promoted the activation of AMPK, decreased the level of acetyl-CoA carboxylase (ACC) and fatty acid synthase (FASN) involved in lipogenesis. Finally, it plays a positive role in inhibiting pancreatic cancer cells proliferation, migration and invasion. The study examined the effects of GA on the viability of pancreatic cancer cell by MTT assay, found that GA can inhibit the growth of pancreatic cancer cells. Wound-scratch assay and scratch assay showed that GA inhibited the migration and invasion capacities of pancreatic cancer cells in vitro [42]. GA activated caspase-3, decreased the expression of Bcl-2 protein and increased the expression of Bax protein, finally causing apoptosis in laryngeal cancer cells [43]. GA also had positive anticancer effects in gastric cancer cells and liver cancer [44, 45]. After treatment with GA, the morphology of liver cancer cell was shrinkage and formed nuclear fragmentation, activating caspases-3 and promoting Bax expression. Finally, it induced apoptosis in liver cancer cells [45]. GA perturbed the proliferation of human cervical cancer cells and enhanced immune function on immunocompromised S180. But the correlation of GA promoting S180 immune function needs to be further studied [46]. A vitro experiment verified that with the increase of GA concentration on cancer cells, GA inhibited the growth of cancer cells but the toxic effect on normal cells also increases. The anti-tumor effect of GA needs to be further proved by animal experiments [47].

2.3 The anticancer effect of *G. biloba* kernel extract

G. biloba kernels called Baiguo in China are the main edible part of the seed, which consist of endosperm and embryo [48]. Ginkgo kernel is consumed as a delicious food in China, Japan and Korea after grilled or boiled [49]. Ginkgo kernels contain 60–70% starch, 10–20% protein, 2–4% lipids, 0.8–1.2% pectin, and about 6% sucrose [50, 51]. Raw or cooked the ginkgo kernel has been shown to cause allergic reactions or death [52]. The medicinal value of ginkgo kernel was overlooked. A few studies shed light to the anticancer effect of kernel. The medicinal value of ginkgo kernel was overlooked. A few studies shed light to the anticancer effect of kernel [53]. However, the role of total G. biloba kernel extract on anticancer was reported recently. A study firstly reported that *G. biloba* kernel extracts exhibited cytotoxic effects in colon cancer and melanoma, characterized by inhibiting cancer cells proliferation and vitality [54]. Melanoma cells are more sensitive to kernel extracts. Meantime, the cytotoxic effect was not found in normal cell line McCoy-Plovdive. However, the anticancer effect of kernel extract needs to be observed in other cancer types, and the molecular mechanism remains to be observed in detail in future.

2.4 The anticancer effect of *G. biloba* flowers extract

G. biloba is an ancient dioecious gymnosperm, which apply to worldwide for landscaping and medical usage. The male flowers with catkin blossom from late March to the middle of April for only three to seven days, varying in different areas of China [55]. The chemical constituents and bioactivities of the flowers contain high contents of nutritional and medicinally relevant components, such as amino acids, vitamins, unsaturated fatty acids, flavonoids, and lactones [56]. The extracts of ginkgo flowers can exhibit anticancer effects. Some phytochemical studies of *G. biloba* flowers enrich the diversity of Ginkgo chemical constituents and broaden its application in phytotherapy. The bioflavonoids from *G. biloba* male flowers promoted cell cycle arrest in the G2/M phase, inhibiting the proliferation of cervical cancer cells [57]. A study showed that biflavonoids bilobetin and isoginkgetin isolated from *G. biloba* flowers exhibited cytotoxic activities on cervical cancer, pancreatic cancer, lung cancer, Lymphoma, and ovarian cancer. The most sensitive cancer cell to these two compounds is cervical cancer. Furthermore, the morphological changes, apoptosis and cell cycle arrest were observed in cervical cancer cell. After treated with bilobetin and isoginkgetin, nuclear condensation together with the decrease on the ratio of Bcl2/BAX and the increase on cleaved-caspase 3, apoptosis rates were observed, indicating that apoptosis was triggered with these two compounds. In addition, cell cycle arrest via promoting G2/M phase arrest was also found in cervical cancer cell treated with bilobetin and isoginkgetin [55].

2.5 The anticancer effect of *Ginkgo Folium* extract

The anticancer effect of *Ginkgo Folium* was studied extensively in recent years. The tumor inhibition effect of *Ginkgo Folium* was demonstrated in mouse S180 mouse sarcoma, which might be due to the elevation on free radical scavenger enzymes [58]. The main reported death way induced by *Ginkgo Folium* is caspase dependent apoptosis that was observed in several cancer types, including cervical cancer [59], colon cancer [60], gastric cancer [61], melanoma [62]. The mechanism responsible for *Ginkgo Folium* induced apoptosis is the disruption on the balance of antiapoptotic protein Bcl-2 and proapoptotic protein BAX, characterized by the decrease on Bcl-2 and the increase on BAX.

Despite of apoptosis, *Ginkgo Folium* can also arrest cell cycle and inhibit cancer cell migration and invasion. The cell cycle arrest induced by *Ginkgo Folium* was due to the suppression on G0/G1 phase in gastric cancer [61, 63]. The suppression on cancer cell migration and invasion were observed in several cancer types through multiple ways. First, upregulation on E-cadherin via lincRNA-p21 mediated suppression on E-cadherin degradation in colon cancer [64]. Second, downregulation on ERK/NF-kB signaling in gastric cancer [65]. Third, inhibition on heat-shock protein 27 (HSP27) mediated by AKT and p38 MAPK pathways in NSCLC [66].

The extracts of *Ginkgo Folium* can combine with herbal formulation to exhibit synergistic effect on anticancer. For instance, it was reported that a new formulation consisted of *Ginkgo Follium* and an herbal mixture Yu Ping Feng San can sensitize cisplatin resistant lung cancer cells through WT1/MVP mediated stabilization on mTOR/AKT pathway [67]. There are few clinical studies on anticancer effect of *Ginkgo*. Considering *Ginkgo Folium* extract has the standard commercial product EGb761, thus, it will be alliable to conduct clinical research with EGb761 to observe whether *Ginkgo* could serve as an adjuvant therapy on anticancer.

3. Conclusions

G. biloba has been used to treat age-related disorders and improve blood circulation. Recently, the extract from ginkgo exocarp, seed, kernel, flowers and Folium showed anticancer effect in various cancer types. The reported researches are mainly focus on the in vitro and in in vivo studies. Clinical studies are need to be further conducted to verify their anticancer effect. Furthermore, the detailed mechanism and the active ingredient responsible for the anticancer effect are still need to be elucidated.

Acknowledgements

This work is supported by the Key Programme of National Natural Science Foundation of China [81730108, 81973635]; the National Natural Science Foundation of China [82174024]; the Natural Science Foundation of Zhejiang Province [LY20H280011]; and the Medical Health Science and Technology Project of Zhejiang Provincial Health Commission [2020367195, 2022508369].

Conflict of interest

The authors declare no conflict of interest.

Author details

Jian-Shu Lou[1,2]*, Die Hu[1,2], Hao-Jie Wang[1,2], Li-Ping Zhao[1,2], Jun-Hu Hu[1,2] and Zhao-Huang Zhou[1,2]

1 School of Pharmacy, Hangzhou Normal University, Hangzhou, Zhejiang, China

2 Key Laboratory of Elemene Class Anti-Cancer Chinese Medicines, Engineering Laboratory of Development and Application of Traditional Chinese Medicines, Collaborative Innovation Center of Traditional Chinese Medicines of Zhejiang Province, Hangzhou Normal University, Hangzhou, Zhejiang, China

*Address all correspondence to: jlouab@connect.ust.hk

References

[1] Lin L, Li L, Chen X, Zeng B, Lin T. Preliminary evaluation of the potential role of β-elemene in reversing erlotinib-resistant human NSCLC A549/ER cells. Oncology Letters. 2018;**16**:3380-3388. DOI: 10.3892/ol.2018.8980

[2] Gong M, Liu Y, Zhang J, Gao YJ, Zhai PP, Su X, et al. β-Elemene Inhibits Cell Proliferation by Regulating the Expression and Activity of Topoisomerases I and IIα in Human Hepatocarcinoma HepG-2 Cells. BioMed Research International. 2015;**2015**:153987. DOI: 10.1155/2015/153987

[3] Han Z, Huang H, Zhang T. Downregulation of DBN1 is related to vincristine resistance in colon cancer cells. Journal of Cancer Research and Therapeutics. 2019;**15**:38-41. DOI: 10.4103/0973-1482.192766

[4] Becker S, Kiecke C, Schäfer E, Sinzig U. Destruction of a Microtubule-Bound MYC Reservoir during Mitosis Contributes to Vincristine's Anticancer Activity. Molecular Cancer Research. 2020;**18**:859-872. DOI: 10.1158/1541-7786

[5] Hong H, Baatar D, Hwang SG. Anticancer Activities of Ginsenosides, the Main Active Components of Ginseng. Evidence-based Complementary and Alternative Medicine. 2021;**2021**:8858006. DOI: 10.1155/2021/8858006

[6] Li X, Chu S, Lin M, Gao Y, Liu Y, Yang S, et al. Anticancer property of ginsenoside Rh2 from ginseng. European Journal of Medicinal Chemistry. 2020;**203**:112627. DOI: 10.1016/j.ejmech.2020.112627

[7] Zeng Z, Zhu J, Chen L, Wen W, Yu R. Biosynthesis pathways of ginkgolides. Pharmacognosy Reviews. 2013;**7**:47-52. DOI: 10.4103/0973-7847.112848

[8] Gertz HJ, Kiefer M. Review about Ginkgo biloba special extract EGb 761 (Ginkgo). Current Pharmaceutical Design. 2004;**10**:261-264. DOI: 10.2174/1381612043386437

[9] Yuan Z, Tian Y, He F, Zhou H. Endophytes from Ginkgo biloba and their secondary metabolites. Chinese Medicine. 2019;**14**:51. DOI: 10.1186/s13020-019-0271-8

[10] Liu L, Wang Y, Zhang J, Wang S. Advances in the chemical constituents and chemical analysis of Ginkgo biloba leaf, extract, and phytopharmaceuticals. Journal of Pharmaceutical and Biomedical Analysis. 2021;**193**:113704. DOI: 10.1016/j.jpba.2020.113704

[11] Strømgaard K, Nakanishi K. Chemistry and biology of terpene trilactones from Ginkgo biloba. Angewandte Chemie (International Ed. in English). 2004;**43**:1640-1658. DOI: 10.1002/anie.200300601

[12] Mei N, Guo X, Ren Z, Kobayashi D, Wada K, Guo L. Review of Ginkgo biloba-induced toxicity, from experimental studies to human case reports. Journal of Environmental Science and Health. Part C, Environmental Carcinogenesis & Ecotoxicology Reviews. 2017;**35**:1-28. DOI: 10.1080/10590501.2016.1278298

[13] Boateng ID, Yang XM. Effect of different drying methods on product quality, bioactive and toxic components of Ginkgo biloba L. seed. Journal of the Science of Food and Agriculture. 2021;**101**:3290-3297. DOI: 10.1002/jsfa.10958

[14] Zhu JP, Gong H, Labreche F, Kou XH, Wu CE, Fan GJ, et al. In vivo toxicity assessment of 4'-O-methylpyridoxine from Ginkgo biloba seeds: Growth, hematology, metabolism, and oxidative parameters. Toxicon. 2021;**201**:66-73. DOI: 10.1016/j.toxicon.2021.08.015

[15] Kirschner R, Okuda T. A new species of Pseudocercospora and new record of Bartheletia paradoxa on leaves of Ginkgo biloba. Mycological Progress. 2013;**12**:421-426. DOI: 10.1007/s11557-012-0849-3

[16] Mahmoudian-Sani MR, Hashemzadeh-Chaleshtori M, Asadi-Samani M, Yang Q. Ginkgo biloba in the treatment of tinnitus: An updated literature review. The International Tinnitus Journal. 2017;**21**:58-62. DOI: 10.5935/0946-5448.20170011

[17] Isah T. Rethinking Ginkgo biloba L.: Medicinal uses and conservation. Pharmacognosy Reviews. 2015;**9**:140-148. DOI: 10.4103/0973-7847.162137

[18] Tanaka K, Galduróz RF, Gobbi LT, Galduróz JC. Ginkgo biloba extract in an animal model of Parkinson's disease: a systematic review. Current Neuropharmacology. 2013;**11**:430-435. DOI: 10.2174/1570159X11311040006

[19] Zuo W, Yan F, Zhang B, Li J, Mei D. Advances in the Studies of Ginkgo Biloba Leaves Extract on Aging-Related Diseases. Aging and Disease. 2017;**8**:812-826. DOI: 10.14336/AD.2017.0615

[20] Zhao Y, Sun Y, Li C. Simultaneous determination of ginkgo flavonoids and terpenoids in plasma: ammonium formate in LC mobile phase enhancing electrospray ionization efficiency and capacity. Journal of the American Society for Mass Spectrometry. 2008;**19**:445-449. DOI: 10.1016/j.jasms.2007.11.015

[21] Wu Y, Wang T, Xin Y, Wang G, Xu LA. Overexpression of GbF3'5'H1 Provides a Potential to Improve the Content of Epicatechin and Gallocatechin. Molecules. 2020;**25**:4836. DOI: 10.3390/molecules25204836

[22] Wang B, Wei PW, Wan S, Yao Y, Song CR, Song PP, et al. Ginkgo biloba exocarp extracts inhibit S. aureus and MRSA by disrupting biofilms and affecting gene expression. Journal of Ethnopharmacology. 2021;**271**:113895. DOI: 10.1016/j.jep.2021.113895

[23] Liu PK, Weng ZM, Ge GB, Li HL, Ding LL, Dai ZR, et al. Biflavones from Ginkgo biloba as novel pancreatic lipase inhibitors: Inhibition potentials and mechanism. International Journal of Biological Macromolecules. 2018;**118**:2216-2223. DOI: 10.1016/j.ijbiomac.2018.07.085

[24] Wang Y, Lv J, Cheng Y, Du J, Chen D, Li C, et al. Apoptosis induced by Ginkgo biloba (EGb761) in melanoma cells is Mcl-1-dependent. PLoS One. 2015;**10**:e0124812. DOI: 10.1371/journal.pone.0124812

[25] D'Apice G, Moschin S, Araniti F, Nigris S, Di Marzo M, Muto A, et al. The role of pollination in controlling Ginkgo biloba ovule development. The New Phytologist. 2021;**232**:2353-2368. DOI: 10.1111/nph.17753

[26] Boateng ID, Yang XM. Ginkgo biloba L. seed; A comprehensive review of bioactives, toxicants, and processing effects. Industrial Crops and Products. 2022;**176**:114281. DOI: 10.1016/j.indcrop.2021.114281

[27] Zhou M, Hua T, Ma X, Sun H, Xu L. Protein content and amino acids profile in 10 cultivars of ginkgo (Ginkgo biloba L.) nut from China. Royal Society Open Science. 2019;**6**:181571. DOI: 10.1098/rsos.181571

[28] Zhao XD, Dong N, Man HT, Fu ZL, Zhang MH, Kou S, et al. Antiproliferative effect of the Ginkgo biloba extract is associated with the enhancement of cytochrome P450 1B1 expression in estrogen receptor-negative breast cancer cells. Biomed Rep. 2013;**1**:797-801. DOI: 10.3892/br.2013.150

[29] Chen Q, Yang GW, An LG. Apoptosis of hepatoma cells SMMC-7721 induced by Ginkgo biloba seed polysaccharide. World Journal of Gastroenterology. 2002;**8**:832-836. DOI: 10.3748/wjg.v8.i5.832

[30] Jiang H, Luan Z, Fan Z, Wu X, Xu Z, Zhou T, et al. Antibacterial, Antibiofilm, and Antioxidant Activity of Polysaccharides Obtained from Fresh Sarcotesta of Ginkgo biloba: Bioactive Polysaccharide that Can Be Exploited as a Novel Biocontrol Agent. Evidence-based Complementary and Alternative Medicine. 2021;**2021**:5518403. DOI: 10.1155/2021/5518403

[31] Ye J, Ye C, Huang Y, Zhang N, Zhang X, Xiao M. Ginkgo biloba sarcotesta polysaccharide inhibits inflammatory responses through suppressing both NF-κB and MAPK signaling pathway. Journal of the Science of Food and Agriculture. 2019;**99**:2329-2339. DOI: 10.1002/jsfa.9431

[32] Zhou G, Yao X, Tang Y, Yang N, Pang H, Mo X, et al. Two new nonacosanetriols from Ginkgo biloba sarcotesta. Chemistry and Physics of Lipids. 2012;**165**:731-736. DOI: 10.1016/j.chemphyslip.2012.08.003

[33] Xu AH, Chen HS, Sun BC, Xiang XR, Chu YF, Zhai F, et al. Therapeutic mechanism of ginkgo biloba exocarp polysaccharides on gastric cancer. World Journal of Gastroenterology. 2003;**9**:2424-2427. DOI: 10.3748/wjg.v9.i11.2424

[34] Cao C, Han D, Su Y, Ge Y, Chen H, Xu A. Ginkgo biloba exocarp extracts induces autophagy in Lewis lung cancer cells involving AMPK/mTOR/p70S6k signaling pathway. Biomedicine & Pharmacotherapy. 2017;**93**:1128-1135. DOI: 10.1016/j.biopha.2017.07.036

[35] Han D, Cao C, Su Y, Wang J, Sun J, Chen H, et al. Ginkgo biloba exocarp extracts inhibits angiogenesis and its effects on Wnt/β-catenin-VEGF signaling pathway in Lewis lung cancer. Journal of Ethnopharmacology. 2016;**192**:406-412. DOI: 10.1016/j.jep.2016.09.018

[36] Cao CJ, Su Y, Sun J, Wang GY, Jia XQ, Chen HS, et al. Anti-tumor Effect of Ginkgo biloba Exocarp Extracts on B16 Melanoma Bearing Mice Involving P I3K/Akt/HIF-1α/VEGF Signaling Pathways. Iran J Pharm Res. 2019;**18**:803-811. DOI: 10.22037/ijpr.2019.1100637

[37] Cao C, Su Y, Gao Y, Luo C, Yin L, Zhao Y, et al. Ginkgo biloba Exocarp Extract Inhibits the Metastasis of B16-F10 Melanoma Involving PI3K/Akt/NF-κB/MMP-9 Signaling Pathway. Evidence-based Complementary and Alternative Medicine. 2018;**2018**:4969028. DOI: 10.1155/2018/4969028

[38] Chen HS, Zhai F, Chu YF, Xu F, Xu AH, Jia LC. Clinical study on treatment of patients with upper digestive tract malignant tumors of middle and late stage with Ginkgo biloba exocarp polysaccharides capsule preparation. Journal of Chinese Integrative Medicine. 2003;**1**:189-191. DOI: 10.3736/jcim20030313

[39] Xu A, Chen H, Wang L, et al. Influence of Ginkgo biloba L. exocarp polysaccharides on serum superoxide dismutase activity and malondialdehyde level in mice under different states. China Journal of Chinese Materia. Médica. 1998;**23**:746-747

[40] Cao C, Su Y, Han D, Gao Y, Zhang M, Chen H, et al. Ginkgo biloba exocarp extracts induces apoptosis in Lewis lung cancer cells involving MAPK signaling pathways. Journal of Ethnopharmacology. 2017;**198**:379-388. DOI: 10.1016/j.jep.2017.01.009

[41] Liu Y, Yang B, Zhang L, Cong X, Liu Z, Hu Y, et al. Ginkgolic acid induces interplay between apoptosis and autophagy regulated by ROS generation in colon cancer. Biochemical and Biophysical Research Communications. 2018;**498**:246-253. DOI: 10.1016/j.bbrc.2018.01.091

[42] Ma J, Duan W, Han S, Lei J, Xu Q, Chen X, et al. Ginkgolic acid suppresses the development of pancreatic cancer by inhibiting pathways driving lipogenesis. Oncotarget. 2015;**6**:20993-21003. DOI: 10.18632/oncotarget.3663

[43] Zhou C, Li X, Du W, Feng Y, Kong X, Li Y, et al. Antitumor effects of ginkgolic acid in human cancer cell occur via cell cycle arrest and decrease the Bcl-2/Bax ratio to induce apoptosis. Chemotherapy. 2010;**56**:393-402. DOI: 10.1159/000317750 Epub 2010 Oct 15

[44] Wu X, Mao G, Zhao T, et al. Isolation, purification and in vitro anti-tumor activity of polysaccharide from Ginkgo biloba sarcotesta. Carbohydrate Polymers. 2011;**86**:1073-1076. DOI: 10.1016/j.carpol.2011.04.069

[45] Yang XM, Wang YF, Li YY, Ma HL. Thermal stability of ginkgolic acids from Ginkgo biloba and the effects of ginkgol C17:1 on the apoptosis and migration of SMMC7721 cells. Fitoterapia. 2014;**98**:66-76. DOI: 10.1016/j.fitote.2014.07.003

[46] Yang X, Qian Z, Chen J, Zhu W, Xie J. Study on antitumor activities of ginkgolic acids from Ginkgo sarcotestas in vitro. Journal of Huazhong Agricultural University. 2004;**27**:40-42. DOI: 10.13300/j.cnki.hnlkxb.2006.04.026

[47] Cao Y, Zhang D, Zheng G, Tang Y, Zhang J. Study on Antitumor and Synergy Effect of "bushen huayu jiedu formula" on Mice Hepatocarcinoma H22. Vol. 27. China: China Academic Publishing House; 2004. pp. 38-40. DOI: 10.13863/j.issn1001-4454.2004.01.022

[48] Lu Y, Hao W, Zhang X, Zhao Y, Xu Y, Luo J, et al. Comparative Study of Physicochemical Properties and Starch Granule Structure in Seven Ginkgo Kernel Flours. Food. 2021;**10**:1721. DOI: 10.3390/foods10081721

[49] Wang HY, Zhang YQ. The main active constituents and detoxification process of Ginkgo biloba seeds and their potential use in functional health foods. Journal of Food Composition and Analysis. 2019;**83**:103247. DOI: 10.1016/j.jfca.2019.103247

[50] Singh B, Kaur P, Gopichand SRD, Ahuja PS. Biology and chemistry of Ginkgo biloba. Fitoterapia. 2008;**79**:401-418. DOI: 10.1016/j.fitote.2008.05.007

[51] Zhang H, Wang Z, Xu SY. Optimization of processing parameters for cloudy ginkgo (Ginkgo biloba Linn.) juice. Journal of food engineering. 2007;**80**:1226-1232. DOI: 10.1016/j.jfoodeng.2006.09.021

[52] Wu CE, Yang JT, Fan GJ, Li TT, Tang ZX, Cao FL. Allergic identification for ginkgo kernel protein in guinea pigs. Food Science and Biotechnology. 2016;**25**:915-919. DOI: 10.1007/s10068-016-0150-3

[53] Chassagne F, Huang X, Lyles JT, Quave CL. Validation of a 16th Century Traditional Chinese Medicine Use of Ginkgo biloba as a Topical Antimicrobial.

Frontiers in Microbiology. 2019;**10**:775. DOI: 10.3389/fmicb.2019.00775

[54] Feodorova Y, Tomova T, Minchev D, Turiyski V, Draganov M, Argirova M. Cytotoxic effect of Ginkgo biloba kernel extract on HCT116 and A2058 cancer cell lines. Heliyon. 2020;**6**:e04941. DOI: 10.1016/j.heliyon.2020.e04941

[55] Li M, Li B, Xia ZM, Tian Y, Zhang D, Rui WJ, et al. Anticancer Effects of Five Biflavonoids from Ginkgo Biloba L male flowers in vitro. Molecules. 2019;**24**:1496. DOI: 10.3390/molecules24081496

[56] Li M, Li B, Hou Y, Tian Y, Chen L, Liu S, et al. Anti-inflammatory effects of chemical components from Ginkgo biloba L. male flowers on lipopolysaccharide-stimulated RAW264.7 macrophages. Phytotherapy Research. 2019;**33**:989-997. DOI: 10.1002/ptr.6292

[57] Li R, Xia Z, Li B, Tian Y, Zhang G, Li M, et al. Advances in Supercritical Carbon Dioxide Extraction of Bioactive Substances from Different Parts of Ginkgo biloba L. Molecules. 2021;**26**:4011. DOI: 10.3390/molecules26134011

[58] Yamashita T, Sato T, Sakamoto K, Ishii H, Yamamoto J. The free-radical scavenger edaravone accelerates thrombolysis with alteplase in an experimental thrombosis model. Thrombosis Research. 2015 Jun;**135**(6):1209-1213. DOI: 10.1016/j.thromres.2015.04.011

[59] Xu Z, Feng Q, Wang M, Zhao H, Lin Y, Zhou S. Green Biosynthesized Silver Nanoparticles With Aqueous Extracts of Ginkgo Biloba Induce Apoptosis via Mitochondrial Pathway in Cervical Cancer Cells. Frontiers in Oncology. 2020;**10**:575415. DOI: 10.3389/fonc.2020.575415

[60] Chen XH, Miao YX, Wang XJ, Yu Z, Geng MY, Han YT, et al. Effects of Ginkgo biloba extract EGb761 on human colon adenocarcinoma cells. Cellular Physiology and Biochemistry. 2011;**27**:227-232. DOI: 10.1159/000327948

[61] Bai Y, Zhao F, Li Y, Wang L, Fang XJ, Wang CY. Ginkgo biloba extract induce cell apoptosis and G0/G1 cycle arrest in gastric cancer cells. International Journal of Clinical and Experimental Medicine. 2015;**8**:20977-20982

[62] Park HJ, Kim MM. Flavonoids in Ginkgo biloba fallen leaves induce apoptosis through modulation of p53 activation in melanoma cells. Oncology Reports. 2015;**33**:433-438. DOI: 10.3892/or.2014.3602

[63] Qian Y, Xia L, Shi W, Sun JJ, Sun YQ. The effect of EGB on proliferation of gastric carcinoma SGC7901 cells. Clinical & Translational Oncology. 2016;**18**:521-526. DOI: 10.1007/s12094-015-1399-3

[64] Chang L, Liu T, Chai Z, Jie S, Li Z, Liu M, et al. lincRNA-p21 Mediates the Anti-Cancer Effect of Ginkgo Biloba Extract EGb 761 by Stabilizing E-Cadherin Protein in Colon Cancer. Medical Science Monitor. 2018;**24**:9488-9496. DOI: 10.12659/MSM.911924

[65] Fu Z, Lin L, Liu S, Qin M, He S, Zhu L, et al. Ginkgo Biloba Extract Inhibits Metastasis and ERK/Nuclear Factor kappa B (NF-κB) Signaling Pathway in Gastric Cancer. Medical Science Monitor. 2019;**25**:6836-6845. DOI: 10.12659/MSM.915146

[66] Tsai JR, Liu PL, Chen YH, Chou SH, Yang MC, Cheng YJ, et al. Ginkgo biloba extract decreases non-small cell lung cancer cell migration by downregulating metastasis-associated factor heat-shock

protein 27. PLoS One. 2014;**9**:e91331. DOI: 10.1371/journal.pone.0091331

[67] Lou JS, Xia YT, Wang HY, Kong XP, Yao P, Dong TTX, et al. The WT1/MVP-Mediated Stabilization on mTOR/AKT Axis Enhances the Effects of Cisplatin in Non-small Cell Lung Cancer by a Reformulated Yu Ping Feng San Herbal Preparation. Frontiers in Pharmacology. 2018;**9**:853. DOI: 10.3389/fphar.2018.00853

Chapter 21

Plant Medicine and Infectious Disease

David Zorngo

Abstract

Our planet since development has experienced a greater perspective of growth. Constituting millions of species exhibiting different kinds of relationships producing both correlational and mutual growth, sums up to the widespread evolutional changes we see today. Mankind as a separate entity within the avalanche of species plays a greater share of the role and thus contributes greatly to the growth and existence of this planet. After having to battle with intraspecies 'fight and survive' relation within his colony conditioning him into psychological, social, and emotional, problems; he unquestionably relates with other species in an interspecies relationship. Though this interspecies relationship does not produce only negative outcomes and raises positive outcomes as well, a great deal of it is a threat to mankind's survival and growth. One interspecies relationship that mankind experiences mutual benefits is that with plants and with species such as those of some virus, bacterial, protozoans, etc., he experiences a parasitic relationship with a lot of negative outcomes. The chapter "Plant and Infectious Diseases," explore the relationship between man and plants that heals him and his relationship with other kinds of species that renders him into illness. It talks about how plants can help us remedy infectious diseases.

Keywords: plants and infectious diseases, plants metabolites, plant medicine, phytomedicine, viral infections, protozoa infections, fungi infections, bacterial infections

1. Introduction

Plants are nature's source of food. Aside from the enormous benefits we derived from plants including shelter and protection, plants are the center of what heals us. Medicinal plants have been with us since the time of our ancestors. Earlier men utilized plants preparations to remedy diseases. They employed archaic means together with instincts, beliefs, observation, taste, and experience to categorized plants as remedies and poisons [1]. Today, the role of medicinal plants as remedies has extended beyond the ways of ancient men. The role of medicinal plants as remedies now hinges extensively on the chemistry of the plant. Based on scientific research, plants are now screened and tested [2]. Phytochemist talks of two groups of compounds in plants. These are the primary plant metabolites and secondary plant metabolites. The primary plant metabolites perform basic life functions and the secondary plant metabolites classify compounds that are important in other aspects such as the ability to destroy or prevent the growth of certain causative agents of diseases [3–5]. The goal of scientists in the field of medicinal plants is to find which plant compound has potency against which causative agents of diseases. Many compounds have proven efficacy in treating many diseases. Some of these compounds serve as stepping stones in the synthesis of synthetic and variants of semi-synthetic compounds. These plants' compounds are with potencies and by screening and testing scientifically their remedies are safe and potent. With recent issues arising from synthetic compounds on the human body both short term and long term, medicinal plants deserve the attention and the urgency of the public as well as scientist. There is no time in history the demands for medicinal plants protection and usage should concern everyone than today. The outbreak of Covid'19 in Wuhan, China, since 2019, has claimed many lives and still claiming lives at the time of this writing. This is not the first of its kind. Infectious diseases keep claiming lives yearly across the globe. With research providing promising evidence of medicinal plants' potencies against many agents of infectious diseases, the world has no reason not to protect plants. Infectious diseases are grouped by the classes of their causative agent which are viral agents, bacterial agents, fungal agents, protozoa agents, helminth, and prions (agents devoid of any nucleic acid) [6–9]. Some plants have proven efficacy against all these agents [10]. With all these broad future expectations of medicinal plants, there are hundreds of medicinal plants on their way to extinction as a result of destructive human activities. This is the era the world should come together to support plants.

2. Plants, man, and infectious diseases

Man and plants as well as infectious agents have existed dating to time immemorable. The relationship between man, plants, and agents causing infectious diseases has not changed to this day. Plants provide us with shelter, nourishment, etc. Infectious diseases caused us infections. When we are infected by any of the infectious agents which you will read on later, we feel sick and experience abnormality in functions and sometimes structure.

Infectious agents have their route of entry or attachment to our body where they cause physiological changes. Some of these changes exhibit clinically on our skin, hands and nails, oropharynx, head and neck, eyes, neurons, heart and lungs, abdomen, musculoskeletal, and genitalia and rectum. Infections present with signs and symptoms some of which are unique to certain infectious agents. Signs include generalized erythema, splinter hemorrhages, finger clubbing, Janeway lesions, vasculitis, dental caries, candidiasis, tonsillar enlargement, lymphadenopathy, red eyes, neck stiffness, delirium, tachycardia, pericardial rub, ascites, joint swelling, discharge from the genitals, etc. [11]. When a man is infected with infectious diseases, the same plants that shelter man, and provide him with nutrients, etc. can again help man to battle infectious diseases.

2.1 Plants and our life (plants as pillar of life)

Imagine you woke up one day to the realization that every plant has died. Now, create a mental picture of this incident. What will the world look like—a world without plants? There will be no food. There will be no shelter. There will be no clean air. There will be a bad water cycle. And soon there will be no animals as well as other organisms. Plants support essentially every life. Together with animals, other organisms, and the abiotic aspect of the ecosystem almost every life is impacted.

Plants are all the organisms belonging to the kingdom Plantae. They are eukaryotes capable of using water, carbon dioxide, and the energy from the sun to produce chemical energy which is stored and, in the process, releases oxygen into the atmosphere which animals and other aerobic organisms depend on for survival. The chemical energy, an end product of photosynthesis, is taken up by animals in the form of food and released through cellular respiration to support life.

Let us step back and analyze well the importance of plants to life. Within the ecology, there exists a sequence of matter and energy transfer from organism to organism. Every organism requires matter and energy for carrying out life processes. These basic requirements have to be transferred from one organism to another hinging on some extent of conservation. This means of matter and energy transfer between organisms is termed the food chain. The food chain is nothing more than feeding relationships between species in a biotic community. These feeding relationships start at the base with a producer, then the primary consumer, the secondary consumer, tertiary consumer, and so on. This trend implies that the producer has to find a way to offer the 'first' matter and energy needed to start the transfer and that is what they do well. The producers make their food which is in turn taken up by the primary consumer. The primary consumers are also in turn taken up by the secondary consumer which in turn are also taken up by the tertiary consumers and so on. The primary producers, the most important aspect of the food chain, arc most often plants (and other autotrophs organisms—algae, cyanobacteria, and chemoautotrophs). Every organism involves in the food chain and food webs (several interrelated food chains) to retrieved energy to carry out its vital process which would have been a fantasy without the producers like plants.

What more? Plants are one of the agents in the oxygen cycle. Plants manufacture the majority of the air we breathe through photosynthesis (the same process through which they give us food.). The human body has water (H_2O) being the majority component that is formed from hydrogen and oxygen (the oxygen we get from plants is part of this oxygen). Aside from plants giving as essential oxygen needed for life, they purified the atmosphere by removing chemicals dangerous to life. The carbon dioxide we breathe out is exchanged for fresh oxygen. At no time in history has there been a rise in the Industrial Revolution than our time. The high demand of the Industrial Revolution presents its mayhem to man and the environment as the result of burning fossil fuel releasing dangerous chemicals into the environment. Despite the frequent burning of fossil fuel and the destruction of vegetation both on land and sea, we still enjoy the relatively stable level of atmospheric oxygen. What can we attribute this to other than the plants that we are still sharing the environment with?

Moreover, plants serve as the habitat for thousands of organisms. In, on, and under plants are thousands of animals that all contribute one way or the other to the existence of the ecosystem. Walk through any forest and you will be amazed at the diversity of life that the forest harbors. Tree kangaroo, giant panda, monkeys, rabbits, foxes, raccoons, squirrels, chipmunks, badgers, moose, bear, bobcats, deer, antelope, lynx, jaguars, elephants are to mentioned but few of wildlife that would have been homeless without the forest. Within the human settlements, plants provide shades moderating temperature, protecting the lands and settlements from wind and water destructions. Again, ornamental plants are employed in almost all human settlements for beautification purposes. Even after cutting plants and destroying their lives they still give us logs from which many products including paper, furniture, houses, and more goodies that make our lives comfortable are retrieved [12].

2.2 Plants as medicine

Aside from all the enormous benefits of plants to mankind, plants remain the center of what heals us. Readers may be surprised to know many conventional drugs are from plants (e.g. **Table 1**). Aspirin, a nonsteroidal anti-inflammatory drug (NSAID) used in inflammation and as an analgesic was from Willow; Digoxin, a cardiac stimulant used in congestive heart failure and cardiac arrhythmia were from Digitalis; quinine from Cinchona, morphine from Papaver, and artemisinin from Artemisia. Across the world especially in Third World countries plant medicine has been integrated into the Primary Health care delivery system. People in Asia, Africa, and Latin America depend to a greater proportion on phytomedicine in the treatment of illness partly caused by the great vast of plant species in their part of the world. No apology should be made for placing plants at the center of man's source of healing.

The use of plants for the treatments of diseases predates the records of human history. History has it that plants were the source of remedies of Pythagoras, Galen, and Hippocrates. The earliest human ancestors discovered the healing potency of plants through factors such as instinct, taste, observation, and experience. By relying on trial-and-error, medicinal plants were differentiated from poisonous plants. However, in many cases, the when and how these medicines were first used was lost in pre-history. Pieces of knowledge of medicinal plants, harmful plants, and their mode of usage were passed from generation to generation through oral transmission. Later, writing replaced the oral transmission mode of conveying knowledge from generation to generation (e.g., the Egyptians Ebers Papyrus). These written pieces of knowledge became the great wealth of knowledge upon which further development and discoveries were made.

Though the ancients men depended on trial and error with the first patients as an experiment in screening their plant medicinal preparations, plants are now screened depending on the modern scientific methods of investigation which comprises of a team of botanists (a scientist specialized in the study of plants), phytochemists (a scientist specialized in the branch of organic chemistry dealing with the chemistry of plants), pharmacologists (a scientist trained in the sciences of drugs) and clinicians (a practitioner of medicine whose work focus more on clinical work other than laboratory experiments).

The potency of plants as medicines depends on their phytochemical constituents. Phytochemist focuses on these compounds which have been divided into Primary Metabolites and Secondary Metabolites. Primary metabolites which include amino acids, lipids, carbohydrates, proteins, and vitamins play physiological roles such as growth, development respiration, storage, and reproduction. Secondary metabolites are organic compounds produced by plants through metabolic pathways derived from the primary metabolite's pathway. These metabolites (secondary metabolites) are not directly involved in the basic life processes of the organism but they are essential in other activities. The identification of secondary metabolites opened the gateway for the use of plants as medicine. These compounds are shown to have biological activities. The secondary plant metabolites are grouped into Alkaloids, Saponins, *Lipids, Phenolics, Terpenes, and *Carbohydrates.

Alkaloids are nitrogenous compounds (at least a nitrogen atom that usually forms part of a heterocyclic ring structure with marked physiological actions in

Popular medicinal plants as a source of modern medicine or bioactive compounds		
Bioactive compounds	**Medical uses**	**Origin**
Acetyldigoxin	Cardiotonic	*Digitalis lanata*
Aescin	Antiinflamatory	*Adonis vernalis*
Ajmalicine	Treatment for circulatory disorders	*Rauvolfia sepentina*
Allantoin	Wound treatment	*Matricaria recutita, Symphytum Officinale,* etc.
Anabesine	Muscle relaxant	*Anabasis sphylla*
Anisodamine	Anticholinergic	*Anisodus tanguticus*
Anisodine	Anticholinergic	*Anisodus tanguticus*
Atropine	Anticholinergic	*Atropine belladonna*
Bergenin	Antitussive	*Ardisia japonica*
Betulinic acid	Anticancerous	*Betula alba*
Caffeine	Central Nervous System stimulant	*Camellia sinensis*
Camphor	Rubecient	*Cinnamomum camphora*
Cocaine	Anaesthetic	*Erythroxylum coca*
Codeine	Antitussive	*Papaver somniferum*
Colchicine	Anticancer	*Colchicum autumnale*
Curcumin	Choleretic	*Curcuma longa*
Deserpidine	Tranquilizer	*Rauvolfia canescens*
L-Dopa	Anti-parkinsonism	Mucana species
Digitalin	Cardiotonic	*Digitalis purpurea*
Digitoxin	Cardiotonic	*Digitalis purpurea*
Digoxin	Cardiotonic	*Digitalis purpurea*
Gossypol	Male contraceptive	Gossypium species
Hyoscyamine	Anticholinergic	*Hyoscyamus niger*
Menthol	Rubefacient	*Mentha species*
Methyl salicylate	Rubefacient	*Gaultheria procumbens*
Morphine	Analgesic	*Papaver somniferum*
Nicotine	Insecticide	*Nicotiana tabacum*
Noscapine	Antitussive	*Papaver somniferum*
Picrotoxin	Analeptic	*Anamirta cocculus*
Podophyllotoxin	Anticancer	*Podophyllum peltatum*
Quinine	Antimalarial	*Cinchona ledgeriana*
Reserpine	Antihypertensive	*Rauvofia serpentina*
Salicin	Analgesic	*Salix alba*
Scopolamine	Sedative	*Datura metel*
Tetrahydrocannabinol (THC)	Antiemetic	*Cannabis sativa*
Theobromine	Vasodilator	*Theobroma cacao*
Thymol	Antifungal	*Thymus vulgaris*

Popular medicinal plants as a source of modern medicine or bioactive compounds		
Bioactive compounds	**Medical uses**	**Origin**
Vinblastine	Anticancer	*Catharanthus roseus*
Yohimbine	Aphrodisiac	*Pausinystalia yohimbe*

Table 1.
Medicinal plants as a source of modern medicine [13].

man and animals). Alkaloids are widely distributed in the Kingdom Plantae especially in angiosperms (higher plants). Alkaloids are rarely found in lower plants. Commonly known plant families in Angiosperm with alkaloids include Papaveraceae, Apocynaceae, Rubiaceae, Berberidaceae, Solanaceae, Convolvulaceae, Ranunculaceae, etc. Example of alkaloids includes Caffeine (central nervous system agent with effects on respiratory and cardiovascular systems.), Vinblastine (an antineoplastic drug from *Catharanthus Roseus*), Nicotine (ganglionic cholinergic receptor agonist), etc.

Saponins are secondary metabolites that contain a high percentage of glycosides (saponin) which can produce stable frothing aqueous solution. Saponins are harmful by their ability to cause hemolysis when injected into the blood but are harmless when taken by mouth. Saponins are proven to possess pharmacological activities including analgesic, antineoplastic, etc.

Lipids are a heterogeneous group of compounds with long-chain fatty acids and glycerol and higher monohydric alcohols. Lipids include fixed oils, fats, waxes, lecithins, phosphatides, etc.; which are relatively insoluble in water but dissolve in organic solvents. Lipids are primary plants metabolites but have been known to possess pharmacological activities.

Phenols probably constitute the largest group of plant secondary metabolites. The phytochemistry of phenols reveals the possession of at least one or more groups of phenol. Phenolic classes of pharmaceutical interest include simple phenolic compounds, tannins, anthraquinones, and their glycosides, coumarins and their glycosides, naphthoquinones, flavone, and related flavonoid glycosides, anthocyanidins and anthocyanins, and lignans and lignin. Phenols have pharmacological properties including antioxidants, anti-inflammatory, etc.

Terpenes are secondary plants metabolites derived from 5-carbon isoprene units. The number of the isoprene units is the basis for terpenes classification. Prefixes such as Hemi, Mono, Sesqui, etc., are used before terpenes to represent the number of isoprene units which in this case are 1, 2, and 3 isoprene units respectively. Hemiterpenes represent a terpene with 1 isoprene unit and so on.

Carbohydrates just like lipids are primary metabolites but form part of a majority of secondary metabolites through glycoxidation linkage. Carbohydrates such as mucilage are used as demulcents employed in ulcer management and inflammatory digestive disorders [14].

2.3 Plants medicine and infectious diseases

At the dawn of civilization, dating back to hundreds of years, snake venom was drunk intending to confer immunity to snake bites. At a similar time, it was found that smearing cowpox on torn skin induces the body to fight against smallpox. Forwarding to 1796, Edward Jenner who is popularly known as the founder of vaccinology in the West was successful in his attempt in the discovery of a solution that will later impact civilization till this day by inoculating a 13-year-old-boy with vaccinia virus (cowpox) and demonstrated immunity to smallpox leading to the discovery of the smallpox vaccine three years later. After this concept underwent medical and technological changes the years ahead, the concept of vaccine and vaccination has been employed across almost every corner of the world and enormous benefits reaped as well.

Despite medical and technological advancement in vaccinology leading to the availability and use of effective vaccines and antibiotics, the concept of infectious diseases still presents a great canker to humanity. To this day that vaccine can be produced in the shortest possible time made possible by the advancement of scientific knowledge leading to research costing millions of dollars, infectious diseases remain an essential problem to the world. Covid'19 outbreak since 2019 has claimed millions of lives across the world daring the elderly and the weak with low immunity as a result of old age, chronic diseases, immunosuppressive drugs, malnutrition, etc., to survive its blow. According to Robbins and Cotran's book, "Pathologic Basis of Disease," Eight Edition, more than 10 million people die each year of infectious diseases [15].

Infectious disease is an impairment of health or a condition of abnormal functioning caused by microorganisms mainly through a specific kind of contact. They can be caught through contact with infected people, infected environments, infected animals, or insect bites. An example includes acquired immunodeficiency syndrome (AIDS), Viral hepatitis, Syphilis, Lyme Disease, Common Cold, Giardiasis, Malaria, Influenza, Measles, Pneumonia, Salmonella infections, Tuberculosis, Whooping cough (pertussis), Rubella, Shingles, Onchocerciasis, Candidiasis, Aspergillosis, Clostridial Infections, etc. Agents responsible for infectious diseases include viruses, bacterial, prions, fungi, helminths, protozoa, etc.

The incessant evidence of the antimicrobial resistance and side effects of synthetic drugs which have been the mainstay of remedying infectious diseases should straighten the line that was once burnt and bring the attention of the global population to the importance of medicinal plants and traditional therapeutic system in remedying infectious diseases.

An attempt to use natural products (plant medicines) to remedy infectious diseases swings on two pivots. The first is to consider factors related to the patients. These factors which must be considered relating to the patients include the patient's previous health histories, susceptibility to infections, chronic diseases, ability to tolerate drug by mouth, age, sex (if female, whether with a child or pregnant). The second factor to consider is that relating to the type of infections and the causal organism.

What follows describes the infectious agents responsible for infectious diseases and further recommends plants medicines for their remedy or which has shown efficacy against such specific infectious agents.

2.3.1 Viruses

Viruses are submicroscopic obligate intracellular infectious agents, which by definition consist of genetic code, either DNA or RNA, enclosed by a protein coat that is sometimes encased in a lipid membrane. Viruses cannot replicate on their own. They, therefore, depend on the host cell's complex metabolic and biosynthetic machinery for their replication. Viruses as infectious agents can infect animals, plants, and microorganisms such as bacteria and archaea. Viruses exist outside their host as virions (also used to describe a fully assembled infectious virus), an inert independent viral particle; nucleic acid, and capsid (and a lipid envelop in some cases). Viruses such as polio and tobacco mosaic virus can even be crystallized. With an infection, the main function of the virion is to deliver the genetic component (DNA or RNA genome) into the host cell so that the genome can be transcribed and translated by the host cell. Viruses are known to be the most numerous types of biological entities. There are millions of species of virus existing with only a few given a detailed description.

Viruses are grouped based on their nucleic acid genome (DNA or RNA and not both), the shape of their capsid (helical or icosahedral), the presence or absence of a lipid envelop, their mode of replication, the preferred cell type for replication (atropism), or the type of pathology.

Viruses are responsible for a great share of human infections including AIDS, Corona Virus Infection, Chicken Pox, Common Cold, Dengue fever, Lassa fever, Herpes zoster, Herpes simplex, measles, SARS, Rabies, Smallpox, Viral meningitis, Viral pneumonia, Viral gastroenteritis, Yellow fever, Cytomegalovirus infection, Ebola hemorrhagic fever, etc. Some viruses are responsible for transient illnesses such as colds and influenza while others are hard to be eradicated from the body. Many viruses have a propensity to cause latent infections by expressing their genome into viral protein. The majority of these viruses belong to the *Herpesviridae* family: Epstein-Barr virus, Varicella-Zoster Virus, etc. Hepatitis B virus is known in several cases to persist in the host cell for a longer duration of time causing latent illnesses which can be reactivated later. The human papillomavirus induced benign warts and cervical carcinoma. The same clinical manifestation can be depicted by different species of virus and the same virus can depict different clinical manifestations depending on factors such as host immune status and age. Viruses can spread through touch, saliva, and through the air, sexual contact, insects (known as vectors), and through sharing of contaminated items [16].

2.3.2 Plant medicines for viral infectious

Viral infection presents a lot of challenges in the health industry. When a living cell is invaded by viruses, they hijack the cell's internal machinery to produce more of their kind in the process destroying a lot of host cells. Viral infections remain an area of medicine for which specific treatments are lacking. In immunocompetent individuals, some viral infections resolve spontaneously on their own. For most viral infections such as those associated with the common cold, treatment involves symptoms relief and not targeting the viral agents per se. Antiviral agents are agents that target the viral agent preventing their replication in the host cell. These agents include plants. *Alchornea cordifolia* is used in Ghana as an antiviral agent [17]. Clausena *anisata* contains carbazole alkaloids that inhibit Epstein-Barr virus early antigen in Ragi cells [18]. *Bridelia ferruginea* contains the flavonoids quercetin, quercitrin, and rutin that have demonstrated antiviral effects against coxsackie, Herpes simplex, measles, parainfluenza, and polioviruses [19]. *Scoporia dulcis* contain scopadulcic acid C which potentiates antiviral effect [20]. Extract of *Momordica charantia* has demonstrated antiviral activity against *Herpes simplex* virus type 1 and the proteins alpha and beta-momorcharin have been reported to inhibit HIV *in vitro*. Other antiviral agents include *Argemone Mexicana* (leave and stem), *Aloe vera, Allium sativum, Acacia nilotica, etc.*

2.3.3 Bacteria

Bacteria are free-living organisms that are found almost everywhere on Earth. Bacteria are prokaryotes, meaning they have a cell wall mostly bound by peptidoglycan, a polymer of glycan and peptides, but lack a distinct nucleus and other organelles due to the absence of internal membranes which distinguish them from eukaryotes. Bacteria are classified based on shape, Gram staining, and need for oxygen. There are three basic shapes. The spherical bacteria are spherical and known as the cocci, the rod-shaped bacteria are known as bacilli (others curved known as the vibrio) and the spiral-shaped bacteria are known as the spirilla. Under gram staining, bacteria can be either classified as gram-positive or gram-negative based on the bacterial cell wall's ability to retain the crystal violet dye during solvent treatment. The gram-positive bacteria retain the dye because of their single thick cell wall and appear purple-brown under the microscope and the gram-negative bacteria do not take up the dye because they have a thin cell wall squash in between two phospholipid bilayer membranes and appear red under the microscope. Bacteria that require oxygen for survival are aerobic bacteria and those that can survive where there is no oxygen are the anaerobic bacteria. Unlike viruses, some bacteria can survive and replicate outside their host. Not all bacteria are harmful. Some bacteria are used in industrial and medicinal processes. Bacteria help in the fixation of nitrogen into the soil from the atmosphere and are vital to the planet's ecosystem. The human body serves as a home for many species of bacteria in a symbiotic relationship. However, several species of bacteria have broken this symbiotic relationship and are pathogenically responsible for many infectious diseases including anthrax, cholera, bacterial meningitis, brucellosis, diphtheria, gonorrhea, Lyme disease, leptospirosis, Pneumococcal pneumonia, syphilis, tetanus, trachoma, tuberculosis, typhoid fever, Q fever, Pertussis, shigellosis, Rocky Mountain Spotted Fever, salmonellosis, tularemia, nocardiosis, campylobacteriosis, etc. [21–23].

2.3.4 Plant medicines for bacterial infections

History has it that antibiotics were limited to substances produced by microorganisms. In 1877 Louis Pasteur discovered that injecting Bacillus anthracis in animals protected them from developing anthrax. Years after Pasteur's discovery, Fleming observed that a colony of Penicillium notatum contaminant on Petri dish inhibited bacteria which lead to the discovery of penicillin. The trend continues leading to the discovery of other compounds. Long before this array of discoveries, nature has already instituted compounds in plants with antibacterial properties waiting to be discovered. Plants' source of antibiotics includes lichen, a thallophytic plant of the division Lichenes that occur as crusty patches or bushy growths on tree trunks, walls, roots, or bare grounds. Lichenes contain usnic acid or vulpinic acid that is known to possessed bacteriostatic properties. Plants belonging to the Order Coniferae have also demonstrated antibacterial activities; essential oils in Juniperus and Pinus spp. possess antibacterial activity. A sulfur-containing amino acid in garlic (alliin) has antibacterial activities. Aloe vera gel and ginger have antibacterial properties. Sesquiterpene ketones in dicotyledons such as hops (humulene and lupulene) and myrrh (furanodiene-6-one and methoxyfuranoguaia-9-ene-8-one; protoanemonine, in *Anemone pulsatilla* and many Ranunculaceae; sulfur-containing compounds in the Cruciferae; plumbagin in Drosera have all demonstrated antibacterial activities [24].

2.3.5 Fungi

Fungi are all the known species of organism belonging to the kingdom Fungi. Fungi include yeast, molds, smuts, mushrooms, and toadstools. Fungi are distinct from green plants. Fungi are eukaryotic organisms and possess thick chitin in their cell walls which separates them from other eukaryotic organisms and ergosterol-containing cell membranes. Fungi can be found almost everywhere on earth. They are with both harmful and beneficial effects. Their characteristics are intermediate between algae and protozoa. They share with plants some characteristics which include possession of cell walls, liquid-filled intracellular vacuoles, microscopically visible streaming of cytoplasm, and they lack motility. Just like bacteria, fungi aid the return of scarce materials to the soil by decomposing animals and plants. Fungi exhibit mycorrhizae association with plants (a symbiotic relationship between the mycelium of a fungus and the roots of a vascular plant) in which they provide plants with some nutrients and water for growth and taking nutrients as well from the plant. Medicines such as penicillin (an antibiotic) were produced from the fungus *Penicillium notatum*. Fungi are also used in the agricultural industry for controlling insect pests on crops. Most species of fungi live in the soil where they can obtain their nutrients, and on living organisms including plants and animals. Fungi again are saprophytic organisms and feed on dead organic matter. Fungi just like animals are heterotrophic organisms (they lack chlorophyll) and depend on the absorption of dissolved organic molecules typically by secreting digestive enzymes into their setting. Despite the enormously beneficial effects of fungi, some fungi are responsible for a wide range of infectious diseases infecting both animals and plants. Fungi are responsible for infectious diseases classified into superficial, cutaneous, subcutaneous, systemic, and opportunistic infections. Superficial diseases involve the skin, hair, and nails. Some fungi invade the subcutaneous while others invade deep tissues destroying internal organs in the immunocompromised host. Opportunistic fungi are generally harmless in their normal environment but become harmful in an immunocompromised host. Infectious diseases caused by fungi include tinea, candidiasis, coccidioidomycosis, aspergillosis, blastomycosis, histoplasmosis, etc. [25].

2.3.6 Plant medicines for fungal infections.

Diterpenes in Taxodiaceae genera under the Coniferae order are known, antifungal agents. Leaves and pericarp of *J. regia* extract pharmacologically demonstrated to be antifungal. *Pterocarpus erinaceus* aqueous and methanolic bark extracts showed *in vitro* antifungal properties [26]. A 10-year human study has shown that the extract of *Senna alata* is an effective antifungal agent for the treatment of *Pityriasis versicolor* [27]. *Vernonia amygdalina* contains sesquiterpene lactones, vernolide, and vernodalol which have demonstrated antifungal activities [28]. *Acacia nilotica* extracts of the root bark and fruits are reported to have antifungal properties particularly against yeasts and *Candida albicans* [29]. Many plants demonstrated antifungal properties and the list is still counting.

2.3.7 Parasitic worms

Unlike the infectious agents discuss so far, parasitic worms also known as helminths are macro-parasites meaning they can be seen with the naked eye. They are highly differentiated multicellular organisms with complex life cycles. In some hosts (definitive hosts) they exhibit sexual reproduction and exhibit asexual reproduction in other hosts (intermediary host or vector). Helminths include the three groups of parasitic worms; nematodes or roundworms, trematodes or flukes, and cestodes or tapeworms. Nematodes are unsegmented worms with elongated rounded bodies pointed at both ends; mostly free-living but some are parasitic. Trematodes have external suckers usually for attaching to a host. Cestodes are ribbon-like flatworms.

While in the infected host, parasitic worms receive nourishment and protection while depriving their host of nutrients. Helminths are transmitted through water, food, soil, and vectors. An infected host can harbor the adult worm, immature stages, or their larval forms. Adult worms in their host produce eggs that can pass out through the stools of their host. Parasitic worms' infection severity depends on the number of parasites harboring in the host. Diseases can also be due to the inflammatory reaction to their eggs and larvae. Helminths are responsible for symptoms such as diarrhea, loss of appetite, fatigue, stomachache, anemia, skin rashes, fever, swellings, weakness, and weight loss [30].

2.3.8 Plant medicines for parasitic worm infections

The leaf extracts of *Adansonia digitata* exhibited anthelminthic activities [31]. *Sorghum bicolor* is considered anthelminthic in India. *Ocimum gratissimum* extracts have shown promising anthelminthic properties by their ability to inhibit glutathione S-transferases from parasitic nematodes [32]. *Momordica charantia* extract also has anthelminthic activity [33]. *Balanites aegyptiaca* also showed anthelminthic properties [34]. Plants are continuously screened and the list keeps on counting.

2.3.9 Protozoa

Protozoa are a group of one-celled eukaryotes minutes organisms either free-living or dependent on the host for support. Protozoa are non-photosynthetic and like animals depend on other matter for nutrients. Protozoa are more related to animals sharing common characteristics which include motility, lack of cell wall, etc. Their locomotive structures include the cilia (hairlike projections from the surface of their cell), flagella (a lash-like appendage that extends from the cell surface.). Some protozoa such as the amoeba moved by forming pseudopodia, a temporal outgrowth that is filled with cytoplasm flowing from the body of the cell. The parasitic protozoa form part of the major causes of infectious diseases ranging from asymptomatic to life-threatening, depending on factors such as the nature of the pathogen and the immune status of the host organism. Parasitic protozoa can be classified based on whether they are responsible for systemic or local infections. Systemic protozoal infections include malaria, sleeping sickness, babesiosis, Chagas' disease, toxoplasmosis, and leishmaniasis. Protozoa such as *Entamoeba histolytica, Giardia lamblia* are responsible for intestinal parasitic infections. Intestinal protozoa infectious are transmitted usually by the fecal-oral route through direct contact with the infected agents by ingesting contaminated food or water [35, 36].

2.3.10 Plant medicines for protozoa infections

The efficacy of plants as a remedy for protozoal infections is remarkable. In the clinical world, plants have been the source of the clinically used antimalarial drugs; quinine from *Cinchona spp.* and artemisinin from *Artemisia annua* with the former being the blueprint for the generation of varieties of synthetic antimalarial agents. Plants agents that have been found to kill or inhibit protozoa infections happen to plants containing phytochemicals such as alkaloids and terpenes. There is a lot of scientific evidence backing the use of alkaloids and terpenes in the treatment of protozoal infections but that does not necessarily mean all plants with alkaloids or terpenes can be used for such purposes. This is because some of those agents might have the efficacy to kill or inhibit the agents but might be harmful in man and should not be considered. Plants with efficacy against protozoa infections include *Cryptolepis sanguinolenta, Holarrhena pubescens, Alstonia boonei (Apocynaceae), Artemisia annua. Cryptolepis sanguinolenta* contained the alkaloid cryptolepine used in the treatment of malaria [37]. The plant has also shown potency in the treatment of amoebiasis [38]. *Holarrhena pubescens* contain conessine which has shown potency in the treatment of amoebic dysentery. *Alstonia* contains alkaloids such as villastonine which have shown an *in vitro* antiplasmodial activity. *Artemisia annua* contained sesquiterpene lactone artemisinin which has shown activity against malarial. Other plants used in protozoal infections include *Cinchona pubescens, Aloe vera, Phyllanthus niruri, Rauwolfia vomitoria, etc.*

3. Threats to plant's life

It would not be doing enough still if our daily mission was to survive a plant life. Though that statement would not be more than fantasy when compared to what we see today, it would have survived mankind himself and his environment and created a livelihood in all his sector but would not still match all the benefits that he reaps from plants. I should say there are more bodies and resources towards the conservation of animal life than there are to survive plants life. Animals are important. They give us pet, food, leather, etc., and forms part of our society and they deserve the efforts to survive and protect them, but, are not plants that give us the ability to live to see our pets, eat meats, and use leather deserves much more attention? We do not need years of research (though they are available) to tell us hundreds of plants species are on the verge of extinction across the globe. Just a few years back, native African plants such as the *khaya senegalensis* were not easy to spot and now, it takes the journey of kilometers into a deep forest zone to spot one or two such plants. And this is happening across all the corners of the globe. If greater urgency and resources are not directed to curb the trend, it will happen earlier than expected—many species of plants will be finally extinct.

In this era where there is a rise in scientific interest in research assaying plants' phytochemicals and their potencies, it would not be long for plants to help us remedy diseases that synthetic products have failed to cure. This is happening and is not a fantasy. HIV-inhibitors named inophyllums have been isolated from *Calophyllum inophyllum*. *Ferula sumbol* has been found to contain coumarins that have shown anti-HIV activity [39]. But if these plants are extinct before they get to the laboratory, what is the hope of the world?

To talk of man involvements as threats to plants' lives, we can consider two separate concepts. One is his physical activities and two, his inactions. His activities include timber exploitations, agriculture, mining, industrialization, urbanization, etc. His inactions are his lack of concern towards the threats to plants' lives.

Man's conscious and unconscious activities threatened the lives of plants and many plants species are battling extinction as a result of such activities. Our desire for timber products instead of other variants is killing plants other than whetting our appetites. Mining, agriculture, and other activities are all gearing towards that path. All these activities result in habitat loss. The homes of these plants are converted into agricultural lands and places for livestock grazing. Industrial production and urbanization are rendering the natural habitats incapable of supporting plants life. Plants that were previously doing well in these habitats are killed in so doing reducing biodiversity.

DOI: http://dx.doi.org/10.5772/intechopen.103701

Man's inaction that endangers plants lives on the other hand is the things he needed to do to immunized his physical activities that throw real danger on the plant's life that he is not doing. We are sending plants to extinction by choosing to do nothing. The logging of trees would not be so destructive as far as we replaced them. We could plant trees to replace those we cut. We could employ reafforestation to immunize deforestation. On an individual level, we could decide to plant trees in our environment as a means of providing shades, beautifying our environment, and in the process, preserving plant life. You could inform someone today of the importance of protecting plants' lives and helping spread the good news. Each and everyone can choose to do nothing or choose to do something. Whatever we choose to do, the process would not be easy. Choosing to protect plants' lives is hard. Doing nothing and watching nature fades away is hard. I am asking you today to choose your hard!

3.1 Recommendations

The journey to protecting plants' lives is everyone's job since everyone is affected positively by the presence of plants. Environmental protection agencies, governmental and non-governmental agencies, individuals, and the whole populace should awake and rethink all the practices that endanger plants species. New bodies aimed at preserving vegetations should be created and already existing ones should be strengthened. Governments, as well as individual philanthropists, should donate towards these bodies making sure they are well equipped to function. Sectors such as the farming sectors that are found of practices that endanger plants' lives should be monitored and those found guilty sanctioned. Frequent campaigned towards plants plantation should be encouraged as well as mass education on the benefits of protecting the vegetations.

Human resources are the center of all the types of resources in the sense that nothing will be meaningful and minimum rewards can be reaped from every resource without trained human resources to channel their course. Aside from preventing plants from extinction, experts should be trained to work and research on plants. Scientists already in the field should be well motivated and channels should be created for others to enter the field.

With the availability of plants and scientists to work on them, plants medicine will propel medicine to a horizon we never anticipated.

4. Conclusions

The above concepts are not claiming all there is to medicinal plants and infectious diseases but it is enough to straighten the logs that were bent years ago. Medicinal plants worked magic for the ancient men and survived them and their generation. If care, enough urgency, and resources are directed towards the preservation of plants, medicinal plants will change the perspective of medicine and impacts generations to come. If we stay adamant and watched as many species of plants suffer extinctions, the world will lose this greater facet of nature and there will be no room to contain the mayhem. Diseases are with us. The world might record new outbreaks of infectious diseases, but with strategic plans that do not exclude interventions geared towards the wellbeing of medicinal plants, any kind of infectious disease can be easily controlled.

Notes/thanks/other declarations

I acknowledge the strength given me by God and my greatest thanks go to Him. And to my brother Cantey Zorngo and sister, Sefa Agartha for the love we share. To Esther Anokyewaa Akoto, you mean the world to me, thank you.

Author details

David Zorngo
Kwame Nkrumah University of Science and Technology, Kumasi, Ghana

*Address all correspondence to: dvdkingson@gmail.com

References

[1] Evans WC. Trease and Evans Pharmacognosy. 15th ed. London: Elsevier Limited; 2002. p. 3

[2] Nanunsha MY, Krauss M, Schonsee CD, et al. Target screening of plant secondary metabolites in river waters by liquid chromatography coupled to high-resolution mass spectrometry (LC-HRMS). Environmental Science Europe. 2020;**32**:142. DOI: 10.1186/s12302-020-00399-2

[3] Hussein RA, El-Anssary AA. Plants secondary metabolites: The key drivers of the pharmacological actions of medicinal plants. In: Builders PF, editor. Herbal Medicine. London: IntechOpen; 2018. DOI: 10.5772/intechopen.76139

[4] Wang S, Alseekh S, Fernie AR, Luo J. The structure and function of major plant metabolite modifications. Molecular Plant. 2019;**12**(7):899-919

[5] Chomel P, Guitonny-Larcheveque M, Fernandez C, et al. Plant secondary metabolites: A key driver of litter decomposition and soil nutrient cycling. Journal of Ecology. 2016;**104**:1527-1541

[6] Vinay K et al. Robbins and Cotran Pathologic Basis of Diseases. 8th ed. London: Elsevier Limited; 2010. pp. 331-332

[7] Mahady GB. Medicinal plants for the prevention and treatment of bacterial infections. Current Pharmaceutical Disease. 2005;**11**(19):2405-2427. DOI: 10.2174/1381612054367481

[8] Introduction to infectious diseases [Internet]. Available from: https://www.bcm.edu/departments/molecular-virology-and-microbiology/emerging-infections-and-biodefense/introduction-to-infectious-diseases

[9] Britannica. The Editors of Encyclopaedia. "list of infectious diseases", Encyclopedia Britannica, 25 July 2016. Available from: https://www.britannica.com/topic/list-of-infectious-diseases-2071204 [Accessed: February 13, 2022]

[10] Dvorkin-Camiel L, Whelan JS. Tropical American plants in the treatment of infectious diseases. Journal of Dietary Supplements. 2008;**5**(4):349-372

[11] Sir Stanley D. Davidson's Principles and Practice of Medicine. 21st ed. London: Elsevier Limited; 2010. pp. 131-133

[12] Why are plants important? Reasons why we need them [Internet]. Available from: https://www.woodlandtrust.org.uk/blog/2018/04/why-plants-are-important/

[13] Veeresham C. Natural products derived from plants as a source of drugs. Journal of Advanced Pharmaceutical Technology & Research. 2012;**3**(4): 200-201. DOI: 10.4103/2231-4040.104709

[14] Evans WC. Trease and Evans Pharmacognosy. 15th ed. London: Elsevier Limited; 2002. p. 131, 133, 191, 289, 333

[15] Vinay K et al. Robbins and Cotran Pathologic Basis of Diseases. 8th ed. London: Elsevier Limited; 2010. p. 332, 333, 334, 335

[16] Sir Stanley D. Davidson's Principles and Practice of Medicine. 21st ed. London: Elsevier Limited; 2010. p. 131, 133

[17] Busia K. Ghana Herbal Pharmacopoeia. revised ed. Accra: STERRI; 2010. p. 25

[18] Ito C, Katsuno S, Itoigawa M, Ruangrungsi N, et al. New carbazole alkaloids from *Clausena anisata* with antitumor promoting activity. Journal of Natural Products. 2000;**63**(1):125-128

[19] Addae-Mensah I. Towards a Rational Scientific Basis for Herbal Medicine: A Phytochemist's Two-Decade Contribution. Accra: Ghana Universities Press; 1992. pp. 22-27

[20] Hayashi T. Biologically active diterpenoids from *Scoparia dulcis* (scrophulariaceae). Studies in Natural Product Chemistry. 2000;**21**(2):689-727

[21] What are bacteria and what do they do? [Internet]. Available from: https://www.medicalnewstoday.com/articles/157973#where-do-they-live

[22] Bacteria [Internet]. Available from: https://en.wikipedia.org/wiki/Bacteria

[23] Bacteria [Internet]. Available from: https://www.genome.gov/genetics-glossary/Bacteria

[24] Evans WC. Trease and Evans Pharmacognosy. 15th ed. London: Elsevier Limited; 2002. p. 432

[25] Vinay K et al. Robbins and Cotran Pathologic Basis of Diseases. 8th ed. London: Elsevier Limited; 2010. p. 335

[26] Nuhu AM, Mshelia MS, Yakubu Y. Antimicrobial screening of the bark extract of *Pterocarpus erinaceus* tree. Journal of Chemical Society of Nigeria. 2000;**25**:85-87

[27] Damodaran S, Venkataraman S. A study on the therapeutic efficacy of *Cassia alata*, Linn. leaf extract against *Pityriasis versicolor*. Journal of Ethnopharmacology. 1994;**42**(1):19-23

[28] Erasto P, Grierson DS, Afolayan AJ. Bioactive sesquiterpene lactones from the leaves of *Vernonia amygdalina*. Journal of Ethnopharmacology. 2006;**106**:117-120

[29] Runyoro DKB, Ngassapa OD, Matee MIN, Joseph CC, Moshi MJ. Medicinal plants used by Tanzanian traditional healers in the management of Candida infections. Journal of Ethnopharmacology. 2006;**106**:158-165

[30] Vinay K et al. Robbins and Cotran Pathologic Basis of Diseases. 8th ed. London: Elsevier Limited. p. 335

[31] Diehl MS, Kamanzi Atindehou K, Téré H, Betschart B. Prospect for anthelminthic plants in the Ivory Coast using ethnobotanical criteria. Journal of Ethnopharmacology. 2004;**95**:277-284

[32] Fakae BB, Campbell AM, Barrett J, Scott IM, et al. Inhibition of glutathione Stransferases (GSTs) from parasitic nematodes by extracts from traditional Nigerian medicinal plants. Phytotherapy Research. 2000;**14**(8):630-634

[33] Lans C. Comparison of plants used for skin and stomach problems in Trinidad and Tobago with Asian ethnomedicine. Journal of Ethnobiology and Ethnomedicine. 2007;**3**:3

[34] Koko WS, Galal M, Khalid HS. Fasciolicidal efficacy of *Albizia anthelmintica* and *Balanites aegyptiaca* compared with albendazole. Journal of Ethnopharmacology. 2000;**71**(1-2):247-252

[35] Protozoan [Internet]. Available from: https://www.britannica.com/science/protozoan

[36] Protozoa [Internet]. Available from: https://en.wikipedia.org/wiki/Protozoa

[37] Boye GL. Studies on antimalarial action of *Cryptolepis sanguinolenta* extract. In: Proceedings of the

International Symposium on East-West Medicine; Seoul, Korea. 1989. pp. 243-251

[38] Tona L, Kambu K, Ngimbi N, et al. Antiamoebic and phytochemical screening of some Congolese medicinal plants. Journal of Ethnopharmacology. 1998;**61**(1):57-65

[39] Evans WC. Trease and Evans Pharmacognosy. 15th ed. London: Elsevier Limited; 2002. p. 432

Chapter 22

Natural Does Not Mean Safe

Onyenmechi Johnson Afonne and Emeka Chinedu Ifediba

Abstract

Medicinal plants are rich sources of natural products, the principal constituents in herbal medicines, utilized for the treatment and prevention of diseases. High consumer expectations for health care, in the face of soaring cost of conventional pharmaceuticals, have popularized herbal medicines in different regions of the world. The consumption of these botanicals and their products has recently gained much impetus with the assumption that since these active principles in them are natural, they are, therefore, safe. Assertive as this idea could be, scrutinizing the perspectives on which it is premised is critical in minimizing probable risk on human health. Most plant parts are repositories of natural toxins, phytosteroids, and bioaccumulated toxicants, all of which are driven by natural processes. Besides intrinsic toxicity possessed by phytotoxins, some innocuous chemicals in medicinal plants can be biotransformed to toxic components. Some chemicals in medicinal plants that are of safety concerns include the endocrine-disrupting chemicals such as phytoestrogens, bisphenol A, and phthalates, among others. The persistent, bioaccumulative, and toxic metals have also been identified in medicinal plants. Some of these chemicals have been found to cause metabolic derangement and carcinogenicity. It is, therefore, imperative that linking natural products to safety should rather be empirical.

Keywords: natural, safe, phytotoxin, phytoestrogen, dioxin, toxic metals

1. Introduction

Herbal medicines are the mainstay of complementary or alternative medicine in most developing and some developed countries [1–3]. The use of herbal medicine in history and in different cultures was premised on the discovery of medicinal plants by trial and error, serendipity, or by the observatory science of zoopharmacognosis [4, 5]. Plants have been used as drug by the primitive man and are presently in high demand with increasing acceptability globally. Currently, the demand for plant-derived products has increased across the world with the Middle East, Latin America, Africa, and Asia accounting for greater than 85% of the populations predominantly relying on herbal medicine for their health care needs [1]. Medicinal plants are a variety of plants with medicinal properties in some or all of its parts. Parts that have prominently contributed to these properties include the seeds, root, leaf, fruit, skin, and flowers [6, 7]. The rich contents of phytochemicals in medicinal plants have provided the basis for their use in herbal medicines. The World Health Organization (WHO) had defined herbal medicines to include herbs, herbal materials, herbal preparations, and finished herbal products that contain, as active ingredients, parts of plants, other plant materials, or combinations thereof [8]. The production of plant secondary metabolites (PSMs) is a common phenomenon in the plant kingdom. These chemicals include a wide range of compounds, such as alkaloids, saponin, flavonoids, anthroquinones, terpenoids, coumarins, lignans, polysaccharides, polypeptides, and proteins [9]. Plant secondary metabolites are known to possess diverse physiological roles. They act as signaling compounds to attract pollinators or seed dispersers and defense against threats such as microbes, insects, predators, and abiotic (radiation, temperature, and drought) stress [9–12]. The presence and diversity of these compounds in plant materials are inducible by natural selection (or processes) and new breeding methods that accentuate these protective/adaptive mechanisms [13]. Most of these products found in medicinal plants surely provide a diverse chemical space for drug discovery and management of many health conditions [14, 15]. The search for these products is attracting interest globally especially from Asia, Africa, or Latin America [16].

The curious expression that PSMs are natural products underpins the belief that as "natural" products, medicinal plants are "safe" or "safer" than conventional medicines. Indeed, some PSMs in medicinal plants are intrinsically toxic [17, 18] or are activated by enzyme systems in humans to toxic compounds [19]. There are also certain classes of PSMs with endocrine-disrupting capabilities [20–22]. This perspective that links natural to safety underscores core health issues in the use of herbal medicines. First, adverse effects resulting from the consumption of herbal medicines are usually not reported since consumers generally regard them as safe and, therefore, would not attribute symptoms to their use [23]. Second, the increased toxicity of conventional drugs when taken concomitantly with these "safe" products can also ensue. The abuse of these natural products is also inevitable, posing an incremental risk of toxicity since consumers usually care less about the quantity (dose) and frequency of herb intake. Besides PSMs, "natural processes," such as adsorption and absorption, introduce environmental toxic substances into plant systems, thereby expanding the profile in the chemical composition of plant species. Environmental changes and pollution effects are major determinants in this regard and are critical in the definition of "nature" and "natural" and the safety attributed to their products. A subset of these xenobiotics is carcinogenic and can also cause metabolic derangement in humans on exposure beyond certain threshold. Regulation governing the production and sale of herbal medicines vary from one country to the other under regulatory categories, such as health foods, dietary supplements, natural health products, and functional foods [8]. These categorizations do not suggest safety in anyway but an approach for control and marketing. Therefore, leveraging on the nominal representation of the word "natural" in defining safety is not only ambiguous but also deceptive. Empirical data have shown that natural does not always mean safe in the premise of utility of medicinal plants for therapeutic consequences.

2. Naturalness of herb constituents

The concept of natural is contested by different perspectives cutting across different fields of learning. However, nature may be considered under different possible definitions: pristine ecology and life processes [24]. The definition of nature as pristine ecology is questionable given the successive cataclysmic evolution that gradually disequilibrated the ecology of the primitive man. Natural as life processes governed by the laws of science (physics, chemistry, and biology) will provide a better platform for this discourse. Therefore, in the light of herbal medicines, the word "natural" suggests essentially that the product is comprised of ingredients produced by nature processes and not the work of man or interference from man. Excitingly, processes suggest activities and reactions that can be conditioned by the environment. The environmental conditions in which a plant grows influence its phytochemical composition and distribution [11, 13]. Second, anthropogenic activities contaminate air and land in addition to agricultural practices (irrigation, fertilization, and pest control), all of which can induce stress to the subsisting plant organisms [12]. The environment and its activities describe nature and could represent natural in this manner since it facilitates life processes. These processes, however, reflect an ecosystem situation and exposure that is far from that of a pristine environment. Safety of constituents of biological organisms, plants inclusive, in such environment should be considered with caution.

3. Safety of herbal constituents

3.1 Natural plant toxins (phytotoxin)

Phytotoxins are toxic plant secondary metabolites employed for defense by the plant kingdom and are also similar to anthropogenic micropollutants in terms of persistence and toxicity [25]. The distribution of these natural products is diverse but present in most plant families used for medicinal purposes [19, 26]. They also differ in biological function and toxicities. Common classes of phytotoxins include the alkaloids, cynogenic glycosides, saponins, furocouramins, lectins, solanines, and chaconine [9]. Sources of some of these chemicals from plant species, such as *Atropa belladonna*, *Datura* spp., *Digitalis* spp., *Papaver somniferum,* and *Strophantus gratus,* are well documented [17, 27]. Apparently, no correlation exists between toxicity and chemical diversity [28], but these toxins might contribute to mixture toxicities and have the potential to overtake anthropogenic chemicals in their overall risk because of constant and ubiquitous production in plants. Since the presence and diversity of these compounds in plant materials are inducible by natural selection [13], medicinal plants with high local abundance often induced by human activity might be of great concern. Phytotoxins cause a variety of adverse effects and pose a serious health threat to man [25] ranging from acute poisoning to long-term health consequences. They mediate their biological activities through mechanisms such as covalent modification of proteins and DNA bases (e.g., furanocoumarins), nonlinam-covalent modification of proteins, and interaction with biomolecules [27]. The common adverse health effects of these phytotoxins in man had previously been reviewed [18, 29] (**Table 1**). Besides phytotoxins with intrinsic toxicity, the metabolic activation of certain inert classes of natural plant products can unmask potential toxicities. Most of these potential herbal toxins are mainly found in chemical classes, such as the pyrrolizidine alkaloids, furanoterpenoids, anthraquinones, bisbenzylisoquinolines, alkenylbenzenes, flavonoids, and alkaloids. Their activation is mainly mediated by hepatic cytochrome P_{450} and in few cases by intestinal bacteria leading to the generation of toxic and reactive metabolites capable of binding to cellular macromolecules/reduction systems with a consequent formation of intermediate complexes and resultant toxicities. A comprehensive review of the activation, mechanisms, and subsequent toxicity of these pretoxic compounds has recently been undertaken by Wang et al. [19] and summarized in **Table 2**.

Class	Common sources	Common toxicity	Mechanism	Sources
Xanthin alkaloids	*Buneriaceae*, *Rubiaceae*, *Theacea*	Stimulate heart rate, force of contraction, and cardiac arrhythmias at high concentration	Inhibits cAMP phosphodiesterase and adenosine receptors	[9, 29]
Furocoumarins	*Leguminosae*, *Rutaceae*, *Apiaceae*, *Moraceae*	Phytophotodermatitis	DNA alkylation	[9, 27]
Lectin proteins	*Leguminosae*	Interferences with digestion and absorption of nutrients	Bind to cell surface	[9, 27]
Cyanogenic glycosides	*Leguminosae*, *Gramineneae*, *Rosaceae*	Diarrhea, convulsion, death in severe case of large acute exposure	HCN produced poisons mitochondrial respiratory chain	[27, 29]
Solanine and chaconine	*Solanaceae*	Hallucinations, hypothermia, fever	Reversible inhibition of cholinesterase	[9, 29]
Sesquiterpen lactones	*Asteraceae*, *Convolvulaceae*, *Rutaceae*, *Umbelliferae*	May be genetoxic	DNA oxidation	[27, 29]
Saponins	*Araliaceae*, *Fabaceae*, *Plantaginaceae*, *Scrophulariaceae*, *Solanaceae*	Diarrhea, excessive salivation	Complex membrane, cholesterol	[27, 29]

HCN, hydrocyanic acid; cAMP, cyclic adenosine monophosphate.

Table 1.
Some phytotoxins and common adverse effects.

3.2 Phytosteroids

Another class of specialized secondary plant metabolites, which can affect human health, is the phytosteroids. These compounds can potentially bind to steroid receptors in animals/humans and, thus, trigger or repress downstream receptor-mediated signaling events [22]. Phytosteroids, usually diverse in structures from endogenous steroid, can act as agonists, antagonists, or agents with both agonist/antagonist activities for steroid receptors [30, 31]. Some of these phytosteroids are the culprit of receptor promiscuity and may also interfere with steroid metabolizing enzymes, gifting this class of compounds a complex modulatory ability on the endocrine and reproductive systems [22]. A prominent subclass of phytosteroids is termed phytoestrogen because of their similarity to the female hormone, estrogen. These estrogen-like substances are the basis for the use of some plants for medicinal purposes [32] and include such classes as isoflavones (e.g., genistein, diadzein, glycitein, and biochanin), lignans (e.g., sesamin, enterodiol, and enterolactone), coumestans (e.g., coumestrol, plicadin, and wedelolactone), and certain classes of phytoalexins (e.g., medicarpin) (**Figure 1**) [33]. Phytoestrogens have been isolated and identified in herbal medicines [34, 35] for the relief of menopausal symptoms and the prevention of osteoporosis and heart diseases [36]. Apparently, they also improve serum triglycerides, total cholesterol, low-density lipoprotein, apolipoproteins A-1

Class	Common source	Toxic metabolites	Induced toxicity	Mechanism
Pyrrolizidine alkaloids	*Boraginaceae*, *Crotalaria*	Pyrrolic esters, necine and necic acids	Hepatotoxicity, pulmonary toxicity	DNA/protein adduct formation
Furan derivatives	*Dioscorea bulbifera*, *Ceratocystis fimbriata Ellis*	cis-Enedial, enedial intermidiates, methofuran	Hepatotoxicity, pulmonary toxicity	DNA/protein adduct formation
Anthraquinones	*Polygoni multiflori*	Quinone intermediates lucidin	Hepatotoxicity	GSH depletion
Epoxy diterpenoids	*Tripterygium wilfordii*		Hepatotoxicity, neurotoxicity	GSH/NAC depletion
Bisbenzylisoquinoline	*Stephania tetrandra*, *Menispermum dauricum*, *Berberis amurensis*	Quinone methide, intermediate, 3-epoxy-3-methylindoline, reactive iminium	Pulmonary toxicity	GSH depletion
Alkenylbenzenes	*Cinnamomum verum*, *Myristica fragrans*, *sweet basil and sweet fennel*	1′-Hydroxymyristicin 1′-sulfooxyestragole	Carcinogenicity	DNA adduct formation
Flavonoids	*Quercus Linn*, *Genus citrus*, *Quercus dentate*	Quinone and quinine, methides, isorhamnetin, 4′-OH-tangeretin	Cytotoxicity	Cell cycle arrest

DNA, deoxyribonucleic acid; GSH, glutathione; NAC, N-acetyl cysteine.
Source: Wang et al. [19].

Table 2.
Potential toxic compounds activated by metabolic systems.

and B, and cell adhesion molecules [37]. Despite these benefits, animal data had also revealed that phytoestrogens have a wide range of adverse molecular, cellular, behavioral, developmental, and reproductive effects at doses and plasma concentrations comparable to that in humans [20, 36, 38, 39]. Based on the estrogenic potential of phytoestrogen, exposure can disturb normal sexual differentiation in fetus and cause menstrual disturbances in females or low sperm counts in males. Owing to the potential interactions between phytoestrogens and the thyroid gland, it is possible that the thyroid function of hypothyroid individuals consuming high levels of phytoestrogen- or goitrogen-rich foodstuffs and supplements may be adversely affected [22]. Exposure to phytoestrogens may have a modest adverse effect on *carotid intima media* thickness (CIMT) progression particularly in postmenopausal women at an increased risk of developing atherosclerosis [37]. The harmful effects of phytoestrogens is a subject of scientific contestation; however, these effects depend on the exposure (type, amount consumed, and bioavailability), ethnicity, hormonal status (age and sex and physiological condition), and health status of the consumer [33]. Besides the phytoestrogens, ligands for receptors of hormones, such as progesterone, thyroid, and gluccocorticoids (**Figure 2**), have also been identified in botanicals [21, 22, 40]. Effects from phytoprogestins (e.g., apigenin), phytoandrogens (e.g., drupanol), and phytocorticoids (e.g., ginsenoside) in medicinal plants are also gaining attention. The promiscuity of these plant-sourced ligands for steroid receptors have been

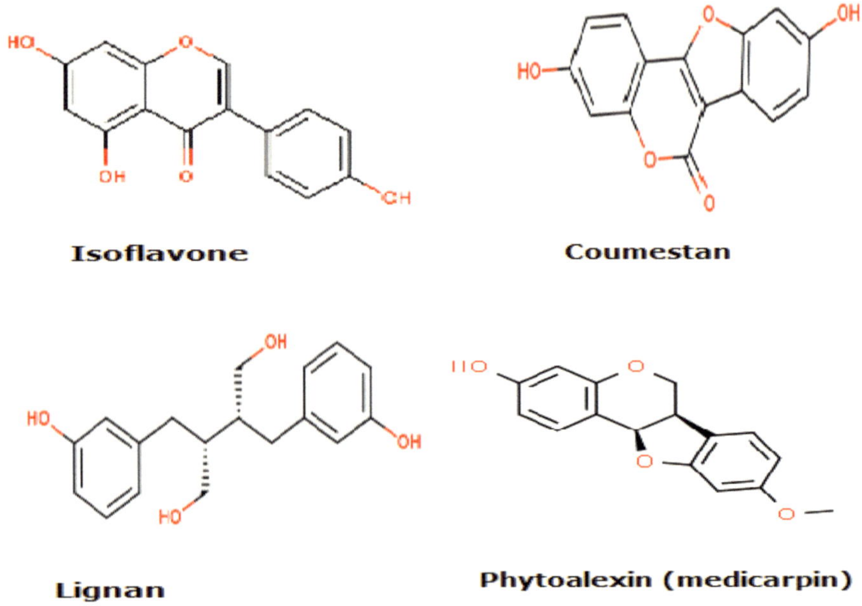

Figure 1.
Structural classes of phytoestrogens. Source: Domínguez-López et al. [33].

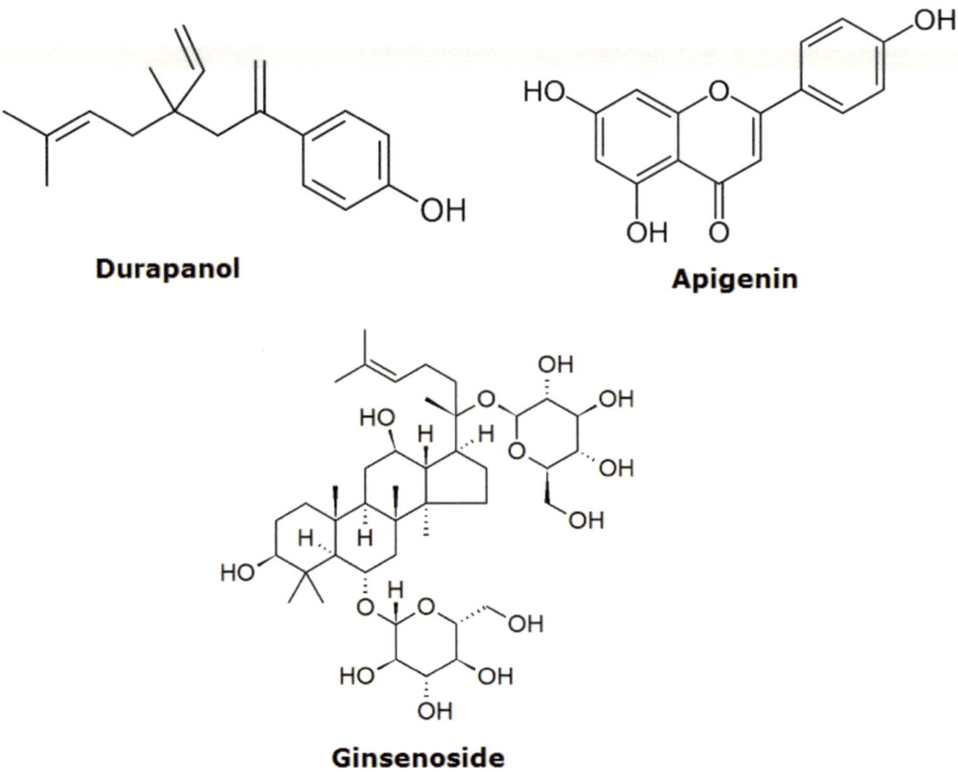

Figure 2.
Other examples of phytosteroids. Source: Dean et al. [22].

reported [22, 41] and have the potential to precipitate side effects leading to cardiovascular disease, stroke, water retention, and weight gain.

3.3 Bioaccumulated toxicants

The abuse of the natural ecosystem by a massive use of materials and energy to meet the demands of the world's growing population has led to a continuous and significant contamination of water, soil, and air. Industrial and agricultural activities are hugely responsible for the release of millions of tons of chemicals known as persistent, bioaccumulative, and toxic (PBT) into the environment. The interactional forces driving the relationship between the three environmental compartments (water, soil, and air) determine the fate of these pollutants, which undoubtedly have become part of nature. Medicinal plants grown in contaminated areas are usually susceptible to concentrating PBT chemicals. Dioxin, dioxin-like polychlorinated biphenyls (PCBs), some indicator PCBs [42, 43], metals [44–46], and phthalates [47–49], among others, are common environmental pollutants that can accumulate in plants in substantial and health-threatening quantities. Exposure to dioxins and dioxin-like substances has been associated with an avalanche of toxic effects during developmental stages, immunotoxicity, and adverse changes in thyroid and steroid hormones and also in reproductive functions [43]. Toxic metals found in botanicals may pose low health risk in one dose of herbal preparations [50] but can have a significant contribution to total body heavy metal burden [51, 52]. Major threats to human health from heavy metals are commonly associated with exposure to lead, cadmium, mercury, and arsenic [53] and have been linked to indicators such as decreased immunity, cardiac dysfunction, fetal malformation, and impaired psychosocial and neurological behavior [52]. Phthalates, globally used as plasticizers readily accumulate in medicinal plants [47, 48], have been found to be potent endocrine disruptors. In addition to endocrine-disrupting abilities, phthalates also possessed teratogenicity, carcinogenicity, and mutagenicity effects [54, 55]. Other toxicants with bioaccumulative capacities in medicinal plants abound. Some of these agents can bind covalently to enzymes and induce the production of reactive oxygen species (ROS), thus leading to negative health effects in humans [56].

4. Naturalness and herbal processing

The preparation of herbal medicines from medicinal plants requires processes such as boiling, roasting, squeezing, and soaking [7, 57]. This is believed to mitigate exaggerated pharmacological actions, alleviate side effects, modify energy properties, mask disagreeable odors, or prolong the shelf life of crude herbs [58]. Herbal processing has been leveraged most of the times as detoxifying processes important for those herbs that are known to contain toxic or undesirable chemical components [59]. For example, steaming and frying may degrade heat-sensitive toxic, while fermentation and aging may result in enzymatic degradation of the toxic ingredients. Despite these positive implications of processing, such practices may also uncover a type of metabolite-deficiency-induced toxicity since the pharmacological potencies of herbal medicinal preparations had been touted as one subserved by synergistic interactions of disparate constituents in an extract [60, 61]. Adjuvants are also often added to enhance therapeutic effects or minimize drug toxicity, thereby broadening the spectrum of clinical application of the processed drugs. Commonly used adjuvants include vinegar, honey, wine, brine, ginger juice, bran, and rice [58, 62]. For example, according to Li et al. [63] approximately 19.4% adverse events, associated with traditional Chinese medicine use between 1949 and 2008 in China, are reported to be ascribable to improper processing. It is believed that adjuvants participate in chemical or physical transformation that improves pharmacological effects, or alter the pharmacokinetic behavior, to provide an enhanced therapeutic effect or counteract drug toxicity [58]. Therefore, concoction, decoction, infusion, and homogenization, among others, are processes that can alter the natural constituents of medicinal plants and thereby introduce a twist in this concept of "natural."

5. Discussion

The safety of medicinal plants has been enmeshed in scientific controversies. While the promoters of "natural is safe" paradigm persisted, different authors had previously justified why natural does not really mean safe in the context of phytotherapy. Most contributions in this regard presented evidence-based toxicity bordering on inherent toxicity of plant constituents [64–66] and herbal–drug interactions [23, 60]. However, the present paper premised this safety concerns on a definition of natural as a process influenced by the immediate habitat of the plant. The impact of the environment and processing procedures are indeed critical players of nature that determine the safety of medicinal plants. However, the general consensus by all authors is that some popular medicinal plant materials contain harmful substances, which may be classified into phytotoxins, phytosteroids, and bioaccumulated toxicants.

6. Conclusion

The folkloric use of medicinal plants has been justified by their constituents of active principles. However, the safety attributable to these natural products is overestimated. There are harmful substances found in plant materials as a result of natural processes. Unfortunately, these processes are reflecting an ecosystem situation and exposure that is far from that of a pristine environment. However, these facts seem to be overshadowed by the views of the "naturalists" who understand nature as pristine, pure, and harmless. Exposure to these natural toxins through herbal preparations and its attendant risks to human health may surge higher under this assumption that if a compound is natural, it is automatically safe. Caution should, therefore, be taken in the use of medicinal plants for treatment of various health conditions against the backdrop of poor regulation of herbal medicines.

We recommend the scientific determination of the safety profile of medicinal plants before use in therapy. In addition, appropriate regulatory agencies should intensify the monitoring of these phytomedicines to ascertain that they meet set regulatory standards, as their being natural does not mean being safe.

Acknowledgements

The authors acknowledge Nnamdi Azikiwe University, Awka, Nigeria, for making her library facilities accessible to the authors for the accomplishment of the book chapter.

DOI: http://dx.doi.org/10.5772/intechopen.104732

Conflict of interest

The authors declare no conflict of interest.

Author details

Onyenmechi Johnson Afonne* and Emeka Chinedu Ifediba
Nnamdi Azikiwe University, Awka, Nigeria

*Address all correspondence to: oj.afonne@unizik.edu.ng

References

[1] Jamshidi-Kia F, Lorigooini Z, Amini-Khoei H. Medicinal plants: Past history and future perspective. Journal of Herbmed Pharmacology. 2018;**7**(1):1-7. DOI: 10.15171/jhp.2018.01

[2] Sánchez M, González-Burgos E, Iglesias I, Lozano R, Gómez-Serranillos MP. Current uses and knowledge of medicinal plants in the autonomous Community of Madrid (Spain): A descriptive cross-sectional study. Complementary Medicine and Therapies. 2020;**20**:306. DOI: 10.1186/s12906-020-03089-x

[3] Liu S, Zhang B, Zhou J, Lei Q, Fang Q, Kennelly EJ, et al. Herbal plants traded at the Kaili medicinal market, Guizhou, China. Journal of Ethnobiology and Ethnomedicine. 2021;**17**:67. DOI: 10.1186/s13002-021-00495-4

[4] Khan H. Medicinal plants in light of history: Recognized therapeutic modality. Journal of Evidence-Based Complementary & Alternative Medicine. 2014;**19**(3):216-219. DOI: 10.1177/2156587214533346

[5] Šantić Z, Pravdic N, Bevanda M, Galić K. The historical use of medicinal plants in traditional and scientific medicine. Medicina Academica Mostariensia. 2017;**5**:1-2

[6] Dwivedi T, Kanta C, Singh LR, Sharma IP. A list of some important medicinal plants with their medicinal uses from Himalayan state Uttarakhand, India. Journal of Medicinal Plants Studies. 2019;**7**(2):106-116

[7] Mbuni YM, Wang S, Mwangi BN, Mbari NJ, Musili PM, Walter NO, et al. Medicinal plants and their traditional uses in local communities around Cherangani Hills, Western Kenya. Plants. 2020;**9**:331. DOI: 10.3390/plants9030331

[8] World Health Organisation. WHO Global Report on Traditional and Complementary Medicine. Geneva: World Health Organisation; 2019. ISBN: 978-92-4-151543-6

[9] Ogori AF. Plant toxins. American Journal of Biomedical Science & Research. 2019;**4**(3):173-175. DOI: 10.34297/AJBSR.2019.04.000793

[10] Bucheli TD. Phytotoxins: Environmental micropollutants of concern? Environmental Science and Technology. 2014;**48**:13027-13033

[11] Yang L, Wen K, Ruan X, Zhao YX, Wei F, Wang Q. Response of plant secondary metabolites to environmental factors. Molecules. 2018;**23**:762. DOI: 10.3390/molecules23040762

[12] Gull A, Lone AA, Wani NU. Biotic and abiotic stresses in plants. In: de Oliveira AB, editor. Abiotic and Biotic Stress in Plants. London: IntechOpen; 2019. pp. 1-6. DOI: 10.5772/intechopen.85832

[13] Clemensen AK, Provenza FD, Hendrickson JR, Grusak MA. Ecological implications of plant secondary metabolites phytochemical diversity can enhance agricultural sustainability. Frontiers in Sustainable Food Systems. 2020;**4**:547826. DOI: 10.3389/fsufs.2020.547826

[14] Mohanraj K, Karthikeyan BS, Vivek-Ananth RP, Chand RP, Aparna SR, Mangalapandi P, et al. IMPPAT: A curated database of Indian medicinal plants. Phytochemistry and Therapeutics. Scientific Reports. 2018;**8**:4329. DOI: 10.1038/s41598-018-22631-z

[15] Hussein RA, El-Anssary AA. Plants secondary metabolites: The key drivers of the pharmacological actions of medicinal plants. In: Builders P, editor. Herbal Medicine. London: IntechOpen; 2018. pp. 11-30. DOI: 10.5772/intechopen.76139

[16] Salmeron-Manzano E, Garrido-Cardenas JA, Manzano-Agugliaro F. Worldwide research trends on medicinal plants. International Journal of Environmental Research and Public Health. 2020;**17**:3376. DOI: 10.3390/ijerph17103376

[17] Nasri H, Shirzad H. Toxicity and safety of medicinal plants. Journal of Herbmed Pharmacology. 2013;**2**(2): 21-22

[18] Bode AM, Dong Z. Toxic phytochemicals and their potential risks for human cancer. Cancer Prevention Research (Philadelphia, Pa.). 2015;**8**(1):1-8. DOI: 10.1158/1940-6207.CAPR-14-0160

[19] Wang YK, Li WQ, Xia S, Guo L, Miao Y, Zhang BK. Metabolic activation of the toxic natural products from herbal and dietary supplements leading to toxicities. Frontiers in Pharmacology. 2021;**12**:1-16. DOI: 10.3389/fphar.2021.758468

[20] Vicdan K, Erdogan D, Özogul C, Elmas C. Effects of dietary phytoestrogens on mouse testis: Evaluation by electron microscopy and Caspase-3 immunostaining. Journal of Turkish-German Gynecological Association. 2007;**8**(3):290-296

[21] Ahmed HMM, Yeh J-Y, Tang Y-C, Cheng WT-K, Ou B-R. Molecular screening of Chinese medicinal plants for progestogenic and antiprogestogenic activity. Journal of Biosciences. 2014;**39**(3):453-461. DOI: 10.1007/s12038-014-9434-z

[22] Dean M, Murphy BT, Burdette JE. Phytosteroids beyond estrogens: Regulators of reproductive and endocrine function in natural products. Molecular and Cellular Endocrinology. 2017;**15**(442):98-105. DOI: 10.1016/j.mce.2016.12.013

[23] Neergheen-Bhujun VS. Underestimating the toxicological challenges associated with the use of herbal medicinal products in developing countries. BioMed Research International. 2013;**9**:1-9

[24] Verhoog H, Matze M, Van Bueren EL, Baars T. The role of the concept of the natural (naturalness) in organic farming. Journal of Agricultural and Environmental Ethics. 2003;**16**:29-49

[25] Gunthardt BF, Hollender J, HungerbuhlerK,ScheringerM,BucheliTD. Comprehensive toxic plants–Phytotoxins database and its application in assessing aquatic micropollution potential. Journal of Agricultural and Food Chemistry. 2018;**66**:7577-7588. DOI: 10.1021/acs.jafc.8b01639

[26] Robertson J, Stevens K. Pyrrolizidine alkaloids: Occurrence, biology, and chemical synthesis. Natural Product Reports. 2017;**34**(1):62-89. DOI: 10.1039/c5np00076a

[27] Wink M. Modes of action of herbal medicines and plant secondary metabolites. Medicines (Basel). 2015, 2015;**2**(3):251-286. DOI: 10.3390/medicines2030251

[28] Clemen-Pascual LM, Macahig RS, Rojas NL. Comparative toxicity, phytochemistry, and use of 53 Philippine medicinal plants. Toxicology Reports. 2020;**9**:22-35

[29] Chandra SJ, Sandhya S, Vinod KR, David B, Sudhakar K, Chaitanya R. Plant toxins—Useful and harmful effects.

Hygeia Journal for Drugs and Medicine. 2012;**4**(1):79-90

[30] Lesovaya E, Yemelyanov A, Swart AC, Swart P, Haegeman G, Budunova I. Discovery of compound A—A selective activator of the glucocorticoid receptor with anti-inflammatory and anti-cancer activity. Oncotarget. 2015;**6**(31):30730-30744. DOI: 10.18632/oncotarget.5078

[31] Toh MF, Sohn J, Chen SN, Yao P, Bolton JL, Burdette JE. Biological characterization of non-steroidal progestins from botanicals used for women's health. Steroids. 2012;**77**:765-773

[32] Saeed IA, Ali L, Jabeen A, Khasawneh M, Rizvi TA, Ashraf SS. Estrogenic activities of ten medicinal herbs from the Middle East. Journal of Chromatographic Science. 2013;**51**:33-39. DOI: 10.1093/chromsci/bms101

[33] Domínguez-López I, Yago-Aragón M, Salas-Huetos A, Tresserra-Rimbau A, Hurtado-Barroso S. Effects of dietary phytoestrogens on hormones throughout a human lifespan: A review. Nutrients. 2020;**12**:2456. DOI: 10.3390/nu12082456

[34] Sulaiman CT, Arun A, Anandan EM, Sandhya CR, Indira B. Isolation and identification of phytoestrogens and flavonoids in an Ayurvedic proprietary medicine using chromatographic and mass spectroscopic analysis. Asian Pacific Journal of Reproduction. 2015;**4**(2):153-156

[35] Haeng LS, Joong KH, Ju LE, Tae CG. The review of the herbal medicines with phytoestrogenic effect. The Journal of Pediatrics of Korean Medicine. 2015, 2015;**29**(2):59-77. DOI: 10.7778/jpkm.2015.29.2.059

[36] Patisaul HB, Jefferson W. The pros and cons of phytoestrogens. Frontiers in Neuroendocrinology. 2010, 2010;**31**(4):400-419. DOI: 10.1016/j.yfrne.2010.03.003

[37] Wolters M, Dejanovic GM, Asllanaj E, Günther K, Pohlabeln H, Bramer W, et al. Effects of phytoestrogen supplementation on intermediate cardiovascular disease risk factors among postmenopausal women: A meta-analysis of randomized controlled trials. Menopause. 2020;**27**(9):1081-1092

[38] Zin SR, Omar SZ, Khan NL, Musameh NI, Das S, Kassim NM. Effects of the phytoestrogen genistein on the development of the reproductive system of Sprague Dawley rats. Clinics. 2013;**68**(2):253-262

[39] Rosenfeld CS. Effects of phytoestrogens on the developing brain, gut microbiota, and risk for neurobehavioral disorders. Frontiers in Nutrition. 2019;**6**(142):1-14. DOI: 10.3389/fnut.2019.00142

[40] Dean M, Austin J, Jinhong R, Johnson ME, Lantvit DD, Burdette JE. The flavonoid apigenin is a progesterone receptor modulator with In vivo activity in the uterus. Hormones and Cancer. 2018;**9**(4):265-277. DOI: 10.1007/s12672-018-0333-x

[41] Austin JR, Kirkpatrick BJ, Rodríguez RR, Johnson ME, Lantvit DD, Burdette JE. Baicalein is a phytohormone that signals through the progesterone and glucocorticoid receptors. Hormones and Cancer. 2020;**11**:97-110

[42] Loutfy N, Mosleh Y, Ahmed MT. Dioxin, dioxin–like PCBs and indicator PCBs in some medicinal plants irrigated with wastewater in Ismailia, Egypt. Polycyclic Aromatic Compounds. 2010;**30**(1):9-26. DOI: 10.1080/10406630903495151

[43] Olatungi OS. Evaluation of selected polychlorinated

biphenyls (PCBs) congeners and dichlorodiphenyltrichloroethane (DDT) in fresh root and leafy vegetables using GC–MS. Scientific Reports. 2019;**9**(538):1-10. DOI: 10.1038/s41598-018-36996-8

[44] Annan K, Dickson RA, Amponsah IK, Nooni IK. The heavy metal contents of some selected medicinal plants sampled from different geographical locations. Pharmacognosy Research. 2013;**5**(2):103-108. DOI: 10.4103/0974-8490.110539

[45] Nkansah MA, Hayford ST, Borquaye LS, Ephraim JH. Heavy metal contents of some medicinal herbs from Kumasi, Ghana. Cogent Environmental Science. 2016;**2**(1):1-9. DOI: 10.1080/23311843.2016.1234660

[46] Viakosen EN, Alade GO. Determination of heavy metals in medicinal plants from the wild and cultivated garden in Wilberforce Island, Niger Delta region, Nigeria. Journal of Pharmacy & Pharmacognosy Research. 2017;**5**(2):129-143

[47] Saeidnia S, Abdollahi M. Are medicinal plants polluted with phthalates? DARU Journal of Pharmaceutical Sciences. 2013;**21**(43):1-4

[48] Manayi A, Kurepaz-Mahmoodabadi M, Gohari AR, Ajani Y, Saeidnia S. Presence of phthalate derivatives in the essential oils of a medicinal plant *Achillea tenuifolia*. DARU Journal of Pharmaceutical Sciences. 2014;**22**(78):1-6. DOI: 10.1186/s40199-014-0078-1

[49] Li Y, Yan H, Yu X. Uptake and accumulation of di-n-butyl phthalate in six leafy vegetables under hydroponic conditions. Food Production, Processing and Nutrition. 2019;**1**(9):1-7

[50] Brima EI. Toxic elements in different medicinal plants and the impact on human health. International Journal of Environmental Research and Public Health. 2017;**14**:1209. DOI: 10.3390/ijerph14101209

[51] Luo L, Wang B, Jiang J, Fitzgerald M, Huang Q, Yu Z, et al. Heavy metal contaminations in herbal medicines: Determination, comprehensive risk assessments, and solutions. Frontiers in Pharmacology. 2021;**11**:595335. DOI: 10.3389/fphar.2020.595335

[52] Olusola JA, Akintan OB, Erhenhi HA, Osanyinlusi OO. Heavy metals and health risks associated with consumption of herbal plants sold in a major urban market in Southwest Nigeria. Journal of Health & Pollution. 2021;**11**(31).1-11

[53] Jarup J. Hazards of heavy metal contamination. British Medical Bulletin. 2003;**68**:167-182. DOI: 10.1093/bmb/ldg032

[54] Wang X, Song M, Guo M, Chi C, Mo F, Shen X. Pollution levels and characteristics of phthalate esters in indoor air in hospitals. Journal of Environmental Sciences. 2015;**37**:67-74

[55] Li K, Ma D, Wu J, Chai C, Shi Y. Distribution of phthalate esters in agricultural soil with plastic film mulching in Shandong peninsula, East China. Chemosphere. 2016;**164**:314-321

[56] Xiang L, Li YW, Wang ZR, Liu BL, Zhao HM, Li H, et al. Bioaccumulation and phytotoxicity and human health risk from microcystin-LR under various treatments: A pot study. Toxins. 2020;**12**:523. DOI: 10.3390/toxins12080523

[57] Alebie G, Urga B, Worku A. Systematic review on traditional medicinal plants used for the treatment of malaria in Ethiopia: Trends and perspectives. Malaria

Journal. 2017;**16**:307. DOI: 10.1186/s12936-017-1953-2

[58] Chen LL, Verpoorte R, Yen HR, Peng WH, Cheng YC, Chao J, et al. Effects of processing adjuvants on traditional Chinese herbs. Journal of Food and Drug Analysis. 2018;**2018**(26):S96-S114

[59] World Health Organisation. WHO guidelines on good herbal processing practices for herbal medicines. WHO Technical Report Series. 2018;**1010**:81-152

[60] Wills RB, Bone K, Morgan M. Herbal products: Active constituents, modes of action and quality control. Nutrition Research Review. 2000;**13**:47-77

[61] Yang Y, Zhang Z, Li S, Ye X, Li X, He K. Synergy effects of herb extracts: Pharmacokinetics and pharmacodynamic basis. Fitoterapia. 2014;**92**:133-147

[62] Chen Z, Ye SY, Zhu RG. The extraordinary transformation of traditional Chinese medicine: Processing with liquid excipients. Pharmaceutical Biology. 2020;**58**(1):561-573

[63] Li RR, Zhang ZJ, Wang ZJ, Wang F, Yuan ST. Literature analysis on toxicity, side effect and adverse reaction of traditional Chinese medicine. Chinese Journal of Experimental Traditional Medical Formulae. 2010;**15**:068

[64] George P. Concerns regarding the safety and toxicity of medicinal plants—An overview. Journal of Applied Pharmaceutical Science. 2011;**1**(6):40-44

[65] Rubin CB, Brod B. Natural does not mean safe—The dirt on clean beauty products. JAMA Dermatology. 2019;**155**(12):1344-1345. DOI: 10.1001/jamadermatol.2019.2724

[66] Dunne FJ. The 'natural health service': Natural does not mean safe. Advances in Psychiatric Treatment. 2009;**15**:49-56. DOI: 10.1192/apt.bp.107.005272

Chapter 23

Rapid Qualitative and Quantitative HPLC/MS Analysis of an *Antioxidant* Couple Consisted of Glutathione and Ascorbic Acid in a Pharmaceutical Product

Stanislav V. Yefimov

Abstract

Vitamin C and glutathione are mostly found together in pharmaceutical products. These two components protect each other from oxidation by forming an antioxidant couple and mutually reinforcing each other's actions. This paper describes a method for determining the activity of the antioxidant couple in pharmaceutical products using HPLC/MS. An Agilent 6125 HPLC equipped with MSD and DAD detectors was used. The first detector is for the detection of glutathione, and the second is for the detection of ascorbic acid. The MS spectrum of glutathione (Glut) was dominated by the signal m / z + = 308.2, which corresponds to the Glut-H + cation. The MS spectrum of ascorbic acid (AA) was dominated by signals m/z + = 177 and 375, which corresponds to the cations AK-H + and 2AK-Na +. The use of HPLC with two detectors (MS and DAD) made it possible to simultaneously determine both components of the antioxidant couple in pharmaceutical products without derivatization and any preliminary sample preparation. The method meets the FDA criteria for accuracy, selectivity, robustness, and reproducibility, and has a low detection limit of both components of the antioxidant couple.

Keywords: *antioxidant* couple, glutathione, ascorbic acid; potency, HPLC/MS; Validation

1. Introduction

In living cells, glutathione protects cells from oxidative damage and maintains redox balance [1]. Vitamin C (ascorbic acid) is one of the powerful reducing agents, it works as a neutralizer of oxidizing free radicals in a living cell [2]. Glutathione and vitamin C often coexist in pharmaceutical products. Both components enhance each other's actions and protect each other from oxidation. This combination is called the antioxidant couple [3].

Determination of the activity of an antioxidant couple in pharmaceutical products is carried out using modern instruments and specially developed methods. In this work, we used HPLC/MS from Agilent [4].

When developing methods of analysis, it is customary to follow the recommendations of the International Conference on Harmonization (ICH), which contains the necessary criteria for validating methods [5]. It is also important for developers to achieve simplicity (fewer stages) and speed of analysis. Both factors affect its cost.

The complexity of the simultaneous analysis of glutathione and ascorbic acid is that Glutathione (**Figure 1**) is relatively poorly visible to UV-VIS detectors. To make it highly visible, chemists are forced to derivatize glutathione by adding a radical containing a benzoic or furan ring through the sulfhydryl group.

Ellman's reagent (5,5'-dithiobis (2-nitrobenzoic acid) [6, 7], O-phthalic aldehyde [8], 4-vinyl pyridine, 4-fluoro-7-sulfobenzofurazan ammonium salt, 4- (aminosulfonyl)-7-fluorobenzofurazan and N- (9-acridinyl) maleimide [9] are used as derivatizing agent. However, the glutathione molecule contains two carboxyl groups and can be ionized at (ESI) and detected by MSD [10, 11], or by HPLC/ MS/MS [12] without derivatization.

The ascorbic acid molecule (**Figure 1**) contains a furan ring and is well detected by the UV-Vis detector. There are some literature data about methods for the determination of ascorbic acid and ascorbates by HPLC in fruits, blood serum, and pharmaceuticals [13–17].

Usually, the UV detector is used [13, 18–20], some authors prefer an electrochemical detector [16]. The tandem of MS and UV-VIS detectors is a useful and effective tool [14, 17, 21, 22].

As a mobile phase for HPLC/MS, methanol and acetonitrile volatile solutions are most popular [14, 17, 21, 22]. The not volatile sodium dihydrogen orthophosphate solutions may be used as a mobile phase for HPLC-UV [13, 16–19].

To simultaneously analyze several components in a pharmaceutical product, chemists select the appropriate detector and suitable chromatography conditions. In the case when the components differ in nature and their concentration is very different, a good result has given the use of two detectors, each of which is focused on the detection of its group of components. In the present study, we used two detectors, one for glutathione and the other for ascorbic acid. This approach allowed us to obtain a satisfactory result of the analysis with a tenfold difference in the concentration of the components and to exclude derivatization.

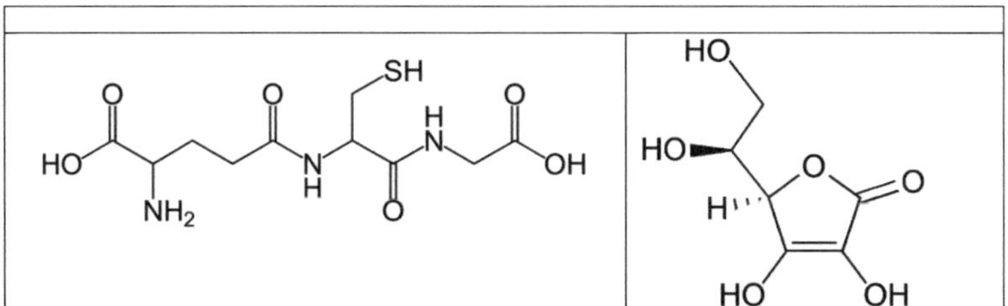

Glutathione. MW:307.3 g/mol

Ascorbic acid. MW: 176.1 g/mol

Figure 1.
Structures of the molecules forming an antioxidant *couple.*

The antioxidant couple analysis method presented in this article was developed for the analysis of nasal spray and injection solution. The specificity, precision, reproducibility, reliability, and selectivity of the method have been validated. The recommendations of the European Medicines Agency [5], as well as the FDA guidelines for the validation of analytical procedures [23–25], were used.

2. Materials and methods

Chemicals. L-ascorbic acid analytical standard from Sigma-Aldrich; formic acid 98-100% analytical grade from Merck; glutathione from European Pharmacopoeia Reference Standard, water HPLC grade purchased from Agilent. All the solvents used were of HPLC grade. Branded pharmaceutical formulation, in form of nasal spray and injection solution, was obtained from commercial sources and used as received, without any further purification.

Samples. All the samples were from a freshly prepared product. The products were tested: Glutathione injection solution, containing 20% of glutathione and 2% of ascorbic acid and, glutathione nasal spray, containing 20% of Glutathione and 3.5% ascorbic acid.

The instruments. The Agilent instrument (Agilent Single Quadrupole LC/MS instrument, 2019) includes the following components: quaternary pump 600 bar maximal pressure; single quadrupole (SQ) mass selective detector (MSD) with electrospray ionization (ESI), 150 V fragmentor, gas flow: 7 L/min, gas temperature 300°C, capillary 4000 V and nebulizer 15 psi; OpenLAB CDS Version 2.2. software. Reversed-phase (RP) column Poroshell 120 EC-C18, 50 × 4.6 mm, particles size 2.7 μm, with guard precolumn. Isocratic elution was performed with mobile phase: 0.1% formic acid water solution and flow rate of 1.0 mL/min.

A qualitative analysis was made using MDS spectrum. Glutathione shows the predominant signal of m/z+=308 which corresponds to the cation Glut-H+. Ascorbic acid (AA) shows m/z+=177, 199, and 375 which corresponds to the AA-H+ cation, AA-Na+ cation, and to the 2AA-Na+ cation respectively.

A quantitative analysis was made based on the standard calibration curve.

Preparation of standard stock solution. An accurately weighed of ascorbic acid and glutathione was dissolved in water. The solution was filtered through a 0.45 μm cellulose acetate membrane filter. The stock solution was stepwise diluted to make a set of standard solutions.

System suitability was tested and validated according to the Centre for Drug Evaluation and Research [24] and Agilent recommendations [25].

Calibration curve. Five standard concentration solutions were tested in the range of glutathione concentrations from 0.1 g/l to 1.0 g/l and AA concentrations from 0.04 g/l to 2.1 g/l. Each point of the calibration curve was the mean of five measurements. Slope (a), intercept (b), and correlation coefficient (r) were calculated by least squares using OpenLAB CDS software. The range of concentrations for which the correlation coefficient was equal to or greater than 0.999 was taken as the working range [24]. For MSD, the type of calibration curve (linear or parabolic) was chosen so that the correlation coefficient was maximum.

Accuracy was expressed as mean absolute recovery and percent relative standard deviation (RSD), for AA and glutathione samples in five copies for each concentration.

The precision of the method was determined by comparing the measurement results of five samples under the same experimental conditions. Intra- and inter-day tests were carried out.

Limits of detection (LOD) **and quantification** (LOQ). LOD is the minimum measurable amount of a substance, LOQ is the minimum measurable amount with acceptable linearity, accuracy, and precision. For a linear calibration curve, LOD is calculated using the formula (1) [5] where (σ) is the standard deviation of the response, and (a) is the slope of the line.

$$LOD = 3.3 * \sigma / a \qquad (1)$$

If the calibration curve is a parabola (y=ax2 +bx + c), then the LOD is the root of the quadratic equation, which is calculated by the formula (2).

$$LOD = (-b + SQRT(b * b - 4 * a * (c - 3.3 * \sigma)))/(2 * a) \qquad (2)$$

The standard deviation of the response (σ) is determined based on the calibration curve as the residual standard deviation of the regression line [5]. The LOQ may be estimated as 3 times LOD.

Repeatability was evaluated in the same tests as for the accuracy and recovery. The measure of repeatability is RSD.

To assess the **specificity** of the method, samples of the pharmaceutical compound and a standard solution of approximately the same concentration of the tested components were compared in terms of tail coefficient, retention time, and the number of theoretical plates. The difference was expressed in RSD.

The r**obustness** of the method was evaluated by the effect of small changes in flow rate, column temperature, and mobile phase composition on the measurement result. The system suitability parameters (T and N) were determined, and the results were compared with acceptable limits.

Statistical analysis. Each experimental point was the average of five measurements. The results $p < 0.05$ were considered statistically significant. Data variation was expressed as standard deviation (SD) and relative standard deviation. A regression analysis based on the Least Squares Method was used to construct a calibration curve. The correlation coefficient (r) and the coefficient of determination (r^2) were calculated.

3. Results

System suitability. The solution of a standard sample with a volume of 1 μl was injected five times. The relative standard deviation of the peak area, retention time, the number of theoretical plates, and tail factor were determined and compared with the acceptable limits (**Table 1**) according to the recommendations [26, 27].

The MS spectra and chromatograms are shown in **Figures 2** and **3**. As we can see in **Figure 2B**, the ascorbic acid DAD signal is clearly visible, while the glutathione peak is barely visible. The situation is the reverse of **Figure 2A**, the glutathione peak is high, and the ascorbic acid peak is very small. As a result of electrospray ionization, glutathione is converted into a single cation m/z+=308 (**Figure 3A**), and ascorbic acid into several cations, including those with m/z+= 177 and 375 (**Figure 3B**).

Linearity, range, and limit of detection. The working range for glutathione was from 0.2 to 1.0 μg, and for AA from 0.5 to 1.0 μg. The limit of detection was calculated based on the standard deviation of the response (σ) and slope (a) according to Eq. (1) for ascorbic acid, and Eq. (2) for glutathione. The results of the LOD calculation are

Test parameters	Mean	S.D.	% RSD	Acceptable limit
AA Peak area (mAU·min)	1,023.90	18.95	1.9	RSD ≤2
Glut. Peak area (counts·min)	2,543,221.44	22,859.33	0.9	RSD ≤2
AA Retention time (min)	0.78	0.00	0.0	RSD ≤2
Glut. Retention time (min)	1.02	0.00	0.2	RSD ≤2
AA Theoretical plates (N)	*30,128.50	4,273.05	1.6	>2,000
Glut. Theoretical plates (N)	*47,000.00	4,242.64	9.0	>2,000
AA Tailing factor (T)	*1.29	0.01	0.6	≤2
Glut. Tailing factor (T)	*1.60	0.01	0.4	≤2

Ascorbic acid (AA) is detected by DAD and glutathione (Glut.) is detected by MSD.
Ascorbic acid standard solution 2.7 μg/μL, injection volume 0.1 μL. Values are presented as mean ±S.D., n = 5, *$p < 0.05$
Glutathione standard solution 0.5 μg/μL, injection volume 1.0 μL. Values are presented as mean ±S.D., n = 5, *$p < 0.05$.

Table 1.
System suitability.

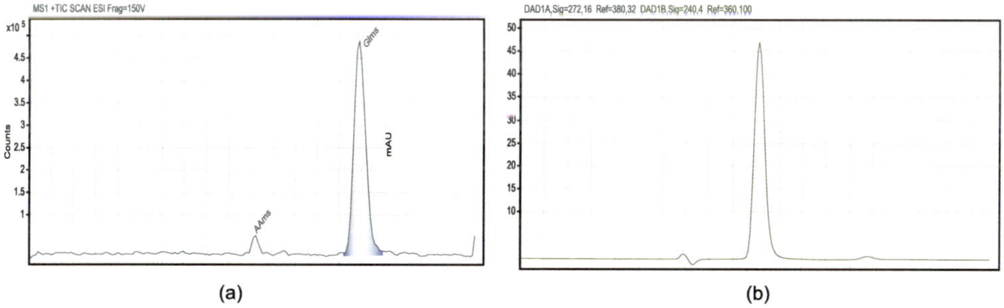

Figure 2.
(a) Chromatogram detected by MSD, hight peak corresponds to glutathione. (b) Chromatogram detected by DAD (272 and 380 nm), hight peak corresponds to ascorbic acid. Concentration of glutathione is 0.62 μg/μL, concentration of ascorbic acid is 0.122 μg/μL; mobile phase is aqua solution of 0.1% formic acid.

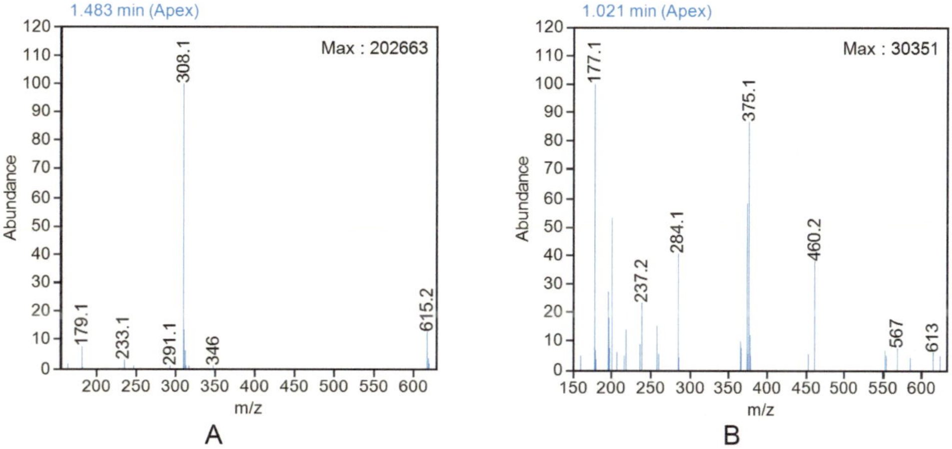

Figure 3.
Extracted spectrum (m/z+ value) of glutathione (A) and ascorbic acid (B). Concentration of glutathione is 0.62 μg/μL, concentration of ascorbic acid is 0.122 μg/μL; mobile phase is aqua solution of 0.1% formic acid.

AA (µg)	Mean Y (n = 5)	Y calc.	ΔY	Glut. (µg)	Mean Y (n = 5)	Y calc.	ΔY
0.0422	150	145	4.8	0.20	1,174,797	1,193,679	−18,882
0.0844	270	271	−1.0	0.33	1,984,510	1,869,527	114,983
0.1266	392	397	−4.8	0.50	2,543,221	2,596,191	−52,970
0.1688	516	523	−6.6	0.67	3,147,655	3,190,815	−43,160
0.211	656	648	7.6	1.00	4,005,954	3,985,687	20,268

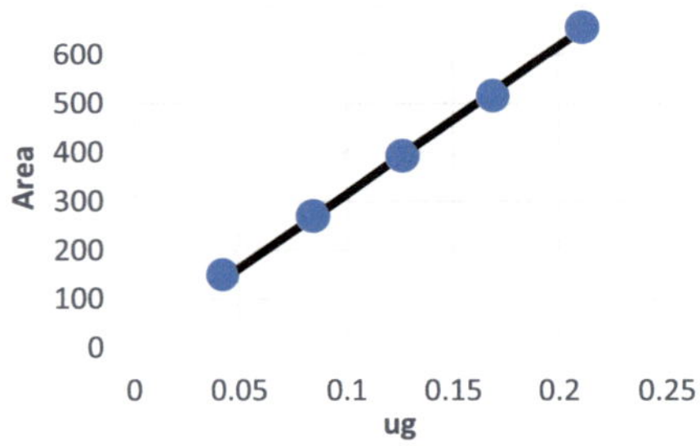

$y = ax + b$

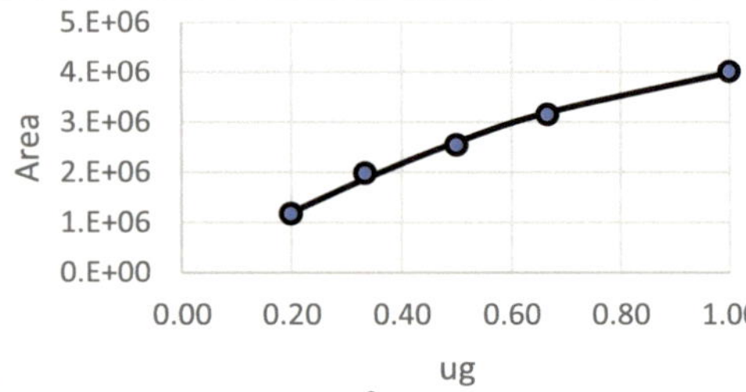

$y = ax^2 + bx + c$

a	2981.04	a	−2,370,063
b	19.4	b	6,334,085
c	—	c	21,664.53
r	0.9991	r	0.99905
Mean ΔY (n = 5)	−1.2	Mean ΔY (n = 5)	4,047.61
S.D. ΔY (n = 5)	6.31	S.D. ΔY (n = 5)	68,145.19
LOD (µg)	**0.01**	LOD (µg)	**0.032**

Ascorbic acid (AA) is detected by DAD and glutathione (Glut.) is detected by MSD. Calibration curves are in the table. Standard errors of the calibration points are represented by the size of the circles ($p < 0.05$).
"x"—the content of AA or Glut. in the sample; "Y"—the peak area; "Y calc."—the calculated peak area; "ΔY"—the residues; "a"—the slope of the regression line; "b"—the intercept; "r"—the correlation coefficient; "S.D. ΔY"—the residual standard deviation of the regression line (σ).

Table 2.
Linearity, range and LOD.

shown in **Table 2**. Linear regression in the case of MSD does not have a good correlation coefficient, so parabolic regression was used for MSD, it gives a satisfactory correlation coefficient ($r \geq 0.999$).

Accuracy/recovery and precision. The accuracy of the method was validated for recovery at 3 different concentrations in five replicate tests. Recovery was determined based on the calibration curve. The results are shown in **Tables 3** and **4**. Interday analysis shows the stability of the AA and Glut samples during the day.

Selectivity analysis (Table 5). Two peaks of both components were compared, one for the standard solution and the other for the drug. It has been shown that the presence of other ingredients in the composition of the drug does not affect the recovery of glutathione and ascorbic acid. In particular, the relative standard deviation of recovery does not exceed 0.72%. Thus, the method is specific to the antioxidant couple.

AA (µg)	Mean recovery (µg)	±SD	RSD (%)	Recovery (%)
1.335	1.316	0.077	6.0	*99
1.780	1.776	0.054	0.0	*100
2.670	2.677	0.092	0.0	*100
♥1.780	1.70	0.010	4.0	*96

Ascorbic acid (AA) is detected by DAD.
Recovery data presents an average value of five independent determinations (n = 5). ♥*The bottom row corresponds to the inter-day analysis. Samples were kept overnight in closed vials at 19°C.* *p < 0.05

Table 3.
Glutathione. Accuracy, recovery, repeatability.

Glut. (µg)	Mean recovery (µg)	SD	RSD (%)	Recovery (%)
0.534	0.54	0.03	5.0	*101
0.84	0.88	0.02	3.0	*105
1.335	1.23	0.00	0.0	*92
♥0.84	0.84	0.03	4.0	*100

Glutathione (Glut.) is detected by MSD.
Recovery data presents an average value of five independent determinations (n = 5). ♥*The bottom row corresponds to the inter day analysis. Samples were kept overnight in closed vials at 19°C.* *p < 0.05.

Table 4.
Ascorbic acid. Accuracy, recovery, repeatability.

Active component, detector	Concentration of active components (µg/µL)	Mean peak area. (Standard) (n = 3)	Mean peak area (Drug) (n = 3)	RSD (%)
Glut.	0.200	1755849	1759024	0.13
AA	0.054	218	220	0.72

Ascorbic acid (AA) is detected by DAD and glutathione (Glut.) is detected by MSD.
Two peaks are compared: one for a standard solution, and the other for a dilute solution for injection containing the following components: glutathione 0.2 g/L, ascorbic acid 0.054 g/L, disodium EDTA 0.001 g/L, NaOH 0.02 g/L, benzyl alcohol 0.015 g/L.

Table 5.
Specificity.

To test for **robustness**, the flow rate, column temperature, and formic acid concentration in the mobile phase were varied. The system suitability parameters (T and N) were determined, they were within acceptable values for all changes in the analysis conditions (**Table 6**). Thus, the method is robust.

4. Discussion

The use of two detectors (MSD and DAD) for the analysis of the antioxidant couple is efficient and extends the range of HPLC analysis. In the tandem of detectors,

Parameter	Ascorbic acid (0.1 μg)				Glutathione (0.5 μg)			
	T	%RSD	N	%RSD	T	%RSD	N	%RSD
Flow rate 1.0 ml/min	1.24	1.5	30,709	1.8	1.59	1.6	44,504	1.9
Flow rate 1.05 ml/min	1.30	1.5	28,320	1.7	1.60	1.7	50,693	1.9
Temperature 22°C	1.24	1.5	30,709	1.8	1.59	1.6	44,504	1.9
Temperature 24°C	1.42	1.7	29,552	1.5	1.81	1.8	43,332	1.7
Mobile phase								
Formic acid 0.10%	1.24	1.5	30,709	1.8	1.59	1.6	44,504	1.9
Formic acid 0.13%	1.21	1.4	30,889	1.6	1.56	1.5	44,651	1.8

Ascorbic acid is detected by DAD and glutathione Is detected by MSD.
T = Tailing factor (mean); N = Theoretical plates (mean); n = 5.

Table 6.
Robustness.

DAD comes first because it is a non-destructive detection method. MSD not only provides information on the qualitative chemical composition of the sample but also in certain situations allows us to determine the quantitative content of the component (glutathione) that is not visible to DAD. The calibration curve for the MSD is not linear, but parabolic, which probably reflects the mutual repulsion of like-charged particles in the gas phase. The use of MSD for quantitative analysis requires further study and justification.

5. Conclusion

The HPLC/MS method has been developed for the determination of the antioxidant couple consisting of glutathione and ascorbic acid in pharmaceutical products. The use of a tandem of DAD and MSD detectors is substantiated. The method has been validated for accuracy, stability, and precision. The method has a low detection limit. The presence of foreign components in samples including sodium hydroxide, disodium EDTA, and benzyl alcohol does not impair the accuracy of the analysis. The method provides a fast, sensitive, accurate, and reproducible means of determining the antioxidant couple in pharmaceuticals. Preliminary special preparation of samples is not required.

Conflict of interest

The authors claim that there is no conflict of interest.

Abbreviations

ACN	acetonitrile
AA	Ascorbic acid
DAD	Diode Array Detector

ESI	electrospray ionization
FDA	Food and drug administration
Glut.	Glutathione
ICH	International Conference on Harmonization
LOD	limit of detection
m/z	mass per charge unit
MSD	mass selective detector
MW	Molecular weight
RP	reversed-phase
SQ	single quadrupole
UV-VIS	Ultraviolet-Visible

Author details

Stanislav V. Yefimov
Pharmetric Laboratory, St. Petersburg, FL, USA

*Address all correspondence to: stanislav@pharmetriclab.com

References

[1] Forman HJ, Zhang H, Rinna A. Glutathione: Overview of its protective roles, measurement, and biosynthesis. Molecular Aspects of Medicine. 2009;**30** (1-2):1-12

[2] Pehlivan FE. Vitamin C: An Antioxidant Agent. InertechOpen. 2017. https://www.intechopen.com/books/vitamin-c/vitamin-c-an-antioxidant-agent [Consulted January 19, 2021]

[3] Meister A. The antioxidant effects of glutathione and ascorbic acid. In: Pasquier C, Olivier RY, Auclair C, Packer L, editors. Oxidative Stress, Cell Activation and Viral Infection. Birkhäuser Basel: Molecular and Cell Biology Updates; 1994. pp. 101-111

[4] Agilent Single Quadrupole LC/MS Instrument. 2019. https://www.agilent.com/en/products/liquid-chromatography-mass-spectrometry-lc-ms/lc-ms-instruments/single-quadrupole-lc-ms/lc-msd [Consulted January 19, 2021]

[5] European Medicines Agency. ICH. Topic Q 2 (R1) Validation of Analytical Procedures: Text and Methodology. 2006. https://www.ema.europa.eu/en/documents/scientific-guideline/ich-q-2-r1-validation-analytical-procedures-text-methodology-step-5_en.pdf [Consulted January 19, 2021]

[6] Raju N, Appala, Sridevi Chigurupati, Raju VV, Appala SS, Kesavanarayanan Krishnan Selvarajan, and Jahidul Islam Mohammad. A simple HPLC-UV Method for the Determination of Glutathione in PC-12 Cells. 2016. https://www.hindawi.com/journals/scientifica/2016/6897890/ [Consulted January 19, 2021]

[7] Florholmen-Kjær Å, Lyså RA, Fuskevåg O-M, Goll R, Revhaug A, Mortensen KE. A sensitive method for the analysis of glutathione in porcine hepatocytes. Scandinavian Journal of Gastroenterology. 2014;**49**(11): 1359-1366

[8] Hou Y, Li X, Dai Z, Wu Z, Bazer FW, Wu G. Analysis of glutathione in biological samples by HPLC involving pre-column derivatization with o-phthalaldehyde. Methods in Molecular Biology. 2018;**1694**:105-115

[9] A Derivatizing Agent for Glutathione Assays. The Protein Man's Blog. 2016. https://info.gbiosciences.com/blog/a-derivatizing-agent-for-glutathione-assays [Consulted January 19, 2021]

[10] Mika A, Skorkowski E, Stepnowski P. The use of different MS techniques to determine glutathione levels in marine tissues. Food Analytical Methods. 2013;**6**: 789-802

[11] Rellán-Álvarez R, Hernández LE, Abadía J, Álvarez-Fernández A. Direct and simultaneous determination of reduced and oxidized glutathione and homoglutathione by liquid chromatography–electrospray/mass spectrometry in plant tissue extracts. Analytical Biochemistry. 2006;**356**: 254-264

[12] Herzog K, Ijlst L, van Cruchten AG, van Roermund CWT, Kulik W, Wanders RJA, et al. An UPLC-MS/MS assay to measure glutathione as marker for oxidative stress in cultured cells. Metabolites. 2019;**9**(3):45

[13] Sawant L, Prabhakar B, Pandita N. Quantitative HPLC analysis of ascorbic acid and gallic acid in Phyllanthus Emblica. Journal of Analytical and Bioanalytical Techniques. 2010;**1**:111

[14] Frenich AG, Torres ME, Vega AB, Vidal JL, Bolaños PP. Determination of ascorbic acid and carotenoids in food commodities by liquid chromatography with mass spectrometry detection. Journal of Agricultural and Food Chemistry. 2005; **53**:197371-197376

[15] Somchai B, Sasiwimon L, Yaneenart S, Supaluk P, Virapong P. Analysis of ascorbic acid and isoascorbic acid in orange and guava fruit juices distributed in Thailand by LC-IT-MS/MS. Food Analytical Methods. 2016; **9**(6):1616-1626

[16] Gazdik Z, Zitka O, Petrlova J, Adam V, Zehnalek J, Horna A, et al. Determination of Vitamin C (ascorbic acid) using high performance liquid chromatography coupled with electrochemical detection. Sensors. 2008;**8**:7097-7112

[17] Mitić SS, Kostić DA, Nasković-Dokić DC, Mitic MN. Rapid and reliable HPLC method for the determination of Vitamin C in pharmaceutical samples. Tropical Journal of Pharmaceutical Research. 2011;**10**(1):105

[18] Racz E, Parlagh-Huszar K, Kecskes T. HPLC Method for Determination of Ascorbic Acid in fruits and Vegetables. Budapest: Technical University; 1990

[19] Watada AE. A high-performance liquid chromatography method for determining ascorbic acid content of fresh fruits and vegetables. Horticulture. Science. 1982;**17**(3):334-335

[20] Lloyd LL, Warner FP, White CA, Kennedy JF. Quantitative reversed phase HPLC analysis of L-Ascorbic acid (Vitamin-C) and identification of its degradation products. Chromatographia. 1987;**24**:371-374

[21] Yefimov SV. Express qualitative and quantitative HPLS/MS analysis of the ascorbic acid in pharmaceutical product. International Journal of Chemical and Pharmaceutical Sciences. 2019;**10**(4): 40-45

[22] Szultka M, Buszewska-Forajta M, Kaliszan R, Buszewski B. Determination of ascorbic acid and its degradation products by high performance liquid chromatography-triple quadrupole mass spectrometry. Electrophoresis. 2014; **35**(4):585-592

[23] FDA Guidance for Analytical Procedures and Methods Validation for Drugs and Biologics Guidance for Industry. 2015. https://www.fda.gov/media/87801/download [Consulted January 19, 2021]

[24] Centre for Drug Evaluation and Research (CDER), FDA. Reviewer Guidance, Validation of Chromatographic Methods. Rockville: FDA. 1994. https://www.fda.gov/media/75643/download [Consulted January 19, 2021]

[25] Evaluating System Suitability CE, GC, LC and A/D ChemStation. Revisions: A.03.0x-A.08.0x. 2019. https://www.agilent.com/cs/library/Support/Documents/a10424.pdf [Consulted January 19, 2021]

[26] Deepak. How to calculate System Suitability in Chromatography. 2013. https://lab-training.com/2013/02/27/how-to-calculate-system-suitability-in-chromatography/ [Consulted January 19, 2021]

[27] Bose A. HPLC Calibration Process Parameters in Terms of System Suitability Test. 2014. https://pdfs.semanticscholar.org/c378/3cd6c88c294be0aecee3b77cfd1eb35789fc.pdf [Consulted January 19, 2021]

Chapter 24

Natural Drugs for Diabetes: Needs of Developing Country

Namrata Dwivedi, Suhel Mehandi, Skand Kumar Mishra and I.P. Tripathi

Abstract

Diabetes mellitus is a metabolic issue and genuine worldwide wellbeing annihilating issue. The plague ascends in the quantity of new pace of diabetes mellitus is perhaps the most disturbing statistic with respect to wellbeing association overall premise. Notwithstanding, customary information could be utilized to help present-day or ordinary diabetes medicines. Here, we distinguish therapeutic plants that have been utilized as medicines for diabetes dependent on Chitrakoot ethnobotanical information. According to individuals' viewpoint, it is demandable and OK to incorporate homegrown concentrates as a component of the clinical intercession that the homegrown medication is viewed as normal and that the training might have been trailed by numerous ages. In this possibility, the utilization of therapeutic plant concentrates to treat a particular sickness was noticed for millennia. Therefore, Natural herbal phyto constitute a potentially important natural resource to provide inexpensive treatment of a disease commonly affecting the population of rural community as well as country. The plants used for diabetes treatment should be tested for pharmacological efficacy to help select the most useful for traditional medicines.

Keywords: diabetes, natural, medicinal plant, pharmaceutical

1. Introduction

Diabetes mellitus is a disease and it is primarily, characterized by lower level of glucose homeostasis ensuing from defects in secretion of insulin, insulin works resulting in impaired metabolism of glucose and other energy-yielding fuels such as lipids and proteins. Present time we faced large increases in the number of people suffering from anti-diabetic potential of medicinal plants more than 115 diabetes. The World Health Organization (WHO) assessed that around 30 million individuals experienced diabetes in 1985 and the number expanded to in excess of 171 million out of 2000. It is evaluated that the number will addition to north of 366 million by 2030 and that immense augmentations will occur in non-modern countries, especially in those individuals developed some place in the scope of 45 and 64 years. Exploratory diabetes in animals has given noteworthy comprehension into the physiological and biochemical craziness of the diabetic state [1]. Different these aggravations have been depicted in hyperglycemic animals. Critical changes in construction and lipid digestion happen in diabetes. In these cases the primary changes are plainly oxidative in nature and are related with advancement of vascular illness in diabetes. In diabetes, expanded lipid peroxidation is likewise connected with hyperlipidemia. The liver, an insulin subordinate tissue that accepts a basic part in glucose and lipid homeostasis, is genuinely affected during diabetes. The liver and kidney partake in the take-up, oxidation and metabolic change of free unsaturated fats, association of cholesterol, phospholipids and greasy oils. During diabetes, a canny change in the obsession and piece of lipids occurs. Despite the staggering movement life that have been settled on in the arrangement and the leaders of diabetes, the contamination Type 2 DM and issues arises by sickness make hardships are extending unabated. Some time later in show contempt for the presence of known underground bug diabetic local medicine in the medication treatment from remedial plants is used with progress to treat this contamination. Various standard plant meds for diabetes are used all through the world [2]. In this manner, treatment with local fixes drugs influences getting β-cells and make balance out change in glucose levels. All things considered, there is not any more natural data on the specific strategies for action in the treatment of diabetes, yet by far most of the plants have been found to contain substances like glycosides, alkaloids, terpenoids, flavonoids, etc. that are regularly involved as having threatening to diabetic effects. The investigation for substitute fixes (from the plant domain) for diabetes mellitus will continue with from one side of the planet to the other as the affliction presents numerous challenges not solely to the specialist yet furthermore to the researcher [3].

2. Background

History of medicine returns essentially to the presence of human advancement. The momentum recognized present day prescription or allopathy has bit by bit made throughout the span of the years by coherent and observational undertakings of specialists regardless, the essential of its improvement stays laid out in standard medicine and medicines. Imbalance in medical care conveyance, especially connected with reasonableness issue, and afterward even more especially in the non-industrial nations has turned into a question of extraordinary worry for world nation Traditional medication can be utilized as a contribution to "present day" drugs research, yet in addition as a wellspring of successful mediations by its own doing [4].

3. Health needs of developing world

The medical condition in the emerging nations however at first sight is by all accounts through their own effort requiring neighborhood remedy and surely from a thin likelihood that is along these lines, involves worldwide concern. The wellbeing inconveniences confronting the growing all around the world, on the off chance that left none acknowledge can push humankind on the opposite side the tipping point with critical phenomenal ramifications for all mankind, showing up and remissive none-neither creating nor created nations. Worldwide conflicts and illegal intimidation make two glaring instances of the unfortunate results [5].

4. Standardization, research and development: current status

The abuse of manufactured drugs with debasements, bringing about higher unfavorable medication response in further developed networks, has propelled humanity to back to nature for more secure cures. Local things are viewed as safeguarded by patients since they are considered to be ordinary. Most medications preceding being supply to buyers go through hard evidence based clinical testing; this is not exactly legitimate for herbs [6]. The inspiration driving WHO rules is to portray principal measures for the evaluation of significant worth, prosperity and suitability of the prescriptions [7].

5. Insulin resistance in type 2 diabetes

Most critical thing we should sees one of the central irregularities type 2 diabetes is insulin opposition. Insulin obstruction has been displayed to be available in prediabetes and at this time of the average history of diabetes, insulin spread is experiential to be expanded, or then again if nothing else, hyperinsulinemia, to make up for the insulin hindrance. Obviously, insulin opposition is a key pathophysiological part of type 2 diabetes and is determinedly associated with cardiovascular wagered factors and sped up atherosclerosis. Insulin is a key of diabetes it's a watchman of glucose work as postal worker. Given the focal control of insulin protection from diabetes, most likely the best fair of treatment for subjects with type 2 diabetes is highlighted developing the insulin responsiveness in vivo. Caloric cutoff and redesignd genuine work are wonderful to additionally foster insulin responsiveness. Amazingly, upkeep of way of life intervention for patients is hazardous in the long run [8].

6. Mechanisms of botanical actions

Regardless the recorded utilization of botanicals to treat diabetes and its related signs, one of the essential issues for this area of study is the deficiency of unquestionable and obvious information on abundancy, and, surprisingly, more basically, a setback of information about distinct mechanism(s) of activity. These are tremendous imperatives, and in gigantic part these cutoff points explain why there is huge doubt concerning the feasibility of local fixes in Western prescription. Regardless, there is creating confirmation around here, and accepting a home grown is displayed to well influence a given part, that will give the thinking to further and more convincing assessments on a particular regular [9].

There is no evidence to date that any of these proposed impacts are dependably noted with any natural upgrade eventually available. Finally, another proposed pathway by which botanicals could work is by direct rule of insulin action in periphery tissues like skeletal muscle and fat tissue. In such way, there is evidence to help the home grown guideline of these cycles. Mechanism of insulin emanation.

7. Medicinal plants relevant to type 2 diabetes

A restricted rundown of chosen botanicals that are accounted for to adjust starch digestion is given in **Table 1**. **Figure 1** showed that the mechanism of insulin secretion. When glucose transport from GLUT 2 transporter [10]. A few botanicals showed against diabetic properties are given beneath.

Scientific name (common name)	Kingdom	Division	Class	Order	Family	Genus	Species
Catharanthus roseus (Sadabahar)	Plantae	Tracheophyta	Magnoliopsida	Gentianales	Apocynaceae	*Catharanthus*	*roseus*
Tebernamontana divericata (Chandni)	Plantae	Tracheophyta	Magnoliopsida	Gentianales	Apocynaceae	*Tabernamontana*	*divericata*
Cascabela thevetia (Kaner)	Plantae	Tracheophyta	Magnoliopsida	Gentianales	Apocynaceae	*Cascabela*	*thevetia*
Momordica charantia (Bitter Melon)	Plantae	Tracheophyta	Magnoliopsida	cucurbitales	Cucurbitaceae	*Momordica*	*charantia*
Dalbergia sissoo (Shisham)	Plantae	Magnoliophyta	Magnoliopsida	Fabales	Fabaceae	Dalbergia	sissoo
Gymnema sylvestre (Gymnema)	Plantae	Tracheophyta	Magnoliopsida	Gentianales	Apocynaceae	*Gymnema*	*sylvestre*
Pennisetum glaucum (Bajra)	Plantae	Magnoliophyta	Monocotyledons	Cyperales	Poaceae	*Pennisetum*	*glaucum*
Saraca asoca (Ashok)	Plantae	Magnoliophyta	Magnoliopsida	Fabales	Caesalpinaceae	*Saraca*	*asoca*
Ginseng (Panax spp.)	Plantae	Tracheophyta	Magnoliopsida	Apiales	Araliaceae	*Panax*	*ginseng*
Cinnamomum cassia (Cinnamon)	Plantae	Tracheophyta	Magnoliopsida	Laurales	Lauraceae	*Cinnamomum*	*cassia*
Allium sativum (Garlic)	Plantae	Tracheophyta	Liliopsida	Liliales	Liliaceae	*Allium*	*sativum*
Ginkgo biloba (Ginkgo)	Plantae	Ginkgophyta	Ginkgoopsida	Ginkgoales	Ginkgoaceae	*Ginkgo*	*biloba*
Aloe vera (Aloe)	Plantae	Magnoliophyta	Liliopsida	Ginkgoales	Aloaceae	*Aloe*	*vera*
Vitex negundo (Nirgundi)	Plantae	Angiosperms	Eudicots	Lamiales	Verbenaceae	*Vitex*	*negundo*
Lantana camara (Gandhaili)	Plantae	Angiosperms	Eudicots	Lamiales	Verbenaceae	*Lantana*	*camara*
Ocimum tenuiflorum (Rama tulsi)	Plantae	Asterids	Asterids	Lamiales	Lamiaceae	*Ocimum*	*tenuiflorum*
Mentha piperita (Pudina)	Plantae	Angiosperms	Eudicots	Lamiales	Lamiaceae	*Mentha*	*piperita*
Acacia catachue (Kaththa)	Plantae	Magnoliophyta	Magnoliopsida	Fabales	Fabaceae	*Acacia*	*catachue*

Table 1.
List of plants having medicinal properties.

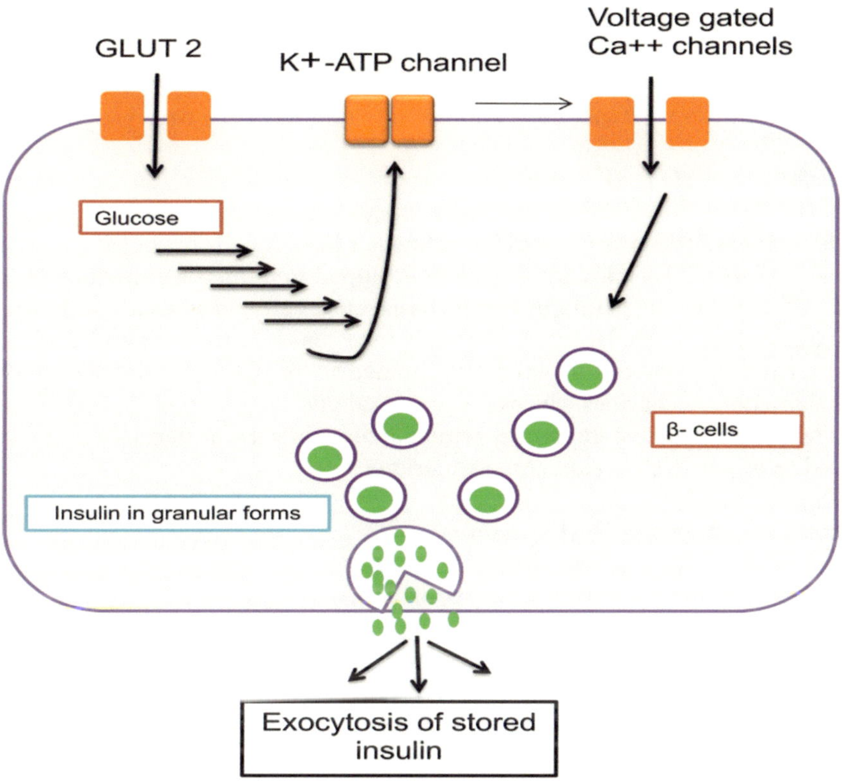

Figure 1.
Mechanism of insulin secretion.

7.1 *Catharanthus roseus* (Sadabahar)

C. roseus is a significant therapeutic plant of family Apocynaceae. Otherwise called Madagascar periwinkle, it is a well known fancy plant found in nurseries and homes. It contains carbs, flavonoids, saponins, and in excess of 400 alkaloids which are utilized in drug, agrochemical, flavor and scent, food added substance and pesticides. Boss alkaloids present in the plants are vinblastin, vincrestine, vindesine, vindelin, tabersonine and so forth [11]. Vinblastin is a alkaloid extracted from leaf part of *C. roseus* used as a anticancerous drug.

7.2 *Tebernamontana divericata* (Chandni)

Tebernamontana divericata (Linn.) is an evergreen plant of family Apocynaceae. Various phytoconstituents like alkaloids, terpenoids, steroids, corrosive have been accounted for in the plant. Restoratively it is utilized to treat infection syphilis, gonorrhea, the runs and jungle fever. It has cell reinforcement, hostile to disease, against ulcer and pain relieving properties. It is likewise utilized as cerebrum, liver and spleen tonic. Alkaloid and terpenoids are the two classes of optional metabolites which are liable for physiochemical and pharmacological properties of living cells. Starting around 1974, 66 distinct alkaloids of *T. divericata* has been distinguished which have been organized in 11 fundamental classes-vincosan, corynanthean, vallesiachotaman, strychnan, Aspidospermatan, plumeran, eburan, ibogan tacaman bis-indole and incidental. Besides, different free revolutionary rummaging proteins, for example, superoxide dismutase, catalase, ascorbate peroxidise, glutathione reductase and phenolic peroxidase have likewise been portrayed from side of the road plants in India.

7.3 *Cascabela thevetia* L. (Kaner)

C. thevetia is a little evergreen plant or bush or little tree. It is a decorative plant and local to tropical America and broadly developed in numerous jungles and sub jungles. All pieces of the plant are viewed as exceptionally poisonous and have cardiovascular glycosides. However in certain investigations they showed antimicrobial exercises. Family Cascabela displays the presence of constituents like terpenoids, cardenolides, polysaccharides, glycosides and alkaloids. Despite their harmfulness, the plant is researched to have numerous remedial uses, in various parts. In India, seed oil is applied remotely to treat skin contaminations.

7.4 *Momordica charantia* (bitter melon)

Unpleasant melon is a conventional plant of Asian beginning that has been a well known organic proposed for treatment of diabetes and diabetes-related inconveniences. The instrument of activity is accepted to be optional to different bioactives, one of which, polypeptide-p, is accounted for to have a design like insulin as found in creatures, and in that capacity, is proposed to have glucose-bringing down impacts. In particular, severe melon organic product contains.

7.5 *Dalbergia sissoo* (Shisham)

D. sissoo (Fabaceae) is a medium to enormous tree of around 25 meters high with dim yellow trunk. It is a significant lumber tree, broadly disseminated in India, Pakistan, Afganistan, Persia, Iraq, Kenya and Tanzania.

7.6 *Gymnema sylvestre* (Gymnema)

G. sylvestre, known as gurmar, is local to Africa, Middle East, and India, and it has verifiable use in the treatment of diabetes and is ordinarily utilized [12]. The gymnema leaf or its concentrate is represented to be the most typically used availability of the plant. Potential antidiabetic compounds fuse oleanane triterpenoid saponins, dammarane saponins called gymnemosides, and a polypeptide called gurmarin. There are wide examinations in animal models. Particularly, the effect of G. sylvestre remove on starch absorption has been prescribed to be assistant to additional creating glucose take-up in periphery tissues and growing insulin release and β cell number in the pancreas.

7.7 *Pennisetum glaucum* (Bajra or pearl millet)

P. glaucum (Bajra or pearl millet) as a staple food in India and Africa is filled in parched and semi bone-dry areas. In India it is developed more than 12 million hectares (11% of absolute cereal creation in the country). It is a rich wellspring of starches, proteins, nutrients and minirals5. As indicated by certain investigations, peripheral layer of millet grain contains high phenolic content, which are likewise present in undeveloped organisms and seed layer of grains6. Also, anti-carcinogenic properties of the spice have been reported. Higher fiber substance of bajra help in decreasing weight and stoppage. It has an exceptionally rich amylase movement, multiple times higher than wheat. Reports likewise uncover that pearl millet has the least glycemic file that could be valuable in overseeing beginning of diabetes. Items dependent on pearl millet can be produced for diabetic licenses. Presence of Omega-3 unsaturated fat in pearl millet makes it helpful in the anticipation of cardiovascular illnesses, diabetes, joint pain and particular sort of diseases.

7.8 *Saraca asoca* (Ashok)

Saraca asoca, is a significant conventional Indian therapeutic plant used to fix different ailments [13]. It is quite possibly the most amazing and sacrosanct trees and tracked down all over Indium. It is reported to contain glycosides, flavonoids, tannins, saponins. Different parts of the tree possess various phytochemicals which are known to cure a number of disorders. Leaves of S. asoca are known to contain carbohydrates, proteins, tannins and saponins and show antibacterial properties. Flowers are reported to treat diabetes, cancer, hemorrhagic dysentery, uterine disorders, bleeding piles. Bark and flowers are also known to exhibit antitumor activity. Dried bark of the plant is rich in tannin, sterol, catechol, organic calcium compounds, aluminum, strontium, iron, magnesium, phosphate, potassium, sodium and silica. It works as blood purifier, prevents skin allergies, improves skin complexion and prevents burning sensations.

7.9 Ginseng (*Panax spp.*)

Ginseng has been a very popular botanical that has been suggested to control diabetes. A review of controlled trials using ginseng extracts. The studies of ginseng (Panax spp.) for efficacy related to cardiovascular risk factors, including blood pressure, lipid profiles, and blood glucose. The overall analysis suggested that ginseng was noted to slightly decrease blood pressure compared with placebo (range: 0–4%), but they observed mixed results for an effect on lipids. Furthermore, they found several studies showing that ginseng lowers blood glucose, but overall they concluded that the results were inconsistent.

7.10 *Cinnamomum cassia* (Cinnamon)

Cinnamon has not only been used historically for the treatment of diabetes but is a supplement that is gaining in popularity, and many cinnamon products are currently available as dietary supplements. However, studies have suggested a positive effect in some settings. The intercession comprised of 1 g/day portion of cinnamon for 90 days and appeared to be successful to altogether bring down precursor glycemia, as evaluated with HbA1c, in the treatment bunch comparative with the benchmark group. Different examinations additionally recommended valuable consequences for glucose and lipids, though different examinations neglected to uncover an impact on glycemia or lipids. Different impacts of cinnamon on cardiovascular gamble factors, for example, antihypertensive impacts have been proposed in preclinical and little clinical preliminaries assessing subjects with metabolic condition.

7.11 *Allium sativum* (Garlic)

Garlic is one of the seriously charming natural cures utilized all things considered. The scope of helpful impacts of garlic is extremely wide and has been generally utilized as an antithrombotic, antihypertensive, cholesterol-bringing down, cell reinforcement, antimutagenic, and antimicrobial specialis. As would be normal for a home grown cure proposed to have such expansive impacts, there has been an enormous measure of examination interest into its activities. Specifically, various preclinical and clinical examinations report the hypotensive impact of garlic, which seems, by all accounts, to be more reliable in creature studies, rather than clinical investigations. The exact instrument of activity by which garlic brings down circulatory strain is not known. Similarly as with other home grown arrangements, the fluctuation in the clinical outcomes might originate from contrasts in garlic arrangements utilized for study or the particular substance of bioactives addressed in the readiness. Some bioactives have been accounted for to incorporate temperamental sulfur-containing compounds, polyphenols, flavonoids, anthocyanins, tannins, and others.

7.12 *Ginkgo biloba* (Ginkgo)

Ginkgo, a popular herbal remedy for centuries in China, has also become popular in Europe and America. One of the proposed indications has been to improve circulation. The focus of several studies has been to evaluate ginkgo leaf extract and measure the modulation of calcium levels in the endothelium and vasodilation. Ginkgo was reported to have a hypotensive effect in preclinical studies. However, other studies have demonstrated that long term intake may not be useful. Clinical data have also suggested that ginkgo may lower blood pressure in healthy subjects over a treatment course of 3 months and within a single treatment for temporary stress-induced hypertension. However, controversy exists as other clinical studies have failed to confirm an effect.

7.13 *Aloe vera* (Aloe)

A. vera has also been used in the medicinal treatment of diabetes in India and the other country Arabian peninsula. The gel, which is found in of the leaves, may contain glucomannan, a fiber whose present these are water-soluble that reportedly has hypoglycemic and insulin-sensitizing actions. Some Preclinical studies have reported inconsistent results. However, small-scale clinical research trials suggested an improvement in fasting glucose levels with the extract. In effect of herbals on glycemia.

7.14 *Vitex negundo* (Nirgundi)

V. negundo deserve from Verbenaceae is a hardy plant and also known as Nirgundi. All parts of this plant possess a wide range of phytochemical secondary metabolites which impart an unprecedented variety of use to the plant. This plant is credited with innumerable medicinal activities like analgesic, antiseptic, alterant, thermogenic, depurative, rejuvenating, ophthalmic, anti-gonorrhoeic, antipyretic, useful in bronchitis, asthma and enlargement of spleen. Its root are tonic, febrifuge, antirheumatic, diuretic and are useful as a demulcent in dysentery, in cephalalgia, otalgia, calic, uropathy wound and ulcers.

7.15 *Lantana camara* (Gandhaili)

Lantana Camara is a poisonous weed otherwise called wild savvy and presently settled in numerous district of the world, including India. Leaves are bubbled and applied for swellings and torment in the body, alkaloidal divisions lower pulse, speed up profound breath and animate gastrointestinal developments, Plant extricates dry spell open minded plant so great Candidates for xeriscaping, Used in society medication for the therapy of malignant growths, chicken pox, measles, asthma, ulcers, swellings, dermatitis, cancers, hypertension, bilious fevers, catarrhal contaminations, lockjaw, stiffness and intestinal sickness. A few examinations exhibit that concentrates from the leaves can be utilized to battle antimicrobial, fungicidal, insecticidal and nematicidal issues. Its capability to fill in as biocide has likewise been represented in a few explores.

7.16 *Ocimum tenuiflorum* (Rama Tulsi)

Ocimum sanctum Linn, a little spice seen all through India, have been suggested for the therapy of bronchitis, bronchial asthma, loose bowels, skin infections, joint inflammation, excruciating eye sicknesses, persistent fever, bug nibble and so forth. Medicinal properties of Ocimum are known for 1000 years to various civilizations of the world. Eugenol is available in the leaves of Ocimum, which are utilized as a home grown prescriptions. Eugenol is utilized as a flavor in the food business, has an assortment of natural action and can fill in as a biomarker. Removed rejuvenating ointments have additionally been displayed to contain naturally dynamic constituents, have insecticidal, nematicidal and fungistatic movement due to presence of prevail medicinal oil comprises, for example, methyl chavicol and methyl cinnamate.

7.17 *Mentha piperita* (Pudina)

Mentha piperita L. is a characteristic crossover that has a few therapeutic properties otherwise called herbal Buena meaning great spice. Pudina is utilized as a tea, color, oil, or concentrate, and applied remotely as a rub or linimentIts development has monetary significance, because of its capacity to create and store natural ointment, whose primary constituent is menthol, utilized in oral cleanliness items, drugs, beauty care products, and food sources. Menthol likewise has high antifungal and antibacterial possibilities, along these lines becoming one of the most requested substances by the fragrances and forces industry.

7.18 *Acacia catachue* (Kaththa)

Acacia catechu belongs to family Febaceae which is also called pea family or legume family due to presence of single chambered legume in all species of this family. *A. catechu* willd is a small to moderate sized plant widely distributed throughout Asia. It contains polyphenolic components, and seeds of this plant are good source of protein. Catechin present in this plant plays a vital role as anti-oxidant. In vivo Catechins are extensively and rapidly metabolized and impart to its anti-oxidant property. It is very famous for its astringent and tanning effect.

Khersal, a crystalline form of cutch sometimes found deposited in cavities of the wood is used medicinally for the treatment of coughs and sore throat. Catechins also have been used for treating fever, diarrhea, leucorrhoea, piles and erysipelas. The bark is said to be effective against dysentery, diarrhea and in healing of wounds. The seeds have been reported to have an antibacterial action. In East Africa, the powdered bark, mixed with sulphate of copper and egg yolk, is applied to cancerous growths.

8. Conclusions

Many are presently accessible in business supplements and are advanced for general medical advantages or for anticipation and therapy of explicit infections. Accordingly, the public's advantage in the likely advantage of organic enhancements on starch digestion is very high. There is lacking proof, in view of as of now accessible information, to effectively suggest the utilization of a specific plant item to treat either high blood glucose or other related hazard factors.. Notwithstanding, there are dynamic examinations in numerous areas for which organic arrangements are steady, and characterized clinical investigations are as yet progressing. We want to anticipate the aftereffects of these painstakingly led examinations. The benefit of a plant extricate is that assuming botanicals are demonstrated to be powerful to further develop digestion and additionally hazard factors on a clinical level, these cures, as a general rule, are usually accessible and thusly might actually help the overall population with respect to stoutness and diabetes. Sadly, albeit the majority of the well known botanicals have a long history in people medication, there is a scarcity of conclusive clinical information, especially as it connects with reliably further developing starch digestion.

Author details

Namrata Dwivedi[1*], Suhel Mehandi[2], Skand Kumar Mishra[3] and I.P. Tripathi[4]

1 Post Doctoral Faculty Biotech Center, Jawaharlal Nehru Krishi Vishwa Vidyalaya, Jabalpur, MP, India

2 Department of Genetics and Plant Breeding, School of Agriculture, Lovely Professional University, Punjab, India

3 Madhav Rao Sadashivrao Golwalkar Collage, Rewa, MP, India

4 Faculty of Science and Environment, MGCGV Chitrakoot, Satna, MP, India

*Address all correspondence to: namratadwivedi5@gmail.com

References

[1] Kayastha BL. Queen of herbs tulsi (Ocimum sanctum) removes impurities from water and plays disinfectant role. Journal of Medicinal Plants Studies. 2014;**2**:1-8

[2] Singh V, Amdekar S, Verma O. Ocimum Sanctum (tulsi): Bio-pharmacological Activities. Web Cen Pharma. 2010;**1**:1-7

[3] Prakash P, Gupta N. Therapeutic uses of Ocimum Sanctum Linn (Tulsi) with a note on eugenol and its pharmacological actions: A short review. Indian Journal of Physiology and Pharmacology. 2005;**49**:125-131

[4] Paul R, Datta K. Animesh, an updated overview on poppermint (Mentha piperita L.). IRJP. 2011;**2**:1-10

[5] Oseane S, Carmen S, Fernandes B, Marcia OMM, Leonardo CF. Yield and composition of the essential oil of Mentha piperita L. (Lamiaceae) grown with biosolid. Brazilian Journal of Plant Physiology. 2005;**17**:345-352

[6] Paula G. Peppermint (Mentha Piperita), Longwood Herbal Task Force, the Center for Holistic Pediatric Education and Research. 2000. Available from: http://www.mcp.edu/herbal/:1-22

[7] Shrivastava A. A review on peppermint oil. Asian Journal of Pharmaceutical and Clinical Research. 2009;**2**:1-4

[8] Liu JH, Chen GH, Yeh HZ, Huang CK, Poon SK. Enteric-coated peppermint-oil capsules in the treatment of irritable bowel syndrome: A prospective, randomized trial. Journal of Gastro. 1997;**32**:765-768

[9] Muhammad AH, Rabia H. A review on acacia catechu willd. Interdisciplinary Journal of Contemporary Research in Business. 2013;**5**:59-54

[10] Ray D, Sharatchandra KH, Thokchom IS. Antipyretic, antidiarrhoeal, hypoglycemic and hepatoprotective activites of ethyl acetate extract of Acacia catechu wild, in albino rats. Indian Journal of Pharmacology. 2006;**38**:408-413

[11] Orwa C, Mutua A, Kindt R, Jamnadass R, Anthony S. Agroforestree Database: A tree reference and selection guide version 4.0. 2009. Available from: http://www.worldagroforestry.org/sites/treedbs/treedatabases.asp

[12] Ahmad N, Hassan MR, Halder H, Bennoor KS. Effect of Momordica charantia (karolla) extracts on fasting andpostprandial serum glucose levels in NIDDM patients. Bangladesh Medical Research Council Bulletin. 1999;**25**:11-13

[13] Shukia R, Sharma SB, Puri D, Prabhu KM, Murthy PS. Medicinal plants for treatment of diabetes mellitus. Indian J Clin Biochem. 2000;**15**:169-177

Section 4

Conservation and Cultivation of Medicinal Plants

Chapter 25

Community Engagement: A Non-Formal Education Approach

Busisiwe G. Ndawonde

Abstract

Medicinal plant sellers primarily rely on trading medicinal plants at various medicinal plant markets as a source of income. Statistically, approximately 4000 tons of medicinal plant material is estimated to be used for medicinal plant purposes yearly. At the same time, the country is having to lose important medicinal plant species such as Warburgia salutaris. Notably, rising rates of unemployment have, additionally, facilitated the harvesting of medicinal plants for selling purposes as an alternative source of livelihood across many communities. The researcher had to intervene with capacity building om sustainable harvesting of medicinal plants. This chapter presents the challenges of propagating medicinal plants and compares indigenous and scientific ways of propagating selected medicinal plant species.

Keywords: medicinal plants, livelihoods, indigenous, propagation, marketing

1. Introduction

The research began in 2010 as a Doctor of Education research project. For ethical considerations and to promote rural community SD, the researcher kept working and collaborating with medicinal plant merchants post data collection sharing with them information on medicinal plant multiplication and cultivation in their respective gardens. One of the motives for growing medicinal plants in home gardens, as will be confirmed in later sections, was to keep women from collecting plants in risky locations distant from their houses. **Figure 1** illustrates such a perspective from which the need analysis was formulated before the engagement.

Figure 1 depicts how socioeconomic and sociocultural factors related to medicinal plant sustenance influence propagation of medicinal plants sustainably in supporting the livelihoods of medicinal plant sellers across generations.

The study invoked a participatory research approach, which has the empirical advantage of allowing participants to freely express their ideas about various methods of doing things at different stages of the study, including indigenous methods of propagation and the culture of medicinal plants. In the main, the study is essentially a cross-sectional analysis of the factors influencing medicinal plant sellers in rural communities of northern KwaZulu-Natal, with a specific focus on medicinal plant conservation.

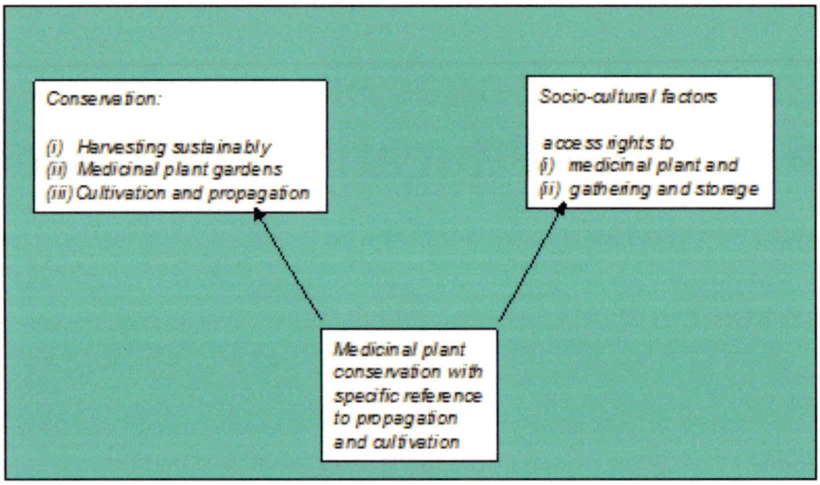

Figure 1.
Factors affecting conservation of medicinal plants.

1.1 Problem statement

There is a belief that science is well taught, conceptualised and learnt in a formal setting [1]. In this way, place (classroom, lecture theatre or science laboratory) is viewed as enabling the conceptualisation of science. There is little recognition of home as a place for learning Life Sciences. As ([2], p. 548) puts it, 'places are much more than just empty geographical spaces' as they contain 'spatialised, timed, sensed and embodied dimensions of nature.' Accordingly, [2] calls for 'place-based models of nature, culture and politics', which are therefore sources 'of facts, identities and behaviours'—incorporating 'notions of culture, local ways of life and human physical and psychological health'. In advocating that science learning often takes place through formal education, to Dib ([3], p. 1), formal education is a place where 'for the most part teachers pretend to teach; students pretend to learn; and institutions pretend to be really catering to the interests of students and that of the society'. He essentially disagrees with non-formal education in which two central elements guide the instructional process, namely (a) 'centralisation of the process on the student, as to his/her previously identified needs and possibilities; and (b) the immediate usefulness of the education for the student's personal and professional growth' ([3], p. 2). Distinguishing between formal and non-formal learning, [1] opine that the former is 'organised and guided by a formal curriculum, which leads to a formally recognised credential such as a high school completion diploma or a degree, and is often guided and recognised by the government at some level, while teachers are usually trained as professionals in some way'. Furthermore, he claims that, while the latter may be loosely organised, it 'may or may not be guided by a formal curriculum', and that it may be guided by either a qualified teacher or alternatively a more experienced leader.

The researcher opted not to walk away from the situation after observing the unsustainable harvesting of medicinal plants as this represented a need to help the sellers understand why and how their practices were impacting the ecosystem. It was determined that warning the sellers about the importance of harvesting plants prudently and considering future generations by taking remedial measures to prevent the extinction of many plants was important. Thus, the notion of sustainability was established, which is simply defined as the smart use of resources and therefore medicinal plant species without negatively affecting the ability of future generations to benefit from the same [4]. In doing so, there was a need to consider the practices of medicinal plants for conserving medicinal plants, hence IKS and Natural Science ways of conserving the plants were integrated.

1.2 Theoretical framework

The theoretical framework of this paper constitutes formal, informal and non-formal education drawing from the Third Space Theory by [5]. The term 'third space' dates back to the popular cultural work of Homi Bhabha, and it essentially refers to the spaces between colliding cultures, a liminal space 'that gives rise to something different, something new and unrecognisable, a new area of meaning and representation negotiation'. In the context of this paper, home is regarded as the first space, while the community (church, print and visual media) is the second space and school is a third space. These were regarded as spaces where education of factors affecting growth of medicinal plants would be studied.

For instance, in its broadest sense, education 'is any act or experience that has a formative effect on the mind, character or physical ability of an individual' and represents 'the entire range of experiences in life through which an individual learns something new via formal, informal and non-formal learning' ([6], p. 75). 'Education, against this background', is defined as 'the deliberate intergenerational transmission of society's acquired knowledge, values and abilities from one generation through institutions and instruction' (formal, informal and non-formal) [6].

The idea of a home task was for the students to explore learning in a place they are familiar with, while offering a space for students to learn from their elders, siblings and one another. However, as a science teacher, I advocate that a formal classroom provides opportunities to explore science using scientific apparatus. This is supported by ([7], p. 15) in attesting that formal education is 'organised, guided by a formal curriculum, leads to a formally recognised credential such as a high school completion diploma or a degree, and is often guided and recognised by government at some level [and] teachers are usually trained as professionals in some way'. I came to my realisation that it is through formal education to accumulate credits that can make one employable. In this context, I relate the role of space and a place as aspects of developmental zones [8]. To me, scaffolding for learning science concepts should be both from parents (home) and society, and as a science teacher, I provide a framework to be followed by each part in building scientific literacy.

In a rather sarcastic tone, [3] posits that formal education is a place where 'for the most part, teachers pretend to teach; students pretend to learn; and institutions pretend to be really catering to the interests of students and of the society.' He disagrees this with non-formal education where the instructional process is guided by two key features namely '(a) centralisation of the process on the student, as to his previously identified needs and possibilities; and (b) the immediate usefulness of the education for the student's personal and professional growth' [3].

Envisioning non-formal education further, ([6], p. 335) sees it as organised education that take place 'outside the formal education system'. In a similar vein, [6] also see non-formal education as 'any organised systematic educational activity carried on outside the framework of the formal school system to provide a selected type of learning to particular sub-group in the population (adults, youth or children)'. Ceschin et al. [6] posit that non-formal education 'may or may not be governed by a formal curriculum', even if it is led by a qualified teacher or a leader with formal experience; that no official credits are awarded in such learning. Further, ([6], p. 336) is of the view that in contrast to formal education, 'non-formal education focuses on needs of special groups such as women or adults'. In the context of the research reported in this paper, using the example of medicinal plants propagation non-formal experiences from home were brought to a science classroom, which is a formal setting.

While ([9], p. 2306) sees non-formal education as 'education that is driven by the objectives of the learners who often participate voluntarily'.

Latchem [8] adopts the UNESCO non-formal education definition, which states as follows:

> *'Any organised and sustained educational activities that do not correspond exactly to the definition of formal education. Non-formal education may therefore take place both within and outside educational institutions, and cater to persons of all ages. Depending on country contexts, it may cover educational programmes to impart adult literacy, basic education for out-of-school children, life skills, work skills, and general culture. Non-formal education programmes do not necessarily follow the 'ladder' system, and may have different duration, and may or may not confer certification of the learning achieved'.*

In terms of informal education, [6] claims that it 'occurs when mentors take responsibility for instructing others in more incidental or spontaneous situations, such as guiding them in learning job skills or in community development activities, without sustained reference to a pre-established curriculum'.

The European Commission (described by ([10], p. 9) as the type of learning that 'come from ordinary life activities relating to work, family or leisure'), which essentially supports the view of [3] on informal education. It is not structured (in terms of learning objectives, learning time or learning assistance) and does not usually result in certification. Informal learning can be purposeful, although most of the time it is unintentional (or 'random')'. However, as ([10], p. 11) opines, 'there is increasing acknowledgement that learning takes place on a continuum and that the boundaries between different forms of education and learning are porous' and that, therefore, the definitions of these terms should not 'suggest a rigid separation between them'. As a result, these unclear lines make it difficult to discern between these three types of schooling. While formal and informal education are typically considered as two sides of the same coin, non-formal education can sometimes be found in both formal and informal settings. As a result, a clear differentiation between the three groups cannot be made on the basis of location, manner of facilitation or assessment. Grade R teaching, for example, in South Africa, early childhood education takes place in a formal environment but is not formally assessed. It can be debated, in this regard, whether the education provided to grade R is formal, casual or non-formal in this scenario, especially because it follows a formal curriculum. In the current state of affairs, few would deny that learning occurs in Grade R. Apprenticeship in home-based care, on the other hand, can take place in any location, but it is examined and part of a certification process.

Ref. [6] also alludes to the fourth type of learning, which he refers to as 'self-directed or collective informal learning'—whereby people 'engage either individually or collectively without direct reliance on a teacher/mentor or an externally organised curriculum'. While realising that this is very important aspect of learning, this paper will not focus on this form of learning.

One of the most distinguishing features of non-formal education is that it usually does not focus on the pursuit of learning outcomes that will only be relevant in the distant future. Non-formal education, according to [7], 'is often considered more engaging, as learners' interests are a driving force behind their participation.' Thus, in the case of the research reported here. As [8] points out, the goal of non-formal education is 'to deliver both skills and jobs for wage-earning and entrepreneurship, along with an opportunity to open the social and political arena for greater access without discrimination and prejudice.'

With regard to the importance of non-formal education, [10] explains that it could, inter alia, be used to 'offer basic education, literacy and numeracy for those unable to gain entry to formal schooling and to provide post-literacy programmes for youths and adults'. Lortan [10] goes further and enunciates the other benefits as follows:

> *'It is needed to educate individuals, groups and entire communities in health, nutrition, family planning, child care and HIV/AIDS management. It is needed to empower communities and encourage and support development, to develop new knowledge and skills in such areas as agriculture, fishing, forestry management, construction, local handicrafts and computing, to provide paraprofessional training, and to help initiate and support local enterprises. It is also sometimes needed to help promote peace and reconciliation, and to facilitate post-conflict reconstruction programmes. ([10], p. 2)'.*

Non-formal education, in contrast to formal and informal education, consists of intentional instructional activities that take place outside of a formally organised educational context. Isaacs [11] agree that the distinctions between different types of schooling originate from the aim and circumstance in which they take place. As a result, these authors distinguish between formal, informal and non-formal education based on the context in which they are delivered. That is, formal education takes place in a formal setting, while non-formal education takes place outside of the formal setting, though it is planned and organised to some extent. Informal education, on the other hand, is haphazard and occurs without prior planning or organization. Informal education often occurs in people's homes, public spaces, social media, and other types of media such as newspapers, radio and television, as well as among peers. Furthermore, most informal education does not include any sort of assessment, whereas formal education takes place in formalised settings and includes formative and summative assessment, as is done in schools. To me, this raises the question of whether teaching, including evaluations, takes place in a location (setting) or in space (opportunity). Agunbiade et al. [12] stated that making science interesting and accessible to students is a major goal of scientific education. Incorporating IK into science teaching and learning helps to achieve this goal by focusing on relevance and sensitivity to learners' cultural backgrounds [4].

2. Research methods

The study used a combination of questionnaires, interviews and field observations, as well as survey and case study research designs. The intervention was mostly in the form of a workshop with a volunteer sub-sample of the survey's initial population. The study used a case study for this chapter. In total, 56 medicinal plant vendors took part in the research. For the purposes of this chapter, the results focus on the 12 medicinal

Challenges
What are the challenges related to the cultivation of medicinal plants in your home gardens
Cultivation
How do you cultivate medicinal plant species

Table 1.
Indigenous and scientific ways of propagating medicinal plants.

plant sellers that were selected based on their willingness to participate further in engagement with medicinal plant propagation and cultivation.

The case study also provides the researcher with a deeper understanding of the dynamics of a situation [11]. In addition, the case study offers a unique example of real people in real-life situations [10]. Case studies look at what it is like to be in a particular situation, and hence they are generally descriptive in nature [10]. In this case, the study aims at gaining insights into how the medicinal plant sellers propagate medicinal plants using indigenous knowledge and medicinal plants from the science literature. The task followed the criteria in **Table 1**.

3. Results

One of the impediments highlighted by the respondents was the plants' water requirements. Water scarcity was considered a serious issue that hampered and derailed the conservation of medicinal plants through cultivation. One of the group's medicinal plant vendors particularly noted the difficulty of getting water for their plants, and their inability to cultivate them on river banks or dams for fear of them being stolen.

One of the respondents' concern was about the plant's water requirements. Water scarcity was a major issue that also hampered medicinal plant conservation through cultivation. One of the group's medicinal plant sellers cited the difficulty to source water for their plants which was compounded by their inability to cultivate them on neither river banks nor dams on account of fearing plant theft.

The medicinal plant vendors mentioned resorted to, from their testimonies, buying water from time to time to irrigate their plants, which consequently leveraged and escalated the cost of plant management. In addition, this ultimately lowered the process their revenue generated from plant sales. Another interesting observation is that medicinal plant vendors are street vendors, which means they leave their homes for prolonged periods to sell medicinal plants on the streets. This means that someone else must care for the plants in their absence given the limited time that they can possibly devote towards the management of plants. Some of the sellers who constituted 2% of the sample complained about their plants being stolen from their homesteads while they are out in the streets selling.

A sizeable number of medicinal plant sellers (31 per cent) reported sluggish growth rates as one of the challenges confronting their business in relation to medicinal plant cultivation, according to **Table 2**. The slow growth rates of some plants acted as a huge impediment to cultivation because they would have nothing to sell while waiting for the cultivated plants to grow. This is consistent with [13] who backs up the concern that some medicinal plant species are slow growers, taking between three and eight years to reach maturity.

Nature of the problem	Percentage (%) of sellers
Poor soil quality	12
Sluggish growth	31
Irrigation and water challenges	17
Limited plant management time	14
Plants occasionally become weedy, e.g., *Calamus* spp.	2
Shortage of seedlings	6
Lack of access to land	4
Theft of plants	2
Limited healing power	12

Table 2.
Problems related to cultivation from 56 observations.

One of the difficulties faced in the cultivation process relates to the attitude that is associated with the healing power of the medicinal plants. One possible explanation for this is that cultivated plants are thought to be inferior to wild collected specimens. This is due to the general belief that the ancestors have a crucial role to play in providing wisdom to traditional healers when it comes to selecting the right plant.

There is ample scientific evidence backing the hypothesis that cultivated medicinal plants are ineffective in treating ailments when compared to wild-collected medicinal plant species. The prevalence of secondary metabolites in medicinal plants is primarily a result of secondary metabolites that the plants require in their natural settings under stress and competition, and which may not be expressed under monoculture circumstances [14]. Fast-growing farmed medicinal plants have lower levels of active components, but wild populations can be older and have higher quantities of active chemicals due to their slower growth rates.

In Botswana, it was observed that cultivated material was undesirable in so far as it fell short of efficacy as material sourced from the wild. Plant activity, on the other hand, can be increased under controlled conditions [14], whereby the medicinal plant activity is stimulated by stressing the plants, causing them to convert their active metabolites into steroids [14]. Consequently, ecological determinants which may include slow germination and sluggish rates of growth, poor soil quality necessary for desirable plant growth, and the concomitant labour required in the weeding and irrigating processes were pinpointed in this analysis as key impediments to the medicinal plant sellers.

Despite the challenges of medicinal plant cultivation, medicinal plant sellers should be encouraged to grow medicinal plants in their own yards [15]. This saves money for medicinal plant sellers as well as the intensive physical effort required when harvesting the plants in the wild.

During the focus group discussions, the participants were also probed in relation to the issues linked with the cultivation of medicinal plants, and some of them reported that they had commenced medicinal plant gardens. They also claimed to have traded their plants for the purposes of buying food and groceries in general, clothing and toys for their children with a white man, who essentially used the same plants as seedlings for propagation. That, nonetheless, was a challenge in and of itself.

'It takes time for the white man with whom we batter medicinal plant seedlings to come and buy our seedlings. However, when he comes we get these toys for our children and groceries for our familie's.

From the discussions evidently, the research participants shared common concerns regardless of their locations. In particular, the storage of medical plants was listed as the biggest issue, the medicinal plants were confronted with in their medicinal plant selling business, yet storage primarily impacts the marketing of the business which consequently influences their profits and therefore revenues. This is because storage affects the volume of sales that these sellers make in their business.

Other obstacles cited by the respondents were water, hygiene and security. Asked about their motivation in the medicinal plant business amid the myriad of challenges, the participants emphasised how the existing and testing challenges had made them stronger and more resilient in their quest to make a profit. Some participants stated that they desperately needed to succeed in order to use their proceeds to pay tertiary fees for their children.

Finally, medicinal plant sellers were asked to initiate and suggest solutions that they believed would help alleviate some of the issues, and the following is what they came up with:

'We require tanks to serve as water reservoirs, as well as sufficient infrastructure to serve as our marketplace'.

On the significance of training, another respondent commented,

'Receiving training is making a big difference since we now understand that harvesting all of the barks around the tree is incorrect. Although we are unhappy with the certificate fees, we are aware that certification reduces unlawful harvesting'.

It was evident from their comments that the medicinal plant selling business was vital to the sustainability and survival prospects of the communities. The government is also addressing some of the issues in the medicinal plant selling industry, such as capacity building in medicinal plant conservation. However, the government alone will not be able to overcome this obstacle.

Thus, to address the first empirical query about the challenges faced by medicinal plant sellers regarding storage, marketing and conservation of medicinal plant species, it was discovered that conservation and marketing were not the only issues that affected the medicinal plant business; other issues that affected the medicinal plant business included crime, sanitation and water scarcity. This necessitates collaboration among different organizations, such as public and private partnerships collaborating with medicinal plant vendors to address the aforementioned difficulties.

4. Conclusion

Taking into account current developments in South Africa that favour IKS and the application of Science and Technology, this study sought to provide further evidence aimed at preserving and preventing the possible extinction of medicinal plant species whose survival chances have, of late, been at the mercy of medicinal plant sellers. The researcher formed collaborations with medicinal plant merchants in order to begin measures to safeguard the medicinal plant selling business's long-term viability. The medicinal plant merchants' participation in medicinal plant cultivation projects was critical in ensuring that they understood their role in maintaining the resources that support their livelihoods. Overall from the results, it was evident that the medicinal plant selling business, like any other business, has unique problems that must be overcome in order for it to be a sustainable endeavour.

Author details

Busisiwe G. Ndawonde
North West University, Potchefstroom Campus, Qualification and Academic Program Planning Unit, South Africa

*Address all correspondence to: busi.ndawonde@nwu.ac.za

References

[1] Eaton SE. Formal, non-formal and informal learning: The case of literacy, essential skills and language learning in Canada. Encyclopedia of Informal Education. 2010:1-36

[2] Seghezzo L. The five dimensions of sustainability. Environmental Politics. 2009;**18**(4):539-556

[3] Dib CZ. Formal, Non-formal and informal education: concepts/applicability. Presented at the "Interamerican Conference on Physics Education", Oaxtepec, Mexico. Published in "Cooperative Networks in Physics Education—Conference Proceedings 173", New York: American Institute of Physics. 1987. pp. 300-315

[4] Bhabha H. The Location of Culture. London: Routledge; 1994. p. 286

[5] Boeren E. Gender differences in formal, non- formal and informal learning. Studies in Continuing Education. 2011;**33**(3):333-345

[6] Ceschin F, Vezzoli C, Zhang J. Sustainability in design: Now! challenges and opportunities for design research, education and practice in the XXI century. In: Proceedings of the Learning Network on Sustainability (LeNS) Conference. Bangalore, India: Greenleaf Publishing; 2010

[7] Ainsworth HL, Eaton SE. Formal, Non-Formal and Informal Learning in the Sciences. 2010. Available from: http://www.eric.ed.gov/PDFS/ED511414.pdf [Accessed: March 26, 2013]

[8] Piaget J. Six Psychological Studies. Vol. 204. New York: Vintage; 1967

[9] Duncan S. Biographical learning and non-formal education: questing, threads and choosing how to be older. Studies in the Education of Adults. 2015;**47**(1):35-48

[10] Lortan C. Principles of mogalakwena community's nomenclature of indigenous plant species of cultural value. Indilinga: African Journal of Indigenous Knowledge Systems. 2016;**15**(3):16-27

[11] Isaacs AN. An overview of qualitative research methodology for public health researchers. International Journal Of Medicine & Public Health. 2014;**4**(4):318-323

[12] Agunbiade E, Ngcoza K, Jawahar K, Sewry J. An exploratory study of the relationship between learners' attitudes towards learning science and characteristics of an afterschool Science Club. African Journal of Research in Mathematics, Science. 2017;**3**(21):271-281

[13] Kumar R. Research Methodology. A Step by Step Guide for Beginners. 2nd ed. London: SAGE Publications; 2005. p. 375

[14] Mader SS, Windelspecht C. Biology. 12th edition. New York: McGraw-Hill; 2013. p. 400

[15] Schippmann U, Leaman DJ, Cunningham AB. Impact of cultivation and gathering of medicinal plants on biodiversity: Global trends and issues. In: Biodiversity and the Ecosystem Approach in Agriculture, Forestry and Fisheries. Satellite event on the occasion of the Ninth Regular Session of the Commission on Genetic Resources for Food and Agriculture. Inter-Departmental Working Group on Biological Diversity for Food and Agriculture. Rome: FAO; 2002. p. 21

Chapter 26

Cultivation Practice of Chinese Medicinal Herbs

Xiahong He, Kuan Yang, Shusheng Zhu, Liwei Guo and Chen Ye

Abstract

An innovative cultivation technique for Chinese medicinal herbs had been practiced in China, which led a new road for medicinal herbs production without input of chemical fertilizer and chemical pesticides. The organic practice was based on the principle of biodiversity for pest control. An example of *Panax notoginseng* (Burk.) F. H. Chen was chosen for explaining cultivation technology under forest. The key technologies for *P. notoginseng* cultivation under forest include forest land selection, land tillage, seedling breeding and transplanting, and on-farm organic management. These technologies can standardize herbs production in large-scale under forest, and the quality and safety of *P. notoginseng* can be effectively improved without applying chemical pesticides and chemical fertilizer in the production process.

Keywords: Chinese herbs, cultivation under forest, biodiversity for pest control, organic production

1. Introduction

For thousands of years, Chinese medicinal herbs were collected from forested mountains, which faded away with the demands of human healthy [1]. People have to choose artificial cultivation in the field and adopted high-yield method for its planting. However, high-yield method betrayed the characteristic of medicinal herb, which caused medical effectiveness and quality to decrease deeply [2]. We explore a new road for medicinal herb cultivation under forest without chemical fertilizer and pesticide. It is based on the principle of biodiversity for pest control.

2. Background and cultivation technology of Chinese medicinal herbs under forest

2.1 The background of Chinese medicinal herbs

Chinese herbs are the important raw material for pharmaceutical production and the material basis for the inheritance and development of traditional Chinese medicine (TCM) for thousands of years. It is also a strategic resource related to the national economy and people's livelihood. As an important support of economic development in many poor areas, it plays a positive role in increasing farmers' income [3]. The clinical value of TCM has progressively been appreciated by the public at home and abroad, particularly the effect shown in the COVID-19 prevention and control, which has demonstrated its unique efficacy and role [4]. With the increasing global population and the complication of disease types, the demand for Chinese herbal medicine continues to rise. It shows a vigorous development trend in the Chinese herbal medicine industry. Historically, the supply of Chinese herbal medicine commodity mainly depends on wild plant resources [1]. Nevertheless, with the soaring demand for medicinal herbs, natural medicinal herbs have been mined out, and artificial farmland cultivation has gradually been adopted. Since the 1950s, China has vigorously developed the production of Chinese herbal medicine, from introduction and trial planting to commercial planting to base cultivation. The planting industry of Chinese herbs has experienced four periods: the germination period, the development period, the growth period, and the prosperity period [2]. However, some problems occurred with the gradual increase in the planting scale and yield of Chinese herbs that require urgent solutions.

First, the quality of Chinese herbs is unstable. At present, the circulation market of Chinese herbs is mixed with different varieties, including wild varieties, semi-wild varieties, wild cultivation, cultivated varieties, genuine land varieties, introduced varieties from different places, etc. [5]. The multichannel sources of TCM lead to its uneven internal quality, which not only increases quality security control difficulty of TCM, but also has a negative impact on the processing of TCM decoction pieces and TCM preparations [6]. The quality of Chinese herbs is affected by various objective elements.

Second, the problem of pesticide residues and excessive heavy metals is prominent. As the market demand for TCM continues to increase, wild medicinal materials have been hollowed out, and its yield has been unable to meet the demand, so most of the medicinal materials have to be cultivated artificially. In the process of cultivation, the high-yield mode of crops was copied for Chinese herbs, and a large number of chemical fertilizers, expansion, and other chemicals were applied, resulting in high yield but low medicinal effective component. The quality of medicinal herbs declined, and the efficacy of Chinese herbs was generally doubted [7]. Moreover, in the large-scale agricultural production of traditional Chinese medicine, pest became severe, and farmers have to apply chemical pesticides in order to guarantee the output, but the lack of scientific management of the field use of pesticides leads to the existence of different degrees of pesticide residue in medicinal herbs [8]. Exogenous harmful residues of medicinal herbs mainly include pesticide residues, heavy metals, polycyclic aromatic hydrocarbons (PAHs), and others [9]. Unreasonable use of pesticides leads to uneven quality of TCM decoction pieces and cannot guarantee their safety [10]. The quality problems of pesticide residues and excessive heavy metals restrict the international development of traditional medicine [11]. The 2020 edition of the Chinese Pharmacopeia has more stringent restrictions on pesticide usage; besides, the European Union, Japan, and South Korea impose severe restrictions on pesticide residues and heavy metals. The Chinese herbal medicine industry will face more serious challenges.

Third, the continuous cultivation disorder of Chinese herbs is serious, and most areas producing genuine medicinal herbs face the risk of having no land to grow [12]. With the increasing demand for Chinese medicine materials, the types and scale of artificial cultivation of that are increasing, but the problem of continuous cropping in cultivation is becoming increasingly prominent, which seriously affects the normal growth and medicinal value and brings great trouble to the development of Chinese medicine [13]. Most of the TCM materials copy the agricultural high-yield mode; however, the reality is that crop varieties have adapted to the high-yield mode after thousands of years of genetic transformation, while the research and development of medicinal herbs are insufficient to support the high-yield mode. Therefore, the application of agricultural high-yield mode has caused major problems such as high yield but low quality, excessive pesticide residues, and continuous cropping obstacles in the production of Chinese herbs. About 70% of the root Chinese medicinal herbs are slow-growing perennial herbs that take many years to reach reproductive maturity; these plants usually experience different degrees of replant obstacles [12, 14]. In addition, most medicinal herbs are not fertilizer-resistant, and soil eutrophication leads to serious obstacles to continuous cultivation. A crop of cultivated land cannot be replanted for several decades, which leads to the serious phenomenon of deforestation for planting Chinese herbs, and most authentic producing areas face the embarrassing situation of having no land to plant, which seriously restricts the sustainable development of the Chinese herbal medicine industry [15, 16].

Around these problems, agricultural scientists in China took the research on large varieties of Chinese herbs such as *Panax notoginseng*, *Panax ginseng*, and *Dendrobium nobile* as a breakthrough point to explore and form a rule that follows the natural growth and development of medicinal herbs, that is, to use under-forest resources to make medicinal materials return to wild forests, and establish the planting mode based on the efficacy of medicinal materials as the first principle, and gradually form a set of perfect theoretical and technical systems to solve the problem of quality decline of Chinese herbs from the source, which provides a strong technical guarantee for the healthy development of the Chinese herbal medicine industry. Theoretical basis of medicinal herbs under forest [17–23].

In the agroforestry system, agroforestry intercropping mode can not only significantly improve the microclimate conditions under forests by reducing soil erosion and wind speed, but also improve soil fertility and crop yield [24]. This pattern can make full use of natural resources and improve the efficiency of land use. Currently, the agroforestry intercropping mode has been successful in walnut/mung bean [25], poplar/soybean [26], jujube/cotton [27], etc. Therefore, the agroforestry intercropping model provides an effective and scientific way to alleviate the shortage of land resources and realize sustainable utilization.

2.2 Cultivation technology of Chinese medicinal herbs under forest

A typical example for explaining planting technology is *Panax notoginseng* (Burk.) F. H. Chen cultivated under forest [28]. *P. notoginseng* belongs to Panax genus, the Araliaceae family. It is one of the most famous Chinese traditional medicinal herbs. It is a rare medicinal herb unique in China and has the functions of promoting blood circulation, dispersing blood stasis, reducing swelling, and relieving pain. As a medicinal herb, *P. notoginseng* has been used for hundreds of years. It was first recorded in Compendium of Materia Medica by Li Shizhen in the Ming Dynasty. The main components of *P. notoginseng* are polysaccharides and saponins and also contain a small amount of flavonoids and volatile oil, as well as trace metal elements and other substances, among which saponins are the main medicinal components. The cultivation of *P. notoginseng* requires very special environmental conditions, including altitude, climate, and soil. Yunnan Province and Guangxi Province are the main planting areas, among which Yunnan province accounts for more than 98% of the total planting area in China [16]. Moreover, Yunnan Province is the authentic production area of *P. notoginseng*, and its yield and quality are better than other those in production areas.

Due to its high medicinal and economic value, *P. notoginseng* has attracted more and more attention. However, pesticides residues and heavy metals overuse, continuous cultivation obstacles, and unstable quality, etc., threaten the development of Chinese medicines. Facing these problems, we had explored the roads under the lead of outstanding phytopathologist Zhu youyong from Yunnan Agricultural University. We have been engaged in the research and promotion of ecological cultivation of high-quality *P. notoginseng* for many years. The previous study of our group showed that Yunnan Pine and Simao Pine have a high canopy density, which is suitable for the shade-demand growth of *P. notoginseng*. The volatiles of pine trees have the effect of pest control. Organic matter formed by the degradation of pine needles is also beneficial to the healthy growth of *P. notoginseng*. In 2015, our group carried out the test for *P. notoginseng* cultivation under the forest of Simao Pine at the altitude of 1500 m ~ 1900 m in the Zhutang Town of Lancang County in Yunnan Province. After 2 years, this innovative cultivation mode achieved success. The technical standards for *P. notoginseng* cultivation under forest were established, and three local standards were issued on June 11, 2020, which promoted poverty reduction in China and was conducive to the rational use of forest resources.

The key technologies for *P. notoginseng* cultivation under forest include forest land selection, land tillage, seedling breeding and transplanting, and on-farm organic management. Using these key technologies can realize the standardization and large-scale production for *P. notoginseng* planting under forest, and the quality and safety of *P. notoginseng* can be effectively improved without applying chemical pesticides and chemical fertilizer in the production process.

2.2.1 Forest land selection

When carrying out the under-forest organic planting for *P. notoginseng*, artificial forestlands and the tree species that have no negative effects on the growth of *P. notoginseng* such as Yunnan Pine, Simao Pine, Huashan pine, Chinese fir, etc., could be selected. The forest canopy density should be 0.7 ~ 0.9 for the growth of *P. notoginseng*, and forest land with slope ≤ 25° could be able to be used for planting because of ecological conservation and.

In addition, the suitable soil for *P. notoginseng* is sandy loam soil or loam soil, and the soil pollutant content should meet the requirements of national standard GB15618. Selected forest land should have not been planted with any crop for at least 8 years so that it meets organic production.

2.2.2 Under-forest land tillage

1. Land preparation. Weeds and small shrubs under the forest should be moved and dead branches and leaves should be cleared. It is important that weeds and shrubs in non-planting areas should be retained as much as possible.

2. Plowing. The soil in the planting area was plowed 2 ~ 3 times with a depth of 20 cm ~ 30 cm by manual or small rotary tillers.

3. Ridging. The ridge direction should be determined according to the natural terrain or tree arrangement: flat land should be ridged according to the direction

of forest tree planting. The slope land should be ridged along the contour line. The ridge surface is arranged in a circular arc, and the distance between the ridge and the tree root is greater than 20 cm. The ridge height is adjusted according to the slope. When the slope is greater than 20°, the ridge height is about 30 cm. When the slope is less than 20°, the ridge height is about 40 cm.

4. Setting up the drainage ditches. Drainage ditch is necessary in rainy season, and it is set up according to different slopes and terrain and leaves a drainage outlet every 15 m ~ 20 m length of the ridge. The drain outlet should be cleaned timely to prevent tree branches or soil accumulation from obstructing the drainage.

2.2.3 Seedling and transplanting under forest

The seedling preparation of *P. notoginseng* for under-forest cultivation includes two steps: seedling and transplanting.

1. Seedling. Seedling refers to sowing healthy *P. notoginseng* seeds on the ridge surface under the forest and using the soil under the forest environment for seedling cultivation. Healthy and high plumpness of seeds should be selected for under-forest seedling, and according to the relevant provisions of GB/T 19630, biological sources that can inhibit the pathogen should be selected to treat the seeds. The sowing time is controlled from mid-November to January of the following year. The sowing method is single seed sowing on demand, with raw spacing not less than 5 cm and the sowing depth is 1.0 cm ~ 2.0 cm. The seeding was covered with fine soil with a thickness of 3 ~ 5 cm, the soil surface was then covered with pine needles with a thickness of 2 ~ 5 cm. Watering after sowing to ensure that the water fully permeates the soil.

2. Seedling transplanting. Seedling transplanting refers to transplanting healthy *P. notoginseng* seedlings to the planting ridge under the forest for 2–3 years of growth. Seedlings with a weight per plant at least 1.5 g, main root diameter of at least 0.9 cm, dormant bud diameter of at least 0.4 cm, and no pesticide residue after pesticide residues detection are transplanted. Seedlings should be transplanted on sunny days during the period of early December to late January of the following year. The transplanting was carried out according to the standards of the (10 cm ~ 15 cm) × (10 cm ~ 15 cm) in row spacing and 3 cm ~ 5 cm in depth. Seedlings should be discharged horizontally and arranged on a line. Make the dormant buds head down and cover the soil with a thickness of 3 cm ~ 5 cm while transplanting. Then the planting ridge surface is evenly and tightly covered with pine needles with a thickness of 2 cm ~ 5 cm. Watering after transplanting to ensure that the water fully permeates the soil.

2.2.4 On-farm management of under-forest P. notoginseng

1. Water management. The water management of under-forest *P. notoginseng* is divided into four stages: ① Before seedling: The soil should be given a good soaking timely after sowing, and the humidity of ridge surface should be observed regularly. It should be watered well in time when the soil moisture content is less than 20%. In the case of too much rainfall, pay attention to drainage and waterlogging prevention.② Seedling germination: After seedling emergence, a small

amount of water should be irrigated many times to ensure that the soil moisture content is not less than 20%. The germination period of *P. notoginseng* overlaps with the dry season in Yunnan. The soil under the forest is loose and the water retention capacity is poor. *P. notoginseng* is easy to dehydrate, which leads to pests and root rot. Therefore, attention must be paid to soil moisture management in production to avoid drought. ③ Rainy season: After entering the rainy season, simple rain shelters should be constructed to avoid excessive soil moisture. When the soil moisture content is less than 20%, the rain-avoidance film can be lifted to accept natural rain showers until the soil is soaked. ④ End of the rainy season and dormant period: The soil also needs to be moist during this period. Soil water shortage will aggravate the problems of root pests and root rot, resulting in a decrease in seedling emergence rate in the next year and affecting the yield of under-forest *P. notoginseng*.

2. Nutrient management. The organic matter under the forest is rich, and no chemical synthetic fertilizer is allowed to be applied throughout the production process of *P. notoginseng*, only light and water management are needed. If the organic content of the soil is less than 2%, organic fertilizer can be appropriately supplemented after the emergence of *P. notoginseng* leaves. The types and selection of organic fertilizer should meet the relevant provisions of GB / T 19630.

3. Ecological prevention and control for diseases. There are several main diseases on *P. notoginseng* in the forest: ① Leaf diseases: rounded spot disease, black spot, powdery mildew, anthracnose disease, etc. ② Root diseases: root rot disease, root-knot nematode disease, vertical blight, quenching disease, etc.

   We conducted the protocol for diseases control: ① Elimination of disease residues. The diseased plants found under the forest should be cleared in time to prevent the spread of pathogens; ② physical prevention and control. Before the rainy season, timely cleaning of the drainage ditch in the plantation for drainage to avoid root rot. Moreover, by building a simple rain shelter on the ridge surface under the forest, it can regulate environmental humidity and play a role in physical prevention and control of diseases. ③ Biological control. Under-forest bases should adopt products such as bio-control bacteria, bio-derived fungicides, and plant elicitors specified in GB/T 19630 for disease prevention or treatment, and the use of chemical pesticides should be strictly prohibited.

4. Weed management. Weeds that affect the growth of *P. notoginseng* on the ridge surfaces (such as *Eupatorium adenophorum)* should be removed promptly, and damage to the *P. notoginseng* root system should be avoided during the removal. Weed that has a shallow root system and does not affect the growth of *P. notoginseng* can be retained to transfer pests.

5. Prevention and control of rat harm. To use natural enemies such as weasel, snakes, etc., to control forest rats; according to the specific forest environment, rat traps, electronic mouse expeller, and other equipment are set up in the rat gathering area or channel to prevent rat harm.

6. Plantation clearance. During the growth of *P. notoginseng*, especially in spring and autumn, there are many dead branches under the forest. When clearing the

plantation, it is necessary to remove the dead branches on the ridge surface, and remove weeds and excessive pine needles that are not conducive to the growth of *P. notoginseng*. From late December to February of the following year is the dormancy period of under-forest *P. notoginseng*, the fallen dead branches and leaves in the forest should be completely removed to keep the ridge clean and healthy, and the dead branches and leaves of aboveground parts of *P. notoginseng* should be cut (cut at >5 cm away from the pine needle).

2.3 Principles of cultivation practice for Chinese medicinal herbs under the forest

Ecological balance principle. Traditional Chinese herbs are mostly grown in the natural ecological system, with high biodiversity, natural growth of medicinal materials, light pests and diseases, high efficacy, and sufficient medicinal power. However, in the high-yield cultivation mode of farmland, the variety of medicinal materials is single, the biodiversity of farmland is reduced, the ecosystem is unbalanced, and the harm of harmful organisms is intensified, resulting in the decrease in quality and safety of medicinal materials. It is an effective way to reduce the harm of diseases and insects and improve the quality of medicinal materials by using the natural law of interspecies mutual restraint. Based on the principle of under-forest biodiversity interaction and ecological balance, the planting of shade-growing Chinese herbs and forest system were effectively combined to construct an efficient, stable, and diverse agroforestry system. On this basis, according to the regularity of occurrence and development of Chinese herbal medicine diseases, the rain-shelter cultivation system of under-forest Chinese herbal medicine can also be constructed. Rain-shelter cultivation can create microclimate conditions that are not conducive to the development of pathogen to achieve physical prevention and control of the plant pathogen [18].

Habitat coupling principle. The cultivation of under-forest Chinese herbs makes full use of the coupling characteristics of forest habitats (light, temperature, water, fertilizer, etc.) and the growth characteristics of Chinese herbal medicines and realizes the genuine and high-quality production of Chinese herbal medicines. The main principles of habitat coupling include: ① light coupling principle. Chinese herbs suitable for under-forest cultivation are shade plants originating from the lower forest vegetation, which are sensitive to strong light [29, 30]. Inappropriate light will affect the growth and quality of Chinese herbs. Under the condition of conventional farmland planting, it is necessary to artificially build a shading shed to simulate its suitable light environment, but it is difficult to simulate to achieve its optimal growth conditions. Under-forest planting of Chinese herbs only uses the light microenvironment naturally formed under forest vegetation, which is more conducive to the growth and quality formation of Chinese herbs [31, 32]. Thermal coupling principle. Chinese herbal medicines are usually sensitive to heat. The artificial shading shed built in farmland has poor buffering capacity for heat, which often leads to heat injury or freezing damage [33, 34]. Due to the shade of trees, the lower layer of forest vegetation has strong buffering capacity for temperature, which can effectively alleviate the stress caused by the fierce change of temperature on the growth of medicinal herbs [35, 36]. ③ Water coupling principle. Forest-shade Chinese herbs growing under the forest have wet-like characteristics. The dry environment is not conducive to their growth. The forest environment can improve the microclimate, slow down the flow of air, and reduce water evaporation, thereby improving the distribution and utilization of water. ④ Nutrient coupling principle. The soil nutrient balance is the material basis for maintaining the primary and secondary metabolic balance of medicinal herbs. At present, the input of organic fertilizer is less and less in the farmland system, and the use of a large number of chemical fertilizers makes the problems of soil acidification and salinization increasingly prominent, resulting in the decline of efficacy, diseases and pests, and continuous cropping obstacles [37, 38]. In the agroforestry system, the roots and leaves of trees can provide a large amount of organic matter for the soil. The decomposition and accumulation of these organic matters can improve the fertility of the soil and provide sufficient nutrient supply for the healthy growth of Chinese herbs [39]. The soil rich in organic matter can also increase the diversity of microorganisms, promote the growth of beneficial microorganisms, and improve the stability of the soil ecosystem and antiviral ability [40]; in addition, understory soils rich in organic matter and microorganisms also produce some disease-resistant substances, which induce plant resistance and effectively reduce the occurrence of diseases [41].

The under-forest ecosystem has rich biodiversity, such as plant diversity, animal diversity, insect diversity, and microbial diversity. Plant–plant, plant-microorganism, plant–animal (insect), and other organisms in the under-forest system form a stable community through complex mutual generation and restriction relationship among the various organisms, which has strong ability to resist natural disasters.

3. Mechanism of cultivation practice for Chinese medicinal herbs under forest

Without chemical fertilizers and pesticides, *P. notoginseng* has been successfully cultivated in forest ecosystems. It was based on the principle of biodiversity for pest control. Most of *P. notoginseng* was cultivated in coniferous forest [*Pinus kesiya* var. *langbianensis*, *Pinus yunnanensis*, *Pinus armandii Franch*. and *Cunninghamia lanceolata* (Lamb.) Hook] (**Figure 1**). The cultivation of *P. notoginseng* under-forest conditions is successful due to the effective use of (i) native environment and biodiversity and (ii) stimulatory allelopathic interactions within the forest system (**Figure 2**).

Forest environment: *P. notoginseng* is shade-loving plant that thrives well under low light intensity and 18–25°C temperature. When the light intensity is >30% of sunlight and temperature is over 30°C, the growth environment becomes harsh for *P. notoginseng*. The environment in the lower layers of forests provides desirable shade and temperature for P. *notoginseng* growth. Compared with traditional cultivation model, this forest cultivation model does not use polyethylene net or straw to provide shade, which greatly reduces the cost. Besides, the leaf litter acts as cover, keeps the soil moist, and maintains suitable temperature for *P. notoginseng* growth.

Soil rich in organic matter and microbes: Long-term decomposition of forest residues improves the soil quality. We found that the physicochemical properties of coniferous forest soil meet the requirements of *P. notoginseng* (pH: 5.5–6.5; electrical conductivity: 60–120 μS cm^{-1}; nutrient contents: 250–360 mg kg^{-1} available N, 10–25 mg kg^{-1} available P, 100–260 mg kg^{-1} available K, and 80–120 g kg^{-1} soil organic matter). Such soil provides adequate nutrients for *P. notoginseng* growth and development of strong root system (**Figure 1**).

Forest soils are generally rich in microorganisms, which reduces the root rot disease and promotes the plant growth by increasing the availability of nutrients. Our laboratory experiments showed that application of microbiome from the forest soil into sick soil improves the germination and growth of *P. notoginseng* and alleviates the soil-borne diseases. Bacteria with strong antifungal activity (*Bacillus* spp., *Pseudomonas* spp., *Streptomyces* spp., *Burkholderia* spp. etc.), against *P. notoginseng* root

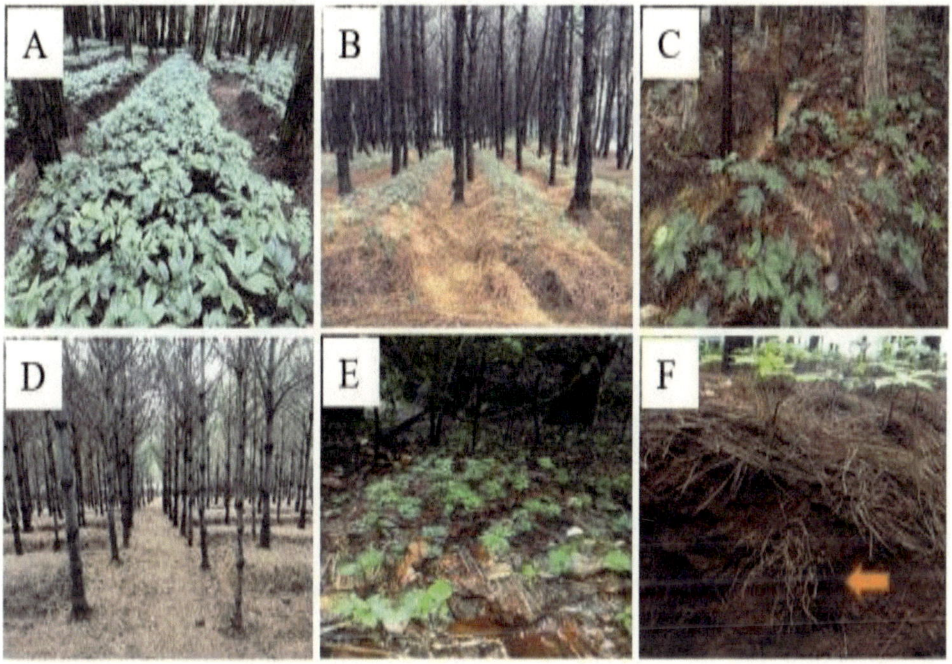

Figure 1.
Cultivation of P. notoginseng *under forest conditions. A.* Pinuskesiya var. langbianensis *forest; B.* Pinus yunnanensis *forest; C.* Cunninghamia lanceolata *(Lamb.) Hook. forest; D.* Pinus armandii *Franch. forest; E. Broadleaf forest; F. The strong roots of* P. notoginseng *in forest soil.*

rot pathogens, have been isolated and identified from forest soil. Besides, the atmospheric nitrogen-fixing microbes (*Bradyrhizobium* spp., *Rhizobium* spp., *Frankia* spp. etc.) are also abundant in forest soils [42].

Allelopathic interactions in forest. Cultivation of *P. notoginseng* under natural forest conditions uses the allelopathy to stimulate the plant growth and prevents the pests and diseases infestation than in monoculture in farmland or greenhouses. The possible pathways for the release of allelochemicals into the environment are: (i) emission of volatile organic compounds (VOCs) from different plant tissue, (ii) leaching from leaves by rain or dew, (iii) decay of plant residues, and (iv) root exudation.

The VOCs of pine tree terpenes (including α-pinene, β-pinene, camphene, etc.) stimulated the growth and reduced the pests and diseases of *P. notoginseng*. Riedlmeier et al. [43] reported that monoterpenes, particularly pinenes, could enhance the systemic acquired resistance in *Arabidopsis thaliana* to the pathogen *Pseudomonas syringae*. Likewise, our results showed that some VOCs from pine needles induce the resistance of *P. notoginseng* to leaf black spot disease (caused by *Alternaria tenuis* Nees). In addition, α- terpineol and terpinen-4-ol are antifungal to growth of fungal pathogens (*Fusarium oxysporum*, *Fusarium solani*, *Cylindrocarpon destructans*, *Phytophthora cactorum*, and *A. tenuis* Nees) (unpublished). It is also observed that leachates from pine needles stimulated the growth and biomass of *P. notoginseng*. Terpenes are one kind of VOCs, from the herbivore damaged plants that attract the predators or parasitoids to attack herbivores [44]. Aldrich et al. [45] reported that an artificial pheromone containing α-terpineol and Terpinen-4-ol emitted from pine could attract the adult predaceous spined soldier bugs, *Podisus maculiventris* (Say).

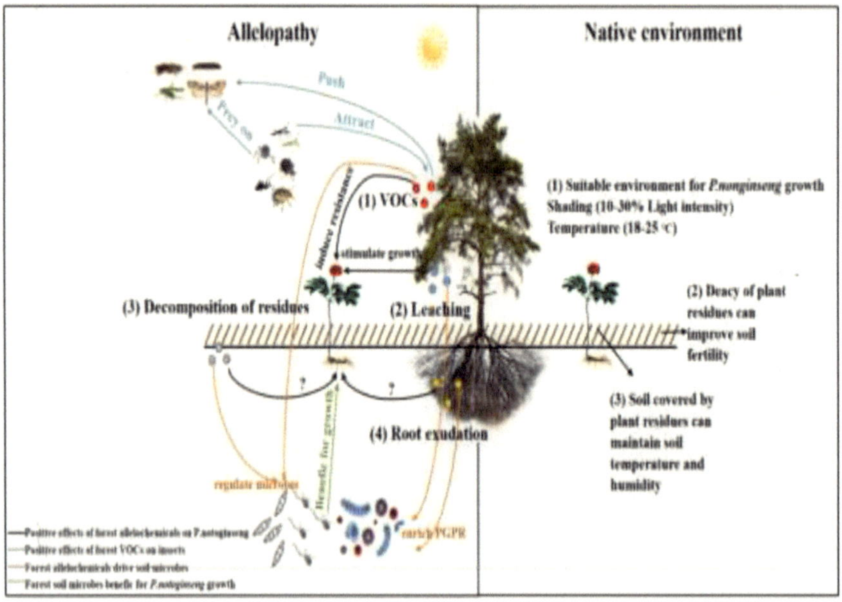

Figure 2.
Mechanisms involved in the cultivation of P. notoginseng *under natural forest conditions [42].*

This confirms that the VOCs from coniferous forests play a positive allelopathic role in pest control.

Cao et al. [46] investigated the diversity of arthropods on *P. notoginseng*, planted in *P. kesiya* var. *langbianensis* forest. The data showed that there were a total of 40 species of arthropods from 33 families, of which the natural enemies were 40%. The Shannon-wiener diversity index of natural enemy subcommunity is significantly higher than the pest subcommunity. Obviously, a high biodiversity of arthropods significantly reduces the damage caused by pests in *P. notoginseng*.

4. Diseases occurrence and control of *P. notoginseng* under forest

Diseases are more sever in Chinese medicinal herbs than in other crops because they grow for longer time and are easily threatened by diseases. However, diseases have not been prevalent in the forest, which contributes to the measures of cultivation under forest described above.

4.1 Round spot disease occurrence characteristics

We had observed the disease from 2016 in the *P. notoginseng* plantations in Lancang County, Pu′er City, Yunnan Province. In rainy season, round, water-soaked spots on the leaves of *P. notoginseng* appeared when it was exposed in rain. Round or nearly round watery spots on leaves are initial symptoms of round spot disease. The lesion appeared transparent when it was viewed in the sun compared with healthy leaf tissue. Then the brown infection spots were observed in the center of the disease spots (**Figure 3A**). Eventually, the lesions gradually expanded, turned brown or grayish brown, and had "wheel marks" (**Figure 3B**). Later, white powdery conidial piles formed on the lesion surface (**Figure 3C**). Finally, multiple lesions merged, causing

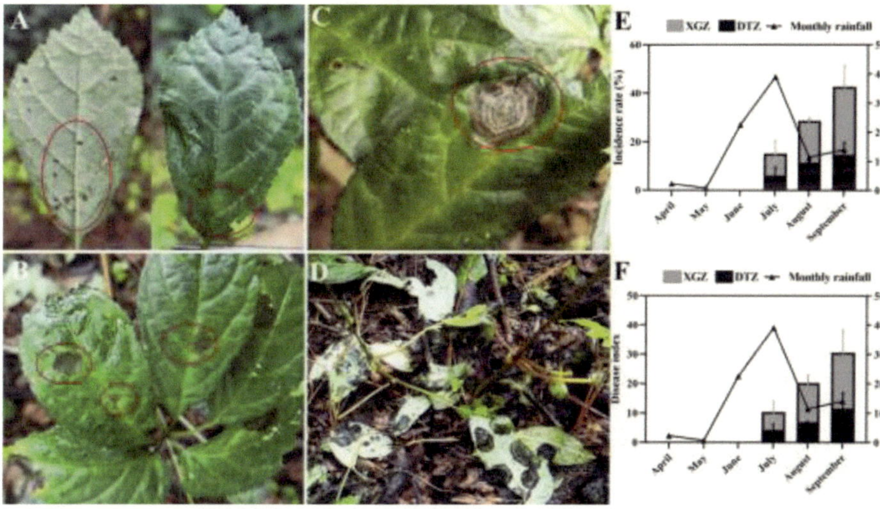

Figure 3.
Symptoms, incidence, and disease index of round spot disease. (A) Watery spots on P. notoginseng *leaves. (B) Watery spots expand to form black wheel-like lesions. (C) Gray white conidia piles form on the lesions. (D) Leaves fall off in the late stage of the disease. (E) Relationship between incidence rate of round spot disease and monthly rainfall in DTZ and XGZ. (F) Relationship between disease index of round spot disease and monthly rainfall in DTZ and XGZ. XGZ: Xiaoguangzha* P. notoginseng *plantation. DTZ: Datangzi* P. notoginseng *plantation.*

the leaves to rot and fall off during rainfall (**Figure 3D**). Based on these characteristics of the disease spots, the disease was preliminarily identified as round spot disease.

The incidence of round spot disease in Lancang County was investigated and monitored. *P. notoginseng* begins to germinate from March to April. From March to June, no round spot disease symptoms were observed (**Figure 3E** and **F**). As of July, round spot disease started to occur. Round spot disease incidence rose in August and September. Lancang County has a subtropical wet summer and dry winter mountain monsoon climate, with distinct rainy and dry seasons. Generally, rainfall is limited in April and May, but begins to increase as of June. **Figure 3E** and **F** shows that round spot disease started to occur after the rainy season.

4.2 Isolation and identification of the causal pathogen of round spot disease

The pathogen causing round spot disease was isolated by single-spore isolation. In total, 30 pathogen strains were isolated from 30 diseased leaves. On PDA, colonies were round, villous, and varied in color from red to gray (**Figure 4A** and **B**). The strains did not produce conidia on PDA; they required water to induce conidia production. Conidiophores produced by thickened hyphae were colorless and bent (**Figure 4F** and **G**). Conidia were solitary, colorless, transparent, and long-arched, with multiple diaphragms (**Figure 4C** and **D**). The tail of the conidia gradually became thinner and the apical cells appeared to be truncated. A long, narrow, accessory filament with septa grew on the side of the apical cell. Notably, thin cilia were observed at the tail of the conidium and the top of the accessory filament (**Figure 4E**). The total length of conidia, including the accessory filament and two cilia, was 171.83–492.92 μm (average, 349.74 μm) (n = 200). Their width, measured at the widest part in the middle of the conidia, was 6.24–13.05 μm (average,

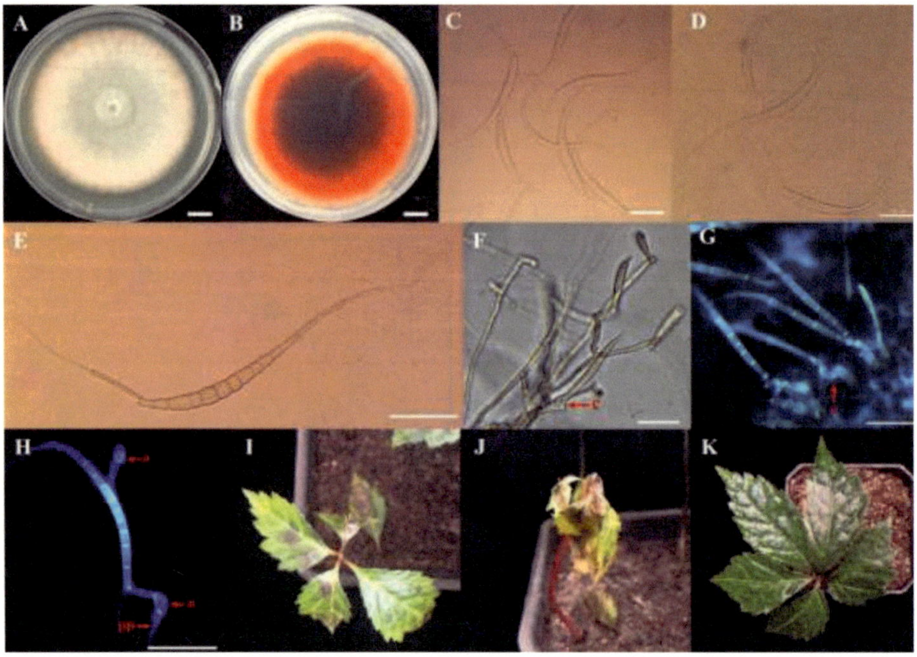

Figure 4.
Morphological characteristics of Mycocentrospora acerina. *(A, B) mycelial colony morphology of* M. acerina *cultured on PDA medium for 7 days at 20°C. (C–E) morphological characteristics of conidia. (F, G) morphological characteristics of conidiophores and conidia. The conidiophores and conidia in panel G were stained with calcofluor white. c: Conidiophore. (H) Conidia on the leaves of* P. notoginseng *germinated to produce an appressorium and penetration peg. A: Appressorium, pp.: Penetration peg. (I) Symptoms on* P. notoginseng *leaves 7 days after inoculation of a conidial suspension. (J) Symptoms on* P. notoginseng *leaves 14 days after inoculation of a conidial suspension. (K)* P. notoginseng *leaves remained healthy for 7 days when being mock-inoculated with sterile water. Scale bars = 10 mm in A–B, scale bars = 50 μm in C–H.*

8.61 μm). Based on the morphology and conidial characteristics, the pathogen was identified as *M. acerina* [47].

The pathogenicity of 10 isolated strains was determined. Seven days post inoculation, all inoculated leaves showed similar lesions, and the symptoms were identical to those in the field (**Figure 4I** and **J**). The control plants remained healthy (**Figure 4K**). The diseased leaves in each treatment were selected for pathogen isolation, and the pathogen was reidentified as *M. acerina*.

4.3 Effects of temperature and wetness duration on conidial germination *in vitro*

Conidial germination was evaluated and observed at all 11 temperatures, except 32°C (**Figure 5A**). Conidia did not germinate within 2 h at all temperatures. At 4, 8, 14, 18, 20, 22, 24, and 28°C, germination started at 4 h. At 6 h, the germination rates at 14, 18, 20, 22, and 24°C all exceeded 30%. At 18 h, the germination rates at 14, 18, 20, 22, and 24°C all exceeded 90%. The highest germination rate was observed at 20°C (97.16%). At 24 h, all conidia at 18, 20, and 22°C had germinated. The germination rate exceeded 90% at 8, 14, and 24°C. Thus, temperatures above 28°C and below 4°C are not conducive to conidial germination, with the optimal temperature for germination between 14 and 22°C.

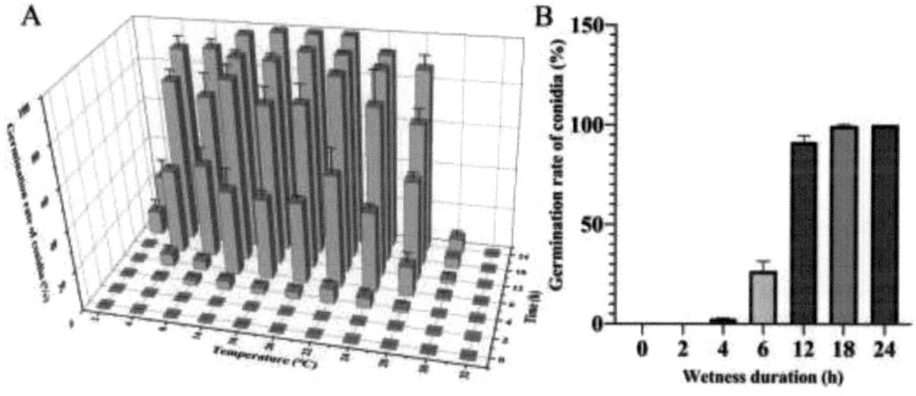

Figure 5.
Effects of temperature and wetness duration on conidial germination in vitro. (A) Average germination rate of conidia at 11 different temperatures and different time points. (B) Average germination rate of conidia under seven different wetness durations.

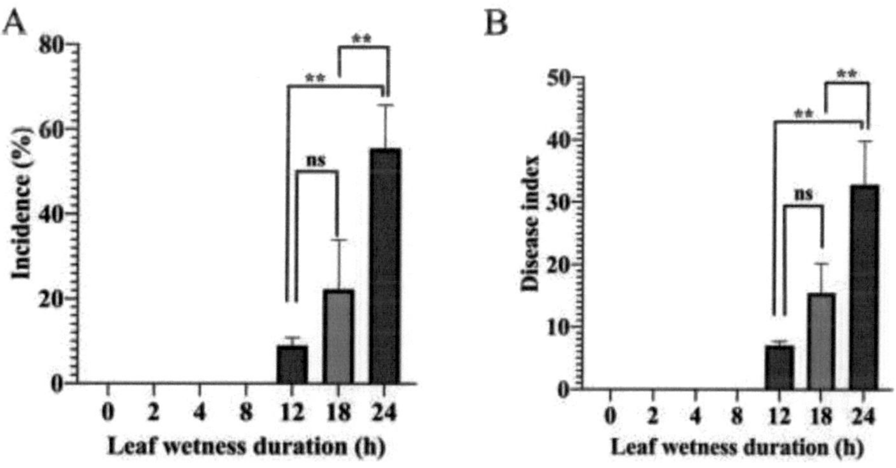

Figure 6.
*Effects of different leaf wetness durations on the occurrence of round spot disease. (A) Incidence and (B) disease index of round spot disease for different leaf wetness durations. *P < 0.05, **P < 0.01; n = 3, ns: no significant difference.*

Free water is a key factor for conidial germination. The effect of leaf wetness duration was first investigated *in vitro*. When the wetness duration was less than 2 h, conidia could not germinate (**Figure 5B**). Between 2 and 24 h, the germination rate increased with increasing wetness duration. All conidia were germinated when a free water film was present for 24 h. Even at 99% relative humidity, in the absence of free water, the conidia did not germinate.

4.4 Effect of *P. notoginseng* leaf wetness duration on conidial infection

To evaluate the effect of leaf wetness duration on conidial infection, in the greenhouse experiment, round spot disease incidence was investigated 10 days after inoculation. When the leaf wetness duration was shorter than or equal to 8 h, no disease spots appeared on the *P. notoginseng* leaf surface. When the leaf wetness duration was longer than or equal to 12 h, the incidence and disease index of round spot disease increased according to the leaf wetness duration (**Figure 4A** and **B**). Round spot disease incidence and disease index at a wetness duration of 24 h were 55.56% and 32.78, respectively, and were significantly higher than those at a wetness duration of 12 h and 18 h (**Figure 6**).

4.5 Infection process of *M. acerina* conidia on *P. notoginseng* leaves

The different infection stages of *M. acerina* conidia on *P. notoginseng* leaves were observed and photographed. For microscopic observation, we used fluorescence staining with calcofluor white. Under excitation with ultraviolet light, conidia and hyphae emit blue fluorescence. The development of conidia on *P. notoginseng* leaves between 0 and 18 h is shown in **Figure 7**. At 6 h, the conidia had grown multiple primary hyphae from cells at different locations. Between 6 and 12 h, the primary hyphae continued to elongate, and at 12 h, some of the hyphal ends were expanded to form an appressorium. At 18 h, lesions had appeared on the leaf surface, which indicated that hyphae had invaded the *P. notoginseng* leaves. The development of conidia on *P. notoginseng* leaves between 24 and 96 h is shown in **Figure 6**. By 24 h, the lesion area had expanded and the lesion became conspicuous, with an appressorium in the center. By 48 h, the lesion center had turned yellow and hyphae on the leaf surface no longer elongated. At 72 h, the lesion was further enlarged and the color of the lesion center changed from yellow to brown. At 96 h, multiple conidia appeared on the lesion surface. The conidia were formed by the mycelium growing and developing in the lesions. The lifecycle of *M. acerina*, from conidial inoculation to the production of conidia, is completed in 4 days (**Figure 8**).

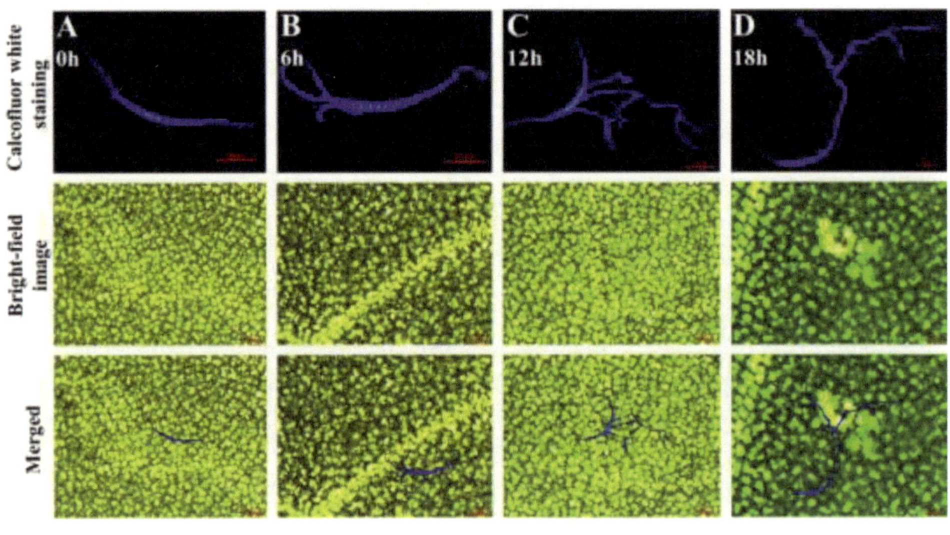

Figure 7.
Development of Mycocentrospora acerina *conidia on* P. notoginseng *leaves. (A–D) conidia were observed on the leaves of P. notoginseng at 0, 6, 12, and 18 h, respectively. The blue color shows* Mycocentrospora acerina *conidia and hyphae stained with calcofluor white stain. The bright-field image shows* P. notoginseng *leaf epidermal cells, and the merged image shows the germination and invasion of* Mycocentrospora acerina *conidia on* P. notoginseng *leaves. Bar = 50 μm.*

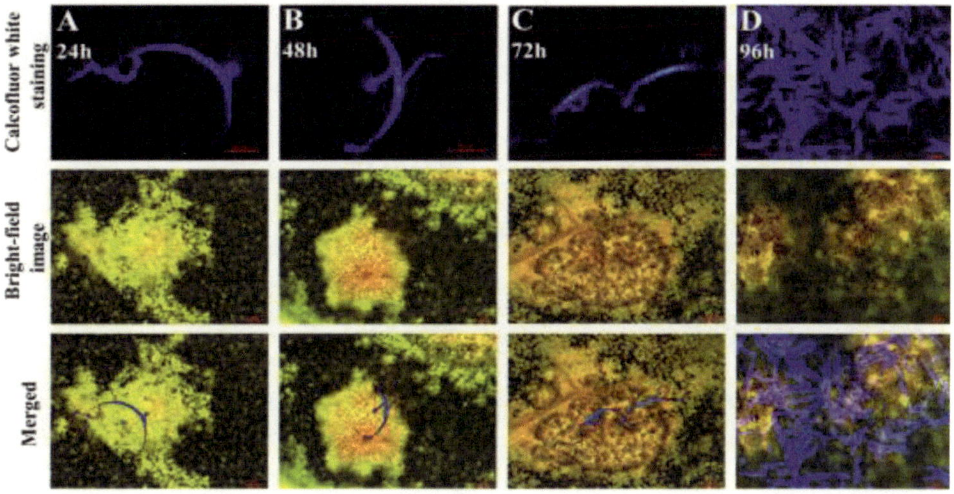

Figure 8.
Development of Mycocentrospora acerina *conidia on* P. notoginseng *leaves. (A–D) conidia were observed on the leaves of* P. notoginseng *at 24, 48, 72, and 96 h, respectively. The blue color shows* Mycocentrospora acerina *conidia and hyphae stained with calcofluor white stain. The bright-field image shows P. notoginseng leaf epidermal cells, and the merged image shows the germination and invasion of* M. acerina *conidia on* P. notoginseng *leaves. Bar = 50 µm.*

4.6 Control of round spot disease by rain-shelter cultivation

In 2020, the rainy season in Lancang County began in June. At the end of June, a rain shelter was built in the *P. notoginseng* field and an open-field control treatment was set up simultaneously. On July 10, the first round spot disease incidence survey was conducted. Neither sheltered nor non-sheltered *P. notoginseng* plants developed the disease (**Figure 9**). However, on July 20, round spot disease started to occur in some areas of the open field. In contrast, the sheltered plants remained healthy. Subsequently, round spot disease began to spread in the open field. By August 10, the average round spot disease incidence in the open field was 18.07%, and the disease index was 8.89. However, the incidence in sheltered plants was still 0.00%. Over time, the disease incidence in the open field increased. As of September 30, the incidence

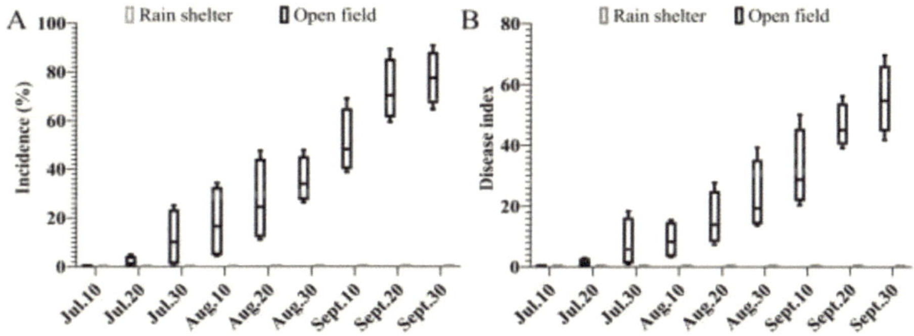

Figure 9.
Effect of rain-shelter cultivation on the incidence rate and disease index of round spot disease. (A) Incidence and (B) disease index of round spot disease in rain-shelter and open-field cultivation.

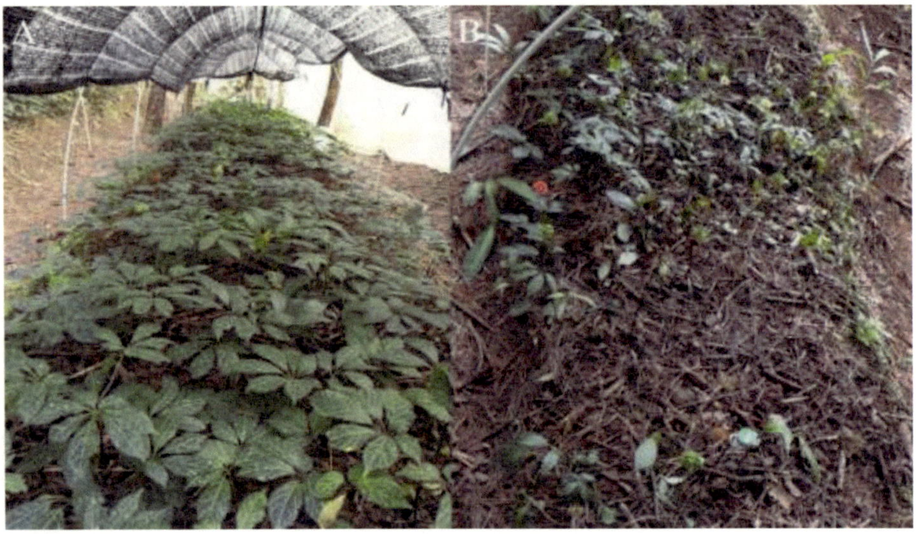

Figure 10.
Effects of rain-shelter cultivation and open-field cultivation on the occurrence of round spot disease. (A) P. notoginseng *plants grown under shelter cultivation remained healthy. (B) Round spot disease occurred in open-field cultivation.*

had reached 77.70%, covering nearly the entire open-field treatment area. However, sheltered plants still remained healthy (**Figure 10**). These data indicated that rain-shelter cultivation has good preventive and control effects on the occurrence of round spot disease, with an average preventive effect of 100%.

5. Conclusion

Cultivation practice of Chinese herbs under forest is a promising technique in the future. It does not occupy arable land, no chemical fertilizer and pesticides, which leads a healthy route for medicinal herbs production.

DOI: http://dx.doi.org/10.5772/intechopen.104859

Author details

Xiahong He[1*], Kuan Yang[2], Shusheng Zhu[2], Liwei Guo[2] and Chen Ye[2]

1 Key Laboratory for Forest Resources Conservation and Utilization in the Southwest Mountains of China, Ministry of Education, Southwest Forestry University, Kunming, China

2 State Key Laboratory for Conservation and Utilization of Bio-Resources in Yunnan, Yunnan Agricultural University, Kunming, China

*Address all correspondence to: hexiahong@hotmail.com

References

[1] Wei JH, Tu OF, LI G, et al. Situation and trends in development of Chinese Medicinal Agriculture in China. Modern Chinese Medicine. 2015;**17**:94-98

[2] Jiang H. The Cultivation of Chinese Herbal Medicine in China Urgently Needs Standardized Development. B07: China Medical News; 2010

[3] Fang YB, Li QX. Analysis and countermeasures of the healthy development of chinese herbal medicine industry in China. Agricultural Outlook. 2021;**17**:123-129

[4] Hu K, Guan WJ, Bi Y, et al. Efficacy and Safety of Lianhuaqingwen Capsules, a repurposed Chinese Herb, in Patients with Coronavirus disease 2019: A multicenter, prospective, randomized controlled trial. Phytomedicine. 2020;**2020**:153242

[5] Huang LQ, Su GQ, Zhang XB, et al. Key points of poverty alleviation of Chinese herbal medicine industry and classification of recommended Chinese herbal medicines. China Journal of Chinese Materia Medicine. 2017;**42**:4319-4328

[6] Wei F, Ma SC. Quality and safety situation of Chinese medicinal materials and supervision thinking. China Food & Drug Administration Magazine. 2019;**2019**:22-29

[7] Shen L, Li XW, Xu J, et al. Cultivation technology system and development strategy of ginseng pollution-free farmland. China Journal of Chinese Materia Medica. 2017;**42**:3267-3274

[8] Yang CG, Zhou T, Zhang XB, et al. Analysis and safety guarantee Suggestions of Chinese medicinal materials. China Journal of Chinese Materia Medicine. 2022;**2022**:1-8

[9] Pytlakowska K, Kita A, Janoska P, et al. Multi-element analysis of mineral and trace elements in medicinal herbs and their infusions. Food Chemistry. 2012;**135**:494-501

[10] Zou XM, Xiao X, Zhou H, et al. Effects of soil acidification on the toxicity of organophosphorus pesticide on Eisenia fetida and its mechanism. Journal of Hazardous Materials. 2018;**359**:365-372

[11] Luo L, Dong LL, Li MZ, et al. RAM research on general standard of pollution-free chinese medicine based on pharmacopoeia algorithm. China Journal of Chinese Materia Medicine. 2019;**44**:2197-2207

[12] Guo LP, Huang LQ, Jiang YX, et al. Soil environment deterioration in Chinese herbal medicine cultivation and its control strategy. China Journal of Chinese Materia Medicine. 2006;**31**:714-717

[13] Fan XC, Liu Q, Xu YW, et al. Research progress on continuous cropping obstacles of Chinese medicinal materials. Sichuan Agricultural Science and Technology. 2021:28-30

[14] Schmidt JP, Cruse-Sanders J, Chamberlain JL, et al. Explaining harvests of wild-harvested herbaceous plants: American ginseng as a case study. Biological Conservation. 2015;**231**:139-149

[15] Guo LP, Zhou LY, Mo G, et al. Traditional Chinese medicine ecological agriculture——The future of traditional Chinese medicine GAP. China Journal of Chinese Materia Medicine. 2015;**40**:3360-3366

[16] Liu H, Yang M, Zhu S. Strategies to solve the problem of soil sickness of *Panax notoginseng* (Family: Araliaceae). Allelopathy Journal. 2019;**47**:37-56

[17] Wang ZH, Wang WP, Liu YB, et al. Investigation and source analysis of root knot nematode disease of *Panax notoginseng* in Lancang County, Yunnan Province. Journal of Yunnan Agricultural University (Natural Science). 2021;**36**:60-68

[18] Yang K, Zhang S, Guo LW, et al. Occurrence of *Panax notoginseng* round spot and control effect of rain shelter cultivation in Lancang County. Journal of Chinese Medicinal Materials. 2020;**43**:2857-2863

[19] Yu ZF, Zhang RJ, et al. Development advantages and key problems of Organic *Panax notoginseng* Industry under Forest. Forest Inventory and Planning. 2019;**44**:177-181

[20] Xiong BJ, Shi R, He S, et al. Effects of secondary metabolites of Panaxnoto ginseng under forest in different cultivation modes. Journal of Shenyang Pharmaceutical University. 2022;**2021**:1-12

[21] Wang Y, He S, Xiong BJ, et al. Effects of different cultivation modes on soil microbial diversity in panax ginseng rhizosphere. Chinese Traditional and Herbal Drugs. 2021b;**52**:5303-5310

[22] Liu JY. Research on Sustainable Development of Underginseng Planting Industry. Chinese Academy of Forestry; 2020

[23] Shu J. Application value of Dendrobium officinale and imitative wild cultivation technique in undergrowth. Modern Agricultural Science and Technology. 2021;**2021**:61-69

[24] Ong C, Black C, Wallace J. Productivity, microcli- mate and water use in Grevillea robusta-based agroforestry systems on hillslopes in semi-arid Kenya. Agriculture Eco-systems and Environment. 2000;**80**:121-141

[25] Sun S, Meng P, Zhang J. Deuterium isotope variation and water use in walnut mung bean complex system in rocky mountainous area of North China. Journal of Ecology. 2010;**30**:3717-3726

[26] Rivest D, Cogliastro A, Bradley R. Intercropping hybrid poplar with soybean increases soil microbial biomass, mineral N supply and tree growth. Agroforestry Systems. 2010;**80**:33-40

[27] Zhang L, Luo M, Han J. Effects of jujube cotton intercropping on soil microflora and metabolic entropy in southern Xinjiang. Journal of Cotton. 2016;**28**:493-503

[28] Yang K, Zhang S, Guo LW, et al. Occurrence of Panax notoginseng round spot and control effect of rain shelter cultivation in Lancang County. Journal of Chinese Medicinal Materials. 2020b;**12**:2857-2863

[29] Xu JT. Application and prospect on the researches of ecological cultivation of Coptis Chinensis. Acta Academiae Medicinae Sinicae. 2004;**26**:601-603

[30] Wang Y, Tan JH, Wang R, et al. Investigation of Understory Medicinal Plant Resources in the Castanopsis hystrix Plantation of Longdong Reservoir, Guangzhou. Forestry and Environmental Science. 2020;**36**:84-90

[31] Li Q, Zhao Y, Zhang Y. Rearch progress of light to medicinal plants and it's implications for ecological cultivation. Research and Practice on Chinese Medicines. 2017;**31**:80-83

[32] Niu H, Wei KH, Xu Q, et al. Effects of different illuminance on growth, physiological characteristics and medicinal components of Anoplecta chinensis. Journal of Plant Resources and Environment. 2020;**29**:26-36+43

[33] Yu LJ. Study on Ginseng Temperature Environment in Greenhouse. Jilin University; 2008

[34] Kong ZQ. Effects of shading on seedling growth of grass coral. Journal of Green Science and Technology. 2019;**2019**:133-135

[35] Zhang SJ, Chen XD, Li YX, et al. Effect of plant communities on the change of soil temperature in Jin Yun Mountain. Journal of Southwest University (Natural Science Edition). 2007;**2007**:162-167

[36] Florian Z, Pieter DF, Jonathan L, et al. Forest microclimate dynamics drive plant responses to warming. Science, New York. 2020;**368**:772-775

[37] Fan QF, Zhang YL, Chen Z. Effects of protected field vegetable cultivation on soil salinity accumulating and pH. Journal of Soil and Water Conservation. 2009;**23**:103-106

[38] Guo LP, Wang TL, Yang WZ, et al. Eecological agriculture: The only way for traditional Chinese medicine agriculture. China Journal of Chinese Materia Medicine. 2017;**42**:231-238

[39] Li JY, Wang QX, Zhang RM. Effects of organic fertilizer and biochar on pakchoi yield and soil nutrient accumulation and utilization in protected vegetable fields. Northern Horticulture. 2019;**22**:16-21

[40] Bonanomi G, Alioto D, Minutolo M, et al. Organic amendments modulate soil microbiota and reduce virus disease incidence in the TSWV-tomato pathosystem. Pathogens. 2020;**9**:379-393

[41] Compant S, Duffy B, Nowak J, et al. Use of plant growth-promoting bacteria for biocontrol of plant diseases: principles, mechanisms of action, and future prospects. Applied and Environmental Microbiology. 2005;**71**:4951-4959

[42] Ye C, Liu Y, Zhang J, et al. α-Terpineol fumigation alleviates negative plant-soil feedbacks of *Panax notoginseng* via suppressing Ascomycota and enriching antagonistic bacteria. Phytopathology Research. 2021;**3**:1-17

[43] Riedlmeier M, Ghirardo A, Wenig M, et al. Monoterpenes support systemic acquired resistance within and between Plants. The Plant Cell. 2017;**29**:1440-1459

[44] Gershenzon J, Dudareva N. The function of terpene natural products in the natural world. Nature Chemical Biology. 2007;**3**:408-414

[45] Aldrich JR, Kochansky JP, Abrams CB. Attractant for a beneficial insect and its parasitoids: Pheromone of the predatory spined soldier bug, Podisus maculiventris (Hemiptera: Pentatomidae). Environmental Entomology. 1984;**13**:1031-1036

[46] Cao NN, Ge WC, Ye C, et al. Composition structure and diversity of arthropod communities on understory planted *Panax notoginseng* in Pinus kesiya var. langbianensis forest. Journal of Southern Agriculture. 2019;**50**:299-306

[47] Wall CJ, Lewis BG. Infection of carrot leaves by Mycocentrospora acerina. Transactions of the British Mycological Society. 1980;**75**:163-165

Chapter 27

Cultivation and Conservation of African Medicinal Plants for Pharmaceutical Research and Socio-Economic Development

Emmanuel Mshelia Halilu

Abstract

Medicinal plants are a huge reservoir of therapeutic agents for the treatment of human and other animals' diseases. This paper highlights the potential of African medicinal plants for pharmaceutical research and socio economic development. The paper also provides an insight on the role of medicinal plants in boosting the economy of African countries. Furthermore, the need for the government and private individuals to invest in the cultivation and conservation of medicinal plants has been discussed. Most importantly, the need to encourage collaboration among African countries towards pharmaceutical research into medicinal plants with the view of developing new drugs for the present and future pandemics have been stated. Therefore, the deliberate research into African medicinal plants may be the saving grace of the African continent against dreaded diseases, for cures yet to be discovered lie mainly in the medicinal plants.

Keywords: conservation, cultivation, COVID-19, drugs, economy and traditional medicine

1. Introduction

A medicinal plant contains either in all or some of its parts or organs substances that can be used for therapeutic purposes or as starting material for the synthesis of pharmaceutically active drugs [1]. In Africa, medicinal plants are the main ingredients used for the preparation of medicaments by the traditional healer. Therefore, due to the frequent utilization of medicinal plants, African Traditional Medicine has played a key role in socio-economic and socio-cultural heritage that services more than 80% of the African populations [2]. Several Africans especially the rural dweller earn their living from the medicinal plant trade [3]. Medicinal plants have formed the basis for the treatment of various diseases in ancient medical practice especially from the recorded history of the Sumerians and Akkadians; and also in Egypt, China, India and Greece [4, 5].

The first recorded history that depicted the importance of the cultivation and conservation of plants is found in the Bible. God created the garden of Eden and carefully put selected plants for specific purposes (Genesis 2:8-9). This story demonstrates the importance of the cultivation of plants; God himself placed our ancestor (Adam) to take care of the garden and there his needs for medicine, food and shelter can be met (Genesis 1:29; 2:8-9).

The cultivation of medicinal plants for pharmaceutical research and development is an area that has received little or no attention from African countries. Medicinal plants are endowed with chemicals substances that have been used and are still in use today for the development of new drugs. Nature has provided mankind with the reservoir of millions of complex/simple bioactive compounds from plants; mainly the secondary metabolites that can be used for therapeutic purposes [6–8]. Therefore, it is evident that cures yet to be discovered (e.g., COVID-19) lie largely in the medicinal plants [9].

Medicinal plants are mainly sourced from the wild. This is no longer sustainable and reliable due to over-harvesting and over-exploitation by the plant collectors and herb sellers [10]. Today, many medicinal plants have gone extinct or are very scarce to find. Therefore, speedy investment in the cultivation of medicinal plants for pharmaceutical research and development beyond the COVID-19 is needed. Cultivation of medicinal plants also provides numerous advantages over wild sources in many ways. The export of cultivated medicinal plants may add to the economy of many African countries [11].

The African continent is enriched with biodiverse varieties of plants which are reservoirs of chemical diversities for the development of new drugs. The African medicinal plants are mainly found in the wild and it has been estimated that there exist about 40,000 to 45,000 plant species on the African continent and out of this; 5000 plant species are thought to have some therapeutic benefits [12]. In Nigeria, there are over 4600 plant species identified, ranking it 11th in Africa for diversity [13]. Therefore, medicinal plants may serve as a huge raw material reservoir, which if harnessed will serve as the driving force towards the revolution of pharmaceutical research and development of the African pharmaceutical industries.

2. The need for cultivation and conservation of African medicinal plants for pharmaceutical research

The emergence of the COVID-19 pandemic has demonstrated that the African continent has made no adequate preparation for the prevention of present and future diseases through systematic advanced biomedical research. Therefore, to prevent future emergencies, there is a need for rapid investment into agro-medicinal plant cultivation. The medicinal plants may provide the following categories of medicinal agents:

a. They provide raw materials for the pharmaceutical industries.

b. They provide compounds that are extremely difficult to be synthesized in the laboratory.

c. They provide some basic compounds whose structures can be modified to become potent drugs.

d. They provide prototype compounds that can be synthesized in the laboratory.

e. The cultivation of medicinal plants provides a constant and genuine source of medicinal plants for the pharmaceutical industries.

In the recent past, there is a growing difficulty in obtaining some medicinal plant species from the wild source due to extinction, scarcity and over-exploitation. Therefore, where there is difficulty in obtaining a medicinal plant; then cultivation of medicinal plants seems to be the best and the most reliable alternative for their conservation. Botanical gardens are important agencies for ensuring their conservation [9].

According to Osemeobo [14] who observed, since the medicinal plants on regular trade are on the decline, stakeholder's participation is required in plant species rehabilitation in the forests. This can be achieved through the establishment of *ex situ* gardens which may sustain the medicinal plant trade.

The continued commercial exploitation of these plants has resulted in receding the population of many plant species in their natural habitat. It is therefore, necessary to initiate systematic cultivation of medicinal plants to conserve biodiversity and to protect endangered species [15].

Medicinal plants harvested from the wild are of immense importance for the well-being of millions of people around the world. They continue to provide both reliefs from illness and a source of income. The loss of habitat, combined with over-harvesting, threatens the survival of many of these plant species.

Furthermore, the rapid extinction of medicinal plants from the wild threatens drug discovery [8]. The more the medicinal plants become extinct, the more difficult it becomes to get these plant species for pharmaceutical research and drug development [8]. The medicinal plants used by the pharmaceutical industries are mostly harvested from the wild [15].

Plants play a pivotal role for the survival of man and other animals [9]. They are the primary producers that sustain all other life forms, regulate air and water qualities, shape ecosystems and control the climate [15]. They provide food, medicine, clothes, shelter and the raw materials from which other products are made. These benefits are widely recognized but poorly understood [9]. Thus, plants are both a vital part of the world's biological diversity and plants are an essential economic resource for human existence [9].

Medicinal plants have been used by mankind for millennia; their use is as old as humanity itself. The range of plant species used for healing purposes is vast. Belinda [9] asserted that "cures as yet undiscovered may exist in plants as yet undescribed". It has been reported by the WHO that over 80% of the World's population depends mainly on plants and plant extracts for health care [16]. It has been estimated that in developed countries like the United States (US), plant drugs constitute about 25% of total drugs. In China and India, they constitute about 80%. It has been estimated that over 250,000 higher plant species occur on earth, with more than 80,000 species reported to have some medicinal values while around 5000 species have specific therapeutic values [15].

Medicinal plants can be classified according to the part used (as a whole plant, root, bark, stem, leaf, fruit, flower and seed), habit (as grasses, sedges, herbs, shrubs, climbers and trees), habitat (as tropical, sub-tropical and temperate) and therapeutic value (as antimalarial, anticancer and anti-inflammatory, antibacterial) [15].

3. Evidence of the need for investment in the cultivation of medicinal plants from the African perspective

The COVID-19 pandemic commenced and most nations of the world swung into action for the search for the cure of the viral infection through several means which include: synthesizing of new drugs, testing already existing drugs and search of new drugs from natural sources. Although, the African countries could not go on to search for cures from other sources; it looked at what is readily available on her continent and made a giant stride towards the utilization of medicinal plants to combat the ravaging COVID-19 pandemic. This effort is evidenced by Madagascar's research institute who developed the Covid-Organics (medicinal plant preparation) derived mainly from *Artemisia annua* and other plants indigenous to Madagascar. Many other African countries including Nigeria have made effort in that regard. As demonstrated from the above, this calls for aggressive pharmaceutical research as it has demonstrated the therapeutic potentials of the medicinal plants of African origin towards the fight against the deadly viral disease (COVID-19). Africa needs to invest in the cultivation of medicinal plants for pharmaceutical research towards the development of drugs. Medicinal plants may be the latent savior for the Africans against present and future pandemics. Africa needs to prepare a head and not wait for other pandemics before it starts searching for a cure. This shows Africa's late response to COVID-19 because it was not prepared. Africa has a great advantage as it houses huge varieties of medicinal plants resources and it is in best position to search for the cure of the future diseases from medicinal plants. Professor Albert Rakoto Ratsimamanga the pioneer of Science in Madagascar stated and declared that "*we (Africa) must move forward at our own pace, we must above all have confidence in ourselves and in the therapeutic virtues of nature. For nature and man are one*" [17].

4. Boosting African economies through medicinal plant cultivation and biodiversity conservation

The cultivation and commercialisation of medicinal plants provide an economic resource for Africa's pharmaceutical industries, which opens business and investment opportunities. There is a need for strong collaboration between the pharmaceutical industry and the academia/research institute to promote sustainable economic growth through the utilization of medicinal plant resources in Africa for drug development and commerce [18].

Several Africans are living in abject poverty who needs to be fed, clothed, housed and employed. The commercialisation of African medicinal plants can be seen as an opportunity to benefit the people on the continent. The industry will create work for the rural and peri-urban unemployed people [18]. This will help the poor to secure a regular income, which in turn helps them to maintain a healthy living condition. Commercial laboratories also play a role in creating, among their employees, an awareness of Africa's rich biodiversity [18]. Cultivation of medicinal plants reduces the pressure on plants in the wild, thereby protecting the diverse flora. Techniques for commercialisation of medicinal plants requires advanced technology and this will encourage collaboration and sharing of ideas in science and technology programmes among African countries. Street and Prinsloo [11] stated that around 80% of South Africans depend on traditional medicine for their primary healthcare needs. They however stated that only a few of the South African medicinal plants have been exploited for their full potential in terms of commercialization. They stated that the exploitation of the South African medicinal plants for the development of new pharmaceutical remains untapped. Marula et al. [3] also reported 78 South African medicinal plants belonging to different plant families currently sold in informal markets which serves as a major source of income to the vulnerable groups living in peri-urban, rural, and marginalized areas. Medicinal plant cultivation if properly harnessed could serve as a major source of income to many Africans.

In Nigeria, in the year 1990, the estimated monetary value of benefits realized from conservation was put at well over $6 billion. In the year 2002, due increase in bio-prospecting and bio-discovery activities and the growth in biotechnology-related industries that utilize indigenous genetic materials as feedstock, the year 2002 estimated benefits of biodiversity to Nigeria was over $8 billion per annum [19]. According to Ibrahim et al. [20], the expected annual profit from the production of 840 liters of eucalyptus oil per annum was N2,273,508.00 and profit after tax of N1,818,806.40 at 20%. This figure indicates how viable medicinal plants can boast the African economy if carefully exploited.

In Ghana, an estimated 951 tons of crude herbal medicine were sold at Ghana's herbal markets in 2010, with a total value of around US$ 7.8 million [21]. In Africa, about 75% of people living with HIV/AIDS patronize Complementary and Alternative Medicine [22]. Cumulatively, the yearly market value of herbal drug products is nearly, USD 43 billion which is far above the total annual budget of several African countries [22]. According to Ndhlala et al. [23], the production of herbal mixtures from medicinal plants has resulted in the growing herbal medicine industry with about 50 to 100 private entrepreneurs in the informal market and has also contributed to the creation of numerous jobs in South Africa. Eziacka et al. [24] reported that the value of the traded medicinal plants has been estimated to be US$300,000 in Johannesburg; US$7.8 m in Ghana; US$1.5 in Gabon and Kenya was US$25,900 [25, 26]. In Tanzania, at Kariakoo Market in Dares Salaam, the value was estimated to US$200,000 [27].

Evidence from outside Africa has shown that medicinal plant can be a huge source of income. In the USA, more than 1500 herbal drugs worth billions USD were sold yearly. In the UK, the yearly expenditure on Complementary and Alternative Medicine was 2.3 billion US dollars [2]. Furthermore, over USD 2.4 billion Traditional Chinese Medicines (TCM) have been sold and USD 400 million worth of TCM have been exported out of China in 1993 [2]. Also, about USD 60 million was realized from the sale of herbs in 1996 in Malaysia and in Europe, North America [22, 28].

5. Impact of medicinal plants on the pharmaceutical industries in relation to economic growth

Medicinal plants have played and are still playing an important role in the pharmaceutical industry. Medicinal plants have contributed immensely to the economic growth of many countries through the sales and production of pharmaceutical products. Paul-Marie [29] reported that the annual global sales of drugs were about 300 billion USD. This includes natural product-derived, semi-synthetic and synthetic drugs. Paul-Marie [29] also reported that the global sale of drugs from natural origin varies but as of 1976 it was estimated to be around 5 billion USD and some years later, it was estimated to be around 20 billion USD. This underscores the contribution of medicinal plants and plant-derived drugs to the economic growth of many countries.

6. The importance of medicinal plants used in traditional medicine in the development of orthodox drugs

Historical experiences with plants as therapeutic tools have helped to introduce single chemical entities in modern medicine. Plants, especially those with ethnomedical uses, have been the primary sources of medicines for early drug discovery. A recent analysis by showed that the uses of 80% of 122 plant-derived drugs were related to their original ethnopharmacological purposes. Current drug discovery from terrestrial plants has mainly relied on bioactivity-guided isolation methods, which, for example, have led to discoveries of the important anticancer agents, paclitaxel from *Taxus brevifolia* and camptothecin from *Camptotheca acuminata* [30]. Plants contain thousands of constituents and are a valuable source of new and biologically active molecules [31].

About 25% of all prescriptions sold in the United States are from natural products, while another 25% are as a result of structural modifications of natural products constituents [6]. Furthermore, Farnsworth [6] claims that 119 characterized drugs are still obtained commercially from higher plants with 74% of them sourced from ethnobotanical information.

One of the most important areas of application of natural products is in the treatment of human and veterinary ailments. Currently, at least 119 chemical substances, derived from 90 plant species, can be considered important drugs that are in use in one or more countries [32]. Although, the use of natural products as medicinal agents presumably predates the first recorded history, as the earliest humans used various but specific plants to treat illness, the treatment of diseases with pure pharmaceutical agents is a relatively modern phenomenon [32]. Nevertheless, the role of traditional medicine in the discovery of potent chemicals is quite crucial. Among some of the earliest successes in developing drugs from natural products, are the reports of isolation of the antimalarial agents such as quinine, quinidine, cinchonine and cinchonidine from *Cinchona succirubra*. Currently, the hydroxychloroquine which is the derivative of quinine under investigation as a potential cure for COVID-19 [33]. Pain relievers such as the morphine from *Papaver somniferum* and acetylsalicylic acid from *Salix alba* [34, 35]. More recently, the vinca alkaloids: vinblastine and vincristine were isolated as antineoplastic agents from the Madagascan periwinkle (*Catharanthus roseus*), and subsequently derivatized to vinorelbine and vindesine, the drugs currently used for cancer treatment [32].

Similarly, a potent antimalarial drug, a sesquiterpenoid endoperoxide, artemisinin was isolated from *Artemisia annua* and is used as a remedy against the multidrug-resistant strains of Plasmodium. This followed the long use of this plant as an antimalarial drug in traditional Chinese medicine. Using the basic structure of artemisinin, semisynthetic compounds such as artemether and dihydroartemisinin were synthesized as potent antimalarial agents with the aim of optimizing the pharmacology of artemisinin. These are now in widespread use around the world [32]. Other drugs that were developed on ethnomedical information include reserpine, an antihypertensive agent from *Rauvolfia serpentina*, Atropine, an anticholinergic from *Atropa belladonna*, digoxin, a cardiotonic from *Digitalis lanata*, Physostigmine, a cholinesterase inhibitor from *Physostigma venenosum* and Ephedrine, a sympathomimetic from *Ephedra sinica* [36].

These few accounts give not only the potential of plants as a source of drugs or as the solid link between folk medicine and drug development but also the necessity of research into medicinal plants [37].

7. Orthodox drugs developed from medicinal plants indigenous to Africa

About 52% of the drugs approved in the U.S. between 1981 and 2002 were from natural products mainly plants [6]. From these drugs, African medicinal plants have provided the drug vincristine (I) and vinblastine (II) from Madagascar periwinkle, combretastatin (III) obtained from the South African bush willow in the 1950 and maytansine (IV) from *Maytenus serrata* isolated in the early 1970s from the Ethiopian plant. This illustrates that, medicinal plants native to Africa are huge potential for the development of therapeutic agents. These drugs are potent anticancer drugs and some

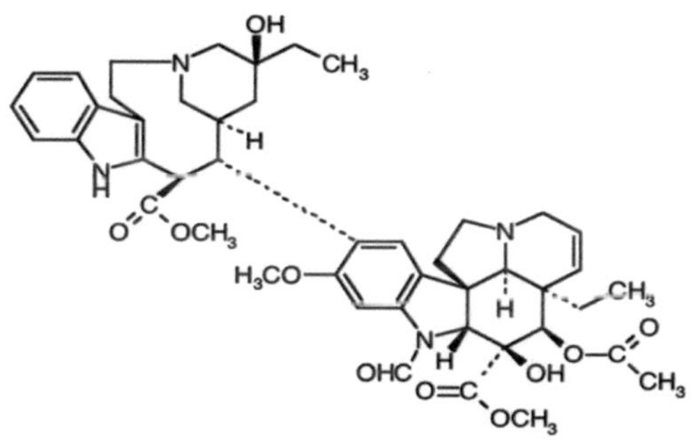

(I)

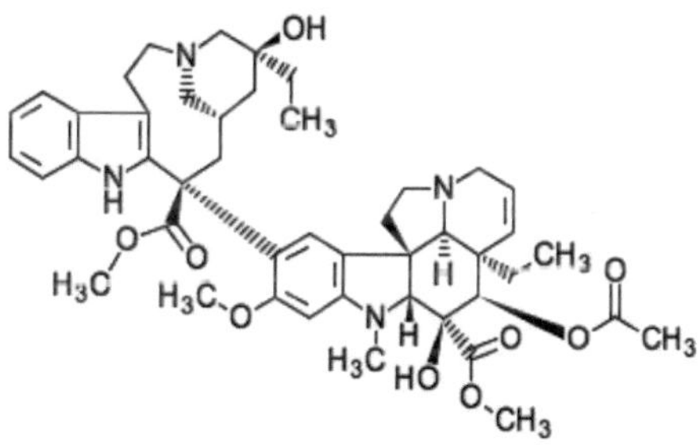

(II)

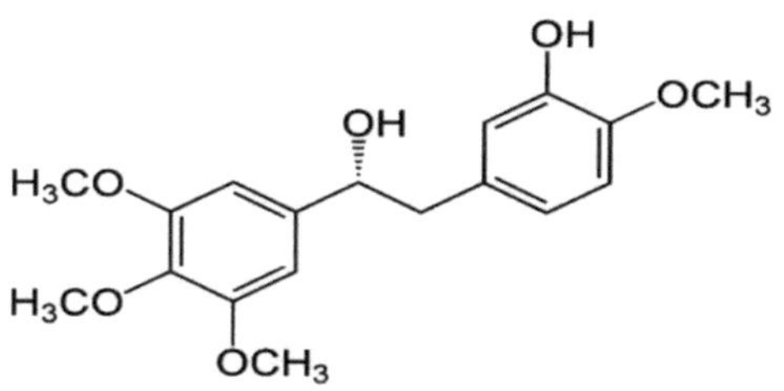

(III)

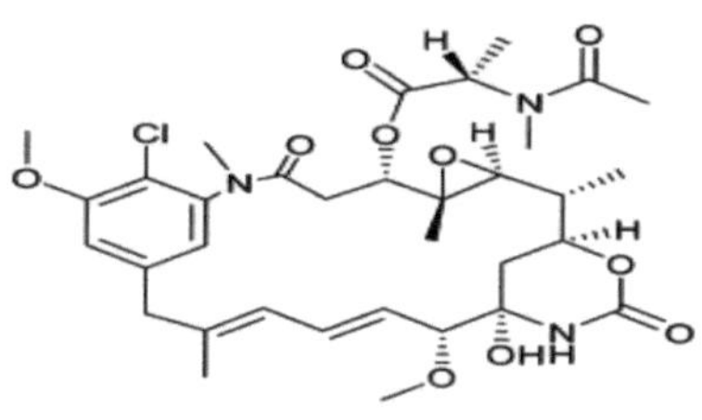

(IV)

Figure 1.
Some bioactive compounds from medicinal plants native to Africa.

Drug Plants source	Plant source	Family
Vincristine	*Catharanthus roseus* (L.) G. Don	Apocynaceae
Vinblastine	*Catharanthus roseus* (L.) G. Don	Apocynaceae
Combretastatin	*Combretum caffrum* (Eckl. & Zeyh.) Kuntze	Combretaceae
Maytansine	*Maytenus serrata* (Hochst.ex A.Rich.) Wilczek	Celastraceae

Table 1.
Plants used for the development of drugs native to African countries.

are still in use today all over the world in different forms as effective anticancer agents (**Figure 1** and **Table 1**) [8].

8. Utilization of African medicinal plants for pharmaceutical research and drug development for the present and the future pandemics

Niprisan is a drug for the treatment of Sickle cell anemia was developed from herbs in Nigeria based on Yoruba Traditional Medicine [38]. Nigeria is home to the largest population of sickle cell anemia patients, estimated to have around 4 million patients with more than 150,000 children born annually with the disease. Despite decades of research, only one FDA-approved drug, hydroxyurea, is available for use in sickle cell anemia [39, 40]. In the late 1980s, in an effort to advance research of traditional herbal medicines, Nigeria's Ministry of Science and Technology established the National Institute for Pharmaceutical Research and Development (NIPRD)–a research body dedicated to identifying, characterizing, developing, and documenting the use of traditional herbal medicines in Nigeria. In May, 2011, three antisickling herbs (*Entandrophragma utile*, *Chenopodium ambrosioides*, and *Petiveria alliacea*) based on Yoruba Traditional Medicine were used at NIPRD to develop Niprisan. At present, three other recipes are currently awaiting development [38]. The Madagascar's research institutes have in the past in collaboration with the National Cancer Institute (NCI) have identified Ipomoeassin and schweinfurthins with potent antiproliferative activities. These compounds were identified from Madagascar's medicinal plants *Ipomoea squamosa* and *Macaranga alnifolia* respectively in the 1990's [41]. More recently the Madagascar's development of Covid-Organics formulated from *Artemisia annua* and other plants by the Malagasy Institute of Applied (IMRA) and the National Pharmacology Research Centre underscore the urgent need for the utilization of African medicinal plants for the research and development of new drugs. These efforts have demonstrated that African medicinal plants can be utilized for the development of many drugs for the treatment of various diseases.

9. Some economically viable medicinal plants of the African origin

Some economically important medicinal plants indigenous to Africa are presented. Street & Prinsloo [11] have reported ten (10) commercially important medicinal plants of South Africa to include: *Agathosma betulina*, *Aloe ferox*, *Aspalathus linearis*, *Harpagophytum procumbens*, *Hypoxis hemerocallidea*, *Merwilla natalensis*, *Pelargonium sidoides*, *Sclerocarya birrea*, *Siphonochilus aethiopicus* and *Sutherlandia frutescens*. Mahomoodally [12] has also reported ten potent African medicinal plants with the potentials to be developed as phytopharmaceuticals to treat infectious diseases. These plants include: *Acacia senegal*, *Aloe ferox*, *Artemisia herba-alba*, *Aspalathus linearis*, *Cantella asiatica*, *Catharanthus roseus*, *Cyclopia genistoides*, *Harpagophytum procumbens*, *Momordica charantia* and *Pelargonium sidoides*. Other plants of economic value include: *Xylopia aethiopica*, *Monodora myristica*, *Aframomum melegueta*, *Khaya senegalensis*, *Pteleopsis suberosa*, *Griffonia simplicifolia*, *Voacanga africana* and *Fadogia agrestis* [21]. According to [41, 42] the most traded species were of plants in Tanzania include: *Zanthoxylum chalybaeum*, *Albizia anthelmintica*, *Zanha Africana*, *Warburgia stuhlmannii* and *Vachellia nilotica*.

In Nigeria, according to [19] the economic viable plants which if harnessed for their fixed can generate a huge amount of revenue include: *Sesame indicum*, *Adansonia digitata, Vitellaria paradoxa* and *Persia americana*.

10. Recommendations

a. Government should invest in the cultivation and conservation of medicinal plants with the view of effective utilization in pharmaceutical research and development of African pharmaceutical industries.

b. There should be an effective collaboration between established African established research laboratories for rapid screening of medicinal plant extracts with reported ethnopharmacological claims on the treatment of viral infections and other diseases.

c. Farmers should be encouraged to cultivate agro-medicinal which can be a good source of revenue, employment and entrepreneurship to the vast majority of African youths.

11. Conclusion

African medicinal plants are a huge reservoir of medicinal agents for pharmaceutical research and development. Cures yet undiscovered lies in the medicinal plants. Our quest for the development of new drugs of African origin may come from the African medicinal plants if concerted effort and commitment from the African heads of government are put towards searching and screening of medicinal plants extracts with established ethnomedicinal claims. The medicinal plants are largely obtained from wild sources where there is no guarantee of constant supply due to over-harvesting, over-exploitation and extinction. Therefore, there is a need for their cultivation and conservation.

Author details

Emmanuel Mshelia Halilu[1,2]

1 Faculty of Pharmacy, Cyprus International University, Nicosia, Turkey

2 Faculty of Pharmaceutical Sciences, Department of Pharmacognosy and Ethnomedicine, Usmanu Danfodiyo University, Sokoto, Nigeria

*Address all correspondence to: emshelia2002@gmail.com

References

[1] Sofowora A. Medicinal Plants and Traditional Medicine in Africa. Third ed. Nigeria: Spectrum Books Limited Ibadan; 2008. pp. 162-179

[2] Elujoba AA, Odeleye OM, Ogunyemi CM. Traditional medicine development for medical and dental primary health care delivery system in Africa. African Journal of Traditional, Complementary and Alternative Medicines. 2005;**2**(1):46-61

[3] Marula TR, Sebua SS, Alfred M. Medicinal plants traded in informal herbal medicine Markets of the Limpopo Province, South Africa. Evidence-based Complementary and Alternative Medicine. 2019;**2019**:11

[4] Samuelsson G, Bohlin L. Drugs of Natural Origin: A Treatise of Pharmacognosy. 6th revised ed. Stockholm, Sweden: Swedish Pharmaceutical Society, Swedish Pharmaceutical Press; 2009. pp. 17-22

[5] Rajandeep K, Karan K, Harpreet K. Plants as a source of anticancer agents. Journal of Natural Product and Plant Resources. 2011;**1**(1):119-124

[6] Farnsworth NR. In: Chadwick DJ, Marsh J, editors. In Bioactive Compounds from Plants. Chichester, UK: John Wiley; 1990. pp. 2-21

[7] Cragg GM, Newman JD. Natural product drug discovery in the next millennium. Pharmaceutical Biology. 2011;**39**(1):8-17

[8] Vicki B. Back to nature: Extinction of medicinal plants threatens drug discovery. Journal of National Cancer Institute. 2008;**100**(12):838-839

[9] Belinda H. Plants for Life: Medicinal Plant Conservation and Botanic Gardens. Botanic Gardens conservation international: Richmond, UK; 2008. pp. 1-5

[10] Van Wyk AS, Prinsloo G. Medicinal plant harvesting, sustainability and cultivation in South Africa. Biological Conservation. 2018;**227**:335-342

[11] Street RA, Prinsloo G. Commercially important medicinal plants of South Africa (a review). Journal of Chemistry. 2013;**2013**:16

[12] Mahomoodally MF. Traditional medicines in Africa: An appraisal of ten potent African medicinal plants. Evidence-based Complementary and Alternative Medicine. 2013;**2013**:1-14

[13] FAO. Nigeria-Country Report to the FAO International Technical Conference on Plant Genetic Resources, Leipzig, Germany. 1996. p. 8

[14] Osemeobo G. Impact of traditional practices on medicinal plant trade In: The rainforest of Nigeria. Geography, Environment, Sustainability. 2010;**3**(3):56-67

[15] Joy P, Thomas J, Samuel M, Baby P. Aromatic and Medicinal Plants. Odakkali, India: Kerala Agricultural University; 1998. pp. 3-22

[16] World Health Organization. Sickle Cell Anaemia Report by Secretariat. Geneva: World Health Assembly; 2000

[17] Razanamparany M. Coronavirus: Madagascar's 'Covid-Organics' Born from Local Traditions. The Africa Report Website; 2020. Available from: https://www.theafricareport.com

[18] Okole BN, Odhav B. Commercialisation of plants in Africa. South African Journal of Botany. 2004;**70**(1):109-115

[19] Federal Republic of Nigeria Fourth National Biodiversity Report Abuja 2010. Nigeria: Federal Ministry of Environment; 2010. p. 12

[20] Ibrahim HM, Abdulrahman AY, Warra AA, Abdullahi K. Entrepreneur in Pharmacognosy: An unexploited area in Nigeria; Gusau. Journal of Entrepreneurship Development. 2019;**1**(1):161-176

[21] Tinde VA, Britt M, Sabine VO. Ghana's herbal market. Journal of Ethnopharmacology. 2012;**140**:368-378

[22] Enwonwu CO. Global Trends in the Use of Complimentary Medicine Proceedings of the 2nd Dr. David Barmes' Memorial Public Health Symposium, 25th March 2003. Brazzaville: The Regional Centre for Oral Health Research & Training for Africa Jos in collaboration with WHO Regional Office; 2003

[23] Ndhlala AR, Stafford GI, Finnie JF, Staden JV. Commercial herbal preparations in KwaZulu-Natal, South Africa: The urban face of traditional medicine. South African Journal of Botany. 2011;**77**:830-843

[24] Eziacka MM, Jeremia RM, Olav JS, Kenneth M, Kitundu B. The value chain of traded productsof medicinal plants in Tanzania: The emerging role of formulators. African Journal of Economic and Management Studies, Emerald Publishing Limited. 2021;**2021**:2040-0705

[25] Delbanco A, Cuni-Sanchez A, Neil DB. Medicinal plant trade in northern Kenya: Economic importance, uses, and origin. Economic Botany. 2017;**71**:13-31

[26] Towns A, Quiroz M, Guinee L, Boer H, Andel T. Volume, value and floristic diversity of Gabon's medicinal plant markets. Journal of Ethnopharmacology. 2014;**155**:1184-1193

[27] Posthouwer C, Veldman S, Abihudi S, Otieno J, Andel T, Boer H. Quantitative market survey of non-woody plants sold at Kariakoo market in Dar Es Salaam, Tanzania. Journal of Ethnopharmacology. 2018;**17**:280-287

[28] Mafimisebi TE, Oguntade AE, Ajibefun IA, Mafimisebi OE, Ikuemonisan ES. The expanding market for herbal, medicinal and aromatic plants In Nigeria and the international scene. Medicinal and Aromatic. 2013;**2**(6):1-9

[29] Paul-Marie L. Medicinal Plant Trade and Opportunities for Sustainable Management in Cape Peninsula, South Africa, Master of Science thesis. Stellenbosch: Department of Conservation Ecology and Forestry Sciences; 2008. pp. 18-19

[30] Kinghorn AD. The discovery of drugs from higher plants. In: Gullo VP, editor. The Discovery of Natural Products with Therapeutic Potential. Boston, MA: Butterworth-Heinemann; 1994. pp. 81-108

[31] Hostettmann K. Biodiversity and bioresources: Conservation and utilization. Pure and Applied Chemistry. 1999;**70**(1):50-56

[32] Newman DJ, Cragg GM, Snader KM. The influence of natural products upon drug discovery. Natural Product and Reproduction. 2000;**17**:215-234

[33] Samia A, Paul K, Zohra SC, Gordon J, Dee DW, Kylie H, et al. Treatment of

hydroxychloroquine, azithromycin, and combination in patients hospitalised with COVID-19. International Journal of Infectious Diseases. 2020;**97**:396-403

[34] Dewick PM. Medicinal Natural Products: A Biosynthetic Approach. 3rd ed. Chichester, UK: John Wiley and Sons, Ltd.; 2002. pp. 8-9

[35] Viktorin M, Sartorius AG. One-hundred-year anniversary of aspirin. The Drug Extracted from the Willow Bark, Göttingen, Germany. Labor Praxis. 1999, 2006;**23**(7/8):82-85

[36] Fabricant SD, Farnsworth RN. The value of plants used in traditional medicine for drug discovery. Environmental Health Perspectives. 2001;**109**(1):65-75

[37] Salim AA, Chin YW, Kinghorn AD. Drug discovery from Plants. In: Ramawat KG, Mérillon JM, editors. Bioactive Molecules and Medicinal Plants. Springer; 2008. pp. 1-25. Available from: http://www.springer.com

[38] Sunday JA, Florence DT, Benjamin UE. Traditional herbal Management of Sickle Cell Anaemia: Lessons from Nigeria (review). Anaemia. 2012;**2012**:9

[39] Steinberg MH. Effect of hydroxyurea on mortality and morbidity in adult sickle cell anaemia. JAMA. 2003;**289**(13):1645-1651

[40] Kumar P, Hassan M, Andrew K, Ronak S, Abdallah SD, Peter AS. The road to commercialization in Africa: Lessons from developing the sickle-cell drug Niprisan. BMC International Health and Human Rights. 2010;**10**(1):S11

[41] Kingston GID. Modern natural products drug discovery and its relevance to biodiversity conservation. Journal of Natural Product. 2012;**74**(3):496-511

[42] Hilonga S, Otieno JN, Ghorbani A, Pereus D, Kocyan A, Boer H. Trade of wild-harvested medicinal plant species in local markets of Tanzania and its implications for conservation. South African Journal of Botany. 2019;**122**:214-224

Chapter 28

Medicinal Plants Threatened by Undocumented Emerging Pollutants: The Sub-Saharan African Viewpoint

John Baptist Nzukizi Mudumbi, Elie Fereche Itoba-Tombo, Seteno Karabo Obed Ntwampe and Tandi Matsha

Abstract

The history of medicinal plants on the African continent is huge, the oldest and probably the most diverse, for there are thousands of spoken languages, in the sub-Saharan African region, that are used during the traditional practices that utilize medicinal plants for healing purposes. However, our lines of research have exhibited a potential unprecedented threat to this remarkable history of African medicinal plants by emerging pollutants, the per- and polyfluoroalkyl substances (PFASs), which are yet to be efficiently and sufficiently reported and documented on in this region. Accordingly, this review chapter reports on sub-Saharan African medicinal plants with the aim of highlighting how undocumented PFASs, in this region, present a huge threat to the extraordinary diversity of these plants and the therapy that they have assisted the low-income populations of this region with for centuries. Thus, we recommend appropriate and regular assessments and monitoring of PFASs, particularly perfluorooctanoic acid (PFOA) and perfluorooctane sulfonate (PFOS) the most studied of these substances and their substitutes, in medicinal plants of the region, for these chemicals have been scientifically proven to be associated to numerous health concerns. The region should also consider properly regulating these compounds.

Keywords: medicinal plants, threats, emerging pollutants, PFASs, sub-Saharan Africa

1. Introduction

Medicinal plants have been in use since ancient times [1]; they carry a long history [2]. These plants are an important mode of combat to serious illnesses and diseases in the world [3]. These crops and their derivatives are used for healing by various populations, and in extreme scenarios, these plants have been chosen as natural alternatives or substitutes to their orthodox counterparts [4]. Reported evidence has indicated that these natural products and their derivatives account for an estimated more than 50% of all the drugs used globally [5]. Available data have previously estimated that 90% of world's rural people use medicinal plants for therapeutic purposes, and according to a recent survey by the World Health Organisation (WHO) 87% of its African member states population rely on traditional medicine, mainly medicinal plants, as their main primary health care source [6–9]. For instance, it has been reported that 90% of the Ethiopians use herbal remedies as their main source of medicines, while up to 80% of South Africans are estimated to be in consultation with healers traditional [6, 7]. Thus, sub-Saharan African medicinal plants in their diverse forms are holistic involving both the body and the mind [6].

Obviously, the history of medicinal plants on the African continent is huge, the oldest, and probably the most diverse [6], for there are over 2000 spoken languages [10], in the sub-Saharan African region, during the use of traditional medicinal plants for healing purposes. In this regard, a variety of medicinal plants is reported to be used for the treatment of ailments in this region of Africa [11]. Hence, it has been reported that sub-Saharan Africa alone has over 50,000 distinct plant species, of which more than 25% of these species is reported to have been used for several centuries in traditional African medicine for the prevention and treatment of illnesses [12]. Recent reports have suggested that the remarkable and enormous biodiversity in medicinal plants in sub-Saharan Africa should not be surprising considering that the continent is geographically located within the tropical and subtropical climate [6, 12, 13]. The region has one of the biggest forests of the world, the Congo basin, which spans across six countries, namely the entire Central African Region (**Figure 1**), i.e., Cameroon, Central African Republic, Democratic Republic of the Congo (DRC), Republic of the Congo, Equatorial Guinea and Gabon. The basin on its own is estimated to have approximately 10,000 species of tropical plants and 30% of these are endemic to the region. This forest, in some extents, provides livelihood to millions of people across this region.

Nevertheless, despite the vast medicinal plants' diversity and highest endemism, sub-Saharan Africa still doesn't have sufficient drugs being commercialized globally [6, 14, 15]. This has been exacerbated by the fact that only a small fraction of medicinal plants, on the African continent, is from commercial cultivated sources, as most of medicinal plants consumed in sub-Saharan Africa and those destined for exportation are mostly harvested from the wild, including forests and national parks; albeit few countries, including Madagascar, Kenya and South Africa, taking initiatives towards commercially producing medicinal plants [16]. Therefore, we can only hope for the continent to efficiently making use of its remarkable medicinal plant potentials to improve the lives of its growing population. Hence, there are positive signs in this regard which have emerged recently. For instance, a WHO reported that by 2018, more than 85% of the total Member States in the WHO African Region have reported having a national policy for medicinal plants and others, compared to Western Pacific Region and the Eastern Mediterranean Region WHO Member States with 65% and 45%, respectively [8].

Additionally, the same report also found that the African region scored the highest percentage (>80%) of countries with national or state level laws and regulations for medicinal plants and others. Certainly, this is a promising path that the African continent has embarked on, even though more still need to be established.

Furthermore, there are several other threats to sub-Saharan Africa's medicinal plant potentials. For example, the literature reviewed has indicated that medicinal plants on the continent are disappearing due to the destruction of its natural habitats in the form of high rates of deforestation, rapid agricultural development, urbanization, and uncontrolled harvesting of these plant materials [6, 7, 12, 17, 18]. Nonetheless, there are threats that have emerged during the last few decades, and

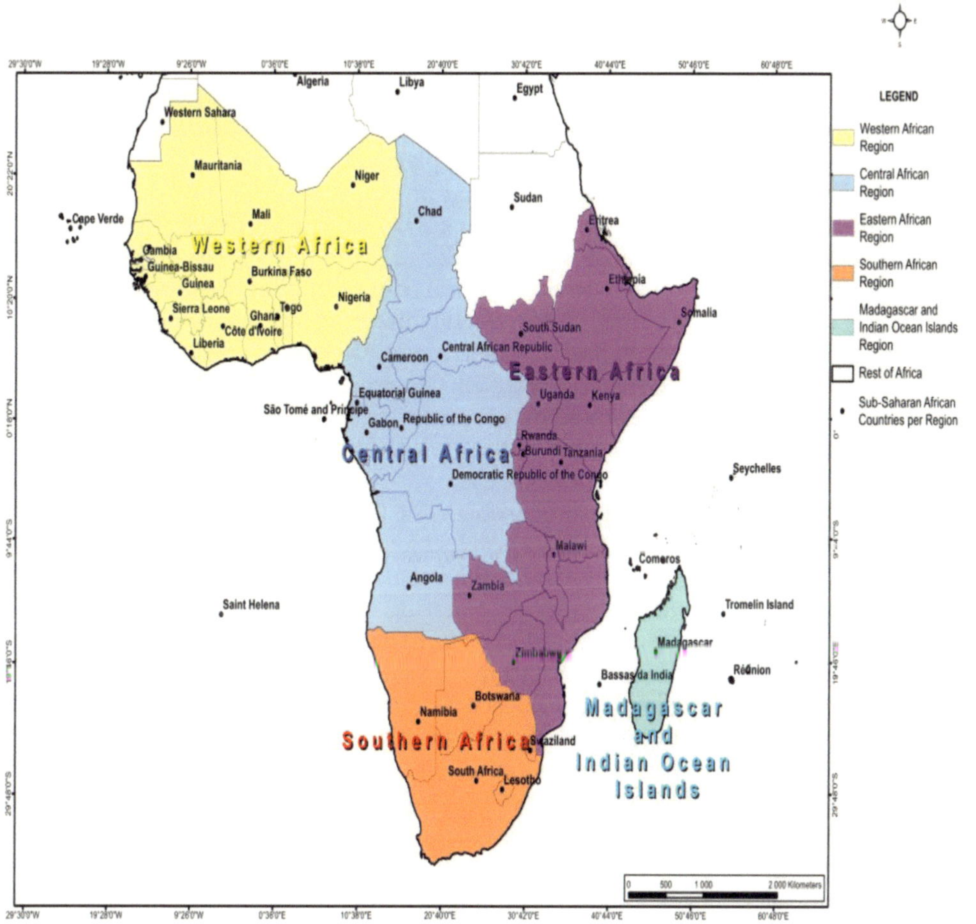

Figure 1.
Sub-Saharan African regions.

which, in our view, have not been reported on, and have thus remained undocumented. They are threats form emerging persistent organic pollutants (POPs), perfluoroalkyl and polyfluoroalkyl substances (PFASs), in particular. Emerging contaminants are contaminants about which we have a new awareness or understanding about how they move in the environment or affect health [19].

2. Persistent organic pollutants: definition and environmental fates

Several international environmental organizations, including the Geneva Inter-Organisation Programme for the Sound Management of Chemicals, the United Nations (UN) under its United Nations Environmental Programme (UNEP), the Food and Agriculture Organization (FAO) and the WHO, have described POPs as chemicals that are stable and persist in the environment, bioaccumulate in organisms and the food chain, are toxic to humans as well as animals, and have chronic effects such as the disruption of reproductive, immune and endocrine systems, as well as being carcinogenic [20–24]. It is believed that these substances can enter the environment through several ways, including release from waste dumps, spillages, industrial and agricultural waste, urban/agricultural runoff and the burning of various materials, thus being distributed in various environmental matrices, including water, air, soils, sediments and living organisms [25–28]. Given the fact that POPs have bioaccumulation potentials and can travel long distances to places far from the points of release by means of waterways, atmospheric exchange and agricultural runoffs, POPs have been detected even in pristine areas such as the Antarctica and the Arctic regions, regions with minimum direct anthropogenic disturbance [25, 28, 29]. In 1997, in order to limit POPs transportation and environmental contamination, the international community decided to work towards the establishment of a convention that would serve as an international, legally binding instrument, to reduce and/or eliminate the release of POPs, as identified in the UNEP Governing Council Decision 19/13C [20]. Consequently, under the Stockholm Convention of POPs (COP-4) for global action, the UNEP, in 1995, listed twelve POPs which are also known as the "dirty dozen", and consisted of Aldrin, dieldrin, dichloro-diphenyl-trichloroethane (DDT), endrin, heptachlor, chlordane, hexachlorobenzene (HCB), mirex, toxaphene, PCDD/Fs i.e., polychlorinated dioxins (PCDDs), polychlorinated dibenzofurans (PCDFs) and polychlorinated biphenyls (PCBs). In this regard, the Convention's Governing Council took a decision 18/32 to begin investigating POPs, and their persistence in the environment, and thus initiate the eradication or restricted use of these substances, and ultimately minimize the contamination of food chain [28–32].

Moreover, the sources of different POPs have been established. For instance, deliberate application to crops and soils is suggested to be the source of agrochemical POPs, while organochlorine pesticides (OCPs) and other industrial chemicals are reported to be intentionally produced for various uses, for example as flame retardants, as ingredients in consumer products, including electronic goods, which generally result in their unintentional release into the environment, some in the form of e-waste [28, 33–36].

In addition, the use of fire-fighting foams, vehicles and the burning of wood, have been mentioned as potential contributors to POP release into the environment in developing countries [28, 35]. Organic pollutants can enter the coastal environment by several processes and once introduced to this environment, they are subject to biogeochemical cycling, sinking, and other environmental processes [28, 37].

Furthermore, evidence suggests that the low rate of escape of POPs into water reservoirs (i.e., streams), or stock of materials and products, is a source of great concern because it could result in exposure that could cause subtle toxicological effects in humans and biota [38–41]. Similarly, an increasing number of materials containing POPs, are used in building materials, in goods and in various consumer products [42, 43]. For POPs contained in consumer products, their low vapor pressure can result in a slow but significant release into the environment [35] which can come from direct volatilization as well as microscale abrasion of plastics [42, 43]. Following release, the fate of the POP compound in the environment is largely based on its physico-chemical properties and the characteristics of the environment [44].

Besides, it has been suggested that the process of environmental transport of these compounds and their detection into food supplies will be augmented if the compound is in the biosolids applied to agricultural lands, in wastewater effluents discharged to surface waters and in landfills adjacent to agricultural lands, and if industrial facilities that use the compound are located near sources of food [45]. The exposure of infants has also been reported as it becomes evident that POPs can be transferred from mother to infant via breast milk, and umbilical cord serum [46–49].

In addition, regardless of the tremendous work that has been done on the African continent regarding reporting and documenting the prevalence of POPs in the African environment over the years [30, 50–53], there is not sufficient evidence on the state of emerging pollutants, such as PFASs, on the continent, compared to the rest of the world; and the reviewed literature has suggested that these undocumented pollutants are a threat to the general African environment [54].

2.1 What are per- and polyfluoroalkyl substances?

There is no general accepted definition of PFASs. However, PFASs are chemicals that fall under the category of new emerging pollutants, for they exhibit properties which are different from traditional pollutants [28] and were anthropogenically synthesized since 1950s by linking a chain of carbon and fluorine atoms together using two major manufacturing methods, namely electrochemical fluorination (ECF) and telomerization technics [55–60]. PFASs are therefore not present in the environment naturally, but are referred to as "forever chemicals", unlike its counterparts such as heavy metals, e.g., compounds such as arsenic (As), mercury (Hg), lead (Pb), cadmium (Cd), chromium (Cr), etc.

These industrial chemicals (i.e. PFASs) contain at least one perfluoroalkyl fraction and have been previously referred to as "perfluorinated chemicals" (PFCs); albeit "PFCs" being a term describing perfluorocarbons, i.e., substances that contain only carbon and fluorine atoms, and having physical properties, such as being oil and water repellent and temperature resistant and reducing friction, and unique chemical functionalities that are fundamentally different from those of many PFASs [59, 60]. Because of these attributes, PFASs have been largely used as part of feedstocks in several manufacturing processes to make consumer and industrial products [60]. Accordingly, the common uses of PFASs have included: (a) non-stick cookware, stain resistant carpets and fabrics, (b) coatings on some food packaging (e.g., microwave popcorn bags and fast-food wrappers), (c) components of fire-fighting foam, (d) many industrial applications, (e) consumer products—for example, products that are stain and/or water resistant, cosmetics, and some cleaning products [19, 60].

Additionally, a common terminology for the nomenclature of PFASs has thus been agreed upon and saw PFASs divided in two classes, namely non-polymeric and polymeric PFASs [60], each with subclasses, groups and subgroups, as depicted on **Table 1**. For more details, there are various references therein [59–64]. In addition, it is currently estimated that more than 5000 known PFAS chemicals exist, with perfluorooctanoic acid (PFOA) and perfluorooctane sulfonate (PFOS) being the most manufactured; and their numbers are expected to increase as industries continue to invent and manufacture new substances [61, 62]. For instance, in 2006, it was reported that the production of these chemicals reached its peak in China, a major trading sub–Saharan African partner, with more than 250 tons/year [58].

2.2 Reasons behind PFASs attention and how people get exposed to them

During the last decades, there has been sufficient evidence on the distribution of PFASs in the environment at large, predominantly in the aquatic and biota environments, but most importantly the attention has been on the fact that these substances have been said to be capable of widely spreading [65]. In this regard, the discovery of PFASs in serum, urine and other tissue samples has prompted researchers wanting to know whether these chemicals can lead to health issues [66]. Similarly, studies have

Per- and polyfluoroalkyl substances (PFASs)		
Non-polymers		Polymers
Perfluoroalkyl substances[ǂ]	**Polyfluoroalkyl substances**[ǂǂ]	
Perfluoroalkyl acids (PFAAs)[a]	Fluorotelomer-based substances[c]	Fluoropolymers
Perfluoroalkyl carboxylic acids/ perfluoroalkyl carboxylates (PFCAs)[a]	Perfluoroalkane sulfonamido Substances[b]	Polymeric perfluoropolyethers (PFPE)
Perfluoroalkane sulfonic acids/ perfluoroalkane sulfonates (PFSAs)[b]	Polyfluoroalkyl ether acids[c]	Side-chain fluorinated polymers
Perfluoroalkane sulfonamides (FASAs)[b]		

[ǂ]*All hydrogen (H) atoms on all carbon (C) atoms in alkyl chain attached to a functional group have been replaced with fluorine (F).*
[ǂǂ]*All H atoms on at least one (but not all) C atoms have been replaced with F.*
[a]*Manufactured by either ECF or telomerization.*
[b]*Manufactured by ECF.*
[c]*Manufactured by telomerization.*
Adapted from [60].

Table 1.
Per- and polyfluoroalkyl substances family.

found that PFASs get exposed to in various exposure pathways, including the numerous products to which the application of PFASs led to their manufacturing, thus causing multiple opportunities for exposure. On the other hand, there are already more than 5000 of these compounds available worldwide, and their number is expected to increase. In addition, PFAS's unique properties have also made them stable in the environment and food sources, ultimately making them to be persistent, i.e., that once they enter the environment PFAS remain in the it for an unknown length of period and take many years to leave the body they have entered [66–68]. The other subject of PFAS's attention is their bioaccumulation characteristic [65].

Moreover, it has been argued that all sources of exposure are not conclusively understood [65], but numerous studies have suggested that people are most likely to be exposed to these compounds by means of drinking and consuming PFAS-contaminated water or food, using products made with PFAS, or breathing air containing PFAS [69–75].

The next pressing subjects of attention as far as PFASs are concerned are PFAS precursors (pre-PFAS) and alternatives to PFASs of concerns. Hence, pre-PFASs are formed by means of biotic or abiotic degradation from other PFASs [60, 76], while concerns over the effect of PFASs, mostly PFOA and PFOS, on humans and the environment led to an interest in exploring suitable alternatives to these substances; and ultimately three types of alternatives to PFASs, namely, (i) substances with shorter per- or polyfluorinated carbon chains, (ii) non-fluorine-containing substances and (iii) non-chemical techniques. Further details on some of the commonly known commercial alternatives PFASs and their potential health impacts are available [76–78]. Short-chain PFASs refer to those with five and seven or fewer carbons that are perfluorinated, while long-chain have six and eight or more perfluorinated carbons [77]. Concerns over PFAS alternatives are to be exacerbated by the expansion of world's biggest economies who are continuously manufacturing these chemicals in hundreds of tons per annum. Examples of commonly known and commercially available PFAS alternatives to long-chain PFASs, and which safety has been questioned are available in the literature, for example, see [76].

Moreover, like all other substances that are bioaccumulative, persistent and toxic in nature, PFASs have been reported to have the potential to cause health problems. As such, epidemiological evidence has suggested associations between perfluoroalkyl exposure and several health outcomes in humans and animals, even though cause-and-effect relationships for humans' cases have remained inconclusive, which have

Plant	**PFASs (ng/g/dw)**				
Cereals	**PFOA**	**PFBA**	**PFPeA**	**PFHxA**	**PFBS**
Corn	2478.44	1448.59	387.68	116.06	0.29
Maize	0.40	37.37	7.65	13.04	<0.05
Rice	1.73	*n/i*	*n/i*	*n/i*	*n/i*
Soybean	3966.62	2378.31	992.62	211.80	<0.02
Wheat	809.75	1102.51	495.77	134.69	0.51
Vegetables					
Cabbage	1.94	17.85	1.79	0.56	*n/i*
Carrot	1468.08	2552.74	852.31	196.85	1.10
Cauliflower	86.08	194.10	78.32	32.79	<0.02
Celery	1119.41	1049.61	324.06	94.30	<0.02
Cucumber	2.60	63	0.85	0.32	15
Lettuce	1038.27	2365.18	281.17	72.19	<0.02
Pepper	39.29	946.46	415.86	74.39	<0.02
Pumpkin	15.09	638.13	64.10	11.65	<0.02
Radish	1879.76	1167.52	426.45	103.31	<0.02
Spinach	2.49	6.70	1.79	3.90	0.17
Tomato	1.70	87	1.30	0.56	13
Welsh onion	360.58	270.39	77.79	30.73	0.07
Yam	110	*n/i*	*n/i*	*n/i*	40
Zucchini	3.20	69	3.10	0.28	11
Fruits					
Grape	1.60	9.80	*n/i*	1	*n/i*
Muskmelon	1	2.90	*n/i*	*n/i*	*n/i*
Peach	1.30	*n/i*	*n/i*	*n/i*	*n/i*
Pear	1	3.70	*n/i*	*n/i*	*n/i*
Sugarcane	110	*n/i*	*n/i*	*n/i*	*n/i*
Watermelon	7.90	3.60	*n/i*	*n/i*	*n/i*

Short-chain PFASs are shown in bold type. Italic and bold are plants that are likely to be find in selected supermarkets in sub-Saharan Africa, but which are only produced in selected countries of the region (e.g., South Africa and Namibia).
n/i: not indicated.
Adapted from [80].

Table 2.
Bioaccumulation of PFASs in edible plants.

implied that more studies are still needed. There are further details on the toxicological profile of perfluoroalkyls [79].

2.3 Prevalence and bioaccumulation of PFASs in plants

PFASs are highly soluble in water, a characteristic that make them to be easily absorbed and translocated in plants. This has become a great centre of interest for researchers wanting to comprehend the phytotoxicity of PFASs. Subsequently, during the recent years, there has been an increase in studies that investigate the prevalence and bioaccumulation of PFASs by plants, including cereals, fruits and vegetables. Thus, high concentration levels of PFASs have been frequently reported in plants near contaminated sites [80–84]. The predominant PFASs have been PFOA, perfluorobutanoic acid (PFBA), perfluoropentanoic acid (PFPeA), perfluorohexanoic acid (PFHxA), and perfluorobutanesulfonic acid (PFBS) in most cases [83–85]. **Table 2** depicts the bioaccumulation of these PFASs in select cereal, fruits and vegetables, some of which are consumed by Africans but not produced locally. It is worth mentioning that the prevalence of these substances in these plants implies exposure to PFASs through the consumption of these crops. More studies are thus required, in this regard, to substantiate this potentiality.

3. PFASs as a threat to sub-Saharan African medicinal plants

For centuries, medicine plants have played a therapeutic role in the lives of millions of people in developing countries worldwide, and in sub-Saharan African regions, in particular. In addition, it has been reported that, due to their bioactive organic chemical compounds content, also referred to as phytochemicals, these plants have been able to play a defensive role against major chronic ailments in both host-metabolic or genetic dysfunctional and infectious diseases, thus making them beneficial for human and animal health [86, 87]. In sub-Saharan African countries (**Figure 1**), millions of people depend on medicinal plants for their primary healthcare therapy for obvious reasons such as, these people are inhabitants who live closer to the natural vegetation such as forests, with an estimated 216,634,000 ha of closed forest [12] and savannas_ the later having been reported to be rich in biodiversity with an estimated 71% of vegetation of these ecosystems being medicinal plants, the easy and free access to these plants, as well as the prohibitive cost of orthodox products [87, 88].

Furthermore, the reviewed literature has reported that many different plant species might be used to treat specific ailment(s) in various sub-Saharan African countries, as well as a particular plant being used for the same kind of illness in two or more countries, thus implying the variety and abondance of these plants in the region and the history that these countries previously shared. For example, a recent article reported on antimalarial medicinal plants used in Benin, Burkina Faso, Cameroon, DRC, Ethiopia, Gabon, Ghana, Guinea, Kenya, Mali, Namibia, Nigeria, Uganda, Senegal, South Africa, Rwanda, Togo, Zambia and Zimbabwe (thus representing all the sub-Saharan regions, see **Figure 1**), with the following plant species used in numerous countries, namely: *Azadirachta indica* (Benin, Burkina Faso, Ghana, Guinea, Ethiopia, Kenya, Nigeria, Togo, Uganda and Zimbabwe), *Nauclea latifolia* (Benin, Cameroon, Gabon, Ghana, Guinea, Kenya, Nigeria, Senegal and Togo), *Carica papaya* (Benin, Ghana, Guinea, Nigeria, Togo, Uganda, Zambia and Zimbabwe), *Cassia siamea* (Benin, Burkina Faso, Ghana, Guinea, Nigeria, Togo,

Zambia and Zimbabwe), *Ficus sur Forssk* (Burkina Faso, Gabon, Guinea, Kenya, Namibia, Nigeria, Togo and Uganda), *Cassia occidentalis* L. (Benin, Kenya, Ghana, Namibia, Nigeria, Zambia and Zimbabwe), *Jatropha curcas* L (Benin, Ghana, Guinea, Ethiopia, Nigeria, Uganda and Zambia), *Maytenus* sp. *nov.* A. (Benin, Guinea, Kenya, Nigeria, Senegal, Sudan and Zambia), *Tamarindus* indica L. (Benin, Ethiopia, Guinea, Kenya, Uganda, Togo and Zambia), *Vernonia amygdalina* (Benin, Ghana, Kenya, Namibia, Nigeria, Uganda and Zambia), *Tithonia diversifolia* A. Gray (Burkina Faso, Guinea, Nigeria, Uganda, Rwanda and Zimbabwe), *Adansonia* digitata L. (Benin, Namibia, Nigeria, Togo and Zambia), *Momordica foetida* Schumach. (Ethiopia, Ghana, Uganda, Zambia and Zimbabwe), *Securidaca longepeduculata* Fresen (Namibia, Nigeria, South Africa and Zambia), and *Flueggea virosa* (Willd.) Voigt (Benin, Kenya, Togo and Uganda), *Ximenia americana* L. (Guinea, Kenya, South Africa and Zambia), and *Zanthoxylum chalybeum* Engl (Kenya, Rwanda, Uganda and Zambia) [11]; and for the management of human immunodeficiency virus (HIV) and other sexually transmitted infections (STIs) in the sub-Saharan region, *Ximenia americana* has been in use (Zambia, Uganda and Kenya), and *Azadirachta indica* (Uganda and Kenya) [89–91]. Similarly, numerous studies have highlighted the anti-diabetic potential of several hundreds of sub-Saharan African medicinal plants [4].

Additionally, a valuable review article has highlighted the commercial importance of African medicinal plants, including 13 species (i.e., *Catharanthus roseus*, *Centella asiatica*, *Coffea arabica*, *Cissampelos pareira*, *Cyclopia genistoides*, *Pausinystalia johimbe*, *Synsepalum dulcificum*, *Sclerochiton illicifolius*, *Strophanthus gratus*, *Physostigma venenosum*, *Thaumatococcus daniellii*, *Voacanga africana* and *V. thouarsii*) which are sources of commercially important chemical constituents, and has, to some extents, represented approximately 10% of commercially developed medicinal plants [13]. The review has further suggested that presently Africa is home to more than 80 beneficial commercial medicinal plant species that are on international markets, and this, in our view confirms the argument that the demand for medicinal plants, including African, is increasing at an alarming rate [7]. Interested readers are encouraged to read this remarkable review article [13] as it depicts a well-informed selection of most popular and important medicinal plants distributed in the different sub-Saharan regions (**Figure 1**).

Nevertheless, albeit the promising prospects of these plants as alluded to, knowledges on African medicinal plants are still very limited in comparison to other societies, such as the Chinese and Indian; this is so because, unlike in China and India where medicinal plants have extensively been researched and documented, studies of African medicinal plants have not been taken seriously. For example, recent evidence from sub-Saharan-southern African region highlighted 257 plant species from this region that are used traditionally for the treatment of viral respiratory ailments, but only one of these plants has this far been tested for its ability to constrain respiratory viruses by means of its ethnobotanical usage [92]; while of the 555 medicinal plants identified to treat inflammation and pain, from the same region, only few have been relatively screened for their anti-inflammatory properties, which prompted the researchers to recommend that further studies be undertaken in that regard [93]. Substantial, this lack of seriousness in this domain has led to information on African medicinal plants either being unavailable or fragmented and, in the end, incompletely documented [12, 13].

Certainly, the challenges that sub-Saharan African medicinal plants are subjected to are numerous [4]. For instance, it has been indicated that there's an urgent need to increase the documentation on sub-Saharan African medicinal plants because of their accelerated losses due to anthropogenic activities [12]. For example, the rate of the loss of natural forest cover or deforestation on the African continent is one of the highest globally [7, 12]. Basically, the global deforestation rate stands at 0.6%, but this rate is at 6.5%, 5.0% and 2.1% in sub-Saharan Africa for countries such as the Cote d'Ivoire, Nigeria and the DRC respectively [12, 94]. Additionally, sub-Saharan African medicinal plants are affected by unsustainable harvesting methods [7, 11, 13, 16, 87], fires, wattle expansion or eradication program and grazing [7, 87], coupled with human settlement expansions, including urbanization, as well as inexistent or weak legislations and/or enforcement failure of existing rules and regulations [16].

Moreover, the most recent challenge threatening the prospects of sub-Saharan African medicinal plants, in our opinion, is the contamination of these plants by PFASs. Hence, unlike in the developed world, where the assessment and monitoring of PFASs prevalence in the natural environment are at an advanced stage [4], it is only recently that PFAS studies from the sub-Saharan African region have started emerging [54]. Thus, during the last two decades there has been reports on PFAS from South Africa, Nigeria, Kenya, Ethiopia, Ghana, Burkina Faso and Ivory coast, Tanzania and Uganda [4, 54, 95, 96]. It is worth mentioning that the continent has over 50 countries, which suggests that PFAS studies are still limited on the continent at large. All available evidence has reported higher level concentrations of specific PFASs in analyzed samples, compared to allowed international standards. For example, higher levels of PFOS and PFOA were reported in tap water from Ghana, but lower in tap and bottled water from Burkina Faso [95]. Similarly, PFASs have been reported in wastewater from wastewater treatment plants (WWTPs) and ultimately in several surface water systems in sub-Saharan Africa, including in South Africa, Kenya, Nigeria, Ghana and Ethiopia [54, 95–97]. Hence, it can be argued that inefficiently treated wastewater represents a risk to plants, including medicinal plants, to which PFAS-contaminated water is or might be applied to. And this is substantiated by the literature that has confirmed that WWTPs are PFAS-contamination hotspots, are considered as the most common point sources of PFASs to surface water [98, 99]. Similarly, available evidence has indicated that the cultivation of medicinal plants at a commercial scale has started emerging from the sub-Saharan African region, with countries such as South Africa, Uganda, Kenya, Tanzania and the DRC having taken the initiatives toward the commercial cultivation of these plants, with high probabilities that surface water (e.g., river water) is used or luckily to be used, like it is the case in South Africa, to irrigate the lands on which medicinal plants are planted with such water, to alleviate the burden of water shortage, for instance. This is a huge potential risk and a threat to medicinal plants.

Furthermore, there are considerable evidence on the prevalence of PFASs in edible plants we have previously alluded to, in the general environment worldwide [80–85], but the state of these substances, in this regard, in the sub-Saharan African region remains largely unknown and undocumented. However, several countries from this region have been commercially trading with world leading economies (e.g., China and USA) from which PFASs have been reported not only in their natural environments, but also in consumer products that are imported from these world greatest economies by their African commercial patterners [58, 79]; this implies the potential prevalence of PFASs in the general environment of this region as previously alluded by Ssebugere et al. [95] who suggested that the likelihood of PFASs in African environments would certainly be due to the uncontrollable and unregulated importation of PFAS-carrier products from these mass manufacturers to the African countries. Further studies are overdue to substantiate these conjectures, which, if confirmed, represent substantial threats to the general African environment.

Similarly, available data further suggest a greater need for investigations to be conducted on the uptake of these compounds by medical plants. In fact, to our knowledge, there is only a single article that has recently reported on the susceptibility of medical plants to PFASs, with the African marigold (*Tagetes erecta* L.) as a typical example [100]. The results from the later study have become a wakeup call, as they suggested medicinal plants as possible conduits of PFASs, including PFOA (94.83 ng/g), PFOS (5.03 ng/g) and PFBS (1.44 ng/g), into humans; and thus represent a huge threat to the entire potential medicinal plants industry of the sub-Saharan African region; and the situation is expected to be exacerbated as the continent embarks on developmental trajectories. Therefore, for this region to remain certain that it maintains its remarkable medicinal plants history and keep its population safe, we are of the opinion that studies, in this regard, should be expanded and diversified in the region, in order for a database of these chemicals on medicinal plants to be efficiently established for the whole of the sub-Saharan African region.

4. Conclusions

The use of medicinal plants to combat diseases and illnesses from which humans suffer is not new. It can thus be said that these plants have a long history. In sub-Saharan Africa the history of medicinal plants is remarkable, huge and divers, transmitted by word of mouth from one generation to another using the thousands of dialects present in the region. Owing it to its tropical and subtropical geographical positions, sub-Saharan Africa is said to be home to an enormous biodiversity of medicinal plants, with over fifty thousand plant species, a quarter of which is well known for their curative potentials. Notwithstanding these possibilities, the region still lacks its own drugs on the global markets due to the limited and/or small-scale type of cultivation of medicinal plants still in practice in the region, coupled with several other challenges that medicinal plants are faced with, including not being sufficiently undocumented, deforestation, conservation inefficiencies, overexploitation or overharvesting, etc. Hence, there isn't any doubt that medicinal plants in sub-Saharan African region are subjected to several encounters. But the most recent of these encounters have been the potential threats from emerging pollutants, i.e., PFASs. These substances are the results of anthropogenic activities unlike their predecessors, the heavy metals, which are naturally find in the environment. To date, there has been over 5000 PFASs manufactured since their dawn in the 1950s. During the manufacturing process that gives life to PFASs, they're given unique properties that make them wanted by several manufacturers of consumer products. Unfortunately, due to these compounds being heavily applied in industrial processes, they have now been detected in different environmental matrices, including water, soil and plants, as well as in animals. PFASs have been even detected in samples from remote areas, far from the places where they were manufactured, with PFOA and PFOS being predominantly studied, owing it to their health concerns. Regardless of PFASs being extensively researched and documented in different parts of the world, the chemicals have remained undocumented in sub-Saharan Africa, to a large extent. This situation is highly concerning in the context of medicinal plants of this region, because PFASs have been proven to translocate and bioaccumulate in plants, and linked to numerous severe diseases, including cancer and diabetes. This state implies that plants, medicinal plants in this case, being a possible pathway through which humans get exposed to these human-made substances. And with medicinal plants being the first line of defense to combat diseases, illnesses and other daily health needs for millions of low-income people from sub-Saharan Africa, there is cause for serious concern. It is therefore recommended that PFAS studies be expanded and diversified in sub-Saharan Africa. Future studies should also investigate the prevalence of novel or the so called PFAS-substitutes in African environments. The region needs trade-agreements and regulations that make provisions for PFASs from countries with the reputation of manufacturing these chemicals and their alternatives. To valorize its current medicinal plant diversity, the region needs to shift from small to large-scale cultivation of medicinal plants. Routine-based assessment and monitoring of PFASs, their precursors and alternatives in general African environments is also recommended, with an emphasis on the cultivation, harvest or collection, and storing of medicinal plants in areas free of any possible contamination.

Acknowledgements

The authors are grateful for the support and assistance received from: Mr. Masibulele Fubesi, Ms. Espérance Byamungu, as well as the staff from the Department of Civil Engineering and Geomatics and all BioERG members for unwavering encouragements.

Conflict of interest

The authors declare no conflict of interest.

Funding

The authors would like to acknowledge the funding assistance from the Cape Peninsula University of Technology, through the University Research Fund (URF)-Cost Centre R484.

Author details

John Baptist Nzukizi Mudumbi[1,2*], Elie Fereche Itoba-Tombo[2,3], Seteno Karabo Obed Ntwampe[2,4] and Tandi Matsha[5]

1 Department of Civil Engineering and Geomatics, Faculty of Engineering and Built Environment, Cape Peninsula University of Technology, Bellville, South Africa

2 Bioresource Engineering Research Group (BioERG), Department of Biotechnology, Cape Peninsula University of Technology, Cape Town, South Africa

3 Department of Environmental and Occupational Studies, Cape Peninsula University of Technology, Cape Town, South Africa

4 School of Chemical and Mineral Engineering, North-West University, Potchefstroom, South Africa

5 Department of Bio-Medical sciences, Faculty of Health and Wellness Science, Cape Peninsula University of Technology, Bellville, South Africa

*Address all correspondence to: jbmudumbi@gmail.com

References

[1] Salmerón-Manzano E, Garrido-Cardenas JA, Manzano-Agugliaro F. Worldwide research trends on medicinal plants. International Journal of Environmental Research and Public Health. 2020;**17**(10):3376

[2] World Health Organization (WHO). General Guidelines for Methodologies on Research and Evaluation of Traditional Medicine. World Health Organization; 2000. Available from: https://scholar.google.co.za/scholar?q=General+Guidelines+for+Methodologies+on+Research+and+Evaluation+of+Traditional+Medicine&hl=en&as_sdt=0&as_vis=1&oi=scholart [Accessed: 21 December 2021]

[3] Miranda JJ. Medicinal plants and their traditional uses in different locations. In: Phytomedicine. Vol. 1. USA: Academic Press; 2021. pp. 207-223

[4] Mudumbi JB, Ntwampe SK, Mekuto L, Matsha T, Itoba-Tombo EF. The role of pollutants in type 2 diabetes mellitus (T2DM) and their prospective impact on phytomedicinal treatment strategies. Environmental Monitoring and Assessment. 2018;**190**(5):1-23

[5] Van Wyk BE, Wink M. Medicinal Plants of the World. UK: CABI; 2018

[6] Mahomoodally MF. Traditional medicines in Africa: An appraisal of ten potent African medicinal plants. Evidence-Based Complementary and Alternative Medicine. 2013;**2013**:1-14

[7] Xego S, Kambizi L, Nchu F. Threatened medicinal plants of South Africa: Case of the family Hyacinthaceae. African Journal of Traditional, Complementary and Alternative Medicines. 2016;**13**(3):169-180

[8] World Health Organization. WHO Global Report on Traditional and Complementary Medicine 2019. World Health Organization; 2019

[9] Villena-Tejada M, Vera-Ferchau I, Cardona-Rivero A, Zamalloa-Cornejo R, Quispe-Florez M, Frisancho-Triveño Z, et al. Use of medicinal plants for COVID-19 prevention and respiratory symptom treatment during the pandemic in Cusco, Peru: A cross-sectional survey. PLoS One. 2021;**16**(9):e0257165

[10] Brenzinger M, Batibo H. Sub-Saharan Africa. In: Atlas of the World's Languages in Danger. Paris: UNESCO Publishing; 2010. pp. 20-25

[11] Chinsembu KC. Plants as antimalarial agents in Sub-Saharan Africa. Acta Tropica. 2015;**152**:32-48

[12] Iwu MM. Handbook of African Medicinal Plants. . Routledge Handbooks Online. Boca Raton: CRC Press; 2014 [Accessed: 16 December 2021]

[13] Van Wyk BE. A review of commercially important African medicinal plants. Journal of Ethnopharmacology. 2015;**176**:118-134

[14] Gurib-Fakim A. Medicinal plants: Traditions of yesterday and drugs of tomorrow. Molecular Aspects of Medicine. 2006;**27**(1):1-93

[15] Atawodi SE. Antioxidant potential of African medicinal plants. African Journal of Biotechnology. 2005;**4**(2):128-133

[16] Moshi MJ, Mhame PP. Legislation on medicinal plants in Africa. Medicinal Plant Research in Africa. 2013;**1**:843-858

[17] Gurib-Fakim A, Mahomoodally MF. African flora as potential sources of medicinal plants: Towards the

chemotherapy of major parasitic and other infectious diseases: A review. Jordan Journal of Biological Sciences. 2013;**147**(624):1-8

[18] Bapat VA, Yadav SR, Dixit GB. Rescue of endangered plants through biotechnological applications. National Academy Science Letters. 2008;**31**(7-8):201-210

[19] Minnesota Department of Health (MDH). Perfluoroalkyl Substances (PFAS) and Health [Internet]. 2021. Available from: https://www.health.state.mn.us/communities/environment/hazardous/docs/pfashealth.pdf [Accessed: 23 December 2021]

[20] Mörner J, Bos R, Fredrix M. Reducing and Eliminating the Use of Persistent Organic Pesticides: Guidance on Alternative Strategies for Sustainable Pest and Vector Management. World Health Organization; 2002. pp. 1-89

[21] Betianu C, Gavrilescu M. Environmental behaviour and assessment of persistent organic pollutants. Environmental Engineering & Management Journal (EEMJ). 2006;**5**(2):213-241

[22] Silva DF, Landgraf MD, Rezende MO. Optimization of a microwave-assisted extraction method for the analysis of the persistent organic pollutant p, p'-DDT in domestic sewage sludge. American Open Chemistry Journal. 2016;**2**(1):14-26

[23] Silva DF. Fast and sustainable determination of persistent organic pollutants from organic fertilizer using optimized microwave-assisted extraction method and gas chromatography-mass spectrometry. Open Access Library Journal. 2015;**2**(11):1

[24] Wang J, Hoondert RP, Thunnissen NW, van de Meent D, Hendriks AJ. Chemical fate of persistent organic pollutants in the arctic: Evaluation of simplebox. Science of the Total Environment. 2020;**720**:137579

[25] Wania F, Mackay D. Global fractionation and cold condensation of low volatility organochlorine compounds in polar regions. Ambio. 1993;**1**:10-18

[26] Si W. Distribution of organic pollutants in water and sediment: An international comparison [doctor of philosophy]. Hong Kong: Department of Biology and Chemistry, City University of Hong Kong; 2008. pp. 1-162

[27] Corsolini S, Ademollo N, Romeo T, Greco S, Focardi S. Persistent organic pollutants in edible fish: A human and environmental health problem. Microchemical Journal. 2005;**79**(1-2):115-123

[28] Mudumbi JBN. Perfluorooctane sulfonate and perfluorooctanoate contamination of riparian wetlands of the Eerste, Diep and Salt Rivers [Masters dissertation]. Cape Peninsula University of Technology; 2012

[29] Taniguchi S, Montone RC, Bícego MC, Colabuono FI, Weber RR, Sericano JL. Chlorinated pesticides, polychlorinated biphenyls and polycyclic aromatic hydrocarbons in the fat tissue of seabirds from King George Island, Antarctica. Marine Pollution Bulletin. 2009;**58**(1):129-133

[30] Olatunji OS. Evaluation of selected polychlorinated biphenyls (PCBs) congeners and dichlorodiphenyltrichloroethane (DDT) in fresh root and leafy vegetables using GC-MS. Scientific Reports. 2019;**9**(1):1-10

[31] UNEP (United Nation Environment Programme). Global status of DDT and its alternatives for use in vector control to prevent disease. In: Stockholm

Convention on Persistent Organic Pollutants Stakeholders' Meeting to Review the Interim Report for the Establishment of a Global Partnership to Develop Alternatives to DDT. United Nations Environmental Program; 3-5 November 2008; Geneva, Switzerland. 2008. Available from: http://chm.pops.int/Portals/0/docs/from_old_website/documents/ddt/Global%20status%20of%20DDT%20SSC%2020Oct08.pdf. p. 31 [Accessed: 31 December 2021

[32] van den Berg H. Global status of DDT and its alternatives for use in vector control to prevent disease. Ciencia & Saude Coletiva. 2011;**16**:575-590

[33] Jones KC, De Voogt P. Persistent organic pollutants (POPs): State of the science. Environmental Pollution. 1999;**100**(1-3):209-221

[34] Lohmann R, Breivik K, Dachs J, Muir D. Global fate of POPs: Current and future research directions. Environmental Pollution. 2007;**150**(1): 150-165

[35] Harrad S. Persistent Organic Pollutants. Chichester, West Sussex, UK: Blackwell; John Wiley & Sons; 2009. ISBN: 978-1-4051-6930-1

[36] Wong MH, Wu SC, Deng WJ, Yu XZ, Luo Q, Leung AO, et al. Export of toxic chemicals—A review of the case of uncontrolled electronic-waste recycling. Environmental Pollution. 2007;**149**(2):131-140

[37] Dachs J, Méjanelle L. Organic pollutants in coastal waters, sediments, and biota: Arelevant driver for ecosystems during the Anthropocene. Estuaries and Coasts. 2010;**33**(1):1-14

[38] Boucher O, Muckle G, Bastien CH. Prenatal exposure to polychlorinated biphenyls: A neuropsychologic analysis. Environmental Health Perspectives. 2009;**117**(1):7-16

[39] Ashwood P, Schauer J, Pessah IN, Van de Water J. Preliminary evidence of the in vitro effects of BDE-47 on innate immune responses in children with autism spectrum disorders. Journal of Neuroimmunology. 2009;**208**(1-2):130-135

[40] Fernie KJ, Shutt JL, Letcher RJ, Ritchie JI, Sullivan K, Bird DM. Changes in reproductive courtship behaviors of adult American kestrels (*Falco sparverius*) exposed to environmentally relevant levels of the polybrominated diphenyl ether mixture, DE-71. Toxicological Sciences. 2008;**102**(1):171-178

[41] Fernie KJ, Shutt JL, Letcher RJ, Ritchie IJ, Bird DM. Environmentally relevant concentrations of DE-71 and HBCD alter eggshell thickness and reproductive success of American kestrels. Environmental Science & Technology. 2009;**43**(6):2124-2130

[42] Kemmlein S, Hahn O, Jann O. Emissions of organophosphate and brominated flame retardants from selected consumer products and building materials. Atmospheric Environment. 2003;**37**(39-40):5485-5493

[43] Webster TF, Harrad S, Millette JR, Holbrook RD, Davis JM, Stapleton HM, et al. Identifying transfer mechanisms and sources of decabromodiphenyl ether (BDE 209) in indoor environments using environmental forensic microscopy. Environmental Science & Technology. 2009;**43**(9):3067-3072

[44] Zhang Q, Xu Z, Shen Z, Li S, Wang S. The Han River watershed management initiative for the South-to-North water transfer project (Middle Route) of China. Environmental Monitoring and Assessment. 2009;**148**(1):369-377

[45] Kelly BC, Ikonomou MG, Blair JD, Morin AE, Gobas FA. Food web–specific biomagnification of persistent organic pollutants. Science. 2007;**317**(5835):236-239

[46] Suzuki G, Nakano M, Nakano S. Distribution of PCDDs/PCDFs and Co-PCBs in human maternal blood, cord blood, placenta, milk, and adipose tissue: Dioxins showing high toxic equivalency factor accumulate in the placenta. Bioscience, Biotechnology, and Biochemistry. 2005;**69**(10):1836-1847

[47] Boda H, Nghi TN, Nishijo M, Thao PN, Tai PT, Van Luong H, et al. Prenatal dioxin exposure estimated from dioxins in breast milk and sex hormone levels in umbilical cord blood in Vietnamese new-born infants. Science of the Total Environment. 2018;**615**:1312-1318

[48] Yu D, Liu X, Liu X, Cao W, Zhang X, Tian H, et al. Polychlorinated dibenzo-p-dioxins, polychlorinated dibenzofurans, and dioxin-like polychlorinated biphenyls in umbilical cord serum from pregnant women living near a chemical plant in Tianjin, China. International Journal of Environmental Research and Public Health. 2019;**16**(12):2178

[49] Bao Y, Zhang L, Liu X, Shi L, Li J, Meng G, et al. Dioxin-like compounds in paired maternal serum and breast milk under long sampling intervals. Ecotoxicology and Environmental Safety. 2020;**194**:110339

[50] De Bon H, Huat J, Parrot L, Sinzogan A, Martin T, Malézieux E, et al. Pesticide risks from fruit and vegetable pest management by small farmers in sub-Saharan Africa. A review. Agronomy for Sustainable Development. 2014;**34**(4):723-736

[51] Olisah C, Okoh OO, Okoh AI. Occurrence of organochlorine pesticide residues in biological and environmental matrices in Africa: A two-decade review. Heliyon. 2020;**6**(3):e03518

[52] Wolmarans NJ, Bervoets L, Gerber R, Yohannes YB, Nakayama SM, Ikenaka Y, et al. Bioaccumulation of DDT and other organochlorine pesticides in amphibians from two conservation areas within malaria risk regions of South Africa. Chemosphere. 2021;**274**:129956

[53] Groffen T, Rijnders J, van Doorn L, Jorissen C, De Borger SM, Luttikhuis DO, et al. Preliminary study on the distribution of metals and persistent organic pollutants (POPs), including perfluoroalkylated acids (PFAS), in the aquatic environment near Morogoro, Tanzania, and the potential health risks for humans. Environmental Research. 2021;**192**:110299

[54] Groffen T, Nkuba B, Wepener V, Bervoets L. Risk posed by per- and polyfluorated compounds (PFAS) on the African continent, with an emphasis on aquatic ecosystems. Integrated Environmental Assessment and Management. 2021;**17**(4):726-732

[55] Fry K, Power MC. Persistent organic pollutants and mortality in the United States, NHANES 1999-2011. Environmental Health. 2017;**16**(1):1-2

[56] Renner R. Growing concern over: Perfluorinated chemicals. Environmental Science & Technology. 2001;**35**(7):154-160

[57] Simons JH, inventor; Minnesota Mining, Manufacturing Co, assignee. Electrochemical process of making fluorine-containing carbon compounds. United States patent US 2,519,983. 22 August 1950

[58] Jiang W, Zhang Y, Zhu L, Deng J. Serum levels of perfluoroalkyl acids

(PFAAs) with isomer analysis and their associations with medical parameters in Chinese pregnant women. Environment International. 2014;**64**:40-47

[59] Organisation for Economic Cooperation and Development (OECD). Working Towards a Global Emission Inventory of PFASs: Focus on PFCAs—Status Quo and the Way Forward [Internet]. 2015. Available from: file:///C:/Users/jbmud/Downloads/4774679%20(2).pdf [Accessed: 08 January 2022]

[60] Buck RC, Franklin J, Berger U, Conder JM, Cousins IT, De Voogt P, et al. Perfluoroalkyl and polyfluoroalkyl substances in the environment: Terminology, classification, and origins. Integrated Environmental Assessment and Management. 2011;7(4):513-541

[61] Organisation for Economic Cooperation and Development (OECD). Towards a New Comprehensive Global Database of Per- and Polyfluoroalkyl Substances (PFAS): Summary Report on Updating the OECD 2007 List of Per- and Polyfluoroalkyl Substances (PFAS) [Internet]. 2018. Available from: https://www.oecd.org/chemicalsafety/portal-perfluorinated-chemicals/countryinformation/european-union.htm [Accessed: 07 January 2022]

[62] Chelcea IC, Ahrens L, Örn S, Mucs D, Andersson PL. Investigating the OECD database of per-and polyfluoroalkyl substances—Chemical variation and applicability of current fate models. Environmental Chemistry. 2020;**17**(7):498-508

[63] Liu J, Avendaño SM. Microbial degradation of polyfluoroalkyl chemicals in the environment: A review. Environment International. 2013;**61**:98-114

[64] Young CJ, Mabury SA. Atmospheric perfluorinated acid precursors: Chemistry, occurrence, and impacts. Reviews of Environmental Contamination and Toxicology. 2010;**208**:1-109

[65] National Institute of Environmental Health Sciences (NIH). Perfluoroalkyl and Polyfluoroalkyl Substances (PFAS) [Internet]. 2019. Available from: https://www.niehs.nih.gov/health/topics/agents/pfc/index.cfm [Accessed: 11 January 2022]

[66] Wang Y, Shi Y, Vestergren R, Zhou Z, Liang Y, Cai Y. Using hair, nail and urine samples for human exposure assessment of legacy and emerging per-and polyfluoroalkyl substances. Science of the Total Environment. 2018;**636**:383-391

[67] Sunderland EM, Hu XC, Dassuncao C, Tokranov AK, Wagner CC, Allen JG. A review of the pathways of human exposure to poly-and perfluoroalkyl substances (PFASs) and present understanding of health effects. Journal of Exposure Science & Environmental Epidemiology. 2019;**29**(2):131-147

[68] Blake BE, Pinney SM, Hines EP, Fenton SE, Ferguson KK. Associations between longitudinal serum perfluoroalkyl substance (PFAS) levels and measures of thyroid hormone, kidney function, and body mass index in the Fernald Community Cohort. Environmental Pollution. 2018;**242**:894-904

[69] Agency for Toxic Substances and Disease Registry (ATSDR). Toxicological Profile for Perfluoroalkyls [Internet]. 2021. Available from: https://www.atsdr.cdc.gov/toxprofiles/tp200.pdf [Accessed: 11 January 2022]

[70] Boone JS, Vigo C, Boone T, Byrne C, Ferrario J, Benson R, et al. Per-and polyfluoroalkyl substances in source and treated drinking waters of the United

States. Science of the Total Environment. 2019;**653**:359-369

[71] Poothong S, Padilla-Sánchez JA, Papadopoulou E, Giovanoulis G, Thomsen C, Haug LS. Hand wipes: A useful tool for assessing human exposure to poly-and perfluoroalkyl substances (PFASs) through hand-to-mouth and dermal contacts. Environmental Science & Technology. 2019;**53**(4):1985-1993

[72] DeLuca NM, Angrish M, Wilkins A, Thayer K, Hubal EA. Human exposure pathways to poly-and perfluoroalkyl substances (PFAS) from indoor media: A systematic review protocol. Environment International. 2021;**146**:106308

[73] Thépaut E, Dirven HA, Haug LS, Lindeman B, Poothong S, Andreassen M, et al. Per-and polyfluoroalkyl substances in serum and associations with food consumption and use of personal care products in the Norwegian biomonitoring study from the EU project Euro Mix. Environmental Research. 2021;**195**:110795

[74] Young AS, Sparer-Fine EH, Pickard HM, Sunderland EM, Peaslee GF, Allen JG. Per-and polyfluoroalkyl substances (PFAS) and total fluorine in fire station dust. Journal of Exposure Science & Environmental Epidemiology. 2021;**31**:930-942

[75] Tang J, Lin M, Ma S, Yang Y, Li G, Yu Y, et al. Identifying dermal uptake as a significant pathway for human exposure to typical semi volatile organic compounds in an e-waste dismantling site: The relationship of contaminant levels in handwipes and urine metabolites. Environmental Science & Technology. 2021;**55**(20):14026-14036

[76] Mudumbi JB, Ntwampe SK, Matsha T, Mekuto L, Itoba-Tombo EF. Recent developments in polyfluoroalkyl compounds research: A focus on human/environmental health impact, suggested substitutes and removal strategies. Environmental Monitoring and Assessment. 2017;**189**(8):1-29

[77] Organisation for Economic Cooperation and Development (OECD). OECD/UNEP Global PFC Group, synthesis paper on per- and polyfluorinated chemicals (PFCs). Environment, Health and Safety, Environment Directorate, OECD; 2013. pp. 1-60. Available from: https://www.oecd.org/env/ehs/risk-management/PFC_FINAL-Web.pdf [Accessed: 19 January 2022]

[78] Jenssen BM, Villanger GD, Gabrielsen KM, Bytingsvik J, Bechshoft T, Ciesielski TM, et al. Anthropogenic flank attack on polar bears: Interacting consequences of climate warming and pollutant exposure. Frontiers in Ecology and Evolution. 2015;**3**:16

[79] Agency for Toxic Substances and Disease Registry (ATSDR). Toxicological profile for Perfluoroalkyls. Atlanta, GA: U.S. Department of Health and Human Services, Public Health Service; 2021. Available from: https://www.atsdr.cdc.gov/ToxProfiles/tp200-c2.pdf [Accessed: 27 January 2022]

[80] Li J, Sun J, Li P. Exposure routes, bioaccumulation and toxic effects of per-and polyfluoroalkyl substances (PFASs) on plants: A critical review. Environment International. 2022;**158**:106891

[81] Brown JB, Conder JM, Arblaster JA, Higgins CP. Assessing human health risks from per-and polyfluoroalkyl substance (PFAS)-impacted vegetable consumption: A tiered modelling approach. Environmental Science & Technology. 2020;**54**(23):15202-15214

[82] Zhang M, Wang P, Lu Y, Lu X, Zhang A, Liu Z, et al. Bioaccumulation

and human exposure of perfluoroalkyl acids (PFAAs) in vegetables from the largest vegetable production base of China. Environment International. 2020;**135**:105347

[83] Wang W, Rhodes G, Ge J, Yu X, Li H. Uptake and accumulation of per- and polyfluoroalkyl substances in plants. Chemosphere. 2020;**261**:127584

[84] Zhou Y, Zhou Z, Lian Y, Sun X, Wu Y, Qiao L, et al. Source, transportation, bioaccumulation, distribution and food risk assessment of perfluorinated alkyl substances in vegetables: A review. Food Chemistry. 2021 Jul;**1**(349):129137

[85] Lesmeister L, Lange FT, Breuer J, Biegel-Engler A, Giese E, Scheurer M. Extending the knowledge about PFAS bioaccumulation factors for agricultural plants—A review. Science of the Total Environment. 2021;**766**:142640

[86] Ugboko HU, Nwinyi OC, Oranusi SU, Fatoki TH, Omonhinmin CA. Antimicrobial importance of medicinal plants in Nigeria. The Scientific World Journal. 2020;**2020**:1-10

[87] Mbinile SD, Munishi LK, Ngondya IB, Ndakidemi PA. Spatial distribution and anthropogenic threats facing medicinal plant *Zanthoxylum chalybeum* in Simanjiro area, Northern Tanzania. Scientific African. 2020;**10**:e00562

[88] Novotna B, Polesny Z, Pinto-Basto MF, Van Damme P, Pudil P, Mazancova J, et al. Medicinal plants used by 'root doctors', local traditional healers in Bié province, Angola. Journal of Ethnopharmacology. 2020;**260**:112662

[89] Chinsembu KC, Syakalima M, Semenya SS. Ethnomedicinal plants used by traditional healers in the management of HIV/AIDS opportunistic diseases in Lusaka, Zambia. South African Journal of Botany. 2019;**122**:369-384

[90] Anywar G, Kakudidi E, Byamukama R, Mukonzo J, Schubert A, Oryem-Origa H. Indigenous traditional knowledge of medicinal plants used by herbalists in treating opportunistic infections among people living with HIV/AIDS in Uganda. Journal of Ethnopharmacology. 2020;**246**:112205

[91] Nagata JM, Jew AR, Kimeu JM, Salmen CR, Bukusi EA, Cohen CR. Medical pluralism on Mfangano Island: Use of medicinal plants among persons living with HIV/AIDS in Suba District, Kenya. Journal of Ethnopharmacology. 2011;**135**(2):501-509

[92] Cock IE, Van Vuuren SF. The traditional use of southern African medicinal plants for the treatment of bacterial respiratory diseases: A review of the ethnobotany and scientific evaluations. Journal of Ethnopharmacology. 2020 Jul;**27**:113204

[93] Khumalo GP, Van Wyk BE, Feng Y, Cock IE. A review of the traditional use of Southern African medicinal plants for the treatment of inflammation and inflammatory pain. Journal of Ethnopharmacology. 2022;**283**:114436

[94] Achille LS, Zhang K, Anoma CJ. Dynamics of deforestation and degradation of forests in the Democratic Republic of Congo from 1990 to 2018. Open Journal of Ecology. 2021;**11**(5):451-461

[95] Ssebugere P, Sillanpää M, Matovu H, Wang Z, Schramm KW, Omwoma S, et al. Environmental levels and human body burdens of per-and poly-fluoroalkyl substances in Africa: A critical review. Science of the Total Environment. 2020;**739**:139913

[96] Melake BA, Bervoets L, Nkuba B, Groffen T. Distribution of perfluoroalkyl substances (PFASs) in water, sediment, and fish tissue, and the potential human health risks due to fish consumption in

Lake Hawassa, Ethiopia. Environmental Research. 2022;**204**:112033

[97] Mudumbi JB, Ntwampe SK, Muganza FM, Okonkwo JO. Perfluorooctanoate and perfluorooctane sulfonate in South African river water. Water Science and Technology. 2014;**69**(1):185-194

[98] Abunada Z, Alazaiza MY, Bashir MJ. An overview of per-and polyfluoroalkyl substances (PFAS) in the environment: Source, fate, risk and regulations. Water. 2020;**12**(12):3590

[99] Stroski KM, Luong KH, Challis JK, Chaves-Barquero LG, Hanson ML, Wong CS. Wastewater sources of per-and polyfluorinated alkyl substances (PFAS) and pharmaceuticals in four Canadian Arctic communities. Science of the Total Environment. 2020;**708**:134494

[100] Mudumbi JB, Daso AP, Okonkwo OJ, Ntwampe SK, Matsha TE, Mekuto L, et al. Propensity of *Tagetes erecta* L., a medicinal plant commonly used in diabetes management, to accumulate perfluoroalkyl substances. Toxics. 2019;7(1):18